CURRENT THERAPY IN ALLERGY, IMMUNOLOGY, AND RHEUMATOLOGY-3

Dear Doctor

Sandoz Pharmaceuticals Corporation is pleased to present you with the new edition of *Current Therapy in Allergy, Immunology, and Rheumatology — 3*, edited by Dr. Lawrence M. Lichtenstein and Dr. Anthony S. Fauci. This edition provides current information on clinical problems with a focus on the therapies for the particular diseases. We trust this informative volume will serve as a valuable reference and useful addition to your medical library.

Sincerely,

Bill Matthews

Your Sandoz Representative

Medical Titles in the Current Therapy Series

Bardin:
 Current Therapy in Endocrinology and Metabolism
Bayless:
 Current Management of Inflammatory Bowel Disease
Bayless:
 Current Therapy in Gastroenterology and Liver Disease
Bayless, Brain, Cherniack:
 Current Therapy in Internal Medicine
Brain, Carbone:
 Current Therapy in Hematology–Oncology
Callaham:
 Current Therapy in Emergency Medicine
Charles:
 Current Therapy in Obstetrics
Cherniack:
 Current Therapy of Respiratory Disease
Dubovsky, Shore:
 Current Therapy in Psychiatry
Eichenwald, Ströder:
 Current Therapy in Pediatrics
Foley, Payne:
 Current Therapy of Pain
Fortuin:
 Current Therapy in Cardiovascular Disease
Garcia, Mastroianni, Amelar, Dubin:
 Current Therapy of Infertility
Glassock:
 Current Therapy in Nephrology and Hypertension
Jeejeebhoy:
 Current Therapy in Nutrition
Johnson:
 Current Therapy in Neurologic Disease
Kacmarek, Stoller:
 Current Respiratory Care
Kass, Platt:
 Current Therapy in Infectious Disease
Lichtenstein, Fauci:
 Current Therapy in Allergy, Immunology, and Rheumatology
Nelson:
 Current Therapy in Neonatal–Perinatal Medicine
Nelson:
 Current Therapy in Pediatric Infectious Disease
Parrillo:
 Current Therapy in Critical Care Medicine
Peat:
 Current Physical Therapy
Provost, Farmer:
 Current Therapy in Dermatology
Rogers:
 Current Practice in Anesthesiology

CURRENT THERAPY IN ALLERGY, IMMUNOLOGY, AND RHEUMATOLOGY-3

LAWRENCE M. LICHTENSTEIN, M.D., PH.D.

Professor of Medicine
The Johns Hopkins University School of Medicine
Baltimore, Maryland

ANTHONY S. FAUCI, M.D.

Director
National Institute of Allergy and Infectious Diseases
National Institutes of Health
Bethesda, Maryland

1988

B.C. Decker Inc • Toronto • Philadelphia

Publisher   **B.C. Decker Inc**   **B.C. Decker Inc**
                     3228 South Service Road   320 Walnut Street
                     Burlington, Ontario   L7N 3H8   Suite 400
                                                                                             Philadelphia, Pennsylvania   19106
Sales and Distribution

United States   **The C.V. Mosby Company**   Asia   **Info-Med Ltd.**
and Possessions   11830 Westline Industrial Drive   802–3 Ruttonjee House
                     Saint Louis, Missouri   63146   11 Duddell Street
                                                                                             Central Hong Kong

Canada   **The C.V. Mosby Company, Ltd.**
                     5240 Finch Avenue East, Unit No. 1   South Africa   **Libriger Book Distributors**
                     Scarborough, Ontario   M1S 5P2   Warehouse Number 8
                                                                                             ''Die Ou Looiery''
United Kingdom, Europe **Blackwell Scientific Publications, Ltd.**   Tannery Road
and the Middle East Osney Mead, Oxford OX2 OEL, England   Hamilton, Bloemfontein 9300

Australia and   **Harcourt Brace Jovanovich Group**   South America   **Inter-Book Marketing Services**
New Zealand   **(Australia) Pty Limited**   Rua das Palmeiras, 32
                     30–52 Smidmore Street   Apto. 701
                     Marrickville, N.S.W. 2204   222–70 Rio de Janeiro
                     Australia   RJ, Brazil

Japan   **Igaku-Shoin Ltd.**
                     Tokyo International P.O. Box 5063
                     1–28–36 Hongo, Bunkyo-ku, Tokyo 113, Japan

---

NOTICE

The authors and publisher have made every effort to ensure that the patient care recommended herein, including choice of drugs and drug dosages, are in accord with the accepted standards and practice at the time of publication. However, since research and regulation constantly change clinical standards, the reader is urged to check the product information sheet included in the package of each drug, which includes recommended doses, warnings, and contra-indications. This is particularly important with new or infrequently used drugs.

Current Therapy in Allergy, Immunology, and Rheumatology-3   ISBN 1-55664-021-8

Library of Congress catalog card number: 85-70619   10 9 8 7 6 5 4 3 2 1

CONTRIBUTORS

SHARON ADLER, M.D.

Assistant Professor of Medicine, UCLA School of
Medicine, Los Angeles; Staff Physician, Harbor-UCLA
Medical Center, Torrance, California
Immunologically Mediated Nephrotic Renal Disease

ELAINE L. ALEXANDER, M.D., Ph.D.

Assistant Professor of Medicine, The Johns Hopkins
University School of Medicine, Baltimore, Maryland
Sjögren's Syndrome

DAVID H. ALLEN, M.B., Ph.D., F.R.A.C.P.

Clinical Lecturer, University of Sydney Medical School;
Consultant Thoracic Physician, Royal North Shore
Hospital, Sydney, Australia
Sulfite Induced Asthma

JOHN A. ANDERSON, M.D.

Clinical Professor, Department of Pediatrics, University
of Michigan Medical School, Ann Arbor; Chairman,
Department of Pediatrics, Henry Ford Hospital,
Detroit, Michigan
Penicillin Allergy

GRANT J. ANHALT, M.D.

Associate Professor, Department of Dermatology, The
Johns Hopkins University School of Medicine,
Baltimore, Maryland
Pemphigus

GERALD B. APPEL, M.D., F.A.C.P.

Associate Professor of Clinical Medicine, Columbia
University College of Physicians and Surgeons; Director
of Clinical Nephrology, Columbia-Presbyterian Medical
Center, New York, New York
Acute Interstitial Nephritis

BARRY G. W. ARNASON, M.D.

Professor and Chairman, Department of Neurology,
University of Chicago, Chicago, Illinois
Multiple Sclerosis

KIRAN K. BELANI, M.D.

Fellow, Department of Pediatrics, Division of Infectious
Diseases, University of Minnesota Medical School,
Minneapolis, Minnesota
Hyperimmunoglobulin E Syndrome

EUGENE R. BLEECKER, M.D.

Associate Professor of Medicine, Division of Pulmonary
Medicine, The Johns Hopkins University School of Medi-
cine, Baltimore, Maryland
Exercise Induced Asthma, Urticaria, and Anaphylaxis

WARREN K. BOLTON, M.D.

Professor of Internal Medicine, University of Virginia
School of Medicine, Charlottesville, Virginia
Immunologically Mediated Nephritic Renal Disease

HOMER A. BOUSHEY Jr., M.D.

Professor of Medicine, University of California School of
Medicine, San Francisco, California
Status Asthmaticus

SUZANNE L. BOWYER, M.D.

Assistant Professor of Clinical Pediatrics, University of
Southern California School of Medicine; Staff Physician,
Division of Rheumatology, Childrens Hospital,
Los Angeles, California
Juvenile Rheumatoid Arthritis

LAURENCE A. BOXER, M.D.

Professor, Department of Pediatrics, University of
Michigan Medical School; Director, Pediatric Hematology
and Oncology, C.S. Mott Children's Hospital,
Ann Arbor, Michigan
Autoimmune Leukopenia

REBECCA H. BUCKLEY, M.D.

J. Buren Sidbury Professor of Pediatrics and Professor of
Immunology, Duke University School of Medicine; Chief,
Division of Allergy and Immunology, Department of
Pediatrics, Duke University Medical Center,
Durham, North Carolina
Common Variable Immunodeficiency

KENNETH D. BURMAN, M.D., Col., M.C.

Professor of Medicine, Uniformed Services University of
the Health Sciences, Bethesda, Maryland; Assistant Chief,
Endocrine Service, Kyle Metabolic Unit, Walter Reed
Army Medical Center, Washington, D.C.
Hashimoto's Thyroiditis

JHOONG S. CHEIGH, M.D.

Associate Professor of Clinical Medicine, Cornell
University Medical College and The Rogosin Institute;
Associate Attending Physician, The New York Hospital-
Cornell Medical Center, New York, New York
Renal Transplant Rejection

ALAN S. COHEN, M.D.

Conrad Wesselhoeft Professor of Medicine, Boston
University School of Medicine; Chief of Medicine, Boston
City Hospital and Director, Thorndike Memorial
Laboratory, Boston, Massachusetts
Amyloidosis

MARIO CONDORELLI, M.D.

Professor and Chairman, Department of Medicine,
University of Naples, 2nd School of Medicine,
Naples, Italy
Acute Rheumatic Fever

KEVIN D. COOPER, M.D.

Director, Immunodermatology and Assistant Professor,
Department of Dermatology, University of Michigan
Medical School and Ann Arbor Veterans Administration
Hospital, Ann Arbor, Michigan
Atopic Dermatitis

THOMAS R. CUPPS, M.D.

Assistant Professor of Medicine, Georgetown University
School of Medicine, Washington, D.C.
Dermatomyositis and Polymyositis
Temporal Arteritis

PEYTON A. EGGLESTON, M.D.

Associate Professor of Pediatrics, The Johns Hopkins
University School of Medicine, Baltimore, Maryland
Asthma in Children

RICHARD EVANS III, M.D., M.P.H.

Professor of Clinical Pediatrics and Clinical Medicine,
Northwestern University Medical School; Head, Division
of Allergy and Immunology, Children's Memorial
Hospital, Chicago, Illinois
Allergic Reactions Caused by Exposure to Animals

ANTHONY S. FAUCI, M.D.

Director, National Institute of Allergy and Infectious
Diseases, National Institutes of Health,
Bethesda, Maryland
Systemic Vasculitis
Takayasu's Arteritis
Acquired Immunodeficiency Syndrome

JOHN I. GALLIN, M.D.

Director, Intramural Research Program, National Institute
of Allergy and Infectious Diseases, National Institutes of
Health, Bethesda, Maryland
Phagocyte Function Disorders

RAIF S. GEHA, M.D.

Professor of Pediatrics, Harvard Medical School; Chief,
Allergy Program, The Children's Hospital,
Boston, Massachusetts
Severe Combined Immunodeficiency Disease

RICHARD J. GLASSOCK, M.D.

Professor of Medicine, UCLA School of Medicine,
Los Angeles; Chairman, Department of Medicine,
Harbor-UCLA Medical Center, Torrance, California
Immunologically Mediated Nephrotic Renal Disease
Goodpasture's Syndrome

BARRY J. GOLDSTEIN, M.D., Ph.D.

Research Fellow, Department of Medicine, Harvard
Medical School; Section of Cellular and Molecular
Physiology, Joslin Diabetes Center; and Department of
Medicine, Brigham and Women's Hospital,
Boston, Massachusetts
Insulin Allergy and Resistance

MALCOLM W. GREAVES, M.D., Ph.D., F.R.C.P.

Professor, United Medical and Dental Schools of Guy's
and St. Thomas's Hospitals; Honorary Consultant, St.
John's Hospital for Diseases of the Skin,
London, England
Physical Urticaria and Angioedema

PAUL A. GREENBERGER, M.D.

Associate Professor of Medicine, Department of Allergy
and Immunology, Northwestern University Medical
School; Attending Staff, Northwestern Memorial Hospital,
Chicago, Illinois
Allergic Bronchopulmonary Aspergillosis

EVA C. GUINAN, M.D.

Instructor in Pediatrics, Harvard Medical School; Clinical
Associate in Pediatric Oncology, Dana-Farber Cancer
Institute, Boston, Massachusetts
Aplastic Anemia

RUSSELL P. HALL, M.D.

Assistant Professor, Duke University Medical Center,
Durham, North Carolina
Dermatitis Herpetiformis

JOHN A. HARDIN, M.D.

Professor of Medicine, Yale University School of
Medicine; Attending Physician, Yale-New Haven
Hospital, New Haven, Connecticut
Mixed Connective Tissue Disease

BARTON F. HAYNES, M.D.

Professor of Medicine and Chief, Division of
Rheumatology and Immunology, Department of Medicine,
Duke University Medical Center, Durham, North Carolina
Cogan's Syndrome

H. FRANKLIN HERLONG, M.D.

Associate Professor of Medicine, The Johns Hopkins University School of Medicine, Baltimore, Maryland
Chronic Active Hepatitis

DOUGLAS A. JABS, M.D.

Assistant Professor of Ophthalmology, The Johns Hopkins University School of Medicine, Baltimore, Maryland
Autoimmune Uveitis

ROBERT E. JORDON, M.D.

Professor and Chairman, Department of Dermatology, University of Texas Medical School; Chief of Dermatology, Hermann Hospital, Houston, Texas
Bullous Pemphigoid

C. RONALD KAHN, M.D.

Director, Elliott P. Joslin Research Laboratory, and Mary K. Iacocca Professor of Medicine, Harvard Medical School; Chief, Division of Diabetes and Metabolism, Brigham and Women's Hospital, Boston, Massachusetts
Insulin Allergy and Resistance

MICHAEL A. KALINER, M.D.

Head, Allergic Diseases Section, National Institute of Allergy and Infectious Diseases, National Institutes of Health, Bethesda, Maryland
Recurrent Idiopathic and Cryptogenic Anaphylaxis

ALLEN P. KAPLAN, M.D.

Professor and Chairman, Department of Medicine, State University of New York, Stony Brook, New York
Hereditary Angioedema

PAUL KATZ, M.D.

Associate Professor and Vice Chairman, Department of Medicine and Chief, Division of Rheumatology, Immunology, and Allergy, Georgetown University School of Medicine, Washington, D.C.
Reiter's Syndrome
Sarcoidosis

A. BARRY KAY, D.Sc., Ph.D., F.R.C.P.

Professor and Director, Department of Allergy and Clinical Immunology, Cardiothoracic Institute; Honorary Consultant Clinical Immunologist, Brompton Hospital, London, England
Asthma Provoked by Exposure to Allergens

BRETT V. KETTELHUT, M.D.

Medical Staff Fellow, Mast Cell Physiology Section, Laboratory of Clinical Investigation, National Institute of Allergy and Infectious Diseases, National Institutes of Health, Bethesda, Maryland
Food Allergy in Adults

JOHN H. KLIPPEL, M.D.

Clinical Director, National Institute of Arthritis, Musculoskeletal and Skin Diseases, National Institutes of Health, Bethesda, Maryland
Systemic Lupus Erythematosus
Lupus Nephritis

JOSEPH H. KORN, M.D.

Associate Professor, Division of Rheumatic Diseases, University of Connecticut School of Medicine, Farmington; Chief, Rheumatology Section and Associate Chief of Staff for Research, Veterans Administration Medical Center, Newington, Connecticut
Ankylosing Spondylitis
Systemic Sclerosis

H. CLIFFORD LANE, M.D.

Senior Investigator, Laboratory of Immunoregulation and Deputy Clinical Director, National Institute of Allergy and Infectious Diseases, National Institutes of Health, Bethesda, Maryland
Acquired Immunodeficiency Syndrome

ALEXANDER R. LAWTON, M.D.

Edward C. Stahlman Professor of Pediatric Physiology and Cell Metabolism, Professor of Microbiology, and Head, Division of Pediatric Immunology and Rheumatology, Vanderbilt University School of Medicine, Nashville, Tennessee
Congenital Immunodeficiency Diseases

RANDI Y. LEAVITT, M.D., Ph.D.

Senior Investigator, Laboratory of Immunoregulation, National Institute of Allergy and Infectious Diseases, National Institutes of Health, Bethesda, Maryland
Systemic Vasculitis
Takayasu's Arteritis

ALAN B. LEICHTMAN, M.D.

Transplant Nephrologist, Eastern Virginia Transplant Program, Sentara Norfolk General Hospital, Norfolk, Virginia
Therapeutic Approach to Renal Transplantation

MICHAEL I. LEVINE, M.D.

Fellow in Nephrology, Columbia-Presbyterian Medical Center, New York, New York
Acute Interstitial Nephritis

LAWRENCE M. LICHTENSTEIN, M.D., Ph.D.

Professor of Medicine, The Johns Hopkins University School of Medicine, Baltimore, Maryland
Insect Sting Allergy in Adults

WILLIS C. MADDREY, M.D.

Magee Professor of Medicine and Chairman of the Department, Jefferson Medical College; Physician-in-Chief, Department of Medicine, Thomas Jefferson University Hospital, Philadelphia, Pennsylvania
Primary Biliary Cirrhosis

GIANNI MARONE, M.D.

Associate Professor of Clinical Immunology, University of Naples, 2nd School of Medicine, Naples, Italy
Acute Rheumatic Fever

PAUL T. McBRIDE, M.S., M.D.

Assistant Clinical Professor, University of Washington School of Medicine; Medical Staff Allergist and Immunologist, Virginia Mason Clinic, Seattle, Washington
Recurrent Idiopathic and Cryptogenic Anaphylaxis

DEAN D. METCALFE, M.D.

Head, Mast Cell Physiology Section, Laboratory of Clinical Investigation, National Institute of Allergy and Infectious Diseases, National Institutes of Health, Bethesda, Maryland
Food Allergy in Adults

LYNNE H. MORRISON, M.D.

Research and Clinical Postdoctural Fellow, Department of Dermatology, The Johns Hopkins University School of Medicine; Senior Clinical Fellow, Department of Dermatology, The Johns Hopkins Hospital, Baltimore, Maryland
Pemphigus

PHILIP M. MURPHY, M.D.

Medical Staff Fellow, Bacterial Diseases Section, Laboratory of Clinical Investigation, National Institute of Allergy and Infectious Diseases, National Institutes of Health, Bethesda, Maryland
Phagocyte Function Disorders

ROBERT NACLERIO, M.D.

Associate Professor, Departments of Otolaryngology, Medicine, and Pediatrics, The Johns Hopkins University School of Medicine, Baltimore, Maryland
Perennial Rhinitis

DAVID G. NATHAN, M.D.

Robert A. Stranahan Professor of Pediatrics, Harvard Medical School; Physician-in-Chief, Department of Medicine, Children's Hospital, Boston, Massachusetts
Aplastic Anemia

HAROLD S. NELSON, M.D.

Professor of Medicine, University of Colorado Health Sciences Center School of Medicine; Staff Physician, Department of Medicine, National Jewish Center for Immunology and Respiratory Medicine, Denver, Colorado
Allergic Rhinitis

CAROL A. NEWILL, Ph.D.

Associate in Immunology and Infectious Diseases, The Johns Hopkins University School of Hygiene and Public Health, Baltimore, Maryland
Allergic Reactions Caused by Exposure to Animals

J. DESMOND O'DUFFY, M.D.

Professor of Medicine, Mayo Medical School; Consultant in Medicine, Mayo Clinic, Rochester, Minnesota
Behçet's Syndrome

ANTHONY D. ORMEROD, M.B., Ch.B., M.R.C.P.

Lecturer, University of Aberdeen; Senior Registrar, Aberdeen Royal Infirmary, Aberdeen, Scotland
Physical Urticaria and Angioedema

ALAN G. PALESTINE, M.D.

Head, Section of Clinical Immunology, Laboratory of Immunology, National Eye Institute, National Institutes of Health, Bethesda, Maryland
Autoallergic Diseases of the External Eye

JOSEPH E. PARRILLO, M.D.

Associate Professor of Clinical Medicine, George Washington University School of Medicine and Health Sciences, Washington, D.C.; Chief, Critical Care Medicine Department, National Institutes of Health, Bethesda, Maryland
Postcardiac Injury Syndrome
Inflammatory Myopericarditis

THOMAS A. E. PLATTS-MILLS, M.D., Ph.D.

Professor of Medicine and Head, Division of Allergy and Clinical Immunology, University of Virginia School of Medicine, Charlottesville, Virginia
Allergic Rhinitis Caused by House Dust and Other Nonpollen Allergens

PAUL G. QUIE, M.D.

Professor, University of Minnesota Medical School, Minneapolis, Minnesota
Hyperimmunoglobulin E Syndrome

ANTHONY T. REDER, M.D.

Assistant Professor of Neurology, University of Chicago, Chicago, Illinois
Multiple Sclerosis

ROBERT E. REISMAN, M.D.

Professor of Medicine and Pediatrics, State University of New York School of Medicine; Attending Physician, Buffalo General and Children's Hospitals and Co-Director, Allergy Research Laboratory, Buffalo General Hospital, Buffalo, New York
Insect Sting Allergy in Children

HERBERT Y. REYNOLDS, M.D.

Professor of Internal Medicine and Head, Pulmonary Section, Department of Medicine, Yale University School of Medicine; Chief, Respiratory Disease Services, Yale-New Haven Hospital, New Haven, Connecticut
Idiopathic Pulmonary Fibrosis

W. NEAL ROBERTS, M.D.

Assistant Professor of Medicine, Virginia Commonwealth University Medical College of Virginia, Richmond, Virginia
Rheumatoid Arthritis

SHAUN RUDDY, M.D.

Professor of Medicine, Microbiology and Immunology; Chairman, Division of Immunology and Connective Tissue Diseases, Virginia Commonwealth University Medical College of Virginia, Richmond, Virginia
Rheumatoid Arthritis

MARC J. SADOVNIC, M.D.

Fellow, Renal Division, University of Virginia School of Medicine, Charlottesville, Virginia
Immunologically Mediated Nephritic Renal Disease

HUGH A. SAMPSON, M.D.

Associate Professor of Pediatrics, The Johns Hopkins University School of Medicine, Baltimore, Maryland
Food Sensitivity in Children

ROBERT T. SCHOEN, M.D., F.A.C.P.

Assistant Clinical Professor, Yale University School of Medicine; Attending Physician, Yale-New Haven Hospital, New Haven, Connecticut
Mixed Connective Tissue Disease

ALAN D. SCHREIBER, M.D.

Professor of Medicine and Chairman, Graduate Group in Immunology, University of Pennsylvania School of Medicine, Philadelphia, Pennsylvania
Autoimmune Hemolytic Anemia

JOHN C. SELNER, M.D.

Clinical Professor of Pediatrics, University of Colorado Health Sciences Center School of Medicine; Director, Allergy Respiratory Institute of Colorado, Denver, Colorado
Chemical Sensitivity

GUY A. SETTIPANE, M.D.

Clinical Associate Professor of Medicine, Brown University Program in Medicine; Director, Division of Allergy, Department of Medicine, Rhode Island Hospital, Providence, Rhode Island
Aspirin Sensitivity in Rhinosinusitis and Asthma

MARJORIE E. SEYBOLD, M.D.

Adjunct Member, Scripps Clinic and Research Foundation, La Jolla, California
Myasthenia Gravis

FERGUS SHANAHAN, M.D., F.R.C.P.(C), M.R.C.P.(UK), M.R.C.P.I.

Assistant Professor of Medicine, UCLA School of Medicine; Associate Director, UCLA Inflammatory Bowel Disease Clinic, Center for Health Sciences, Los Angeles, California
Ulcerative Colitis and Crohn's Disease

N. RAPHAEL SHULMAN, M.D.

Chief, Clinical Hematology Branch, National Institute of Diabetes, Digestive and Kidney Diseases, The National Institutes of Health, Bethesda, Maryland; Clinical Professor of Medicine, Georgetown University School of Medicine, Washington, D.C.
Idiopathic Thrombocytopenic Purpura

MARTHA SKINNER, M.D.

Professor of Medicine, Boston University School of Medicine; Visiting Physician, Boston City Hospital, Boston, Massachusetts
Amyloidosis

RAYMOND G. SLAVIN, M.D.

Professor of Internal Medicine and Microbiology, Saint Louis University School of Medicine, Saint Louis, Missouri
Hypersensitivity Pneumonitis

DOROTHY D. SOGN, M.D.

Chief, Allergy, Asthma, and Immunology Branch, Allergic and Immunologic Diseases Program, National Institute of Allergy and Infectious Diseases; Staff Physician, The Clinical Center, National Institutes of Health, Bethesda Maryland
Drug Reactions

PETER G. SOHNLE, M.D.

Professor, Department of Medicine, Medical College of Wisconsin; Chief, Section of Infectious Diseases, Veterans Administration Medical Center, Milwaukee, Wisconsin
Chronic Mucocutaneous Candidiasis

NICHOLAS A. SOTER, M.D.

Professor of Dermatology, New York University School of Medicine; Attending Physician, University, Bellevue, and Manhattan Veterans Administration Hospitals, New York, New York
Chronic Urticaria
Cutaneous Vasculitis

KURT H. STENZEL, M.D.

Professor of Medicine and Biochemistry, Cornell
University Medical College and The Rogosin Institute;
Attending Physician and Chief, Division of Nephrology,
The New York Hospital-Cornell Medical Center,
New York, New York
Renal Transplant Rejection

FRANCES J. STORRS, M.D.

Professor of Dermatology, Department of Dermatology,
Oregon Health Sciences University School of Medicine,
Portland, Oregon
Contact Dermatitis

TERRY B. STROM, M.D.

Associate Professor of Medicine, Harvard Medical
School; Staff Physician, Brigham and Women's and
Beth Israel Hospitals, Boston, Massachusetts
Therapeutic Approach to Renal Transplantation

TIMOTHY J. SULLIVAN III, M.D.

Associate Professor of Internal Medicine and
Microbiology, Department of Internal Medicine; Head,
Allergy and Clinical Immunology, Parkland Memorial
Hospital, University of Texas Southwestern Medical
Center, Dallas, Texas
Systemic Anaphylaxis

RICHARD J. SUMMERS, M.D.

Assistant Professor of Medicine, The Johns Hopkins
University School of Medicine, Baltimore; Associate
Professor of Medicine and Pediatrics, Uniformed Services
University of the Health Sciences, Bethesda, Maryland
Allergic Reactions Caused by Exposure to Animals

MANIKKAM SUTHANTHIRAN, M.D.

Associate Professor of Medicine, Cornell University
Medical College and The Rogosin Institute; Associate
Attending Physician, The New York Hospital-Cornell
Medical Center, New York, New York
Renal Transplant Rejection

ALAIN TAÏEB, M.D.

Assistant des Universités, Université de Bordeaux II;
Assistant des Hôpitaux, Service de Dermatologie, Hôpital
des Enfants, Centre Hospitalier Universitaire de
Bordeaux, Bordeaux, France
Atopic Dermatitis

STEPHAN TARGAN, M.D.

Professor of Medicine, UCLA School of Medicine;
Director, UCLA Inflammatory Bowel Disease Clinic,
Center for Health Sciences, Los Angeles, California
Ulcerative Colitis and Crohn's Disease

JOHN H. TOOGOOD, M.D., F.R.C.P.(C), F.C.C.P.

Professor of Medicine, University of Western Ontario
Faculty of Medicine; Director, Allergy Clinic, Victoria
Hospital, London, Ontario, Canada
Asthma in Adults

PAUL P. VANARSDEL Jr., M.D.

Professor of Medicine and Head, Section of Allergy,
University of Washington School of Medicine; Attending
Physician, University Hospital, Seattle, Washington
Drug Reactions

ROBERT WALKER, M.D.

Fellow in Pulmonary Medicine, Cardiopulmonary
Division, Hospital of the University of Pennsylvania,
Philadelphia, Pennsylvania
Acquired Immunodeficiency Syndrome

GEORGE W. WARD Jr., M.D.

Associate Professor of Medicine, Division of Allergy and
Clinical Immunology, University of Virginia School of
Medicine, Charlottesville, Virginia
*Allergic Rhinitis Caused by House Dust and Other
Nonpollen Allergens*

HARRY J. WARD, M.D.

Assistant Professor of Medicine, UCLA School of
Medicine, Los Angeles; Medical Director, Renal
Transplant Section, Harbor-UCLA Medical Center,
Torrance, California
Goodpasture's Syndrome

ETHAN WEINER, M.D.

Assistant Professor, Division of Rheumatic Diseases,
University of Connecticut School of Medicine,
Farmington, Connecticut
Systemic Sclerosis

ROBERT A. WOOD, M.D.

Assistant Professor of Pediatrics, The Johns Hopkins
University School of Medicine, Baltimore, Maryland
Asthma in Children

KIRK D. WUEPPER, M.D.

Professor of Dermatology, Oregon Health Sciences
University of Medicine, Portland, Oregon
Erythema Multiforme

KIM B. YANCEY, M.D.

Associate Professor, Department of Dermatology,
Uniformed Services University of the Health Sciences;
Consultant, Dermatology Branch, National Institutes of
Health and Department of Dermatology, Bethesda Navy
Hospital, Bethesda, Maryland
Herpes Gestationis

PREFACE

In our preface to the first two editions of this book we noted our impression that we were experiencing a rapid growth in the relevance of immunologic research and principles to the practice of medicine. In the three years since the previous edition, this has become even clearer, particularly with the enormous attention, both professional and public, given to the acquired immunodeficiency syndrome, which has increased the prominence of immunology as a basic scientific and clinical discipline. The book continues to focus on clinical immunology and its close relatives, allergy and rheumatology.

We have attempted to make this edition responsive to the rapid growth of information and to have it continue to serve two major purposes. The first is rapid publication, providing timely information to the clinician rather than forcing him to rely on more standard texts, which are issued only once or twice a decade. The second need recognized by this book arises from the fact that most of the standard immunology texts and, certainly, most general medicine texts, do not focus on the therapy of the diseases in question. In this volume, as in previous volumes, we have asked the authors to deal with pathogenic and diagnostic concepts only as they pertain to therapy and to focus on defining the clinical problems clearly, detailing precisely how to treat these diseases in all of their various manifestations. In response to the comments of our readers and reviewers, we have changed the format of this edition to include a limited set of relevant references. We hope this will improve the usefulness of this volume. We have provided no rigid guidelines to the authors for describing the therapy of the diseases discussed in this book. There are moderate variations in therapeutic approach among investigators and institutions, and indeed, some approaches that are new and innovative. We have called upon the most prominent clinical investigators, experts in each of the diseases covered, to provide their own up-to-date therapeutic advice.

Because of this approach, the success of this volume depends almost entirely on the fund of knowledge, judgment, and clinical experience of the authors. We are pleased that once again we have been able to persuade eminent experts from a variety of medical specialties to share these attributes with us.

We would like to acknowledge again the assistance of our publisher, Mr. Brian C. Decker, as well as the editorial assistance of Ms. Margaret Askey and Ms. Ann C. London. Our major debt continues to be to the scientists who have been willing to provide us and the profession with their insights into the treatment of allergic, immunologic, and rheumatologic diseases.

Lawrence M. Lichtenstein, M.D., Ph.D.
Anthony S. Fauci, M.D.

CONTENTS

Allergic Rhinitis 1
Harold S. Nelson

Allergic Reactions Caused by
Exposure to Animals 5
Richard Evans III
Richard J. Summers
Carol A. Newill

Allergic Rhinitis Caused by House Dust
and Other Nonpollen Allergens 8
George W. Ward Jr.
Thomas A. E. Platts-Mills

Perennial Rhinitis 14
Robert Naclerio

Asthma Provoked by Exposure to
Allergens 21
A. Barry Kay

Asthma in Adults 25
John H. Toogood

Asthma in Children 31
Peyton A. Eggleston
Robert A. Wood

Aspirin Sensitivity in Rhinosinusitis
and Asthma 36
Guy A. Settipane

Exercise Induced Asthma, Urticaria,
and Anaphylaxis 39
Eugene R. Bleecker

Sulfite Induced Asthma 42
David H. Allen

Status Asthmaticus 44
Homer A. Boushey Jr.

Chemical Sensitivity 48
John C. Selner

Food Sensitivity in Children 52
Hugh A. Sampson

Food Allergy in Adults 56
Brett V. Kettelhut
Dean D. Metcalfe

Chronic Urticaria 60
Nicholas A. Soter

Physical Urticaria and Angioedema 62
Anthony D. Ormerod
Malcolm W. Greaves

Hereditary Angioedema 66
Allen P. Kaplan

Penicillin Allergy 68
John A. Anderson

Drug Reactions 77
Dorothy D. Sogn
Paul P. VanArsdel Jr.

Insect Sting Allergy in Adults 81
Lawrence M. Lichtenstein

Insect Sting Allergy in Children 87
Robert E. Reisman

Systemic Anaphylaxis 91
Timothy J. Sullivan III

Recurrent Idiopathic and Cryptogenic
Anaphylaxis 98
Paul T. McBride
Michael A. Kaliner

Systemic Lupus Erythematosus 101
John H. Klippel

Rheumatoid Arthritis 106
Shaun Ruddy
W. Neal Roberts

Juvenile Rheumatoid Arthritis 115
Suzanne L. Bowyer

Reiter's Syndrome 121
Paul Katz

Sjögren's Syndrome 125
Elaine L. Alexander

Ankylosing Spondylitis 130
Joseph H. Korn

Systemic Sclerosis 135
Ethan Weiner
Joseph H. Korn

Dermatomyositis and Polymyositis 140
Thomas R. Cupps

Mixed Connective Tissue Disease 145
Robert T. Schoen
John A. Hardin

Systemic Vasculitis 149
Anthony S. Fauci
Randi Y. Leavitt

Cutaneous Vasculitis 155
Nicholas A. Soter

Temporal Arteritis 157
Thomas R. Cupps

Takayasu's Arteritis 161
Randi Y. Leavitt
Anthony S. Fauci

Behcet's Syndrome 165
J. Desmond O'Duffy

Cogan's Syndrome 170
Barton F. Haynes

Dermatitis Herpetiformis 173
Russell P. Hall

Herpes Gestationis 176
Kim B. Yancey

Atopic Dermatitis 177
Kevin D. Cooper
Alain Taïeb

Contact Dermatitis 182
Frances J. Storrs

Pemphigus 186
Lynne H. Morrison
Grant J. Anhalt

Bullous Pemphigoid 189
Robert E. Jordon

Erythema Multiforme 190
Kirk D. Wuepper

Immunologically Mediated Nephrotic
Renal Disease 192
Sharon Adler
Richard J. Glassock

Acute Interstitial Nephritis 198
Gerald B. Appel
Michael I. Levine

Renal Transplant Rejection 201
Kurt H. Stenzel
Jhoong S. Cheigh
Manikkam Suthanthiran

Lupus Nephritis 204
John H. Klippel

Goodpasture's Syndrome 209
Harry J. Ward
Richard J. Glassock

Hypersensitivity Pneumonitis 212
Raymond G. Slavin

Idiopathic Pulmonary Fibrosis 214
Herbert Y. Reynolds

Allergic Bronchopulmonary
Aspergillosis 220
Paul A. Greenberger

Sarcoidosis 223
Paul Katz

Multiple Sclerosis 228
Barry G. W. Arnason
Anthony T. Reder

Myasthenia Gravis 231
Marjorie E. Seybold

Autoimmune Uveitis 235
Douglas A. Jabs

Autoallergic Diseases of the
External Eye 239
Alan G. Palestine

Ulcerative Colitis and Crohn's
Disease 242
Fergus Shanahan
Stephan Targan

Chronic Active Hepatitis 251
H. Franklin Herlong

Primary Biliary Cirrhosis 254
Willis C. Maddrey

Acute Rheumatic Fever 258
Gianni Marone
Mario Condorelli

Postcardiac Injury Syndrome 263
Joseph E. Parrillo

Inflammatory Myopericarditis 268
Joseph E. Parrillo

Idiopathic Thrombocytopenic
Purpura 274
N. Raphael Shulman

Autoimmune Hemolytic Anemia 280
Alan D. Schreiber

Autoimmune Leukopenia 285
Laurence A. Boxer

Aplastic Anemia 289
Eva C. Guinan
David G. Nathan

Phagocyte Function Disorders 293
  Philip M. Murphy
  John I. Gallin

Common Variable Immunodeficiency . . . 301
  Rebecca H. Buckley

Severe Combined Immunodeficiency
Disease 305
  Raif S. Geha

Congenital Immunodeficiency
Diseases 308
  Alexander R. Lawton

Hyperimmunoglobulin E Syndrome 313
  Paul G. Quie
  Kiran K. Belani

Amyloidosis 316
  Martha Skinner
  Alan S. Cohen

Hashimoto's Thyroiditis 322
  Kenneth D. Burman

Insulin Allergy and Resistance 327
  Barry J. Goldstein
  C. Ronald Kahn

Chronic Mucocutaneous Candidiasis 331
  Peter G. Sohnle

Immunologically Mediated Nephritic
Renal Disease 334
  Marc J. Sadovnic
  Warren K. Bolton

Therapeutic Approach to Renal
Transplantation 339
  Alan B. Leichtman
  Terry B. Strom

Acquired Immunodeficiency
Syndrome 343
  Robert Walker
  H. Clifford Lane
  Anthony S. Fauci

ALLERGIC RHINITIS

HAROLD S. NELSON, M.D.

Rhinitis is a common affliction that varies in severity, producing nearly disabling symptoms in some patients while in others producing such mild symptoms that they are not easily distinguished from heightened awareness of the normal mucus production of the nose. The types of rhinitis also present a broad spectrum: Seasonal allergic rhinitis is usually clearly distinguishable, but perennial rhinitis may be separated less precisely into a group of disorders having an allergic basis, a group that is nonallergic but clearly is associated with other allergic or potentially allergic conditions, and finally the group formerly called vasomotor rhinitis. The latter could more accurately be called merely nonallergic, noneosinophilic rhinitis since little is known of its cause or mechanisms. The importance of distinguishing among these types of rhinitis is that they affect the therapeutic approach. Clearly allergen avoidance and allergy immunotherapy are indicated only for rhinitis that truly has an allergic basis. Nonallergic rhinitis associated with asthma, eczema, or seasonal allergic rhinitis does not benefit from an allergen directed therapy, but often responds more satisfactorily to pharmacotherapy than does nonallergic rhinitis not sharing these associations.

CLASSIFICATION OF RHINITIS

Seasonal allergic rhinitis is characterized by symptoms of nasal and ocular pruritus, repetitive sneezing, watery rhinorrhea, and nasal obstruction occurring during a particular season corresponding to the appearance in the air of an allergen to which the subject can be demonstrated to be sensitive. Significant seasonal allergic rhinitis in the absence of skin test reactivity to the suspected allergen has not been convincingly demonstrated.

Perennial allergic rhinitis, in areas where the occurrence of frost insures a season without significant outdoor aeroallergens, is primarily due to sensitivity to animal dander and insect allergens, particularly those from the house dust mite but perhaps more often than appreciated also those from the cockroach. The importance of indoor molds in the etiology of perennial allergic rhinitis is suspected in some instances when damp areas exist in homes, but few studies have attempted to document their clinical importance. Ingestant allergens have been even less well studied, but the usual opinion is that they are of little importance as a cause of rhinitis beyond infancy and early childhood.

Perennial nonallergic eosinophilic (atopic) rhinitis is a condition that has only slowly been recognized, although the pace has been accelerated by several recent studies. It has been known for over 50 years that patients with nonallergic asthma have associated rhinitis and hypertrophic sinusitis with a tendency toward nasal polyp, and that their nasal secretions, like their sputum and blood, are characterized by an excess of eosinophils. Nasal biopsies, or examination of tissue removed at the time of sinus surgery has regularly shown an eosinophilic infiltration of the tissue. It is a reasonable assumption that the same nonallergic rhinitis, characterized by eosinophilic infiltration of the tissues and eosinophilia of the secretions, can occur alone as well as in conjunction with the other atopic diseases, such as seasonal allergic rhinitis, bronchial asthma, and atopic eczema. Also, just as patients with atopic eczema and bronchial asthma may have positive skin test results that are not clinically relevant to their disease, so too may patients with this atopic form of nonallergic rhinitis. Finally, as evidence has been presented that in patients with atopic diseases there may be enhanced mediator release in response to nonimmunologic stimuli, it should not be surprising that patients with nonallergic atopic rhinitis may experience symptoms suggesting the release of histamine, with itchy eyes and nose, sneezing, and rhinorrhea of a degree seen in seasonal allergic rhinitis.

Perennial nonallergic noneosinophilic (nonatopic) rhinitis formerly was termed vasomotor rhinitis, with the proposal that these patients experienced symptoms as a result of an excessive parasympathetic response to various noxious nonimmunologic stimuli. Although these patients do respond with symptoms to irritating odors and temperature changes, so too do virtually all patients with rhinitis. Since there is no convincing evidence that these patients' symptoms are caused by autonomic mechanisms or even that they constitute a single disease entity, a new term is needed that more accurately reflects the state of our knowledge. In general, the response of these patients to pharmacotherapy is not as favorable as it is in patients with the other types of rhinitis. However, there are a few well categorized conditions that might be separated from this group, such as the rhinitis of pregnancy and hypothyroidism, and rhinitis medicamentosa due to either the topical use of decongestants or systemically administered medications. These conditions offer the prospect of a more successful resolution.

THERAPY OF ALLERGIC RHINITIS

The therapies of allergic and nonallergic rhinitis may be justifiably considered together. Measures directed toward allergens—avoidance and immunotherapy—are appropriate only in cases of rhinitis in which a significant allergic component has been demonstrated. Usually the treatment of rhinitis includes a major component of pharmacotherapy, and here the drugs employed are the same, although the response to the drug varies with the type of the rhinitis.

Avoidance

The first consideration in the treatment of allergic rhinitis should be an attempt to avoid completely or decrease the exposure to the offending allergen. Although, with the exception of family pets, complete elimination is seldom possible, substantial reduction in exposure often can be accomplished. In most pollen seasons the periods of peak counts are of limited duration, and these counts are generally highest during the midday or afternoon. Pollen concentrations are considerably reduced indoors, particularly if air conditioning is employed allowing windows and doors to remain closed. For these reasons patients with pollen induced seasonal allergic rhinitis often can avoid excessive symptoms by not undertaking outdoor recreational activities during the times of highest pollen counts. Although the season for the dry spore molds, such as *Alternaria* and *Cladosporium,* is more prolonged than it is for most pollens, peak counts are again encountered during dry windy summer afternoons, allowing for some reduction in exposure by modification of activities at these times. The spores that particularly characterize periods of dampness and rain—basidiospores and ascospores—are especially numerous during the early morning hours. If they are suspected of causing allergic problems (a determination more dependent on history than testing because of the general lack of relevant extracts), closing windows at night, through the use of air conditioning if necessary, would be expected to effect a major reduction in exposure.

The most important allergens causing perennial allergy, and the major components of "house dust," are animal danders and allergens derived from the house dust mite. The latter is ubiquitous except in the drier portions of the country, such as the Rocky Mountains and the southwest. An additional significant component—cockroach allergen—is encountered in areas where these insects are prevalent, such as the inner city areas of the north and the warmer portions of the country. Since house dust mites tend to accumulate in bedding, upholstered furniture, and adjacent carpeting, some control of allergen exposure is possible. When this has been undertaken in a thorough manner, a significant decrease in symptoms of asthma in children has been reported. The role of air cleaning devices in the avoidance of house dust mite allergen is not clear, since the allergen occurs predominantly in relatively large fecal pellets, which would be expected to rapidly fall from the air by gravity. Thus, local reservoirs, such as pillows, mattresses, and bed covers, appear more likely to be an important source than the allergen floating in the air.

Dander from pets, particularly cats and dogs, is a major perennial allergen. Clearly complete avoidance should be possible, but emotional ties or the presence of pets in the homes of others often frustrates avoidance measures. It should be possible to "animal proof" the bedroom by excluding the pet from this room and keeping the door and heating ducts closed. There are no data that indicate whether under these circumstances the use of a room air filtering device in the bedroom would be a worthwhile additional measure. There is evidence that with the continued access of the pet to the bedroom, the concentration of allergen in the furnishings would negate any impact of the use of air filtration on the total allergen load. If less than complete elimination of the family pet is possible, the more restricted the area in which the animal is allowed and the less furniture and carpeting to which it has access, the better.

The role of indoor mold allergy in producing allergic rhinitis is unclear. Damp areas in the house that cause symptoms should be dehumidified if possible, and if humidifiers are employed, care should be taken that they are cleaned regularly and do not become a source of spore aerosols.

For all patients with rhinitis, nonimmunologic irritants are a problem. Some can be avoided, and tobacco smoking within the home or workplace should be eliminated. It should also be possible, at least within the family, to avoid the use of strongly scented toiletries and cleaning products.

Pharmacotherapy

Antihistamines

Competitive antagonists of the H_1 receptor have been the traditional basic treatment for allergic and nonallergic rhinitis. The older preparations have been grouped into six classes in part with the expectation that changing from one class to another might evade the tolerance that develops to this group of drugs. Recently it has been demonstrated that the tolerance is probably related to the histamine receptor and is not specific for the class of agent that induced it.

It has been suggested that subjects be provided with multiple samples of antihistamines to determine which they find most effective. However, several studies employing representatives from each of the antihistamine classes have confirmed a general pattern that the alkylamines, represented by chlorpheniramine and brompheniramine, are preferred by the largest number of subjects, and that hydroxyzine in the doses commonly employed appears to be slightly more effective than chlorpheniramine but also causes slightly more side effects, making it generally less satisfactory. A limited number of studies suggest that azatadine may also cause relatively few side effects.

The side effects of the traditional antihistamines are primarily of two types. There are direct central nervous system effects, which sometimes include stimulation, restlessness, and nervousness but much more often are characterized by drowsiness or incoordination. The second major group of side effects are related to anticholinergic actions of these drugs and include dryness of the mouth, urinary retention, impotence, and blurring of vision. Tolerance to the central nervous system side effects develops rapidly, and by 4 to 10 days the incidence of drowsiness in many studies is similar to that with placebo. Tolerance to the desired antihistaminic properties also develops by 3 weeks, but this does not appear to be as profound in degree as the central tolerance, effectively improving the therapeutic ratio for these drugs. Recently, antihistamines have been developed that are nonsedating because they do not cross the blood-brain barrier. Furthermore, these drugs are free of anticholinergic action, thus avoiding some of the other side effects of the traditional antihistamines. Of this group, only terfenadine is currently approved for use in the United States, but approval of astemizole appears likely in the near future.

Antihistamines block some, but not all, of the symptoms of allergic rhinitis. They effectively relieve pruritus, sneezing, and rhinorrhea, whereas they are largely ineffective for nasal congestion. Among the reasons offered for the latter is the demonstration that vasodilation in the nose is mediated largely by H_2 receptors. This has led to the suggestion that combined treatment with H_1 and H_2 antagonists might enhance symptomatic relief, and indeed the effectiveness of this combined treatment has been demonstrated both with nasal allergen challenge and in the course of seasonal allergic rhinitis. The use of H_1 and H_2 antagonists has not achieved widespread popularity, probably because of the availability of highly effective alternatives, such as topically applied corticosteroids. The availability of relatively pure H_1 antagonists, such as astemazole, has demonstrated that histamine is important in the production of symptoms in nonallergic as well as allergic rhinitis. The decision whether to try antihistamine therapy is best made based on the basis of the types of symptoms the patient is experiencing, rather than by the perception whether the symptoms have an allergic basis.

Pharmacokinetic studies in adults have revealed unexpectedly long serum half-lifes for a number of antihistamines. Hydroxyzine, chlorpheniramine, and brompheniramine all have serum half-lifes of approximately 24 hours, suggesting that once daily dosing at bedtime with nonsustained release formulations should be adequate for the relief of symptoms. This dosing schedule has the advantage that maximal serum levels, and therefore sedation occurs while the patient is asleep. The use of single bedtime dosing, in addition to a gradual build-up of the dosage over 1 to 2 weeks, may allow the use of an inexpensive medication effectively with minimal side effects. In children the serum half-lifes of these drugs are about 12 hours, perhaps accounting for the relatively larger dosages of antihistamines employed in children but also making single daily dose therapy in children impractical. The new nonsedating antihistamine terfenadine has a half-life somewhat shorter than that of the preparations just listed, and twice daily dosing appears to be appropriate. Astemizole, on the other hand, possesses pharmacokinetic properties of a different order, with a calculated half-life of 104 hours and with suppression of skin test reactions persisting for several months after the discontinuation of therapy.

In comparative trials, usually of only 1 or 2 weeks duration, terfenadine, 60 mg twice daily, has produced control of symptoms equivalent to that with dosages of chlorpheniramine of 6 to 16 mg per day but with a lower incidence of side effects. It has not been demonstrated by controlled trials that the equal effectiveness and the reduced side effects would continue with prolonged therapy after central nervous systems tolerance has developed to chlorpheniramine. In one study that compared terfenadine and astemizole over several months in the treatment of seasonal allergic rhinitis, there appeared to be a definite decline in the effectiveness of terfenadine relative to placebo in the latter part of the study. Clearly more long term, controlled studies of terfenadine are needed, especially considering the marked cost differential between terfenadine and conventional antihistamines such as chlorpheniramine.

It is frequently stated that the antihistamines are more effective when administered on a regular basis, rather than being taken as needed for the relief of already existing symptoms. Since these drugs are competitive antagonists, this proposition is reasonable, although untested. Another argument for the regular use of the older preparations is that tolerance develops to the central nervous system side effects, improving their therapeutic ratio.

Decongestants

The drugs employed as decongestants are nonselective alpha-adrenergic agonists capable of constricting blood vessels elsewhere in the body. For that reason the preferred route of administration would be topical application to the nasal mucosa. Long acting topical decongestant therapy is recommended for the treatment of nasal congestion associated with viral respiratory infections, to promote drainage during acute infections of the paranasal sinuses and middle ears, and to facilitate penetration during the first few days of topical corticosteroid therapy in patients with marked nasal obstruction. The limitation to their use is the well recognized development of rebound obstruction, probably due to the induction of down regulation of the alpha-adrenergic receptors.

Orally administered alpha-adrenergic decongestants are also available, both as single drugs and in combination with antihistamines. They produce well recognized side effects of tremor, restlessness, and agitation and can cause hypertension and urinary retention. Hypertension particularly has been reported with phenylpropanolamine, which appears to have a very narrow therapeutic range. Pseudoephedrine, the other commonly employed drug, has been implicated less frequently. Nevertheless a recent review concluded that there were inadequate studies to insure the safety of oral decongestant therapy in patients with hypertension.

There also are few studies that have addressed the effectiveness of these drugs as decongestants during the course of long term administration when some degree of alpha-adrenergic tolerance may be presumed to have developed. A reduction in nasal airway resistance was demonstrated following a dose of 60 mg of pseudoephedrine, but it persisted for only 2 hours. The sympathomimetics, however, have one advantage, and that is that their side effects tend to be directly opposed to those of the older antihistamines, making the combination attractive from the standpoint of reduced side effects.

Cromolyn Sodium

A nasal solution of 4 percent cromolyn sodium, administered four to six times daily, has been demonstrated to provide moderate relief of the symptoms of seasonal allergic rhinitis. As would be anticipated for a nasal spray, it does not alleviate eye symptoms. Cromolyn nasal solution also has been tested in patients with perennial rhinitis, in whom it produced a modest reduction in symptoms in those with positive skin test results but no better results than placebo in patients with negative skin test results, even in those who had profuse nasal eosinophilia. The topically applied steroid sprays have consistently demonstrated marked superiority over cromolyn in comparative trials and appear to be the preferred treatment except in patients with significant local side effects from the topical use of steroid preparations or those with marked "steroid phobia." Antihistamines have been demonstrated to be as effective as cromolyn and have the advantage of less frequent dosing, control of eye symptoms, and usually less cost. Therefore, in patients tolerating antihistamines, they would appear to be the preferred initial treatment.

Cromolyn also is available as a 2 percent solution for use in the eyes. Again there is the inconvenience of six time daily use, but this preparation does provide good control of ocular symptoms as well as some effect on nasal symptoms and thus may complement topical nasal steroid therapy in the treatment of seasonal allergic rhinitis in patients whose ocular symptoms are prominent.

Corticosteroids

Two formulations of nasal steroids are available: beclomethasone dipropionate as a micronized powder in a freon propelled vehicle and flunisolide as a propylene glycol solution delivered by a pump spray. The initial dosage of the former is usually four discharges into each nostril daily, and these can be delivered as one spray four times daily or two twice daily without affecting efficacy. Flunisolide therapy frequently has been initiated with two sprays into each nostril three times daily, but the dosage may be decreased to twice daily sprays without loss of control. In these dosages the two topically applied corticosteroids appear to be of similar efficacy. Both have some tendency to cause mucosal bleeding, but a particular problem with flunisolide for some patients is nasal burning, sufficient in a few patients to cause them to discontinue the medication.

Both drugs are very effective in seasonal allergic rhinitis, although symptom control is seldom complete. They do not relieve eye symptoms. Furthermore, there is a delay of several days for maximal effect. If marked nasal obstruction is present, they may be ineffective because of lack of access to the nasal mucosa, and initiation of therapy with 3 to 5 days of prednisone, 40 mg per day, or the topical use of a decongestant spray before each dose of corticosteroid for the same period may be necessary. Several studies suggest that antihistamines and topical corticosteroid therapy are complimentary; there are no similar data for cromolyn and topical corticosteroid therapy.

It is clear that the topical corticosteroid therapy is more effective in "atopic (or nonallergic) eosinophilic rhinitis" than in rhinitis that is not related to the atopic diseases. Thus, a positive family history of atopic diseases, positive skin test results, pale swollen mucosae, or the presence of eosinophils in the nasal secretions all were predictors of a likely favorable response to topical corticosteroid therapy. The absence of these markers indicated perhaps at best a 24 percent chance of improvement. Despite this unpromising likelihood of a response, since these are generally patients who have failed to respond to other medication, a 2 week, carefully evaluated trial is indicated.

In patients with recurrent sinusitis or nasal polyps, the treatment of the associated nasal symptoms with topical corticosteroid therapy had been reported to diminish recurrences.

Miscellaneous Treatments

The vehicle of the flunisolide spray—propylene glycol—as well as saline nasal sprays and washes have been reported to diminish symptoms of perennial rhinitis, and in some cases this has been accompanied by an improvement in histopathologic findings.

The anticholinergic properties of the older antihistamines were thought to contribute to their efficacy by exerting a drying effect. Ipratropium bromide, a recently introduced anticholinergic, has been tried in selected cases of nonallergic perennial rhinitis characterized by marked rhinorrhea, with some decrease in symptoms.

Immunotherapy

Immunotherapy is reserved for last because that is its proper role in the treatment of allergic rhinitis. This is not a reflection of a lack of efficacy. Placebo controlled studies have clearly demonstrated that injection of extracts of pollens, animal danders, and house dust mite produce not only a decrease in clinical symptoms on natural exposure but also immunologic changes, which include a progressive decline in the levels of IgE specific for the substances being injected. Thus, unlike the other treatment modalities mentioned, allergy immunotherapy offers the promise of actually reversing the sensitized state.

Why then is the use of allergy immunotherapy deferred until other forms of therapy have first been tried, and failed? The reason is the rigorous requirements placed upon the physician and the patient if allergy immunotherapy is to succeed: First the physician must determine that the symptoms are truly allergic—that the nature and timing of symptoms, the patient's exposure, and the patient's degree of sensitivity strongly suggest a causal relationship. Next the allergen must be specifically identified; this often is possible with pollens but rarely is possible with molds. Then potent extracts of these substances must be injected, ultimately at high concentrations, which carry the danger of serious or rarely even fatal reactions. The requirement on the patient's part is the investment in time and money over several years if lasting results are to be obtained. Anyone working in the field of allergy has to be concerned about the frequency with which immunotherapy is undertaken without these requisites being satisfied and the number of patients who report no decrease in symptoms after an investment of several years and many hundreds of dollars. Under present circumstances allergy immunotherapy should be reserved for clear-cut allergy, to well defined allergens, in patients who have responded poorly to symptomatic therapy and have a prolonged season or perennial symptoms.

There are allergy extract preparations that have not yet been approved for release and that to some extent might restore the previous balance between symptomatic and allergy injection therapy. These are the modified extracts, allergenic extracts that have been treated to reduce their allergenicity, with preservation of their immunogenicity. These extracts hold the promise, should they obtain government approval, of allowing allergy immunotherapy to be offered with greater safety and with many fewer injections. These advantages, together with the fact that of the available modes of therapy of allergic rhinitis, only allergy immunotherapy can promise to correct the underlying abnormality, would make injection therapy a much more attractive alternative than it presently is.

SUGGESTED READING

Hillas J, Booth RJ, et al. A comparative trial of intra-nasal beclomethasone dipropionate and sodium cromoglycate in patients with chronic perennial rhinitis. Clin Allergy 1980; 10:253–258.

Howarth PH, Holgate ST. Comparative trial or two non-sedating H_1 antihistamines, terfenadine and astemizole, for hay fever. Thorax 1984; 39:668–672.

Long WF, Taylor RJ, et al. Skin test suppression by antihistamines and the development of subsensitivity. J Allergy Clin Immunol 1985; 76:113–117.

Murray AB, Ferguson AC. Dust-free bedrooms in the treatment of asthmatic children with house dust or house dust mite allergy: a controlled trial. Pediatrics 1983; 71:418–422.

Sibbald B, Hilton S, et al. An open cross-over trial comparing two doses of astemizole and beclomethasone dipropionate in the treatment of perennial rhinitis. Clin Allergy 1986; 16:203–211.

Turkeltaub PC, Norman PS, et al. Treatment of seasonal and perennial rhinitis with intranasal flunisolide. Allergy 1982; 37:303–311.

Wohl J-A, Peterson BN, et al. Effect of the nonsedative H_1 receptor antagonist astemizole in perennial allergic and nonallergic rhinitis. J Allergy Clin Immunol 1985; 75:720–727.

ALLERGIC REACTIONS CAUSED BY EXPOSURE TO ANIMALS

RICHARD EVANS III, M.D., M.P.H.
RICHARD J. SUMMERS, M.D.
CAROL A. NEWILL, Ph.D.

Animals have interacted with man in his environment for milleniums. It is estimated that there are 100 million pets in the United States. At least two thirds of all United States households own, or have owned, a pet or farm animal. Dogs and cats are the most common household pets. However, in recent years rodents, such as gerbils, guinea pigs, and hamsters, as well as other exotic animals have gained in popularity.

Not only are people exposed to animals in the home, but there is a large occupational force of more than 90,000 workers in the United States who are exposed to animals in the laboratory. Although many different species of animals are used in research, laboratory animal handlers are most commonly exposed to rodents.

This article deals with the management of human allergic reactions that result from exposure to animal allergens. The reactions include allergic rhinitis and asthma that result from airborne exposure to the allergens and urticaria following direct contact.

PATHOPHYSIOLOGY

In the past the source of the animal allergen in furred animals has commonly been accepted to be hair and dander. However, recent evidence indicates that the tissue or tissue fluid source of allergen varies from animal to animal. There are a number of allergens identifiable by immunochemical analysis in the hair, dander, serum, and urine from different species. In cats and dogs the major allergen is in the saliva. The major source of allergen in rodents is urine, while in horses the hair and dander contain the most allergen. In most other animals the allergen source is unknown. Although animal serum albumin is frequently allergenic in humans, the clinical significance of this has not been determined.

Some cat and dog serum proteins are immunogenically cross reactive with human serum IgE antibodies. This is also true of rodent serum proteins and probably of other mammalian serum proteins. It is not known whether this is of medical importance.

Respiratory reactions occur when the foregoing allergens become airborne. The mechanism by which these particles elicit an allergic reaction in humans has been examined in detail in relation to sensitivity to cat. The major cat allergen, cat allergen 1 (CA-1), is present in saliva and has been found on airborne particles in sizes ranging from less than 1 micron to larger than 10 microns. Recent advances in bioengineering technology have led to the development of a small volumetric air sampler that can be worn on the lapel in the work or home environment. The filter of this device can be analyzed immunochemically to provide both a qualitative and a quantitive measurement of various airborne animal allergens. It has been determined that the quantities of CA-1 allergen found during natural exposure in a room containing living cats correlate with the amount of CA-1 delivered by bronchoprovocation required to elicit a decreased FEV_1 in cat allergic subjects.

CLINICAL MANIFESTATIONS

Although dogs are the most common household pets, allergic symptoms from exposure to cats are more common among pet allergic persons. This is probably related to the greater domestic closeness of these animals to their owners, thus leading to more cat allergen exposure.

Although there is a broad range of time between first exposure to an animal and the onset of clinical illness, symptoms of allergic rhinitis from exposure to laboratory animals among persons exposed to these animals in the workplace occur after an average of 2 years of contact with the antigen. An estimated 30 to 40 percent of these persons eventually develop asthmatic symptoms. As the severity of the asthma increases, many of these individuals eventually are forced to seek another occupation away from laboratory animals.

DIAGNOSIS

As in other allergic diseases, the general principles of diagnosis based on a detailed history confirmed by a diagnostic test apply to allergy to animals as well. A history of allergic symptoms with intermittent exposure to an animal species is the most obvious and easiest to interpret. Often patients do not appreciate the association between their long term daily allergic symptoms and a history of prolonged day to day exposure to a household pet. Sometimes it is necessary to separate the patient and the pet in order to convince the individual that there is truly a relationship between the symptoms and exposure to the pet.

The physician must be careful to explain to the pet owner that it may require 1 or 2 months to reduce the airborne animal allergen load in a house to a level below that eliciting symptoms. Otherwise the allergic person may believe that he is not actually allergic to the pet if the animal is removed from the environment only for a short period. The history obtained following separation may be more definitive when the patient is away from home for an extended period on a business or pleasure trip.

Occasionally a pet allergic individual begins to have increased allergic symptoms following a move into a house previously occupied by an owner with a pet. Animal sensitive individuals should query the sellers about pets prior to purchasing a previously owned home.

Once a careful history appears to incriminate animal allergens as the etiology of the allergic symptoms, the confirmatory test of choice in suspected animal allergy is the direct allergen skin test. Cat extracts have been standardized to CA-1, thus providing a good skin test material. However, the other animal allergen skin tests have not been standardized. Most animal allergens are prepared from the whole pelts of the animals and do not all contain adequate amounts of the relevant allergens for diagnostic purposes. This may account for a poor correlation between the history and skin test results. Although widely utilized, in vitro diagnostic tests, such as the measurement of serum specific IgE antibody, are rarely useful, because these tests have not been standardized and also lack the relevant allergens.

TREATMENT

When the allergic symptoms are due to an animal allergy, avoidance is the most satisfactory therapeutic approach when symptom amelioration is the single goal. Many asthmatic patients have been relieved of daily symptoms of their disease merely by removal of the offending pet from the home. Cat allergen induced asthma is a classic example of this.

This approach is not always practical, however. There are a variety of reasons why people keep pets, and sometimes these are more compelling than the desire to be free from allergic symptoms.

Although avoidance is usually relatively easy for a pet owner, such a therapeutic approach can be difficult when the livelihood of such individuals as veterinarians, the vision impaired, animal laboratory personnel, and scientific investigators is dependent upon working with animals. A variety of protective devices such as air filters and personal protective equipment are available. However, it is not known whether these devices actually ameliorate symptoms induced by animal allergen exposure.

Pharmacotherapy of allergic symptoms resulting from animal exposure is similar to the treatment of symptoms resulting from contact with other allergens. Individuals who can predict their animal exposure should be taught to premedicate themselves prior to the exposure. We have had success with the intraocular (two drops in each eye) or intranasal (two sprays in each nostril) use or inhalation (two inhalations by mouth) of cromolyn sodium about 30 minutes prior to animal exposure and then four times a day throughout the duration of the exposure.

Immunotherapy

As of this writing, there have been four published blinded trials of immunotherapy in persons allergic to animals. Animal extracts for injection that have been studied include cat and dog. Three of the clinical trials have shown decreased sensitivity to the relevant allergens by bronchoprovocation; the fourth, a conjunctival provocation study, demonstrated less sensitivity as well. Three of the four trials measured skin sensitivity quantitatively and found a reduction in reactivity following allergen injection therapy. Two of the four investigations evaluated the effects of animal immunotherapy on symptoms. In both studies symptomatic improvement was evident in the treated subjects, who were able to tolerate animal exposure for longer periods before developing ocular and pulmonary symptoms.

Immunotherapy with animal allergens is not different from treatment with pollen allergens in terms of the immunologic responses. Specific IgG antibody titers rise as increased allergen dosages to patient tolerance are attained.

Immunotherapy with animal allergens is conducted in the same manner as that for pollen allergens. Because of the whole pelts utilized, commercially available animal extracts often contain large amounts of serum proteins. Although never described in this form of therapy, serum sickness-like reactions are a theoretical possibility. However, the possibility of such a reaction becomes even more remote when the quantity of animal serum proteins is less than 100 micrograms per injection.

Animal injection therapy has the greatest appeal to that group of occupationally exposed patients who suffer from significant symptoms in the presence of optimal pharmacotherapy. Although we are currently engaged in a clinical trial with rat allergic subjects using an extract known to contain lesser amounts of serum protein and larger amounts of relevant urinary allergens (i.e., alpha-2-euglobulin and prealbumin), it is premature to recommend this form of treatment for allergy to laboratory animals.

SUGGESTED READINGS

Ohman JL Jr, Findlay SR, Leitermann KM. Immunotherapy in cat-induced asthma. Double-blind trial with evaluation of in vivo and in vitro responses. J Allergy Clin Immunol 1984; 74:230–239.

Sundin B, Lilja G, Graff-Lonnevig V, Hedlin G, Heilborn H, Norrlin K, Pegelow K-O, Lowenstein H. Immunotherapy with partially purified standardized animal dander extracts. J Allergy Clin Immunol 1986; 77:478–487.

Swanson MC, Agarwal MK, Reed CE. An immunochemical approach to indoor aeroallergen quantitation with a new volumetric air sampler: studies with mite, roach, cat, mouse, and guinea pig antigens. J Allergy Clin Immunol 1985; 76:724–729.

Taylor WW, Ohman JL Jr, Lowell FC. Immunotherapy in cat-induced asthma: double-blind trial with evaluation of bronchial responses to cat allergen and histamine. J Allergy Clin Immunol 1978; 61:283–287.

Valovirta E, Koivikko A, Vanto T, Viander M, Ingeman L. Immunotherapy in allergy to dog: a double-blind clinical study. Ann Allergy 1984; 53:85.

Vanto T. Sources of allergens in animals. Allergy 1985; (Suppl 3):51–53.

ALLERGIC RHINITIS CAUSED BY HOUSE DUST AND OTHER NONPOLLEN ALLERGENS

GEORGE W. WARD Jr., M.D.
THOMAS A. E. PLATTS-MILLS, M.D., Ph.D.

Patients with allergic rhinitis present with a variety of nasal symptoms, including sneezing, running nose, congestion, pressure, soreness, "sinus headaches," and postnasal drip. In those who do not recognize a specific season or a specific precipitating factor for their symptoms, the form of the symptoms is not very helpful in deciding whether the symptoms are "allergic."

Traditionally patients with perennial nasal symptoms have been divided into three groups: those with nasal disease such as chronic sinus infection, nasal polyps, or granulomatous disease; those with vasomotor rhinitis due to abnormalities or alterations of autonomic control of blood vessels in the nasal mucosa; and a large group of patients who have perennial nasal inflammation because they are allergic to foreign proteins that are present for much of the year. However, there is considerable overlap among these groups; nasal disease does not exclude an allergic basis and a positive skin test result does not establish that the symptoms are due to a particular allergen. In most areas pollens and fungal spores are present in the outside air only for limited periods of the year, and therefore the commonest source of perennial allergens is the patient's own house. The major sources of indoor allergens are dust mites, animal dander, and fungi. However, it is important to recognize that arthropods such as moths, beetles, and cockroaches also can contribute to house dust. Although most indoor allergens are perennial, some show marked seasonal variations; in particular, dust mite allergen shows a seasonal increase from August to December in much of the Southeastern United States.

Although some patients recognize a specific site in the house as the source of the allergen they are sensitive to (e.g., a damp basement, the cat, or a small animal), more commonly they have little awareness of the relationship between house dust and the chronic symptoms. The symptoms of perennial rhinitis are similar to those of hay fever, but there are differences; itching of the back of the throat and ears is more common in seasonal rhinitis, and it is unusual to have to treat conjunctivitis in patients who have dust mite sensitivity alone.

The management of a patient with perennial rhinitis always requires an assessment of the history and general health and a physical examination, because rhinitis can be a presenting symptom of systemic disease and because the drugs used may have side effects. Certain records are essential before starting treatment. It is important to seek a history of reversible airway obstruction or other lung disease and to measure the peak expiratory flow rate, because patients with persistent allergic or nonallergic rhinitis may develop asthma. In addition, the occasional patients with cystic fibrosis presenting with nasal congestion and polyps (usually in children) and those with granulomatous disease or systemic inflammatory disease (e.g., Sjögren's syndrome) presenting with nasal soreness or blockage need to be identified. The blood pressure must be known because nasal decongestants can increase blood pressure. Urinalysis is essential before starting any form of steroid treatment. It is also wise to obtain a blood count both to check for the presence of eosinophilia and because blood dyscrasias can occur as a rare complication of antihistamine treatment. All children should have a growth chart, because even local steroid therapy can have some systemic effects and a growth chart may be the first clue to an otherwise unsuspected overdosage.

Further assessment of a patient depends on the general health status, the severity of symptoms, and the response to initial treatment. Options that need to be considered include fiberoptic rhinopharyngoscopy, sinus x-ray examination, and measurement of serum immunoglobulin levels. Rhinopharyngoscopy is useful in excluding disease in patients with unexplained nasal bleeding or unilateral blockage and in defining nasal polyps. The results may also be useful in reassuring the patient about the absence of other disease, however, at present we do not consider it part of the routine initial assessment of perennial rhinitis. Sinus x-ray examination similarly can be useful in defining marked mucosal thickening in patients who may benefit from more prolonged antibiotic therapy with or without a short course of oral steroid therapy. Sinus x-ray examination should be considered in patients who have severe pain, fever, and a purulent discharge and is also indicated in those who respond poorly to other treatment. In the patient with inconclusive skin test results and a poor response to treatment, it is well worth measuring serum IgE, IgG, and IgA levels. Low levels of IgE suggest an absence of an allergic etiology, whereas low levels of the other immunoglobulins may suggest increased use of antibiotics and even immunoglobulin in occasional cases. Although there are reports of IgG subclass deficiency in patients with recurrent sinusitis, it is not clear that this represents an indication for intravenous gamma globulin therapy. By contrast, normal or increased IgE levels with normal IgG and IgA levels often lead to further evaluation by skin testing and consideration of desensitization.

Our approach to treating perennial rhinitis is outlined in Table 1. Because the condition is likely to continue for some years, it is best to escalate treatment slowly. On the other hand, it is easy to underestimate the misery caused by rhinitis, and it is important to explain early that there is a range of treatments that can be used if they prove necessary. In general, we do not

TABLE 1

TABLE 1 Treatment of Perennial Allergic Rhinitis

Persistent nasal symptoms in an otherwise healthy person
  Sneezing and running: oral antihistamines; adjust dosage to reduce sedation or try other antihistamines with or without nasal decongestant
  Predominant blockage: oral decongestant with antihistamine

Continuing moderate symptoms (>6 months)
  Allergic history and skin tests: consider allergen avoidance
  Consider sinus x-ray examination
  Administer nasal cromolyn sodium or beclomethasone
  Continue oral antihistamine therapy if acceptable

Severe symptoms or local treatment inadequate or unacceptable
  Full allergy history and skin testing obligatory: serum IgE and possible RAST testing.
  If problem is sufficient and patient suitable, explain allergen avoidance and outline strategy; visit house if possible
  Continue local treatment; combined cromolyn and flunisolide

Symptoms unrelenting
  Reconsider diagnosis: e.g., chronic nasal infection, sinus infection, polyps, salicylate sensitivity, IgG or IgA deficiency, granulomatous disease, occupational allergy
  Consider emotional reasons for failure to recognize or accept treatment
  Consider desensitization treatment combined with local treatment and oral antihistamine therapy

use challenge tests because in our experience they do not add to the information available from the history or skin testing.

DRUG TREATMENT OF PERENNIAL RHINITIS

Antihistamines

The antihistamines on H_1 inhibitors given orally can reduce nasal discharge, itching, and sneezing, but only rarely do they control rhinitis completely. Most H_1 inhibitors cause drowsiness that may interfere with driving or working, and thus patients must be warned. Antihistamines may produce more side effects in geriatric patients and can produce additive depressant effects with alcohol and other central nervous system depressants. Most H_1 inhibitors have demonstrable anticholinergic activity, which is thought to be responsible for their sedative effects and their effectiveness against seasickness; this effect also causes dry mouth in some patients.

Recently a new antihistamine has been released, terfenadine, which has no anticholinergic effect and causes little or no sedation. Terfenadine is chemically different; being lipophilic, it does not cross the blood-brain barrier and has essentially no central nervous system sedative side effects. This preparation has been particularly helpful in patients whose occupations or activities demand alertness for safety. Terfenadine at present has three problems: It is expensive, it is not yet

available as a tablet combined with a decongestant, and it is less potent than full doses of other antihistamines. However, many experimental protocols are using higher dosages, e.g., 120 mg twice daily, which also appear to be safe, and such dosages may well be recommended in the future.

In some patients the sedative effects of other antihistamines decrease with time; however, even if they persist, the patient becomes much better at coping with them and learning when to take the tablets. Antihistamines are most effective when used early, as soon as symptoms appear. Individual patients respond differently to different antihistamines, and it is always worth trying several different types. In addition to drowsiness, antihistamines occasionally give rise to insomnia, nervousness, tremors, or gastrointestinal disturbances. They should be used with caution in patients with a history of epilepsy, narrow angle glaucoma, stenosing peptic ulcer, symptomatic prostatic hypertrophy, and bladder neck obstruction. Table 2 lists the different classes of antihistamines with their relative tendencies to cause central nervous system stimulatory effects, "antihistaminic activity," anticholinergic activity, and indications for use.

Nasal Decongestants

A variety of drugs are used specifically as local nasal decongestants, including ephedrine, oxymetazoline, and xylometazoline (e.g., Afrin and Dristan). Similar drugs are also marketed in combination with antihistamines that act locally (e.g., 4-Way Nasal Spray). It is not clear that antihistamines are active locally, but they may have an effect because of their weak local anesthetic effect. When they are taken locally, the great disadvantage of decongestants is rebound congestion. If patients are not warned of this effect, they will react by taking more of the local spray until they become "addicted," with a very uncomfortable nose with sensations of burning, soreness, or dryness—i.e., rhinitis medicamentosa. It must be remembered that all nasal sprays have an irritant effect and also include a preservative that may itself irritate the mucosa.

Rebound congestion is not a problem when the same drugs are taken orally, and many patients with mild rhinitis respond well to decongestants alone (e.g., Sudafed) or to combination tablets including an antihistamine. Oral sympathomimetic preparations can cause systemic side effects. They can increase the blood pressure, they interact with antidepressant drugs, and they should be avoided in cases of hyperthyroidism or diabetes. Nonetheless the combination tablets are an effective and important form of treatment for rhinitis. Suitable combination tablets are available as either over the counter or prescription drugs, e.g., Drixoral, which is dexbrompheniramine with pseudoephedrine (available over the counter) and Bromfed, which is bromphenira-

TABLE 2   Drugs with H₁ Receptor Activity

Class and Examples	Trade Names*	Usual Adult Dosage	CNS Sedation	Antihistaminic Activity	Anticholinergic Activity	Comments
Ethanolamines						
Diphenhydramine	Benadryl	25–50 mg q6h				Diphenhydramine also used
Clemastine (Rx)	Tavist	1.34–2.68 mg bid,tid	Marked	Moderate	Marked	in motion sickness; has
Dimenhydrinate	Dramamine	50–100 mg q4–6h				local anesthetic effect
Ethylenediamines						
Tripelennamine (Rx)	PBZ	25–50 mg q4–6h	Relatively	Mild to	Mild, if any	Gastrointestinal side effects
Pyrilamine	Triaminic	25 mg q8h	mild	moderate		are common; tripelenna-
						mine has potential for IV
						abuse; pyrilamine used as
						sleeping aid
Alkylamines						
Chlorpheniramine	Chlor-Trimeton	4 mg q4–6h				Possibly some central ner-
Brompheniramide	Dimetane	4 mg q4–6h	Mild	Marked	Moderate	vous system stimulation;
Pheniramine (Rx)	Triaminic TR	25 mg q8h				classic antihistamines to
						date
Piperidines						
Azatadine (Rx)	Optimine	1–2 mg q12h				Cyproheptadine is scrotonin
Cyproheptadine (Rx)	Periactin	4 mg q6–8h	Mild to	Moderate	Moderate	antagonist and used also
Diphenylpyraline (Rx)	Hispril	5 mg q12h	moderate			in cold urticaria
Phenothiazines						
Promethazine (Rx)	Phenergan	12.5–50 mg q4–6h				Usually used for motion
Trimeprazine (Rx)	Temaril	2.5 mg q6h	Marked	Marked	Marked	sickness, antiemetic, anti-
						tussive; promethazine has
						antiserotonin activity; tri-
						mepraxine is antipruritic
Piperazines						
Hydroxyzine (Rx)	Atarax, Vistaril	10–50 mg q6h		Hydroxyzine		Hydroxyzine also used as
Cyclizine	Marezine	50 mg q4–6h	Mild	moderate	Mild	sedative and tranquilizer,
Meclizine (Rx)	Antivert	25–100 mg daily in		Others		antiemetic; others used for
		divided doses		mild		motion sickness
Others						
Terfenadine (Rx)	Seldane	60 mg bid‡	Essentially	Moderate	Very little	Lipophilic; do not readily
Astemizole†	—	—	none	to marked		cross blood-brain barrier;
						longer duration; greater
						affinity to H₁ receptor

Rx; prescription required.
*Many of these drugs also are available in sustained action, delayed release forms and in combination with decongestants.
†Not yet available in the United States.
‡Has been used safely in experimental studies in doses up to 180 mg.

mine, 4 mg, with pseudoephedrine, 60 mg (a prescription drug). For the patient the practical advantages of a single oral tablet are considerable.

Disodium Cromoglycate or Cromolyn Sodium

Disodium cromoglycate originally was marketed in a powder form for inhalation into the lung. Attempts to provide a similar spinhaler for the nose were not successful because in many patients the powder would not penetrate beyond the anterior nares. Subsequently disodium cromoglycate has been marketed as a 2 percent solution in nonpressurized spray form, which is effective but requires administration four to six times per day. This spray appears to be useful in hay fever, but in cases of perennial rhinitis the need for frequent application is a problem. Although patients tolerate frequently repeated sprays for the hay fever season, they are often unwilling to persist for the whole year. The dose of disodium cromoglycate spray is approximately 2 mg (the spincap is 20 mg) and a higher concentration may well be more effective. It also may be effective in combination with local steroid therapy (see next section).

The mode of action of disodium cromoglycate has been widely discussed. It appears to have a definite mast cell stabilizing effect that can reduce allergen induced histamine release. However, there are good reasons for believing that it may have a more general effect in stabilizing membranes to reduce mediator release from macrophages, neutrophils, or both. The most important feature of the drug is the very low incidence of side effects; systemic side effects are rare.

Local Steroid Therapy

Systemic steroid therapy provides effective short term treatment for perennial rhinitis as well as seasonal hay fever, but there are few occasions when systemic steroid therapy is justified for perennial rhinitis. Steroids can be used occasionally in the management of rhinitis medicamentosa, for controlling severe or prolonged episodes of sinusitis or for a particularly severe episode (for instance, during or after moving to a new house). The danger is that the patient will demand repeated courses or repeated depot injections and that the treatment will become continuous.

Because of the effectiveness of steroids, many attempts have been made to design steroid preparations that would be active when administered directly to the nose or lung. Beclomethasone dipropionate is very active locally, and it is rapidly metabolized so that it has little systemic effect. The use of 300 μg per day locally (that is, one dose in each nostril three times daily) is as effective as 5 to 10 mg of prednisone per day orally. The systemic effect of 300 μg of beclomethasone per day nasally is estimated to be approximately equivalent to that with 0.5 to 1.0 mg of prednisone per day. Thus, although the nasal administration of beclomethasone is preferable to systemic steroid therapy, it is not completely without a systemic effect and if abused, particularly together with inhaled steroids for asthma, occasionally can cause significant adrenal suppression. The local administration of steroids is effective treatment for nasal blockage, secretion, and sneezing and may be effective when used once or twice daily. As with all steroids, potentiation of infection is a risk, but this appears to be rare in the nose. Even Candida infection, which can occur in the throat with inhaled beclomethasone, is not recognized as a problem in the nose.

In many patients who undergo nasal steroid therapy, small blood vessels in the anterior part of the nasal mucosa dilate. This is not an indication for stopping treatment unless bleeding becomes a problem, which is rare. However, a proportion of patients develop a sore dry nose, which in up to 20 percent of the cases may necessitate stopping the drug. This effect appears to be due in part to the propellant or the preservative, since it also can occur with placebo sprays. In these cases it is worth trying an alternative steroid spray, steroid drops, or disodium cromoglycate. Flunisolide nasal spray, equally effective, has the advantage that it is not in a pressurized canister. In addition to avoiding the possible effects of freon, this allows the addition of other drugs, e.g., cromolyn sodium powder, ten capsules per container to

the flunisolide. Although this has not been recommended by the manufacturers, it is simple to do and it appears to be helpful.

Steroid nasal drops are the medical treatment of choice for nasal polyps whether associated with allergy or not (betamethasone, 0.1 percent, approximately 50 μg per drop, two drops in each nostril three times daily). As with all nasal applications, the key problem with drops is their distribution. It is not possible to apply nasal drops by tilting the head backward when the patient is standing or sitting upright. To apply drops to the whole nose, the patient should lie supine with his head over the end of a bed completely upsidedown. After applying drops the patient should stay in this state for at least 1 minute. As with all potent steroids applied topically, nasal drops may be effective on an alternate day or even twice weekly basis. Drops have less tendency to cause a sore nose but have disadvantages because they are slightly less readily accepted than nasal sprays and the betamethasone is absorbed systemically.

Ipratropium Bromide (Atropine)

Atropine-like drugs can dry mucosal surfaces, but systemic use is not justified or effective for rhinitis. There are several preparations of atropine-like drugs in use for bronchodilation, but such preparations rapidly lose effectiveness for rhinitis. Recently a related anticholinergic drug, ipratropium bromide, has been released in the United States for use in obstructive lung disease. The same drug is in use for rhinitis in Europe and may be a useful adjunct to therapy.

Desensitization Treatment

Desensitization treatment (or immunotherapy) should be considered only when the patient is definitely sensitive to a well defined allergen, there is good reason to believe that exposure to that allergen is responsible for symptoms, and avoidance measures have not produced sufficient improvement. In addition, there are patients whose jobs require mental alertness and in whom antihistamines, cromolyn, or local steroid therapy are not effective or cause unacceptable side effects. Desensitization also should be considered in these patients.

House dust extracts were first used for desensitization in 1920 and appeared to be effective for both asthma and perennial rhinitis. The major constituents of house dust are now well recognized, and potent extracts of both mite and cat allergens are available. In addition, it has been established that mite and cat extracts can be effective in immunotherapy. In using aqueous mite extracts, the approach to desensitization is the same as that for pollen allergens. The extracts can be very potent, and fatal anaphylaxis has occurred with mite extracts.

There seems to be no justification for carrying out desensitization outside a clinic capable of resuscitation measures. Our experience with desensitization for perennial rhinitis has been similar to that for hay fever; that is, 60 to 70 percent of the patients experience significant improvement in 6 months.

ALLERGEN AVOIDANCE

Effective allergen avoidance depends to a large degree on accurate diagnosis. A careful history often suggests that the relevant allergens are domestic in origin, and there are good diagnostic skin test extracts for most of the allergens that contribute to house dust. This is certainly true for cat dander and house dust mites, although there is still some doubt about fungal allergen extracts. Patients are often allergic to several allergens in the house. It is important not to give the impression that removing one item will indicate whether it is relevant or that vacuum cleaning the mattress for a few weeks will indicate whether mites are involved. If there are multiple allergens in the house, removing one, even if it is important, will not give clear information because the patient's symptoms will continue. The best approach is to consider the overall problem—if necessary, including a visit to the house. If avoidance is thought to be worth trying, a progressive policy to reduce allergens should then be outlined.

Domestic Animals

Most highly atopic patients who live with a cat, dog, guinea pig, mouse, or rabbit in the house will become allergic. Animals that live outside are much less of a problem. Any patient who has perennial rhinitis and positive results on immediate skin tests should be strongly urged to remove the relevant animal. It must be stressed that because it usually takes 6 weeks or more to remove cat or dog dander from a house, a short term trial of removing the animal is useless.

Dust Mites

Dust mites grow best at 18 to 28° C and with a relative humidity higher than 65 percent. They are thought to live usually on human skin scales or fungi on the skin scales, but they can eat a variety of different organic materials. The major allergens produced by dust mites accumulate and become airborne in the form of fecal particles.

Even before the discovery of the importance of dust mites by Spieksma and Voorhoorst in 1964, it was common practice to advise patients about methods of reducing house dust. These methods include regular vacuum cleaning of the mattress, carpets, and curtains

in the bedroom together with regular washing of bed clothes. Some patients benefit from this kind of advice, but more often the results are poor. Furthermore, studies using measurements of dust mite allergen in dust suggest that this kind of precaution (even if followed) effects only modest reductions in allergen levels. On the other hand, dust mite allergen levels in hospitals are often very low—less than 2 percent of the levels in houses— and dust mite allergic patients generally improve in the hospital. The implication is that dust mite avoidance could work but would require more aggressive changes in a house than are normally recommended. Reduction of mite allergens can be achieved by removing the sites in which mites live (e.g., carpets in living rooms as well as bedrooms, feather pillows, nonwashable comforters, thick clothes, soft toys), denaturing the allergen and killing the mites by washing in hot water (hotter than 55° C), using specific chemical acaricides, and removing mite feces and other debris by regular vacuum cleaning or damp wiping of surfaces.

There is no satisfactory acaricide at present. A complex insecticide called Paragerm has been used in France, but the smell is offensive and may require leaving the house. An antifungal agent, Pimaricin, is being used in trials in Europe. Pirimiphos methyl is a potent acaricide that is relatively nontoxic and will kill mites in carpets and furniture, but it is not currently available in the United States.

Our present policy is to recommend a complete change in the patient's bedroom—that is, replace carpets with linoleum or wood, wash all bedding regularly in hot water (weekly or every 10 days), cover the mattress with an impervious plastic cover, remove all soft toys and upholstered furniture, and keep clutter to a minimum. The rest of the house should be vacuumed regularly with a machine that has an effective filter. If patients do cleaning work, they should wear a mask. Soft furniture and curtains also should be vacuumed regularly. Polished floors are ideal, and in some climates carpets can be beaten in the sun. Mite allergic patients should avoid living in basements. In Northern Europe carpets are more essential and the sun is not reliable; these areas await a suitable domestic acaricide.

Fungi

Although fungi undoubtedly can cause allergic symptoms, it is difficult to assess their general importance as a cause of perennial rhinitis. Measuring viable fungal spores in a house is possible using a culture plate, but measuring allergen levels is not. As has been pointed out, the number of varieties of fungi is so great that it is difficult to exclude fungal allergy. Nonetheless the quantities of fungal allergens in a house almost certainly can be reduced by some simple measures. Removal of house plants from all (or most) rooms in the house is essential. Obvious sites of fungal growth must be carefully cleaned or removed, e.g., shower curtains, bathroom windows, damp walls, and areas with dry rot. Most of the fungi implicated in allergy are fungi imperfecta, which appear as black or greenish stains. Finally measures taken to reduce the accumulation of dust mite allergens will reduce both the production and accumulation of fungal allergens. Both mites and fungi require humid conditions. However, many fungi flourish in colder conditions than mites; under really humid warm conditions different fungi may overgrow mite cultures.

Control of Airborne Allergens

Normal houses have dust particles in the air, but most are less than 5μm in diameter. The allergens that we know most about are carried on large particles, for example, pollen grains, (approximately 20 μm in diameter) and mite fecal particles (10 to 40 μm in diameter). In addition, many important fungal spores are "large." In still air, particles of this size fall within 10 to 15 minutes. As for dust mite allergens, the quantity of allergen that becomes airborne is a tiny fraction of the total amount present in carpets or bedding and is detectable only during domestic activity. Because of this, the major exposure to allergens probably occurs during activity, and face masks, a good vacuum cleaner—and someone else to do the housework—are useful.

Filtering the incoming air may be helpful in preventing seasonal pollen or fungal allergens from entering the house but is largely irrelevant for allergens produced within the house. Obviously if an allergen falls within 10 to 15 minutes, filtering the inside air will have little effect on exposure, e.g., to dust mite feces. However, there is some evidence that cat allergen can be airborne in the form of small particles (i.e., less than 2 μm in diameter), which do not fall rapidly. It is therefore possible that a high efficiency particulate air filter in the room could help such a patient, and it is unwise to be too dogmatic about such filters. However, the first approach with all house dust allergens is to reduce the sources and the reservoirs of dust in the house and thus reduce the amount that becomes airborne during domestic activity.

Noninhaled Allergens

Two groups of noninhaled allergens are worth considering in troublesome and unexplained cases of perennial rhinitis; food antigens and dermatophyte sensitivity. Our understanding of the role of diet in asthma and perennial rhinitis remains totally unsatisfactory. Many patients think that some aspects of the diet make nasal blockage worse, but this has been difficult to confirm objectively. In particular, neither skin tests nor serum assays for IgE antibodies to cow's milk proteins have proved reliable. Nonetheless some patients appear to benefit from diets that avoid cow's milk proteins, egg

proteins, coloring, and preservatives. If the patient is enthusiastic, we provide dietary advice both to achieve complete avoidance and to make sure that the patient does not develop vitamin or calcium deficiency. Avoidance diets for rhinitis should not be considered in growing children. The idea that dermatophytes, particularly Trichophyton, can contribute to rhinitis was widely accepted by allergists in the 1930s. Recently we have seen several patients with perennial rhinitis (or asthma) who had obvious signs of dermatophyte infection, positive immediate skin test results to Trichophyton extract, and detectable serum IgE antibodies. Some of these patients improve with effective treatment of the local infection. In view of the simplicity of treatment with antifungal ointment, e.g., Lotrimin, it seems wise to inspect these patients for signs of topical fungal infection.

CONCLUSIONS

When a patient presents with nonseasonal rhinitis, it is worth using antihistamines with or without oral decongestant treatment. If the problem remains troublesome, a detailed history and examination are required. Assessing the evidence for an allergic basis requires a history, skin testing, and possibly a total serum IgE determination. Some advice about avoidance may be obvious at this point. However, most patients should be offered a trial of one of the more potent nasal sprays, that is, disodium cromoglycate or beclomethasone dipropionate. If the patient tolerates oral antihistamine therapy, it should be continued. Either type of nasal spray may be effective; the steroid has the advantage of less frequent dosage, but the disadvantages are that a few more patients develop a sore nose (about 20 percent) and there is a small risk of contributing to systemic side effects.

If the patient is inadequately controlled after 3 to 12 months and the physician is convinced that the symptoms are really a problem (a difficult decision that may well require an assessment of the social situation), allergen avoidance should be pursued. This is often the point at which the patient is first seen by a specialist. It is important to spell out the policy and make it clear that all changes need not be made at once. Unless the physician is convinced of the diagnosis, it is impossible to persuade the patient to change the bedroom, to give away the pets, or even to buy a new vacuum cleaner. It is often much easier to convince the patient if someone has visited the house. Not only can one get an accurate record of the state of the house, but it is also an extremely effective way of educating the patient and explaining the purpose of changes. Although sufficient allergen avoidance to abolish symptoms is difficult, it is often possible to reduce the problem to the level at which either pharmacologic treatment or desensitization treatment becomes effective. Successful education of patients allows them to decide how much change is justified by their symptoms. With a combination of nasal treatment, oral antihistamine therapy, desensitization, and allergen avoidance, 80 to 90 percent of the patients with perennial allergic rhinitis should be adequately controlled.

SUGGESTED READING

Kirkegaard J, Mygind N, Molgaard F, Grahne B, Holopainen E, Malmberg H, Brondbo K, Rojne T. Ordinary and high-dose ipra-tropium in perennial nonallergic rhinitis. J Allergy Clin Immuno 1987; 79:585–590.

Mygind N. Nasal allergy. 2nd ed. London: Blackwell Scientific Publications, 1979.

Platts-Mills TAE, Hayden ML, Chapman MD, Wilkins SR. Seasonal variation in dust mite and grass pollen allergens in dust from the houses of patients with asthma. J Allergy Clin Immunol 1987; 79:781–791.

Platts-Mills TAE, Tovey ER, Mitchell EB, Moszoro H, Nock P, Wilkins SR. Reduction of bronchial hyper-reactivity during prolonged allergen avoidance. Lancet 1982; 2:675–678.

Settipane GA, ed. Rhinitis. Providence, RI: The New England and Regional Allergy Proceedings, 1984.

PERENNIAL RHINITIS

ROBERT NACLERIO, M.D.

When a patient complains of nasal symptoms for more than 2 hours per day for more than 9 months of the year, we refer to his problem as perennial rhinitis. Unfortunately the nasal response to illness is limited, and many different disease processes result in the same symptoms: nasal congestion, rhinorrhea, or sneezing. It behooves the practitioner, therefore, to define the etiology of perennial rhinitis prior to instituting treatment. Before discussing the management of patients with perennial rhinitis, the approach used to define the etiology of the problem will be summarized.

A carefully obtained history defining where, when, and by what means symptoms are provoked is essential. Emphasis should be placed on relating the onset of symptoms to life events (e.g., change of occupation, moving to a new house, acquiring a pet) and on defining the symptoms by the number of episodes of nose blowing or sneezing, the characteristics of secretions (clear versus purulent), the presence of a postnasal drip, the presence or absence of pain, and the characteristics of air flow obstruction. The characterization of symptoms serves as a baseline to which therapeutic interventions are directed. The history should also detail the description of medicines consumed. Although patients easily discuss their use of orally administered prescription medicines, they infrequently mention the use of over the counter medicines, such as aspirin, or topically applied medicines, such as beta-blockers used to treat glaucoma. Inquiries about the sense of smell assist in determining the severity and location of the air flow obstruction. Severe nasal obstruction causes a decrease in the sense of smell, which is frequently perceived as a loss of taste. A history of surgery assists in defining nasal obstruction that developed gradually after a rhin-

oplasty or dental extraction or that resulted from a metastatic lesion from a previously resected carcinoma or from hypothyroidism occurring after thyroidectomy. Trauma can cause septal deviations or shearing of the olfactory nerve at the cribriform plate. Clear rhinorrhea following trauma may indicate a cerebrospinal fluid leak.

Finally questions should be directed toward disturbances of sleep. Snoring secondary to nasal obstruction may be a social problem, but sleep apnea and its physiologic sequelae can profoundly affect the patient. When obtaining the details of the history of a patient with perennial rhinitis, note the manner in which the patient relates the details. Patients frequently become fixated on their nasal complaints; thus, appreciating any psychologic stress will have a profound effect on the results of treatment. After a careful history, proceed with an equally careful physical examination.

The physical examination does not begin with the placement of a nasal speculum; a complete ear, nose, and throat examination is necessary. The presence of unilateral otitis media with effusion in an adult should make the clinician suspicious of a nasopharyngeal mass. Inspection of the oral cavity might show infected tooth roots as a cause of sinusitis. Bite lines in the buccal mucosa and the presence of bruxism indicate nervous tension. Enlarged neck nodes may be secondary to a primary neoplasm in the nasopharynx. Exophthalmos or limitations in ocular motility can result from diseases within the paranasal sinuses. Likewise, areas of hypesthesia can indicate previous surgery or underlying malignant disease.

Start the nasal examination by grossly visualizing the exterior contour of the nose. Asymmetry indicates prior trauma or an expanding mass. Next examine the nasal vestibule for evidence of folliculitis or compromise of the nasal valve, the area of greatest air flow resistance between the external environment and the alveolus. The valve can be compromised by loss of cartilaginous strength in the elderly person or by relapsing polychondritis. An edentulous upper alveolus causes the upper lip to hang and may also be a cause of compromise of the nasal valve.

After assessing the nasal valve and the external

nasal configuration, a nasal speculum is inserted. The opening of a bivalved nasal speculum enlarges the nasal vestibule and may dramatically improve breathing, directing attention to the etiology of the problem. By looking through the nasal speculum, the mucosa as well as internal structures can be assessed. The mucosa may demonstrate unexpected granulomatous disease or papilloma. Pooled secretions under the inferior turbinate point to the need to investigate for the immotile cilia syndrome. After observing both nasal cavities, a decongestant should be applied topically to permit better visualization of the nasal cavity and to help determine the contributions of the mucosa and bone or cartilage to nasal obstruction. A slow or negative response of the nasal mucosa to a decongestant indicates the presence of hyperplastic mucosa.

After decongestion has been achieved, be sure to visualize the area of the anterior edge of the middle turbinate. This area is the region of greatest nasal air flow and the area of greatest particle impaction; hence this area may be the first region affected by environmental influences. This concept is supported by the fact that adenocarcinomas secondary to the inhalation of hard wood dust start in this region. Since the majority of air entering the nose flows over the anterior edge of the turbinates, passes up over the middle turbinate, and then descends into the nasal pharynx, a septal spur along the floor of the nasal cavity would contribute minimally to nasal obstruction, whereas an anterior nasal deflection at the level of the middle turbinate would have a more profound effect. Anterolateral to the middle turbinates are the openings to the frontal, maxillary and anterior ethmoidal sinuses. Nasal polyps usually originate in this region. Visual inspection, however, does not distinguish a tumor from an inflammatory polyp, and a biopsy may be indicated. Likewise, unilateral polyps should arouse suspicion of a tumor. Congenital deformities of the turbinates or the presence of concha bullosa can also be seen; they predispose to sinusitis.

Whereas use of a nasal speculum combined with the topical use of a decongestant permits visualization of about one third of the nasal cavity, small fiberoptic telescopes permit visualization of the entire nasal cavity. Most telescopic examinations add little additional information, but the ease of performing the examination, high patient acceptance, and the early identification of a tumor justify all the negative examinations. Besides tumors, fiberoptic endoscopy detects septal spurs, which compromise the middle meatal region, as well as inflammation affecting the openings of the sphenoidal sinuses. In children the contribution of adenoids to nasal obstruction can be appreciated without the need for x-ray evaluation, and unilateral choanal atresia may be seen.

The physical examination contributes to understanding the role of structural abnormalities, including tumors, in nasal obstruction and sinusitis. However, when the history and physical examination are completed, the paranasal sinuses are the only area not fully evaluated. Sinus x-ray examinations or a CAT scan evaluates the sinuses, but they might not be necessary if the cause of the perennial rhinitis has already been established. Other laboratory evaluations, such as a complete blood count, eosinophil count, quantitative immunoglobulin determinations, sedimentation rate, thyroid function tests, and RAST or skin testing, are ordered as indicated.

Before discussing the management of perennial rhinitis, several issues deserve comment. Despite a thorough evaluation, a specific diagnosis cannot always be achieved. Patients may be given a diagnosis of vasomotor rhinitis, which I try to avoid, since it offers little information and can lull the clinician into not thinking further about the patient's problem. Perennial rhinitis may result from multiple causes, making it difficult to establish the relative importance of each to the patient's symptoms. For example, plain sinus x-ray findings have been found to be abnormal in over 50 percent of the subjects with perennial allergic rhinitis, raising questions about the best approach to these patients. Another frequently encountered problem is that the cause of the rhinitis may change over time. An example is occupation induced disease. Initially the employee may have problems only at work. These may progress to off hours; eventually even stopping exposure at work may not resolve the problem. Finally, if a diagnosis cannot be established, the clinician may need to attempt a therapeutic trial of a medicine to assist in understanding the patient's disease.

Unfortunately the number of therapeutic options is limited: antibiotics, corticosteroids, antihistamines, decongestants, nasal cromolyn administration, and salt water douches. The remainder of this article focuses on applying these therapeutic options in patients with and without diagnoses.

AVOIDANCE

Elimination of the offending agents from a patient's environment has the greatest potential for complete resolution of symptoms, but the clinician must identify all the offending factors. This approach works best when perennial rhinitis is secondary to allergic disease caused by perennially present antigens, such as animal dander, dust, or molds. Because most perennial antigens are located in the home, details regarding the home environment must be obtained. Measures directed at reducing household exposure must include all relevant antigens, because partial elimination is rarely effective. The bedroom, the room where most patients spend the majority of their time, should be made free of clutter. Clutter collects dust, of which dust mites are a major component. The dust mites feed off human epithelial scales and organic debris. Pillows and mattresses should be vacuumed twice weekly or encased in protective linings. All bedding should be washed in hot water. Removing house plants from the bedroom and eliminating mold from basements and around shower stalls can reduce exposure to mold, another perennial antigen. Pets may be the direct etiology of the problem, or they may carry pollens in their coats into the inside of a house. Electrostatic precipitators effectively reduce airborne particles, but the aerodynamics of dust mite antigen and most pollens cause them to settle quickly from the air, limiting the effectiveness of this approach. Disturbing the reservoir of particles (for example, sitting on a sofa) causes them to become airborne in the immediate environment of the patient. Twice weekly vacuuming of beds, sofas, and carpets is helpful. Masks help reduce the exposure of patients who must clean their homes.

Multiple seasonal allergies are another cause of perennial problems. Air conditioners in cars and houses reduce pollen exposure and help patients with seasonal allergies. Besides household and outdoor exposure, the work place or hobbies should be considered as a source of offending substances. Laboratory animal exposure also can be a cause of perennial rhinitis. Both topical and systemic administration of medications can contribute to the problem. If another medication can be substituted safely, the source of the problem can be easily identified in this instance. Food as the sole cause of perennial rhinitis occurs infrequently; however, inquiries about unusual food habits occasionally may reveal the source of the problem. Elimination of chocolate and caffeine from the diet helps patients with common migraine, which often presents as "sinus headaches."

Although avoidance cannot always be absolute, a reduction in exposure can enhance the therapeutic efficacy of other modes of treatment. However, extreme fanaticism about eliminating all potential environmental hazards can create psychologic problems as well as lead to nutritionally inadequate diets.

PHARMACOLOGIC TREATMENTS

Antihistamines and Decongestants

The effectiveness of antihistamines in treating allergic rhinitis cannot be disputed. Clinically their greatest efficacy is in the relief of sneezing, itching, and rhinorrhea; they have little effect on nasal congestion. Their use in the treatment of perennial rhinitis is primarily in patients with perennial allergic rhinitis, but occasionally they show efficacy in those with rhinorrhea as the predominate symptom, an effect probably related to their anticholinergic properties. In treating patients with rhinorrhea, choose an antihistamine from the ethanolamine class because they have the greatest anticholinergic activity, e.g., diphenhydramine. Anticholinergic activity causes dryness, one of the common side effects of antihistamines, and can be associated with urinary retention in males with enlarged prostates. Antihistamines have a longer half-life than is usually ap-

preciated, possibly explaining why their continuous use provides greater efficacy than whenever-necessary dosing. Giving these medicines at bedtime frequently avoids sedation, which is the most common complaint, and the long half-life may lead to daytime efficacy.

The use of nonsedating antihistamines is another approach to decreasing sedation, which affects about 10 percent of the patients. Terfenadine, a nonsedating antihistamine, is currently marketed in the United States. In clinical trials its potency in the usual dosage (60 mg twice daily) was equivalent to that of chlorpheniramine (4 mg three times daily) but caused no more sedation than placebo. It was shown to be as efficacious as 8 mg of chlorpheniramine in the treatment of perennial rhinitis. However, the cost of terfenadine is high. In 1985 the average wholesale price to the pharmacist was $43.86 for one hundred 60 mg tablets, whereas one hundred 4 mg tablets of generic chlorpheniramine maleate cost $0.80. Another nonsedating antihistamine, astemizole, is currently undergoing clinical testing. It may have increased efficacy because of additional antiallergic properties. Astemizole's half-life, however, is measured in days, which may be a disadvantage. Other nonsedating antihistamines are currently undergoing development. Besides sedation and dryness, side effects include hyperreactivity or gastrointestinal discomfort.

Another phenomenon that patients frequently describe regarding antihistamines is their loss of efficacy with continued usage. For unknown reasons, switching to an antihistamine of a different class occasionally alleviates this problem. The availability of over the counter antihistamines makes rare the patient with perennial rhinitis who has not tried these medicines prior to seeking help from a physician. A history of usage avoids prescribing an antihistamine that failed or caused unacceptable side effects. The long clinical experience with these medications makes them safe for the prolonged treatment of a lifelong disorder.

Since antihistamines have limited efficacy in the treatment of nasal congestion, they are frequently combined with systemically effective decongestants. Another reason given for combining the two medications is the hope that the stimulant effect of the decongestant will counteract the sedation induced by antihistamines. The decongestants most commonly used are pseudoephedrine hydrochloride and phenylpropanolamine. In the treatment of perennial allergic rhinitis, the combination of antihistamine and decongestant is helpful, and the single pill is preferred by the patient. Patients who are allergic to multiple pollen allergies benefit more than those with allergies to perennial antigens, such as molds, and animal dander, because the latter patients have a greater problem with congestion than with rhinorrhea or sneezing. Patients with perennial nasal congestion without known allergies can be treated with only the decongestant. The dose of pseudoephedrine hydrochloride ranges from 30 to 120 mg. The larger the dose, the greater the amount of decongestion but also the greater the incidence of stimulant side effects, and hypertensive patients should have the blood pressure monitored. Systemically effective decongestants work after a few doses or not at all; thus prolonged therapeutic trials are unnecessary. These medicines, like antihistamines, are first line medications in the treatment of perennial rhinitis.

Topically as well as systemically administered decongestants are alpha-adrenergic stimulants. The topically administered decongestants are much more efficacious in achieving nasal decongestion than their oral counterparts. For example, oxymetazoline has an onset of action within minutes and a 10 to 12 hour duration of action. The main disadvantage of these stimulants is the development of rhinitis medicamentosa, the development with continued usage of a progressively shorter duration of action, until almost continual application provides no efficacy. The tendency for this to occur is greatest when the duration of the condition for which the medicine is taken exceeds several weeks. Thus, patients with perennial rhinitis are likely candidates to develop this side effect. With a strong caution to the patient, topically administered decongestants have some indications. Patients with perennial allergic rhinitis who respond to topical steroid therapy but who have sufficient nasal congestion to inhibit access of the drug to the nasal mucosa benefit by predosing with a decongestant. Patients with acute exacerbations of sinusitis benefit from the topical addition of a decongestant to antibiotic treatment. Some patients with perennial nasal obstruction unresponsive to other treatment may benefit from a single dose at bedtime. All these patients must be carefully instructed about the possibility of developing rhinitis medicamentosa.

If rhinitis medicamentosa is the cause of perennial rhinitis, the key to successful treatment is the identification of the pathologic event that initiated the process. Chronic sinusitis, allergic rhinitis, or a traumatic deformity can predispose to this condition. After defining the underlying cause, the key to therapy for rhinitis medicamentosa is withdrawal of the decongestant. A period of 2 weeks of abstinence from the decongestant will resolve the problem. Unfortunately, during this 2 week period, nasal congestion becomes severe and the patient tends to return to the decongestant. The use of a short course of systemic steroid therapy or the gradual substitution of topical steroid for topical decongestant therapy seems to assist in the withdrawal process.

Cromolyn Sodium

Cromolyn sodium is purported to be a mast cell stabilizer and therefore should be of significant benefit in the treatment of allergic disease. Well designed clinical trials have demonstrated clinical efficacy in the treatment of seasonal allergic rhinitis. However, its clinical utility in the management of perennial rhinitis appears to be limited because of its frequent dose schedule (four to six times per day) and the need to begin

treatment preseasonally. The drug is well tolerated, with few side effects.

Ipatroprium

Cholinergic imbalance is considered to be the cause of vasomotor rhinitis. There is, however, little evidence to support or refute this statement. Ipatroprium bromide, a potent, topically applied anticholinergic drug with little systemic absorption, has been available in Europe and is currently undergoing clinical trials in the United States. It appears to exert its greatest efficacy in the class of patients described as "drippers" and has little or no benefit in those with allergic rhinitis or viral infections. Another problem is that the drug appears to lose effectiveness with prolonged usage.

Saline Solutions

Saline solutions are used postoperatively by surgeons to remove crusts and dried mucus from the nasal cavity. These solutions have been used in other types of nasal complaints because some patients find them soothing. They are useful in cold induced rhinorrhea, i.e., patients whose nasal mucosa responds to dry and cold environments. Humidification of the house and covering the nose with a scarf while outdoors in the winter, however, are more practical treatments. If humidifiers are used in the house, they need to be cleaned regularly, since they can become a reservoir for fungi, which can induce symptoms in patients with mold induced allergic rhinitis. Saline solutions can be either purchased or made at home. The formula for one homemade solution is ½ teaspoon of salt, ½ teaspoon of baking soda, and 1 teaspoon of Karo syrup in 6 ounces of water. The patient needs to be instructed carefully in the preparation of these solutions, since excess salt can create hypertonic solutions, which adversely affect the nasal mucosa. Spray bottles, as opposed to droppers, provide the best distribution of the solutions. Refrigeration helps retard bacterial growth, but spraying cold water into the nose hurts, so the patient needs to warm the solution prior to application. The limited cost of saline solutions and their safety, if prepared correctly, make them a useful adjuvant in some patients.

Topical Corticosteroid Therapy

In the United States the introduction of steroids for the topical treatment of rhinitis in the 1960's greatly assisted the clinician in the management of patients with allergic rhinitis and some patients with idiopathic perennial rhinitis. Prior to that time systemic corticosteroid treatment was known to be of value, but the risks of complications from long term use outweighed their benefit. The topical application of steroids was an attempt to achieve site specific efficacy without systemic side effects. Decadron Turbinaire, the first available topically administered steroid for nasal use, was effective, but minimal systemic absorption limited its widespread acceptance. The more recent formulations of flunisolide and beclomethasone, which have no detectable effect on early morning cortisol levels, have permitted topical steroid therapy to play an important role in the management of perennial rhinitis.

Before discussing how to use topical steroid therapy it is helpful to understand why these preparations fail. A common reason for failure is that nasal congestion can be so severe that the medicine never penetrates to the site of the problem. This can be circumvented by topical premedication with a decongestant or by beginning with a short systemic course of steroids and substituting topical medication as the patient begins to respond. Another reason for failure is patient expectations. Many patients expect nasal sprays to work within minutes, but topically applied steroids become effective over days to weeks. Patients with perennial problems usually require a greater amount of time to achieve efficacy than patients with seasonal allergies.

Other problems are related to the delivery system. Since steroids are not water soluble, they must be dissolved in polyethylene glycol (flunisolide) or made into a suspension with freon (beclomethasone). These preparations cause local irritation, their major side effect. Flunisolide causes more stinging, whereas beclomethasone causes more sneezing. The solutions seem to have better distribution, and an occasional patient who obtains no benefit from a freon preparation may benefit from the solution. Flunisolide seems more moisturizing, whereas beclomethasone is more drying. These effects of the vehicle may be a factor in choosing a preparation for a particular patient until steroid preparations in less irritating aqueous preparations are developed. Decadron Turbinaire appears more potent and occasionally helps a patient who has been unresponsive to either flunisolide or beclomethasone.

Another problem with the topical application of steroids is that in only 20 percent of the patients associated eye symptoms are relieved by this form of treatment; thus there will be the need for additional medications. Although this is a disadvantage in seasonal allergic rhinitis, it is not a major problem with perennial rhinitis, since eye complaints usually are not a major component of the symptom complex. Before beginning the topical use of steroids, the patient needs to be assured about the lack of systemic side effects, told about the local irritations, and informed that instantaneous relief is not to be expected.

Begin treatment with the usual recommended dosages: flunisolide, two sprays in each nostril twice daily, and beclomethasone, one spray in each nostril three times daily. The patient should return to the office in about 2 weeks so that the physician can assess efficacy, evaluate any irritant effects, and discuss long term use of the medication. If there is no evidence of efficacy despite appropriate usage, one might consider increasing the dosage or switching the preparation. If a patient with perennial problems shows evidence of efficacy, one needs to consider the chronicity as well as the variability in the degree of symptomatology, the goal being to use as little medication as possible. The patient should try to taper the medication dosage if there is an excellent response. Remember that although the medication gradually achieves efficacy, its effects may be prolonged. Thus, reduce the dosage no more frequently than at weekly intervals and do not reduce the dosage prior to anticipated periods of exacerbations. Any local irritation apparent on physical examination should be followed closely, as an occasional patient may develop a septal perforation. If the patient is tolerating the medication well, he will usually continue to do so without problems. Patients are usually followed at 6 month intervals but are told to report any episodes of persistent bleeding.

A question frequently asked is what to do about the medication when the patient acquires a viral respiratory tract infection. Opinions regarding this vary, but I usually maintain the patient on topical steroid therapy. I believe that the risk of increasing nasal congestion from the primary disease as a result of stopping the local medication increases the incidence of secondary bacterial complications and that the benefit of continuing the steroid treatment outweighs any theoretical adverse effect on the response to the virus.

Topically applied steroids have been a great advantage to the clinician in treating perennial rhinitis, since they are effective in the majority of patients with positive skin test results and they benefit some of the patients with idiopathic perennial rhinitis. Another group of patients who benefit are those with nasal polyps, because the period between recurrence of nasal polyps appears to be prolonged if topical steroid therapy is begun postoperatively.

Antibiotics

No article on perennial rhinitis would be complete without mentioning the use of antibiotics. Unfortunately a short format permits only a highlighting of some facts and observations of particular relevance. First, patients with perennial rhinitis have a high incidence (about 55 percent) of abnormal sinuses, as indicated by x-ray examination, and the incidence would be even greater if CAT scanning were performed to detect abnormalities. Many of the patients with x-ray evidence of abnormalities benefit from the addition of antibiotics to their current treatment.

Chronic sinusitis rarely presents as a dramatic illness with fever but rather as a persistence of low grade nasal complaints; it should be considered when clinical deterioration occurs in a patient who previously was doing well on treatment or when a patient does not respond as expected. The choice of the first line antibiotic should be based on the common organisms within a community. An inadequate dosage may cause this approach to fail. For example, amoxicillin reaches its best sinus mucosa tissue levels in adults at a dosage of 500 mg, not 250 mg. Another common reason for failure is organisms that are resistant to the first choice of antibiotics. If a patient does not respond to the initial empiric choice of an antibiotic, a culture should be obtained. Since intranasal cultures do not correlate with cultures from within the maxillary sinus, an antral puncture is needed to obtain a proper culture. The material obtained should be cultured for aerobes, anaerobes, and fungi. Depending on the locale, the incidence of fungal sinusitis can be as high as 10 percent. In immune compromised hosts, cultures are particularly important and should be obtained early.

Some patients who respond initially but fail soon after the medication is terminated respond to a prolonged course of antibiotics. Although this is arbitrary, if a patient is maintained on an antibiotic for 6 weeks and then relapses, a surgical consultation is indicated. Also consider the possibility of an immune defect, while realizing that all immune defects do not lead to catastrophic illness. For example, about 1 in 200 patients with atopic disease have an IgA deficiency. Although most of these patients compensate for this defect with other classes of antibodies, some have problems with chronic recurrent infections. An occasional patient with recurrent infections realizes a reduction in symptoms and less frequent acute exacerbations with a once daily dose of an antibiotic. Flare-ups during continuous low dose antibiotic treatment can be managed by increasing the number of doses of the antibiotic or by switching to another antibiotic.

Another role for antibiotics in perennial rhinitis is in the treatment of *Staphylococcus aureus* carriage that presents as a low grade folliculitis. Short courses of antistaphylococcal antibiotics or topically applied antibiotic ointments usually treat the folliculitis but frequently are followed by recurrence. The literature suggests that rifampin may provide a more prolonged benefit. Another approach is the topical use of antibiotic solutions. A typical mixture might include 40 mg of neomycin with 200,000 units of polymyxin B in 1 liter of normal saline. Ampules containing these antibiotics can be purchased from Burroughs Welcome.

Antibiotic use plays an important role in the management of perennial rhinitis.

Immunotherapy

Immunotherapy, repeated injections of known allergens, is used only in the treatment of perennial allergic rhinitis. Since immunotherapy is covered in another section in this book, only a few philosophic comments regarding the use of this treatment are given here. First, this form of treatment is specific for the offending antigen. Nonspecific effects have not been demonstrated. The clinician must thoroughly define all offending antigens prior to instituting therapy, since immunotherapy takes months for maximal benefit to be achieved. Patients started on long courses of treatment will surely be disappointed if the treatment is only partially effective because a relevant antigen was omitted from the immunotherapy solution. Second, its efficacy, although clearly demonstrated for pollen allergens, has not been well studied for fungi and animal dander. Third, whether immunotherapy is more or less effective than pharmacologic treatment is probably more of academic interest than of practical concern; therefore the decision to choose one form rather than another becomes more a matter of patient and physician preference. Weekly injections are costly and time consuming to maintain and may be associated with adverse allergic reactions, whereas daily medication causes problems with compliance and can be associated with adverse reactions. However, both types of therapy are not mutually exclusive. For instance, patients given immunotherapy who are having exacerbations of symptoms during the peak of a pollen season may benefit from the addition of antihistamines or topical steroid therapy. Finally, immunotherapy can effectively treat patients with perennial allergic rhinitis, but proper administration requires a clinician experienced in its usage.

SURGERY

Surgery can cure nasal air flow obstruction secondary to mechanical factors or assist in the management of some patients with perennial rhinitis by improving the air way and providing better access for topical therapy. When the patient gives a history of trauma and there is nasal obstruction limited to one side, the patient will invariably benefit from surgery. The more difficult judgments relate to patients with both perennial rhinitis and a moderately deviated septum; a therapeutic trial of medical treatment for the perennial rhinitis assists in making the decision. If medical management leads to an acceptable result, any surgical consideration can be delayed. However, if the patient improves but still has sufficient difficulty to warrant further treatment, surgical intervention is indicated. In the latter situation the patient needs to fully appreciate that the goal of the surgery is to improve the nasal air way and that surgery will not eliminate mucosal disease.

Septal perforations, the major causes of which are prior surgery, trauma, and substance abuse, do not cause obstruction but can be the source of chronic nasal crusting and bleeding. After identifying the cause, surgical closure of the perforation or coverage with a plastic obturator may be indicated.

Recurrent acute and chronic sinusitis are major causes, as well as complications, of perennial rhinitis. If patients with these conditions fail medical management, several surgical procedures exist to correct the problem. A CAT scan evaluation prior to surgical intervention helps in choosing the best approach. A coronal scan without contrast medium allows excellent visualization of the middle meatus and defines the pathologic disorder. An occasional person with recurrent sinusitis has a septal spur that protrudes into the medial meatus and causes the problem. Since most sinus disease begins in the anterior ethmoids, this region must not be omitted from the surgical plan. Swelling and disease in the middle meatus can compromise drainage through the frontal recess (the opening to the frontal sinus), the natural ostia of the maxillary sinus, and the anterior ethmoids. More severe disease will spread to the posterior ethmoids and eventually to the sphenoidal sinuses. In most cases the changes in the maxillary and frontal sinuses (the sinuses most easily evaluated by routine sinus x-ray examination) are secondary changes. This statement is not intended to ignore the fact that a dental abscess may lead to sinusitis but is directed to emphasize the more common situation. It also helps to explain why certain surgical procedures fail.

A Caldwell-Luc operation enters the maxillary sinus through the anterior maxillary wall after an incision is made in the gingivobuccal fold. The contents of the sinus are removed, and a nasoantral window is created under the inferior turbinate. The operation eliminates disease within the sinus and creates an opening for ventilation, but it does not eliminate the usual cause of the problem, blockage of the natural ostium. It was thought that the Caldwell-Luc operation would bypass this problem until the discovery was made that mucociliary clearance in the maxillary antrum is toward the natural ostium. Mucus carried toward the natural ostium collects there until it falls toward the floor of the antrum to be transported again toward the ostium. With the advent of fiberoptic telescopes, this process can be visualized through the artificial nasoantral window. Many of the failures therefore are the result of an inadequate understanding of the disease process. When disease occurs in both the maxillary sinus and the ethmoid, an ethmoidectomy must accompany the Caldwell-Luc procedure. Some of the changes in the maxillary sinuses can be reversed by clearing and enlarging the natural ostium, further supporting the concept that changes in the maxillary sinus can be a secondary phenomenon. Fiberoptic telescopes for operating in the sinuses also provide the surgeon with better visualization of the nasal cavity and paranasal sinuses. This improved visualization leads to more precise surgical innervation with fewer complications. Other surgical procedures, such as frontal sinus obliteration, have specific indications, and the interested reader is referred to the otolaryngology literature for more information.

Nasal obstruction is not always the result of a septal deviation or mucosal congestion. The nasal valve located in the anterior naris can be the cause of the problem. This area can be compromised by curling of the lower lateral cartilages, loss of cartilaginous support, or hypertrophy of the anterior portions of the inferior or middle turbinates. The surgical approach to this problem is individualized and based on delineation of the anatomic features. The anterior portion of the turbinates can be resected, weak cartilage can be supported, and curled lower lateral cartilages can be resected. Many types of surgical approaches for the treatment of hypertrophied turbinate mucosa have been described, ranging from complete resection of the bone and its overlying mucosa to destruction of the mucosa by freezing (cryosurgery) or cauterization. Total turbinectomy can be followed by problems with chronic nasal crusting, adhesions, or a paradoxic situation in which the absence of air flow obstruction is associated with the subjective feeling of obstruction. A satisfactory explanation of the latter phenomena is lacking. Cryosurgery and cauterization are followed by a 1 month period of marked nasal crusting and then an improvement in air way function. Unless the underlying cause of the mucosal hypertrophy is identified, the improvement is not permanent, and subjective complaints will begin to return 6 months to 1 year after surgery.

The last surgical procedure related to perennial rhinitis is vidian neurectomy. The vidian nerve contains both the parasympathetic and the sympathetic nerve supplies to the nasal mucosa. This operation has been used for the treatment of vasomotor rhinitis in Europe and in the treatment of some patients in Japan with perennial allergic rhinitis who were unresponsive to medical management, but it has never gained popularity in the United States.

Surgery aimed at eliminating sinus disease and improving the airway can play an integral role in the overall management of perennial rhinitis.

SUMMARY

Perennial rhinitis refers to the year-round subjective complaints of rhinorrhea, nasal congestion, or irritation. This symptom complex is the end result of many different disease processes; thus, the clinician must approach this problem with a detailed history, making every effort to identify a precipitating factor. An equally careful physical examination must be performed to assist in understanding the relationship between structure and function. It is as remiss for the surgeon to miss an underlying allergic diathesis as for the allergist to miss a structural abnormality that is precipitating recurrent bouts of sinusitis in a patient with allergic rhinitis. After the problem is identified, treatment is directed toward the cause as well as toward providing symptomatic relief. Avoidance or reduction of exposure to allergens and environmental inhalants should be one goal. Pharmacologic measures include antihistamines, decongestants, corticosteroids, antibiotics, and saline solutions. Surgery may help the patient with chronic nasal obstruction or sinusitis, since sinusitis and perennial rhinitis frequently occur together. When patients with perennial allergic rhinitis stop responding to treatment, one should consider sinusitis as a possible cause. Because the allergic diathesis is so common, one must avoid the tendency to make this the final diagnosis without a thorough evaluation. Other factors, such as the immotile cilia syndrome and IgA deficiency, may complicate and alter the management of patients with perennial rhinitis. Despite a thorough evaluation, some patients remain without a diagnosis and have to be treated symptomatically. One must not stop considering such a patient's problems and must not create a psychologic cripple who becomes paranoid about his environment. Diagnosing and treating patients with perennial rhinitis constitute a challenge to the skills of the physician and surgeon.

SUGGESTED READING

Harding SM, Heath S. Intranasal steroid aerosol in perennial rhinitis: comparison with an antihistamine compound. Clin Allergy 1976; 6:369–372.

Hillas J, Booth RJ, Somerfield S, Morton R, Avery J, Wilson JD. A comparative trial of intranasal beclomethasone dipropionate and sodium cromoglycate in patients with chronic perennial rhinitis. Clin Allergy 1980; 10:253–258.

Kennedy D, Zinreich J, Rosenbaum A, Johns M. Functional endoscopic sinus surgery. Arch Otolaryngol 1985; 111:576–582.

Norman PS. An overview of immunotherapy: implications for the future. J Allergy Clin Immunol 1980; 65:87–96.

Turkeltaub PC, Norman PS, Johnson JD, Crepea S. Treatment of seasonal and perennial rhinitis with intranasal flunisolide. Allergy 1981; 37:303–311.

Welsh PW, et al. Efficacy of beclomethasone nasal solution, flunisolide, and cromolyn in relieving symptoms of ragweed allergy. Mayo Clinic Proc 1987; 62:125–134.

ASTHMA PROVOKED BY EXPOSURE TO ALLERGENS

A. BARRY KAY, D.Sc., Ph.D., F.R.C.P.

The term asthma describes a broad clinical spectrum ranging from mild, readily reversible bronchospasm to severe chronic intractable obstruction to air flow. The disease is difficult to define, since reversibility of airway obstruction may be impossible to demonstrate on certain occasions. For instance, the mild episodic asthmatic may be free of symptoms and have normal lung function for prolonged periods of time, whereas in acute severe asthma, airway obstruction may persist for several days before reversibility can be demonstrated. Nonspecific bronchial hyperreactivity is also a cardinal feature of the disease, but whether this is primary or secondary to mediator release or tissue damage is controversial.

It is well known that a number of events such as exposure to specific allergen, exercise, or infection are associated with exacerbations of asthma. Anxiety and psychologic triggers also are often implicated, but the precise role of emotional factors is poorly defined. Similarly there is scanty knowledge of the mechanisms by which infection leads to airway narrowing. On the other hand, a considerable amount of information has accrued regarding the events surrounding episodes of asthma elicited under controlled clinical conditions, such as allergen inhalation, various exercise procedures, isocapnic hyperventilation at rest, breathing cold air, the ingestion of certain foods, food additives and drugs, and the inhalation of agents such as histamine, methacholine, sulfur dioxide, and ozone.

THE ROLE OF ATOPY AND THE ATOPIC STATE

The contribution of atopy and the atopic state to asthma has given rise to some confusion. An atopic individual can be defined as one who gives positive immediate responses to skin prick tests to common inhalant allergens regardless of whether symptoms are present. The demonstration of immediate skin responses in a single individual is not by itself particularly helpful in the identification of triggering factors. Genetic studies suggest that atopy and asthma are inherited independently but that the inheritance of atopy, in many subjects, increases the expression of clinical asthma.

Allergic asthma is due to the inhalation of specific antigenic materials to which the individual has made an IgE antibody response. Common environmental inhaled allergens are particularly important. In the United Kingdom the feces of the house dust mite (Dermatophagoides pteronyssinus) is thought to play a major role in the initiation and potentiation of asthma and rhinitis in sensitized subjects. Other common allergens include grass and tree pollens and various animal danders, particularly those of cats, horses, and laboratory animals. The interaction of antigen with specific IgE bound to the membrane of mast cells (and possibly other mediator cells) leads to the release of a variety of spasmogenic, vasoactive, enzymatic, and chemotactic mediators, which in turn account for many of the features of the asthmatic response.

Allergens have certain characteristics. For instance, they are water soluble, often have a molecular weight of approximately 20 kd, and are usually proteins or glycoproteins with a relatively large particle size (i.e., between 15 and 20 microns). They are deposited largely in the upper airways. Allergens do not seem to have a unique chemical structure, and it is probable that their capacity to evoke an IgE response is determined more by their accessibility to antibody forming cells than by the possession of unusual antigenic determinants. The sites of IgE formation to inhaled allergens are predominantly in the upper airways.

The precise contribution of specific allergen(s) to the clinical features in an individual patient are usually suspected from the clinical history. For instance, house dust mite induced asthma is often associated with symptoms of rhinitis and is precipitated by activities such as bedmaking and exposure to old, dusty, or damp premises, which produce optimal conditions for the breeding of *D. pteronyssinus*. Allergy is usually prominent when the clinical features of asthma are episodic and correspond with the grass pollen season, or less commonly with high tree pollen counts. The role of animals, such as cats and horses, is usually obvious from the clinical history. The diagnosis of allergen induced, IgE mediated asthma has to be substantiated by a positive reaction to a skin prick test or, if this is not possible, a radioallergosorbent test (RAST) using the appropriate allergen. Other allergens such as molds or foods are sometimes important factors in individual patients. It is important to stress that allergy may be a trigger for asthmatic attacks for a relatively short period in the natural history of the disease. Allergen induced asthma is most common in childhood, but subjects may either "grow out" of their wheeziness or proceed to develop a more chronic form of the disease in which allergy seems to become less important.

Measurements of the total serum IgE concentration are of little use in the day to day management of asthma. On the other hand, a low total IgE level (i.e., less than 50 IU per ml) may be helpful evidence against an allergic basis for the disease. The range of IgE levels found in normal healthy nonatopic individuals is less than 0.1 to 150 IU per ml. The range of IgE levels found in clinical practice is very large, and the level is sometimes greater than 30,000 IU per ml. These high values are rarely seen in bronchial asthma unless they are accompanied by other conditions, such as atopic dermatitis or helminthic disease.

FOOD INDUCED WHEEZE

A number of foods are known to be associated with attacks of asthma, particularly milk, eggs, and nuts. In many instances these are classic anaphylactic types of reactions, specific IgE antibodies being readily detectable by skin prick tests or RAST. A number of patients have been described with milk induced wheeze who have had no evidence of either specific IgE or IgG4 antibodies but yet have had reproducible symptoms in a blind placebo controlled challenge situation. These individuals developed milk induced airway obstruction that was blocked by prior administration of sodium cromoglycate or oral doses of beclomethasone. The increases in airway resistance were accompanied by a rise in concentrations of circulating mast cell associated mediators. These situations seem to be another example of nonimmunologic release of mast cell associated pharmacologic mediators. It is of interest that in this situation, as with exercise, sodium cromoglycate appears to block mast cell degranulation as the result of a nonspecific stimulus.

OCCUPATIONAL ASTHMA

The term occupational asthma is generally restricted to asthma induced by agents inhaled at work caused by a specific hypersensitivity reaction. Evidence for a specific immunologic response has been obtained for some but not all its causes.

The occupations in which exposure to biologic agents occurs include agriculture, food manufacture, forestry, laboratory animal usage, and the commercial exploitation of microbes, both as animal (and human) food sources and for their products—particularly antibiotics and proteolytic enzymes. In these occupations the causative agents are inhaled as dusts, but exposure to biologic derivatives may also involve a vapor, of which the most important example is the pine wood resin colophony used as a soft solder flux in the electronics industry, which evaporates at its temperatures of use.

The chemical agents that induce hypersensitivity reactions are more limited in number, but exposure to them may be widespread. Three important examples of such chemical agents are the complex platinum salts, isocyanates, and acid anhydrides.

AVOIDANCE

Avoidance is the first principle of therapy and is relatively easy with respect to pet and hobby related exposures, provided patients are willing to cooperate. Sometimes boarding a pet with friends for a month or so will convince a family to get rid of the pet, if the patient improves significantly. Avoidance is more difficult with employment related activities, as in veterinarians, bakers, and individuals exposed to allergens in industry, in whom relocation to another work area or a change in job may be required. Every effort must be made, however, to remove the individual from the asthma provoking environment. Noxious industrial exposures should be corrected by proper ventilation and other industrial hygiene measures, which must be discussed with the officials of the involved industry.

In the home environment a number of relatively simple measures can help the patient avoid indoor allergens: for example, getting rid of feather pillows (using synthetic materials instead), covering the mattress with air-tight materials, taking up dusty carpets (also an area where mites locate), frequently changing the furnace filter, and careful cleaning with a wet dust mop to reduce dust exposure to a minimum. In addition, during pollen seasons, keeping the windows closed and installing an air conditioner in the patient's bedroom will reduce pollen exposure.

PHARMACOLOGIC MODULATION OF THE ASTHMATIC RESPONSE

Many drugs are available for the treatment of asthma. In general, medication is required for both the prevention of recurrent attacks and the relief of acute wheeze. The precise therapeutic requirements in individual patients vary considerably and may necessitate the use of three or more different preparations to achieve good control. For these reasons it is essential that the clinician have a basic knowledge of the mode of action of the various drugs currently available in order that they can be prescribed to full advantage. It is often useful to obtain objective measurements of the degree of airway reversibility over a period of time. This can be undertaken by self-monitoring of the peak expiratory flow rate. This procedure is useful both in diagnosis and in assessing the severity and response to treatment. Even though several drugs might have to be used at any one time, it is desirable for these to be kept to a minimum and for the physician to spend a considerable amount of time educating the patient about the disease, the correct usage of the various medicines, and the differences between drugs used for prevention and relief. Although it is important to identify triggers such as specific allergens and exercise, it has to be appreciated that the etiology of asthma is, by and large, poorly understood and that procedures such as hyposensitization do not hold much promise of a cure except in the mildest cases of seasonal asthma.

The drugs currently prescribed for the treatment of asthma can be broadly divided into bronchodilators (beta-adrenoceptor agonists, methylxanthines, and anticholinergics), corticosteroids, and disodium cromogylcate (and analogues).

Beta- (Beta$_2$-selective) Adrenoceptor Agonists (Sympathomimetics)

The beta$_2$-selective agonists (such as salbutamol, terbutaline, and fenoterol) have replaced nonselective beta-agonists such as isoprenaline and isoetharine, which are now virtually obsolete. Beta-agonists can be used either by inhalation (as a pressurized aerosol or nebulizer) or orally or intravenously in selected cases. Beta-agonists are extremely effective bronchodilators and appear to act principally by causing direct relaxation of the bronchial smooth muscle of both the large and the small airways. These agonists also inhibit the release of pharmacologic mediators from human lung fragments and dispersed pulmonary mast cells, as well as decreasing airway microvascular permeability. They also may inhibit cholinergic neurotransmission as well as increasing mucociliary clearance.

Inhaled beta-agonists are rapidly effective and without significant side effects. When given orally or intravenously, they may produce symptoms related to beta$_2$-receptor stimulation in other tissues (muscle tremor, tachycardia, metabolic effects such as hypokalemia). Although tachyphylaxis to beta-agonists in human bronchial smooth muscle preparations has been demonstrated in vitro, there is little evidence for beta-receptor tolerance in the airways of asthmatics in vivo when conventional doses of beta-agonists are used.

Beta-agonists are particularly useful for "relief" of wheeze but also can be used regularly (usually four times daily) for "prevention" and are very effective in protecting against exercise induced asthma. In acute severe asthma beta-agonists given in high doses by nebulizer are as effective as intravenously administered beta-agonists or aminophylline and are therefore the preferred bronchodilator treatment in this situation.

Methylxanthines (Theophyllines)

Methylxanthines such as theophyllines are widely used for the stabilization of asthmatic individuals and the emergency treatment of acute severe attacks. Their precise mode of action in asthma is in doubt.

Theophyllines and their analogues are most effective when administered parenterally, orally, or rectally. They cannot be given by inhalation because they are too irritating. Slow release formulations are useful for treating nocturnal wheezing, since therapeutic concentrations over hours may be achieved.

A major disadvantage of theophyllines is the low therapeutic-toxic ratio. Attempts usually are made to maintain plasma theophylline levels between 10 and 20 μg per ml. However, at levels above 20 μg per ml nausea, vomiting, headache, and palpitations often occur. High concentrations result in convulsions, arrhythmias, and sometimes death. There are considerable differences among individuals in the clearance of theophyllines, and this makes it difficult to predict plasma concentrations and emphasizes the importance of measuring plasma levels. The absorption and metabolism of theophyllines are also influenced by smoking, diet, liver disease, cardiac failure, viral infections, chronic airway disease, and drugs such as erythromycin and cimetidine.

Anticholinergics

Generally speaking, anticholinergic drugs such as ipratropium bromide (Atrovent) are most effective in older nonatopic asthmatic patients in remission or in older bronchitic patients with asthmatic features. These compounds are not such good bronchodilators as beta-agonists, but they may have additive effects when combined with beta-agonists. They also have been used with effect in the management of acute severe asthma. They act by inhibiting reflex induced bronchoconstriction and are most effective in the large airways. Unlike beta-agonists, they probably have no effect on mast cells and vascular permeability.

Corticosteroids

Intermittent or long term treatment with corticosteroids is the mainstay of the therapy of moderate to severe asthma. The introduction of locally acting, inhaled corticosteroids in the mid-1960s was a major therapeutic advance because it enabled many patients, previously dependent on oral corticosteroid therapy, to receive medication by inhalation and so minimize generalized side effects.

A wide range of preparations is available. The relative potencies of selected corticosteroids (in terms of their anti-inflammatory effects) are as follows: hydrocortisone, 10 mg; prednisolone, 5 mg; triamcinolone, 4 mg; betamethasone, 0.75 mg; and dexamethasone, 0.75 mg. Hydrocortisone has the shortest biologic half-life (12 to 24 hours), whereas dexamethasone and betamethasone have longer half-lives (longer than 48 hours). The use of drugs with a shorter half-life has the advantage of allowing the hypophysis-pituitary-adrenal axis time to recover between doses. Prednisolone is the most commonly used corticosteroid because of its enhanced anti-inflammatory action, its intermediate half-life, and the fact that it can be taken orally. Most of the circulating prednisolone is bound to plasma proteins (transcortin and albumin), but the small protein free fraction is thought to be the active component.

In asthma corticosteroids can be administered either orally, by inhalation, or intravenously. Oral candidiasis occurs in 5 to 10 percent of the individuals who take inhaled corticosteroids, and aphonia (due to a direct effect on the larynx and not candidiasis) is a rare complication. When the dosage of inhaled corticosteroid exceeds 1 mg per day, hypophysis-pituitary-adrenal suppression and generalized side effects may be observed as with orally administered preparations. Some individuals require a combination of both oral and inhaled corticosteroid administration for optimal results. It is preferable to give steroids orally as a single dose in the morning, ideally on alternate mornings to reduce side effects. Before starting oral corticosteroid therapy it is important to establish objective evidence of benefit by a formal "trial," usually by giving 30 to 40 mg of prednisolone daily for 2 weeks and recording changes in peak flow.

Corticosteroids may be indicated in asthma at any age and irrespective of whether the asthmatic is atopic or nonatopic. Steroids have undoubted value in chronic asthma and are often life-saving. Short courses of oral prednisolone therapy (e.g., prednisolone, 30 mg daily for 6 days) can be administered by the patients themselves at times of destabilization. Thus corticosteroids are for "prevention" and have no immediate bronchodilator effect. They must be used continuously, and the dosage must be titrated to the individual patient's needs.

Sodium Cromoglycate

Sodium cromoglycate (cromolyn, Intal) inhibits allergen induced bronchoconstriction in man and passive cutaneous anaphylaxis in the rat. On this basis its principal mode of action was ascribed to inhibition of mediator release from mast cells (it is marketed as a "mast cell stabilizer"). Recently some doubt has been cast on mast cell stabilization as its principal mode of action, since, for instance, high concentrations of the compound are required to inhibit histamine release from immunologically challenged human chopped lung preparations. Furthermore, a number of compounds have been developed that are several orders of magnitude more potent than sodium cromoglycate in rat passive cutaneous anaphylaxis, but these have been uniformly disappointing in clinical trials.

In selected cases the drug is highly effective as a prophylactic agent in bronchial asthma, although it is difficult to predict effectiveness. Children and young adults appear to derive most benefit, but the compound is worthy of evaluation in older asthmatics, especially those with a clear history of allergen induced wheeze. The drug has a remarkable safety record with few side effects apart from some local irritation and very occasional anaphylactic reactions. The drug is administered either by dry powder inhaler, by pressurized inhaler, or by nebulization. Sodium cromoglycate inhibits both immediate and late phase allergen induced bronchoconstriction, as well as exercise induced asthma and certain forms of food induced wheeze.

Other "Mast Cell Stabilizers"

Ketotifen (Zaditen) is also marketed in Europe and elsewhere for oral use as a mast cell stabilizing agent. This compound has not been shown to be appreciably better than placebo in a number of clinical trials, and the marginal efficacy observed in some individuals is probably attributable to its mild antihistaminic properties. It causes considerable drowsiness and cannot be recommended for routine use.

More recently nedocromil sodium (Tilade) has been introduced as a prophylactic antiasthma agent. It is chemically related to sodium cromoglycate and is said to have ''anti-inflammatory'' (corticosteroid sparing) properties as well as effects on mast cells. Its true place in the management of asthma is yet to be established.

IMMUNOTHERAPY

Although there is no absolutely convincing evidence from controlled double blind clinical trials that immunotherapy is effective for patients with asthma, the practice is still popular in certain parts of the world. In the United Kingdom this form of treatment has been virtually abandoned because of severe reactions and the number of deaths directly attributable to injection immunotherapy. In fact, hyposensitization can be performed in the United Kingdom only in centers that have immediate access to cardiopulmonary resuscitative fa-cilities, and patients must wait for 2 hours after each injection. Although immunotherapy conceivably may have a place in allergic asthma in selected individuals, it always has to be borne in mind that the pharmacotherapy of the disease is extremely effective. The situation regarding immunotherapy is continuously under review, but the patients who do respond to this form of therapy will have to be defined more clearly.

SUGGESTED READING

Buckle DR, Smith H, eds. The development of anti-asthma drugs. London: Butterworths, 1984.
Clark TJH, Godfrey S, eds. Asthma. 2nd ed. London: Chapman & Hall, 1983.
Kay AB, ed. Asthma: clinical pharmacology and therapeutic progress. Oxford: Blackwell Scientific Publications, 1986.
Kay AB, ed. Allergy and inflammation. London: Academic Press, 1987.
Kay AB, Austen KF, Lichtenstein LM, eds. Asthma: physiology, immunopharmacology and treatment. London: Academic Press, 1984.
Kay AB, Goetzl EJ, eds. Current perspectives in the immunology of respiratory diseases. Edinburgh: Churchill Livingstone, 1985.

ASTHMA IN ADULTS

JOHN H. TOOGOOD, M.D., F.R.C.P.(C), F.C.C.P.

To properly treat a patient with chronic asthma, the prerequisites cited in Table 1 must be met. All decisions about therapy are founded on these data.

TREATMENT

Three goals of treatment are common to all patients with asthma. These are to reduce exposure to identifiable ''trigger'' factors, both specific (i.e., allergic) and nonspecific (e.g., frosty air, tobacco smoke), to reverse or prevent bronchospasm using bronchodilator drugs, and to reduce the degree of nonspecific airway reactivity. The latter reflects, in part at least, the degree of airway inflammation. Regular treatment with a glucocorticoid, cromolyn, beta-agonists, theophylline, or immunotherapy (in appropriately selected cases) can each reduce nonspecific airway reactivity in addition to the effects that are more immediately perceptible, such as the bronchodilator action of beta-agonists or theophylline.

In patients with allergic asthma it is also important to reduce the exposure to inhalant allergens. Rigorous environmental control of house dust can significantly improve nonspecific airway reactivity in asthmatics and reduce morbidity and the requirement for antiasthmatic drugs as well as the long term costs of treatment.

It is convenient to consider the details of asthma therapy in terms of different levels of disease severity.

Chronic Asthma: Mild

Definition: No acute or chronic disability. Symptoms less frequent than daily. Prompt response to bronchodilator inhalant. No nocturnal asthma.

TABLE 1 Diagnostic Prerequisites

Accuracy of asthma diagnosis?
Priority ranking in problem list?
Severity of pulmonary impairment?
Importance of allergic versus nonspecific ''triggers''?
Clinical course: progressing, stable, labile?
Current therapy and drug intolerances?
Personality, life style, social circumstances?
Expected results from therapy?

Plan:

1. Eliminate any identifiable cause (e.g., the cat in the house).

2. Albuterol, two puffs (200 μg) to relieve tightness of chest. Repeat every 2 hours as needed.

3. For predictable risk situations (e.g., exercise induced asthma or occasional exposure to a known environmental allergen), premedicate with albuterol or cromolyn. The former is the more effective. Repeat four times daily for the duration of the exposure (e.g., a weekend stay in a "catty" household).

Chronic Asthma: Moderate

Definition: Inhaled bronchodilator required almost daily. Nocturnal attacks. Restriction of life style by exertional dyspnea or by periodic asthma exacerbations.

Plan:

1. Eliminate identifiable trigger factors, specific and nonspecific.

2. Give sustained action theophylline preventatively twice daily. Adjust the dosage to achieve a therapeutic blood level (55 to 110 μmol per liter). If the patient is symptom free with blood levels less than 55 μmol per liter, do not push the dosage higher.

3. As an alternative, the patient should inhale cromolyn, 20 mg four times daily. This is the preferred regimen for children.

4. Give beclomethasone dipropionate, 0.4 to 0.8 mg per day in four divided doses (or equivalent dose of budesonide, flunisolide, or triamcinolone). The patient should inhale the drug slowly over 5 to 10 seconds and breath-hold for 5 to 10 seconds after full inspiration.

5. To relieve "breakthrough" asthma symptoms, the patient inhales 200 μg of albuterol. Repeat every 2 hours as needed. If albuterol is required more than six times per day, this indicates the need for a change in the treatment plan. The physician should be contacted. If, on the other hand, the need for albuterol approximates zero, discontinue theophylline and continue the beclomethasone (except when compliance with the beclomethasone regimen is unsatisfactory).

6. To correct, or avert, disabling exacerbations, give prednisone, 40 to 60 mg per day for 5 to 7 days, in two to four divided doses. Reduce to zero over about 3 weeks. A 2 to 4 day burst may suffice if the asthmagenic challenge was short lived. Abrupt withdrawal after a short burst is safe.

Chronic Asthma: Severe

Definition: Life style restricted by exertional dyspnea despite regular use of bronchodilators, cromolyn, or inhaled steroids in conventional doses. Bursts of prednisone are required more than three times per year to correct acute relapses.

Plan:

1. Use aggressive prednisone therapy to correct disability, and determine the maximal reversibility of the obstructive impairment. Continue administration of 40 to 60 mg per day, if tolerated, until improvement plateaus. In older adults who have some chronic obstructive pulmonary disease associated with the asthma, this usually requires 1 to 3 weeks. Monitor the response objectively if possible by daily peak expiratory flow rate measurements at home or periodic spirometry in the office or hospital. After "plateauing," taper to a maintenance dosage level over 3 to 4 weeks.

2. Cotreat with sustained action theophylline twice daily. If low "trough" blood levels indicate a fast metabolizer, shift to three times daily dosing and increase the per diem dosage cautiously.

3. Increase the inhaled steroid dosage, e.g., to ≥ 1.0 mg per day of beclomethasone and have the patient inhale the drug via a spacer. A large volume spacer such as the Inspir-Ease (about 700 ml) can double the intrapulmonary delivery of the drug. Titrate the oral and then the inhaled steroid dosage to determine the minimal dosages of each required to prevent disability and maintain symptom control. Provided minimal doses are used, there is no contraindication to the combined use of inhaled and oral steroid therapy (usually high dose inhaled and low dose, alternate day oral). Some patients with labile severe asthma may require as much as 1 year of careful follow up and dosage manipulation to achieve stable and optimal disease control.

4. Inhale albuterol immediately before each beclomethasone treatment. This improves the air flow and helps prevent the reflex cough that may be triggered if beclomethasone is inhaled too rapidly. Ipratropium may confer additional advantage in the older asthmatic with associated chronic obstructive pulmonary disease. Use extra doses of albuterol to relieve breakthrough symptoms of bronchospasm. Ipratropium is also effective but takes about 20 minutes to act.

5. In a very few cases it may be necessary to administer nebulized albuterol at home, using an air compressor and mask (2.5 mg dissolved in about 2.0 ml of diluent, inhaled two to four times daily).

6. Cotreatment with cromolyn, administered via spincaps or a metered dose inhaler, does not add materially to the results that can be obtained with inhaled steroids alone. However, in labile asthmatics refractory to other treatment, especially those with atopic allergy, 1 percent cromolyn solution may be added, two to four times daily. The rationale for this treatment lies in its well documented safety record, the reliable delivery system, and the drug's capacity to reduce nonspecific airway reactivity with long term use.

Acute Asthma: Mild

Definition: Transient nondisabling bronchospasm.
Plan: Any of the inhaled beta-agonist drugs listed

TABLE 2   Beta-agonist Bronchodilators

Albuterol	Isoproterenol
Epinephrine	Orciprenaline (metaproterenol)
Fenoterol	Terbutaline

TABLE 3   Characteristics of High-Risk Asthmatics Seen in Emergency Room

Previous life-threatening attack

Very labile asthma or gradually deteriorating air flows

Long delay before seeking medical attention

Pulsus paradoxus

PEFR $<$ 100 liters per minute or FEV_1 $<$ 0.7 liters

Inadequate response 1 hour after nebulized albuterol administration ($\triangle$PEFR $<$ 60 liters per minute or $\triangle FEV_1$ $<$ 0.4 liter)

Respiratory alternans or paradoxic inspiratory diaphragmatic movement

Diminishing consciousness; increasing exhaustion

$PaCO_2$ normal, rising, or elevated

Presence of pneumothorax or mediastinum

in Table 2 are effective. Albuterol is the most efficient in terms of prompt action, sustained action, and minor adverse effects. Epinephrine is least efficient.

If mild dyspneic attacks consistently fail to respond within 3 to 5 minutes to inhaled albuterol, they are probably not the result of asthma; functional dyspnea should be considered. If such attacks continue to recur despite explanation and reassurance, selected patients may benefit from relaxation breathing exercises, using autohypnosis techniques or a yoga type of regimen.

Acute Asthma: Moderate

Definition: The symptomatic response to bronchodilators is not sustained. Potentially disabling, recurrent exacerbations.

Plan:

1. Abort exacerbations of infective asthma or asthmatic bronchitis by a burst of steroid administered systemically early in the illness: 20 mg of prednisone twice daily for about 5 days, reducing to zero after 10 days (longer, if necessary, depending on the severity of the attack). Use oral and inhaled bronchodilator administration concomitantly.

2. The infections that trigger these exacerbations are mostly viral. If an antibiotic is considered necessary, tetracycline, ampicillin, amoxicillin, trimethoprim sulfa, and erythromycin are reasonable choices. However, erythromycin increases the risk of theophylline toxicity.

If a satisfactory response is not obtained after 1 week, repeated courses of antibiotic usually do not improve the situation. The persisting wheezy bronchitis commonly indicates the need for more aggressive steroid treatment, e.g., another week of prednisone, 20 to 40 mg per day.

Acute Asthma: Severe

Definition: Increasingly severe asthma, despite frequent (often excessive) bronchodilator use at home. Disabled.

Plan:

1. Treat with oxygen and nebulized 0.6 percent albuterol solution (2.5 mg inhaled at a flow rate of 6 to 8 liters per minute over 5 to 10 minutes). If no response occurs in 30 minutes, repeat the albuterol treatment. In partially responsive cases, repeat as needed at 1 to 4 hour intervals. Check blood gas levels (off oxygen). Criteria for admission to hospital are shown in Table 3.

2. Cotreatment with theophylline intravenously may increase the toxicity of the treatment without a comparable increase in benefit. In patients presenting with a history of recent theophylline ingestion, withhold intravenous therapy with theophylline until a failure to respond to combined albuterol-corticosteroid treatment clearly establishes the need for theophylline and the results of a theophylline blood level measurement are at hand.

3. Steroids should be used routinely for severe asthma. Because the steroid response is slow to appear (6 to 9 hours), bronchodilators must be used as well. Give 250 mg of hydrocortisone intravenously immediately and repeat every 8 hours (or 750 mg running continuously over 24 hours); 150 mg of methylprednisolone per 24 hours is equally effective and has less mineralocorticoid activity. Larger doses confer no additional benefit and occasionally may cause disastrous complications.

4. If narcotics and tranquilizers are avoided and aggressive bronchodilator-steroid-oxygen treatment is pursued, the need for assisted ventilation in uncomplicated asthma is rare.

COMPLICATIONS

Beta-agonists

Muscle tremor can be minimized by using an inhaled rather than an oral formulation or substituting ipratropium inhalant.

The question of patients "abusing" their bronchodilator inhaler merits special attention. The increasingly frequent use of the metered dose inhaler usually signals a dangerous deterioration in ventilatory function due to beta-adrenergic tachyphylaxis or an increasing inflammatory component in the airway obstruction. Warnings about the danger of ''inhaler abuse'' are inappropriate in these circumstances. Steroids can reverse the problem and are urgently needed. Restoration of the airways' responsiveness to adrenergics may begin within 1 hour. However, the widespread mucus plugging of small airways may take 1 week or more to fully resolve. Patients who have experienced such dangerous relapses should be committed to regular steroid treatment or given a home supply of prednisone with instructions outlining the indications for use and details of dosage.

Theophylline

Theophylline commonly leads to gastric reflux and occasionally reflux esophagitis. When patients with active systems of reflux are given prednisone, ranitidine or cimetidine should also be prescribed preventatively to inhibit gastric acid secretion. If the patient is symptomatic, add alginic acid compound (Gaviscon) three times daily after meals and at bedtime.

Insomnia, irritability, or nausea responds to lowering of the theophylline dosage. Major complications are avoidable if blood levels are kept below 110 μmol per liter. Erythromycin inhibits theophylline metabolism, and so do virus infections. Together or singly, these factors may trigger dangerous toxic effects. Avoid erythromycin in asthmatic patients taking theophylline.

Mood Altering Drugs

Narcotics are contraindicated for asthma treatment. Tranquilizers are inappropriate for asthma and occasionally are dangerous. Typically, anxiety resolves spontaneously as severe asthma is brought under control with bronchodilators and steroids.

Steroid Induced Bone Disease

To minimize the risk of steroid osteoporosis (and other systemic complications), follow the guidelines listed in Table 4. Postmenopausal women starting regular steroid therapy should maintain a high calcium intake (milk, cheese, supplemental calcium if necessary), ingest 800 IU of vitamin D daily, and exercise regularly outdoors. Estrogens, if started soon after the menopause, prevent excessive bone loss.

Treat patients with symptomatic vertebral fractures

TABLE 4 Prevention of Systemic Complications of Steroid Therapy

Use prednisone in preference to slowly metabolized steroids e.g., dexamethasone

Use the single dose, alternate morning regimen

Titrate dose to minimal effective level

Replace some or all the prednisone with inhaled steroid

Give calcium supplement (to reduce osteoporosis)

with calcium supplements, vitamin D, and enough codeine to facilitate walking (weight bearing stress is essential for bone repair). After appropriate metabolic assessment, selected patients may benefit from estrogens (to decelerate bone loss), vitamin D (to increase calcium absorption), hydrochlorothiazide (to reduce urinary calcium loss), or fluoride (to stimulate bone formation). Monitor to avoid hypercalcemia. Fluoride's safety remains uncertain.

Steroid Withdrawal Syndrome

Abrupt or accelerated withdrawal of systemic doses of steroids, after a long period of regular usage, may precipitate disabling arthralgia, joint swelling, cellulitis, peripheral edema, lethargy, anorexia, and nausea—so-called ''pseudorheumatism.'' The syndrome responds well to indomethacin and may be avoided altogether if the steroid dosage is tapered slowly, using an alternate day regimen.

Use of Steroids in Asthmatics at Risk from Tuberculosis

When starting steroid treatment, routine isoniazid treatment is not indicated for asthmatic patients with a positive skin test to tuberculin unless they have clinically active tuberculosis or have recently converted to skin test positive status. Combined antituberculosis chemotherapy and beclomethasone has been used successfully in patients with active tuberculosis and asthma.

Treatment of the Pregnant Asthmatic

Treat the asthma to ensure optimal control. Topically active drugs such as beclomethasone, cromolyn, albuterol, or ipratroprium are preferred. Systemic steroid treatment should be used as needed because the risk of steroid induced adverse effects to the fetus or mother appears to be negligible, whereas uncontrolled asthma increases the incidence of maternal complications, premature delivery, and perinatal fetal morbidity and mortality.

Preoperative Preparation of the Steroid Dependent Asthmatic

Anyone presenting for surgery with a history of use of oral or inhaled steroid therapy during the preceding year should receive 100 mg of cortisone acetate (20 ml) intramuscularly 24 hours preoperatively, as well as a repeat dose in 8 hours and 1 hour preoperatively. If the blood pressure drops, give hydrocortisone, 100 mg intravenously immediately. Repeat every 6 to 8 hours to prevent hypotensive crises. If emergency surgery is necessary, 4 mg of dexamethasone given intravenously 1 hour preoperatively is preferable to cortisone because it acts more quickly.

Inhaled Steroids

High dose inhaled steroid therapy in adults, or conventional dosage in children, may suppress hypophysis-pituitary-adrenal axis function. Also steroids inhaled in conventional dosages may perpetuate adrenocortical hypofunction caused by earlier systemic steroid treatment. To minimize the problem, titrate the dosage to determine each patient's minimal needs.

A common complication of inhaled steroid treatment is reflex cough triggered by deposition of the drug in the central airways and carina region. To resolve the problem, peripheralize the dose by having the patient inhale the drug more slowly or via a spacer or by pretreatment with an inhaled beta-agonist. A 10 day burst of prednisone may be required in some cases to restore accessibility of the distal airways to the inhaled drug and thus eliminate the cough.

Dysphonia (huskiness) complicating inhaled steroid therapy is caused by dyskinesia of the muscles that control vocal cord tension. Therefore antifungal therapy is inappropriate. To alleviate or avoid huskiness, reduce deposition of the drug around the larynx by reducing the daily dosage, inhaling via a spacer, or reducing the speed of inspiration. Acute or chronic laryngeal stress, common in switchboard operators, sports coaches, and singers, aggravates the problem. Rigorous voice rest may be needed. Resumption of therapy with the drug is usually well tolerated if laryngeal stress is avoided.

To minimize the incidence of oropharyngeal candidiasis, the patient should inhale the steroid via a spacer, avoid concomitant prednisone or antibiotic use as much as possible, and rinse the mouth after each treatment. Conversion from four times to twice daily dosing will largely eliminate thrush but may also reduce the drug's antiasthma efficacy. Esophageal candidiasis

is an unusual complication that illustrates the interaction of multiple risk determinants.

Systemic steroid treatment is preferable to inhaling steroid for the long term treatment of allergic bronchopulmonary aspergillosis. Asthmatics who have epithelialized cavities, cysts, or bronchiectatic segments may be at risk of mycotic superinfection if inhaled steroid therapy is used. In the immunocompromised patient, avoid any form of steroid therapy, oral or inhaled, or use it with great caution because of the risk of opportunistic infection.

Complicated Problems

Multiple factors may interact to produce complications in a particular patient. To deal effectively with the problem, it is necessary to unravel these interactions. The data in Tables 5 and 6 and Figure 1 summarize the latter process in a young man with an array of complications that had led to a therapeutic impasse. Table 5 lists his presenting complaints. Figure 1 displays a flow chart of their pathogenesis. Constructing such a chart helps the physician to plan an effective strategic approach. The treatment plan and clinical results are shown in Table 6.

BEYOND DRUGS

Every patient with asthma brings three basic needs to the therapeutic encounter:

1. The need for an explanation of the mechanism of the symptoms and their prognostic significance. This explanation must be expressed in terms that are understandable to the patient, given his or her concepts of bodily function and disease. These concepts vary with social class and with cultural background and they may be radically different from those of the physician.

TABLE 5 Presenting Complaints*

1. Frequent "chest colds" (? pneumonia); constantly taking antibiotics for >6 months
2. Continuous nystatin for oral thrush for >6 months
3. Low substernal dysphagia, heartburn, bloating
   Endoscopic diagnosis: candidiasis of esophagus; no response to nystatin
4. Frightening "choking" attacks—about three per day
5. Cough, gagging, vomiting attacks, two or three each hour, triggered by any deep inhalation or by inhalation of an antiasthmatic drug (including albuterol)
6. Tight chest (but afraid to inhale albuterol)
7. Nose plugged, mouth breathing, anosmia
8. Unable to work for 4 months, depressed, anxious

*Complex drug interactions causing adverse reaction are: theophylline + BDP + antibiotics + salbutamol (see Figure 1).

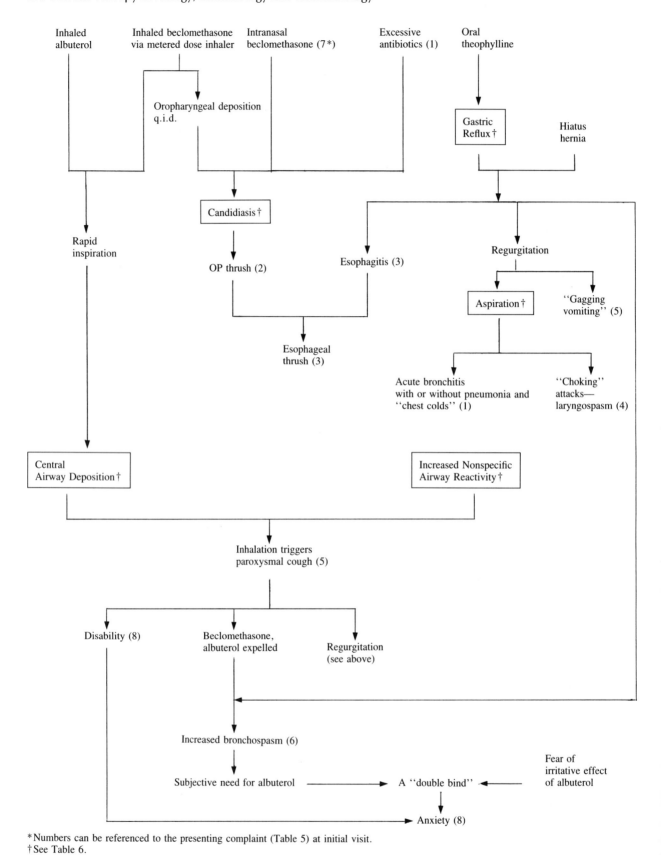

*Numbers can be referenced to the presenting complaint (Table 5) at initial visit.
†See Table 6.

Figure 1 Pathogenesis of presenting complaints that lead to a therapeutic impasse.

TABLE 6 Treatment Plan*

1. Control reflux and aspiration:

   Quit theophylline. Substitute oral doses of albuterol. Elevate head of bed. Cimetidine b.i.d. + alginic acid compound q.i.d. (+ antacid p.r.n.)

2. Eliminate candidiasis:

   Avoid antibiotics (which stimulate Candida growth). Treat "chest colds" symptomatically only. Inhale beclomethasone via spacer (reduces oropharyngeal deposition 90%). Rinse mouth after each treatment.
   Quit intranasal beclomethasone. Use antihistamine orally instead. Switch beclomethasone dosage from q.i.d. to b.i.d. (Conserves antifungal host defences at mucosal surface.)

3. Shift aerosol deposition away from upper airways, trachea, carina:

   Eliminate high velocity impact on pharynx, larynx (by using spacer). Slow inhalation to 25 liters per minute—slower if necessary (to peripheralize inhaled drugs).
   Breath-hold 10 seconds after inhaling beclomethasone (to maximize antiasthmatic effect).

4. Reduce nonspecific airway reactivity:

   Continue beclomethasone.
   Time.

Result:

At 2 months:	Improving. Nonspecific airway reactivity still high.
At 5 months:	Much improved. Working.
At 14 months:	Unrestricted vigorous exercise. No longer taking antacids.
At 24 months:	Doing very well on beclomethasone and albuterol spray q.i.d. via spacer. Antihistamine/decongestant p.r.n. for rhinitis. Prednisone weeks = 3/104. No antibiotics or nystatin in 2 years.

*Goals 1 to 4 can be referenced to the items enclosed by a rectangle in Figure 1.

2. The need to be assured that there are things he or she can do to control the illness.

3. The need to believe that the therapist is supportive and caring.

In meeting these needs, the good physician forges the "patient-physician" relationship—and the latter is at least as important as any drug for long term therapeutic success.

A system of regular clinical follow up strengthens the patient-physician bond. Furthermore, it shifts the emphasis of the therapeutic plan from intervention to prevention, from correcting illness to maintaining wellness. The process of follow up also teaches the physician a great deal about the natural course of chronic asthma and how to deploy the various modalities of treatment to the greatest advantage of each patient.

SUGGESTED READING

Dolovich J, Hargreave FE, Wilson WM, Greenbaum J, Powles ACP, Newhouse MT. Control of asthma. Can Med Assoc J 1982; 126:613–618.
Littenberg B, Gluck EH. A controlled trial of methylprednisolone in the emergency treatment of acute asthma. New Engl J Med 1986; 314:150–152.
Mawhinney H, Spector SL. Optimum management of asthma in pregnancy. Drugs 1986; 32:178–187.
Rebuck AS, Chapman KR. Asthma. 1. Pathophysiologic features and evaluation of severity. Can Med Assoc J 1987; 136:351–354.
Rebuck AS, Chapman KR. Asthma. 2. Trends in pharmacologic therapy. Can Med Assoc J 1987; 136:483–488.
Siegel D, Sheppard D, Gelb A, Weinberg PF. Aminophylline increases the toxicity but not the efficacy of an inhaled beta-adrenergic agonist in the treatment of acute exacerbations of asthma. Am Rev Respir Dis 1985; 132:283–286.

ASTHMA IN CHILDREN

PEYTON A. EGGLESTON, M.D.
ROBERT A. WOOD, M.D.

Asthma is a common childhood disease, affecting literally millions of children. It is responsible for more than 20 percent of school absences and for a major proportion of pediatric admissions to emergency rooms and hospitals. At the same time our current understanding of its pathogenesis and the effectiveness of available drugs allows the physician to help most children encountered. This review deals separately with the treatment of acute attacks and long term therapy.

ACUTE ASTHMA ATTACKS

When a child presents with an acute asthma attack, a limited but carefully directed history and physical examination should precede therapy. Important points in the history of this attack include the precipitant, the duration, the specific medications already taken (especially their dosage and timing), and the fluid balance. It is also important to ask about the course of previous attacks and their response to therapy and to be aware of other illnesses.

The physical examination should also be brief and directed at assessing the severity of the respiratory distress and detecting the complications of the attack. Signs associated with more severe obstruction are listed in Table 1. When present, they indicate a need for more aggressive therapy and for laboratory tests to confirm the physician's impression. A peak expiratory flow rate

TABLE 1   Acute Asthma Attacks: Signs of Severe Obstruction

Intercostal, suprasternal retractions

Sternocleidomastoid contraction

Pulsus paradoxus greater than 20 mm Hg

Obvious cyanosis

Significant agitation or lethargy

Quiet chest in an otherwise distressed patient

can be determined in most school aged children to assess obstruction and should be used to monitor the course of treatment. Arterial blood gas levels should be obtained in all children with significant respiratory distress. The more common complications of acute asthma are atelectasis, pneumomediastinum, and pneumonia; pneumothorax is uncommon. A chest x-ray examination is indicated when these conditions are suspected by findings on the physical examination or when the attack is severe or unresponsive to therapy.

Treatment is begun with beta-adrenergic agonists. Aqueous epinephrine (0.01 cc per kg) is traditional, but much better drugs and delivery systems are available. Epinephrine crystalline suspension (Susphrine, 0.005 cc per kg) or terbutaline (0.01 cc per kg) may provide considerably longer clinical effects, but tachycardia and tremor are still significant and the child still receives a painful injection.

Administration of adrenergic drugs by aerosol offers a number of advantages. Effective bronchodilation is achieved with much smaller doses of medication. Side effects are reduced, while the onset and duration of action are similar. Of even more importance to the patient, aerosol therapy does not hurt. Nebulizers should be powered by wall oxygen delivery in the emergency room to avoid occasional transient hypoxemia, but relatively inexpensive portable compressor-nebulizer units or ultrasonic nebulizers are available for office and home use (Maximyst, Mead-Johnson; Pulmonaide, Devilbiss). Older children may inhale the nebulized solution through a T tube, and an infant may be treated sitting in the mother's lap with a mask attached to the nebulizer.

The available nebulized drugs are listed in Table 2. The recommended doses listed are for adults, but these can be varied easily by mixing the listed dose in 3 ml of saline, nebulizing it constantly for 5 minutes,

TABLE 2   Aerosol Solution of Adrenergic Drugs

Preparations		Dose	Duration of Action
Isoproterenol (Isuprel)	10 mg/ml	0.1 to 0.5 ml	1 hour
Isoetharine (Bronkosol)	10 mg/ml	0.2 to 0.5 ml	1 hour
Metaproterenol (Alupent)	50 mg/ml	0.2 to 0.3 ml	4 hours
Albuterol (Proventil)	5 mg/ml	0.5 ml	4 hours
Terbutaline (Brethine)	1 mg/ml	0.5 ml	4 hours

and letting the patient's varying tidal volume automatically adjust the dose.

Up to three doses of an adrenergic agonist may be used over the first hour of therapy. However, if the wheezing does not improve significantly with the first dose, it is much less likely to improve with a second, and very unlikely to improve with a third. Thus one gives aminophylline, 7 mg per kg, as a liquid, uncoated tablet, or intravenous bolus, followed in 20 to 30 minutes by the second adrenergic agonist dose. Most children with asthma will have taken theophylline already. Their dose will rarely be adequate to produce a serum concentration greater than 10 μg per ml, but it is still appropriate to give a reduced dose of perhaps 3 to 4 mg per kg or to eliminate the dose altogether if previous serum levels have been therapeutic. If there is a question about the theophylline dosing, a blood level measurement is indicated.

When wheezing resolves and the child is discharged, one must be aware that the airway is still unstable and partially obstructed. Oral administration of a bronchodilator, such as theophylline, 20 mg per kg per day, or metaproterenol, 2 mg per kg per day, should be given daily for the next 5 to 7 days. If the response to treatment has been questionable, if an attack has recurred, or if the child was taking steroids for a long period, prednisone treatment should be given for 7 days at a dosage of approximately 0.5 mg per kg per day (20 to 40 mg in most school aged children) given as a single morning dose. A follow-up visit should be scheduled in about 2 weeks to discuss prolonged therapy.

The decision to hospitalize a child should be made if there is severe obstruction with little response to the first adrenergic dose, if improvement is not complete after 3 to 4 hours of therapy, or if one is dealing with an infant with a less than complete response. Most children suffering an attack that has recurred within 48 hours should be hospitalized.

The most important treatment offered to a child hospitalized with status asthmaticus is careful observation. Everything else—theophylline, adrenergic aerosols, corticosteroids, and even oxygen—can be given easily at home. Children with status asthmaticus (acute asthma unresponsive to outpatient therapy) are at significant risk of respiratory failure, although with today's aggressive therapy, this occurs in less than 1 percent of admissions.

To ensure adequate observation, the vital signs should be recorded hourly for the first 8 hours of hospitalization. In some hospitals this requires admission to an intensive care unit, but usually this intensive observation can be accomplished in a room close to the nursing station. Because the intensity of most attacks decreases within the first 8 hours, intensive observation can be short.

Basic laboratory studies for a child hospitalized for an acute asthma attack include a chest x-ray examination (25 percent are abnormal), arterial blood gas analysis, and peak expiratory flow rate measurement. Electrolyte

TABLE 3 Respiratory Scoring System

	0*	1	2
PaO$_2$ (mm Hg)	70–100	≤70 in room air	≤70 in 40% oxygen
Cyanosis	None	In room air	In 40% oxygen
PaCO$_2$ (mm Hg)	<40	40–65	>65
Pulsus paradoxus (mm Hg)	<10	10–40	>40
Use of accessory muscles of respiration	None	Moderate	Marked
Air exchange	Good	Fair	Poor
Mental status	Normal	Depressed or agitated	Coma

* Interpretation or respiratory scoring system: 0–4 = no immediate danger, 5–6 = impending respiratory failure, 7 or greater = respiratory failure.

levels, a complete blood count, and urinalysis should be carried out if clinically indicated. The blood count, predictably, will show granulocytosis, especially if adrenergic drugs have been given, and ketonuria and an elevated specific gravity are typically found on urinalysis.

Table 3 outlines a useful definition of respiratory failure developed by Downes. Severely ill children with impending respiratory failure should have an electrocardiographic monitor and an arterial catheter in place for repeated blood gas sampling. An anesthesiologist or critical care specialist should be consulted to help plan for support should the child progress to respiratory failure.

Therapy should continue as begun in the emergency room. Fluids should be administered intravenously, usually on the basis of an assumed mild fluid deficit; as the urine specific gravity falls, fluid therapy can be reduced. Aminophylline is administered as a 7 mg per kg bolus dose followed by a constant infusion of 1.2 mg per kg per hour. The bolus may be omitted or adjusted downward if the serum level is found to be adequate; a change of 1 mg per kg will change the peak serum level 2 μg per ml. This dose should be diluted in 50 ml of saline and administered over 20 minutes. To adjust the infusion rate, it is useful to know that a 50 percent change in infusion rate usually changes the steady state theophylline concentration by a factor of 2. The administration of aerosolized adrenergic agonists should be continued, using metaproterenol or albuterol at 2 to 4 hour intervals. Corticosteroids need not be given to every child, but any child who is steroid dependent or in impending respiratory failure should be dosed immediately (Table 3), as should any child who has not improved within 8 hours. Hydrocortisone may be given as a 7 mg per kg bolus, followed by 15 mg per kg per day, and methylprednisolone may be given as a 1 mg per kg bolus followed by a dosage of 2 mg per kg per day. Higher dosages than these have not been shown to be more effective.

Supplemental oxygen and antibiotics should be administered as indicated. Humidified oxygen, 7 liters per minute administered by nasal cannula or mask, is indicated if the Po$_2$ value is less than 70 mm Hg while breathing room air. Antibiotics are indicated for clear-cut infections but not for mild fever (which may be expected if the attack was precipitated by a cold) or for leukocytosis or pulmonary infiltrates without other signs of infection.

Currently, respiratory failure and impending failure are treated with either frequent nebulized adrenergic agonists (every 20 minutes) or with isoproterenol administered intravenously at a starting dose of 0.1 μg per kg per minute, increasing by 0.1 μg per kg per minute every 15 minutes until respiratory effort improves or until the heart rate increases beyond 200 beats per minute. A second intravenous line is maintained and electrocardiographic monitoring is required. All other intravenous medications are continued. Mechanical ventilation should be instituted if isoproterenol fails to reverse the respiratory failure.

When an attack is controlled and the patient is improving, discharge plans begin. Oral theophylline therapy is begun at a dosage extrapolated from intravenous requirements (24 hour aminophylline dose times 0.85 divided by the dosing interval for the oral preparation). Aminophylline therapy is then abruptly stopped; if a slowly absorbed theophylline is given, wait 4 hours to discontinue intravenous aminophylline therapy. Oral prednisone therapy is given as a single morning dose of 1 mg per kg per day with a planned 7 to 10 day taper. Oral adrenergic agonists are frequently started and inhaled adrenergic agonists are continued if needed using a metered dose inhaler or nebulizer. An outpatient return visit should be scheduled in 2 weeks.

LONG TERM ASTHMA MANAGEMENT

The general goals of prolonged therapy are to prevent acute attacks and daily wheezing, and to foster independent management by the child and his family. These must be specifically adapted to the child's expectations and those of the family. For instance, freedom from exercise induced wheezing has little value for a sedentary family but may be of major importance to one that is sports oriented. Goals must also be adapted to the family's intellectual and economic ability to effect the necessary changes.

The majority of children require little medical evaluation to confirm a diagnosis of asthma, especially if there is evidence of allergic disease (rhinitis, eczema, gastrointestinal food allergy) or a family history of allergy or if obstruction is obviously labile (easily induced or reversed with medication). The differential diagnosis in the wheezing child is limited but should be reviewed for all patients, especially when dealing with a wheezing infant, when there is a history of x-ray documented pneumonia, foreign body aspiration, regurgitation, or choking with meals, or when there is evidence of malabsorption, failure to thrive, or digital clubbing. All infants and any children with a suspicious history or physical examination findings should undergo chest x-ray examination and any abnormality should be evaluated further.

Multiple visits are usually needed to understand the individual pattern of the patient's asthma, with special attention to the following points:

1. Natural history: Onset of symptoms, trend of severity (most children go through a period in which asthma becomes increasingly severe).

2. Symptom pattern: Is there occasional severe obstruction with asymptomatic intervals? Are mild attacks frequent, and if so, how frequent? Is there persistent daily dyspnea?

3. Precipitants for attacks: Allergens? Colds? Sinusitis? Weather changes? Exercise? Irritants (smoke, cooking odors, pollutants, perfumes)? Emotion? Aspirin? Most children can identify multiple precipitants.

4. Previous evaluation and treatment: Toxicity and effectiveness of drugs.

5. Personal adjustment to asthma: Denial and underreporting (the "asymptomatic" child with abnormal findings on examination)? Fear of attacks?

6. Impact on the child: Hospitalization, school loss, activity, and personality limitations.

7. Socioeconomic impact on the family: Parental stability, maturity and intelligence, economic resources, and the disease's impact on these economics.

Just as much time should be spent during these visits teaching the family how to adapt to necessary changes and providing them with enough information about medication to allow some independent management. Literature is available from the Allergy and Asthma Foundation of America (Suite 303, 1302 18th Street N.W., Washington, D.C. 20336) and from the American Lung Association that is particularly useful in fostering self-management in the older child.

Rationally, precipitants should be avoided when possible. It is important to identify the most important precipitants first and then begin to work on solutions. For instance, the smoking parent should stop smoking, at least around the child. Many times exposure can be anticipated and extra medication administered.

Chronic maxillary sinusitis is not uncommon in asthmatic children as young as 2 years of age. It may worsen chest symptoms when present and symptoms have been reported to improve with antibiotic treatment. It should be suspected in any child with chronic purulent rhinitis or an unexplained exacerbation of asthma. Radiographic confirmation of the diagnosis is important, as is follow-up. Amoxicillin (30 to 40 mg per kg per day) for 2 to 3 weeks is the treatment of choice.

Allergy management is important, as over 80 percent of asthmatic children are atopic. Allergy testing should be performed using skin tests or RASTs to identify specific allergens that may be problematic. Specific recommendations for allergen avoidance should be based on a careful history as well as allergy testing, and time should be spent in developing solutions to identified problems. This may be as straightforward as wearing a mask or damp bandanna when cutting grass or as difficult as identifying and solving a mold problem in a basement or bathroom. Many families have such emotional ties to their pets that it seems that the child may be given away first; a compromise such as keeping the pet outside or in one room sometimes can help. House dust is an ubiquitous allergen and is almost impossible to eliminate, but by removing fuzzy cloth materials, including wall to wall carpet from the child's bedroom, covering the mattress, and reducing the humidity, the major dust antigen can be reduced.

Although the exact role of immunotherapy in the management of asthma remains unclear, it should be considered in any child being given continuous drug therapy. Antigens should be selected on the basis of the history and skin or RAST testing. It should be approached as a trial, and if no benefit is seen at the end of 1 year, it should be stopped.

Asthma, like many other chronic illnesses, is associated with emotional problems. Attacks may be precipitated by stress, and emotional illness, especially chronic anxiety, may make asthma difficult to treat. On the other hand, the chronic disability, the necessary restrictions, the financial drain, and the terrifying acute attacks disrupt family routines and cause severe strains on the patient and his family. A supportive sympathetic approach by the physician with an awareness of these factors is essential to manage the asthmatic child adequately. Only occasionally is formal psychotherapy needed, but it should be pursued as actively as any other aspect of therapy when indicated.

It is usually impossible to avoid precipitants thoroughly enough to have a major impact on symptoms, and drugs must be used to decrease the level of bronchial responsiveness to these precipitants. The pattern of drug use should be individualized on the basis of the patient's history. A suggested schedule is given in Table 4.

Theophylline and adrenergic agonists are currently

TABLE 4 Patterns of Chronic Asthma

Category	Description	Therapy
Intermittent	Attacks may be severe and last several days, occur no more often than once a month. Between attacks, child is asymptomatic.	Intermittent
Frequent mild	Attacks occur daily or every few days, but are usually self-limited and mild. Sometimes frequent mild coughing may be the only manifestation. Physical examination and spirometry may be slightly abnormal.	Continous low dose
Severe	Daily continuous wheezing with frequent attacks and activity limitation. Physical examination and spirometry are abnormal.	Continous high dose

the drugs of choice for long term asthma management. Theophylline is becoming less attractive because of its narrow therapeutic index and complex pharmacokinetics. Treatment is begun with 20 mg per kg per day (high dosage) or 10 mg per kg per day (low dosage). We see little reason to vary the starting dosage with age (except in infants less than 1 month old in whom it should not exceed 10 mg per kg per day), since interindividual clearance varies so widely and since the dosage ultimately must be adjusted in accordance with serum levels. Many slowly absorbed preparations are available, and the ultimate choice of a specific preparation depends on intangibles such as the availability of an appropriate dose for a given patient (for example, 200 versus 250 mg tablets) or the need to give a beaded preparation with an infant's food. The daily dosage should then be divided by the number of doses planned—never more than three times a day for slowly absorbed preparations. The patient and parent should be warned of mild toxic effects expected (personality changes, headaches, stomach aches) and told to call if these occur. The physician should be aware that severe toxic effects (usually seizures) may occur without milder toxic effects.

Serum theophylline concentrations are monitored to prevent toxic reactions, not to improve disease control; a child on low dose therapy with an adequate symptomatic control does not need monitoring. Serum

levels are indicated in the following situations: always with high dose therapy to avoid dangerously high but asymptomatic levels; sometimes when toxic symptoms appear, but usually the dose can simply be reduced without assessing the blood level; and sometimes when compliance is in question. In our laboratory, salivary levels correlate closely with serum levels and are usually used for monitoring outpatients. We obtain specimens at the time of expected peak concentrations, that is, 6 hours after a slowly absorbed dose or 1 hour after a rapidly absorbed dose. In outpatients, we try to maintain levels less than 15 μg per ml so that toxic effects are less likely to occur during the stress of a febrile illness or during erythromycin therapy.

Beta-adrenergic agonists are rapidly assuming a therapeutic role equal to theophylline. They may be substituted when theophylline side effects appear with low doses or low serum levels (about 10 percent of the cases) or when infants will not tolerate the bitter taste of theophylline. They are added to theophylline for acute attacks or when control of daily symptoms cannot be gained with theophylline alone. Their major disadvantages are their rapid pharmacokinetics and the lack of serum assays to monitor compliance.

Currently available preparations are listed in Tables 2 and 5. Side effects include tremor, tachycardia, and occasional central nervous system effects (either sedation or excitation). We treat with aerosolized preparations whenever possible for the same reasons mentioned before. Aerosolized solutions may be delivered at home by a compressor-nebulizer unit (Maximyst, Pulmonaide) or by a freon powered metered dose inhaler. The metered dose inhaler is a convenient alternative but must be used with precautions against overuse. As a rule, we give no more than two refills of the metered dose inhaler and do not give them at all to patients with questionable compliance. Toddlers can use them effectively with the aid of a reservoir (Aerochamber, Inhal-Aid, Inspirease), which eliminates the need to coordinate inspiration with the metered dose inhaler jet.

In children who require a second bronchodilator on a regular basis, a trial of cromolyn is indicated. The major disadvantages are its cost, ineffectiveness as a bronchodilator, and the significant numbers of patients whose asthma is not affected at all. Initially the unusual delivery system (Spinhaler) also limited its usefulness, but nebulizable solutions and a metered dose inhaler are

TABLE 5 Beta-adrenergic Agonists for Long Term Management

	Tablets	Liquid	Dose
Oral			
Metaproterenol	10, 20 mg	10 mg/tsp	2–4 mg/kg/day
Terbutaline	2.5, 5 mg	NA	0.3–0.4 mg/kg/day
Albuterol	2, 4 mg	2 mg/tsp	0.3–0.4 mg/kg/day
Metered dose inhaler			
Metaproterenol	0.65 mg/puff		1–2 puffs qid
Terbutaline	0.20 mg/puff		1–2 puffs qid
Albuterol	0.09 mg/puff		1–2 puffs qid

now available. The major reason for including it in our regimen is that approximately one in every three or four patients responds dramatically to the drug.

Although corticosteroid therapy traditionally has been reserved only for children with the most severe disease, the use of inhaled steroids has significantly increased in recent years because of their low incidence of side effects. Before initiating any steroid therapy, bronchodilators should be used in maximally tolerated doses, chronic sinus infection should be excluded, and allergen management should be optimal. The child's parents and the older child should be aware of the subtle side effects and how to avoid them, and they should be apprised of the physician's plan for using the drug. In general, we have three plans for steroid use:

1. When acute attacks have been poorly controlled, we give a dosage of 0.5 to 1.0 mg per kg of prednisone, in four doses on the first day, a single morning dose on the second day, and then on a rapidly tapering single daily dose for the next 7 days.

2. We may treat for several months with inhaled steroids or with prednisone, 10 to 20 mg every other day, to control symptoms in a pollen season or to try to gain symptomatic control.

3. Finally, a small proportion of patients with continually abnormal pulmonary function test or physical examination results despite high dose bronchodilator therapy require supplemental steroids for long periods. This can usually be accomplished with an inhaled agent such as beclomethasone (100 to 200 μg four times daily). Some patients cannot be treated successfully, such as the infant who is not well enough coordinated to inhale the drug and the older child who refuses to take the drug at school. The reservoirs mentioned earlier are helpful with some toddlers to be dosed with parents' help. If compliance is in question, the child may be

TABLE 6   Contingency Plan for Home Treatment

Begin treatment early in attack.
Notify physician if a step fails or if step 3 is required.
  Step 1
    Theophylline—increase dose or add extra dose of
                  short acting preparation
  Step 2
    Add adrenergic drug
    Oral: metaproterenol 0.5–1 mg/kg qid
          or albuterol   0.075 mg/kg qid
    or inhaled (see Tables 2 and 5)
  Step 3
    Add prednisone, 0.5 mg/kg/day for 7 days

better treated with a supervised morning dose of prednisone. Any child taking long term corticosteroid therapy should be seen semiannually to re-evaluate growth and to reassess the steroid dosage. An ophthalmologic examination and a morning serum cortisol level should be included annually for all children taking systemic steroid therapy.

Finally, families need to be given contingency plans for initiating treatment at home for acute attacks. One such plan is given in Table 6.

SUGGESTED READING

Newhouse MT, Dolovich MB. Current concepts: control of asthma by aerosols. N Eng J Med 1986; 315:870.
Rachelefsky GS, Siegel SC. Asthma in infants and children; treatment of childhood asthma. J Allergy Clin Immunol 1985; 76:409–425.
Seigel SC. Adrenal corticosteroids in the treatment of asthma. Clin Rev in Allergy 1983; 1:123.
Szefler SJ. Practical considerations in the safe and effective use of theophylline. Pediatr Clin North Am 1983; 30:943–954.

ASPIRIN SENSITIVITY IN RHINOSINUSITIS AND ASTHMA

GUY A. SETTIPANE, M.D.

The triad of aspirin intolerance, asthma, and nasal polyps frequently is associated with severe nonallergic steroid dependent asthma, usually found in adults. This type of asthma involves the bronchospastic type of aspirin intolerance, not the urticaria-angioedema type. In many cases only two parts of the triad are present, asthma and aspirin intolerance, which usually occur within 1 year of each other. Nasal polyps frequently occur about 10 years later. The mean age at onset of the asthma and aspirin intolerance parts of the triad is about 31 years. However, the cumulative frequency increases with age so that in patients over 40 years old, the frequency is over 6 percent.

The characteristics of this triad are listed in Table 1. The important features are the familial occurrence, the marked eosinophilia, the pathogenic mechanism involving arachidonic metabolism, and the frequent association with chronic sinusitis. Symptoms of aspirin intolerance may begin with severe rhinorrhea followed by acute bronchospasm. Occasionally, both the broncho-

TABLE 1 Characteristics of the Bronchospastic Type of Aspirin Intolerance

Found in asthmatic patients

Correlated with nasal polyposis and chronic sinusitis

Similar age onset as asthma

Severe rhinorrhea with aspirin reactions

Increased frequency in older age groups

Familial occurrence

Eosinophils in nasal smear

Elevated total (blood) eosinophil count

NSAID cross reaction

No specific IgE (antiaspiryl)

Normal total IgE

Desensitization possible to aspirin

Pathogenic mechanism: prostaglandins

TABLE 3 Nonsteroidal Anti-inflammatory Drugs

Cyclo-Oxygenase Inhibitors

Aminophenazone	Indomethacin
Aspirin	Mefenamic acid
Benzydamine	Naproxen
Diftalone	Nictindole
Ditazole	Noramidopyrine
Fenoprofen	Piroxicam
Flumizole	Sulindac
Ibuprofen	Tolmetin

spastic and urticarial types of aspirin intolerance may occur in the same patient. The pathogenesis of the urticarial type is unknown, but it is not thought to be associated with an IgE mechanism. The frequencies of aspirin intolerance in various medical conditions are listed in Table 2.

TREATMENT

The most important treatment for aspirin intolerance is avoidance of aspirin or aspirin-like drugs. Nonsteroidal anti-inflammatory drugs cross react with aspirin in aspirin intolerant patients (Table 3). These drugs are inhibitors of the cyclo-oxygenase pathway of arachidonic metabolism. This inhibition may result in a preference for the lipo-oxygenase pathway, resulting in increased production of leukotrienes LTC4, LTD4, and LTE4 (SRS-A), which produce bronchospasm. Also a decrease in prostaglandin E occurs, and this allows the

TABLE 2 Frequency of Aspirin Intolerance in Various Conditions

Type of Population	Frequency of Aspirin Intolerance (%)
Chronic urticaria	23–28
Nasal polyps	14–23
Asthma	4–19
Rhinitis	≃1.4
Normal	≃0.3

Note: The low frequencies are associated with studies in which the data were obtained by history alone, whereas the higher frequencies are associated with aspirin challenge studies.

bronchospastic effects of PGF and leukotrienes to predominate. A similar mechanism involving arachidonic acid and prostaglandins in the formation of nasal polyps has not been defined at this time.

The cyclo-oxygenase inhibitors listed in Table 3 cross react with aspirin in intolerant patients practically 100 percent of the time. Nonacetylated salicylates usually do not cause adverse reactions similar to those of aspirin in intolerant individuals. However, an occasional isolated case report has noted a cross reactivity resulting in adverse reactions. There are hundreds of over the counter drugs that contain aspirin, and sensitive patients should be familiar with them.

Some noncyclo-oxygenase inhibitors such as acetominophen and the yellow dye tartrazine occasionally have been reported to cross react with aspirin in intolerant individuals.

Acute reactions after the accidental ingestion of aspirin or nonsteroidal anti-inflammatory drugs usually constitute a medical emergency. These reactions may begin with severe rhinorrhea followed rapidly by acute bronchospasm and even shock; an occasional patient may have acute urticarial angioedema with or without respiratory distress. These severe reactions should be treated promptly with epinephrine 1/1000, 0.1 to 0.5 ml, which could be repeated in 30 to 60 minutes. Less severe reactions may be treated with aerosolized beta-agonists such as albuterol or metaproterenol in repeated doses. If symptoms persist, aminophyllin in intravenous doses sufficient to achieve or maintain therapeutic blood levels may be used. Cyanosis should be treated immediately with oxygen (2 to 5 liters per minute via nasal catheter or 34 percent by Venturi mask). Hypotension should be treated with intravenous fluid administration, volume expanders, dopamine hydrochloride, or norepinephrine bitartrate. In prolonged reactions the intravenous administration of methylprednisolone, 125 mg, or Solu-Cortef, 100 to 200 mg, may prevent status asthmaticus.

The treatment of asthma in aspirin intolerant patients frequently requires corticosteroids for the control of respiratory symptoms. Otherwise, the standard form of asthmatic treatment consisting of oral doses of theophylline and aerosolized beta-agonist mediation should be initiated.

Since these patients frequently have associated chronic sinusitis or nasal polyps, treatment also should be directed to the upper airway. Through the rhinosinobronchial reflex, acute or chronic sinusitis and nasal polyps can aggravate asthma, and successful treatment of the upper airway disease may decrease the asthma. Sinusitis should be treated vigorously with antibiotics and oral and nasal administration of decongestants.

The usual infections found in sinusitis result from *Haemophilus influenzae* and *Streptococcus pneumoniae,* and these respond well to amoxicillin, 500 mg three times daily. Antibiotic treatment should be given for at least 2 weeks. Erythromycin and sulfur preparations may be used in selected patients. In patients in whom infection persists, surgical treatment of sinusitis may be necessary. Successful control of the sinus condition frequently results in a decrease in asthma; this is manifested by a decrease in the maintenance steroid dose necessary in steroid dependent asthma.

Medical and surgical polypectomy also may result in a decrease in symptoms of asthma. Shrinking or removal of nasal polyps may decrease the bronchospastic stimulation effect of the rhinosinobronchial reflex. Despite medical or surgical treatment, nasal polyps frequently recur. The recurrence incidence after surgical polypectomy is about 40 percent. Surgical polypectomy does not aggravate or precipitate asthma. In a series of patients whom we studied there was no change in pulmonary function test results and methacholine challenges before and after polypectomy. We did report a decrease in the steroid requirement within 6 months following polypectomy.

At present I believe that the treatment of choice is a 10 day course of systemic corticosteroid therapy beginning with 50 mg of prednisone orally. This short burst of corticosteroids should not produce a clinically significant suppression of the pituitary-adrenal axis. Afterward the patient may be maintained on topical beclomethasone or flunisolide therapy, realizing that long term topical use of these medications may result in suppression of the pituitary-adrenal axis. Such new products as topically applied fluocortin butyl may help to avoid these complications, since this steroid has not been found to have a significant pituitary-adrenal effect. The drug is still undergoing clinical investigation and has not yet been released to the practicing physician in the United States.

Steroid injection of nasal polyps has been used with some success by expert otolaryngologists. However, injection of steroids into the nasal turbinates and polyps has resulted in 10 instances of vision loss, five of which were permanent as of 1981. Steroid emboli were demonstrated in the retinal vessels in six cases. This type of treatment for nasal polyps should be reserved for use by the very skilled otolaryngologist, if used at all.

Even with systemic and topical corticosteroid therapy, nasal polyps frequently may recur, and periodic bursts of systemic corticosteroid therapy may have to be administered. When systemic corticosteroid treatment has no effect or is contraindicated, surgical polypectomy may be done.

Patients with nasal polyps deserve an allergy evaluation even though a large percentage are nonatopic. If clinically relevant IgE mediated disease is found, a course of hyposensitization may be given, especially in those with recurrent polyposis. IgE mediated disease is not the cause of nasal polyps, but it may contribute to episodes or exacerbation.

In patients with nasal polyps and no history of aspirin intolerance, other diseases should be ruled out, such as cystic fibrosis (those who are 16 years old or younger), Kartagener's syndrome (bronchiectasis, chronic sinusitis, and, frequently, situs inversus) and Young's syndrome (sinopulmonary disease, azoospermia, and nasal polyps).

Desensitization with aspirin to decrease asthma and sinusitis has not been satisfactory. Selected patients with aspirin intolerance and resistant arthritis may be candidates for desensitization. These arthritic symptoms should be severe enough to warrant the inherent risk associated with desensitization procedures, as outlined by Stevenson and his colleagues. Desensitization is initiated immediately following aspirin challenge studies. The 1 day challenge procedure is useful when aspirin sensitivity is not suspected and the patient has limited time (Table 4).

The usual procedure in the patient with a history of aspirin intolerance is the 3 day aspirin challenge (Table 5). It is important to remember that one must start with a 3 mg aspirin dose in patients with a history of severe reactions. If aspirin is continued over the ensuing days, the patient will continue to be desensitized to aspirin. However, in certain patients the aspirin reaction may again break through even though the desensitized patient is taking aspirin daily. The refractory period after a positive aspirin challenge usually is 2 to 4 days if aspirin administration is not maintained daily. Desensitization to aspirin also desensitizes the patient to

TABLE 4   One Day ASA Challenge*

Time	ASA Dosage (mg)	Cumulative Dosage (mg)
8 AM	30	30
10 AM	60	90
12 AM	100	190
2 PM	325	515
4 PM	650	1,165
6 PM	End†	

*From Stevenson DD. Oral challenge: aspirin, NSAID, tartrazine and sulfites. NER Allergy Proc 1984; 5:111–118.

†If a reaction does not occur, patient is not ASA sensitive. If FEV$_1$ ↓ ≥25%, then 7 or >days later carry out placebo challenge to confirm specificity. One day challenge is useful when ASA sensitivity is not suspected and patient has a limited time.

SUGGESTED READING

Mabry RL. Visual loss after intranasal corticosteroid injection. Arch Otolaryngol 1981; 107:484–486.

Samter M, Beers RF Jr. Intolerance to aspirin: clinical studies and considerations of its pathogenesis. Ann Intern Med 1968; 68:975–983.

Settipane GA. Asthma, aspirin intolerance and nasal polyps. In: Settipane GA, ed. Current treatment of ambulatory asthma. NER Allergy Proceedings, Providence, Rhode Island, 1986: 136–141.

Settipane GA. Nasal polyps. In: Settipane GA, ed. Rhinitis. NER Allergy Proceedings, Providence, Rhode Island, 1984: 133–140.

Settipane GA, Klein DE, Lekas MD. Asthma and nasal polyps. In: Myers E, ed. New dimensions in otorhinolaryngology. Head and Neck Surgery. Amsterdam: Excerpta Medica, 1985: 499.

Stevenson DD, Pleskow WW, Simon RA, Mathison DA, Lumry WR, Schatz M, Zieger RS. Aspirin sensitive rhino-sinusitis asthma: a double-blind crossover study of treatment with aspirin. J Allergy Clin Immunol 1984; 73:500–507.

Stevenson DD. Oral challenge: aspirin, NSAID, tartrazine and sulfites. NER Allergy Proc 1984; 5:111–118.

Table 5   Three Day ASA Challenge*

Time	Days		
	1	*2*	*3*
8 AM	placebo	ASA 30(3) mg	ASA 150 mg
11 AM	placebo	ASA 60 mg	ASA 325 mg
2 PM	placebo	ASA 100 mg	ASA 650 mg

*From Stevenson DD. Oral challenge: aspirin, NSAID, tartrazine and sulfites. NER Allergy Proc 1984; 5:111–118.
1. Discontinue antihistamines; cromolyn and sympathomimetics.
2. Increase corticosteroids for 3 days prior to challenge to produce FEV $>$ 70% or a value of 1.5 liters per minute.
3. History of severe reactions: start challenge at 3 mg ASA (20% of time).

other nonsteroidal anti-inflammatory drugs. Presently the use of nonacetylated salicylic acid in desensitizing procedures is being investigated.

EXERCISE INDUCED ASTHMA, URTICARIA, AND ANAPHYLAXIS

EUGENE R. BLEECKER, M.D.

This article deals with the treatment of exercise induced asthma as well as two less common forms of physical allergy: exercise induced anaphylaxis and urticaria. A brief review of the pathophysiology of each is presented to serve as a basis for the development of a rational approach to the management of these disorders. Because of recent emphasis on health and physical fitness, the incidence of these exercise related syndromes has increased and they have received renewed attention by the medical community. Thus, our understanding of their diagnosis, pathogenesis, and treatment has improved.

EXERCISE INDUCED ASTHMA

A common and important trigger for bronchial asthma is physical exertion. Exercise induced bronchospasm is characterized by decreases in expiratory flow rates and increases in airway resistance that are often associated with pulmonary hyperinflation. An asthmatic complains of dyspnea and cough, usually accompanied by audible wheezing, 5 to 10 minutes after beginning strenuous exercise. Exercise induced asthma occurs in 70 to 80 percent of asthmatics when appropriately stressed, and it is an example of the generalized increase in nonspecific airway reactivity that is characteristic of this disease. Patients with severe asthma or adults with chronic obstructive lung disease often avoid the levels of physical activity that would trigger this response. However, in individuals with mild asthma, especially children and young adults, this phenomenon may be the primary clinical manifestation of the disease.

When a specific diagnosis of exercise induced asthma cannot be made by evaluating clinical symptoms, standardized laboratory challenge procedures are available to test for the presence and assess the severity of this disorder. Thus, exercise induced asthma represents an important symptom complex that may be a major disabling manifestation of asthma or an unrecognized cause of exercise induced dyspnea.

The initial stimuli for exercise induced asthma appear to be drying and cooling of the respiratory tract by the high levels of ventilation produced by strenuous exercise. Although the precise mechanisms by which these changes cause bronchospasm are unknown, it has been hypothesized that changes in airway surface fluid osmolarity and respiratory heat exchange could trigger air flow obstruction by one or more of the following mechanisms: the release of mediators of immediate hypersensitivity, alterations in airway epithelial permeability, activation of autonomic neural reflex pathways, or changes in bronchial blood flow. Knowledge of these potential mechanisms and the important role of airway surface water and heat loss explains some of the questions that have existed about the pathogenesis of exercise induced asthma and provides a basis for its management.

For example, activities such as swimming in a warm humid environment would be less likely to produce bronchospasm than cross country skiing or jogging outdoors in cold, dry winter conditions. Breathing through the nose or a mask would tend to humidify and warm inspired air more than mouth breathing and therefore be less asthmagenic. Also brief periods of exercise lasting 1 to 2 minutes, even if vigorous and intense, produce little change in respiratory function, whereas exercising for more than 6 to 10 minutes does not seem to increase the severity of exercise induced bronchospasm. In fact, some asthmatic patients with mild disease are able to prevent the development of bronchospasm by continuing to exercise, e.g., ''run through their asthma.'' This finding as well as the development of mild transient bronchodilation during exercise may be the result of systemic release of catecholamines and the effects of sympathetic stimulation on bronchial smooth muscle tone.

The primary strategies in the management of exercise induced bronchospasm are to prevent its development or to reduce the severity of postexertional bronchospasm to levels that will not produce symptoms or adversely affect exercise capacity. This can be accomplished by modifying the activity that triggers air flow obstruction and by treatment with appropriate pharmacologic agents. Asthmatics should not be told to avoid exercise, since this approach may be especially difficult and is usually unnecessary. In addition, therapy is effective, and even small reductions in postexertional bronchospasm may significantly lessen the impact of this condition on the maintenance of a normal life style.

A brief warm-up period at submaximal exercise levels should be included before beginning strenuous exercise. Activities should be selected that do not require prolonged maximal exertion in cold, dry environmental conditions. An asthmatic may be able to perform outdoor activities in the summer such as jogging, but during the winter one may need to substitute swimming or other indoor sports. If these activities cannot be avoided, attempting to humidify and warm inspired air by breathing through the nose, placing a scarf over the mouth and nose, or wearing a cold weather mask may be helpful. In addition, asthmatics should avoid exercise under conditions in which they may be exposed to airborne pollutants, such as ozone and sulfur or nitrogen dioxide. These exposures may increase airway reactivity and worsen postexertional bronchospasm.

Although reducing the magnitude of the stimulus for exercise induced asthma is important, the major approach in its management is the use of pharmacologic agents to prevent or diminish the severity of postexertional bronchospasm. One should realize that even a moderate reduction in the bronchospastic response can be important, since asthmatics with relatively normal baseline pulmonary function usually do not become symptomatic until the forced expiratory volume in 1 second (FEV_1) falls by more than 20 percent.

The preferred pharmacologic approach for the treamtent of exercise induced asthma is therapy with inhaled beta-sympathomimetic drugs or cromolyn. When these drugs are administered locally as aerosols to the respiratory tract, both partially or completely prevent the development of postexertional bronchospasm with virtually no systemic side effects. $Beta_2$-sympathomimetic drugs alter exercise induced asthma either by producing bronchodilation that overcomes the bronchoconstrictor effects of exercise or by other actions, such as preventing the release of inflammatory mediators in the lungs. In fact, inhibition of exercise induced asthma can be partially separated from the bronchodilator effects of beta agonists.

The most effective agents in this class of drugs appear to be albuterol and fenoterol, which can prevent exercise induced asthma for several hours; other sympathomimetics such as terbutaline and metaproterenol have a shorter duration of activity. These drugs have a rapid onset of action, and inhalation therapy should be administered 15 to 30 minutes prior to exercise. It can be repeated 1 to 2 hours later if necessary, but overdosage should be avoided. Regular treatment with these drugs should be employed for the overall management of an individual's asthma, but it is not necessary for the treatment of exercise induced bronchospasm that is the only manifestation of asthma.

Cromolyn is not a bronchodilator, and its mechanism of action may be related to its capacity to stabilize mast cells or basophils, thereby preventing mediator release, or to the proposed effects of this drug on autonomic neural reflex pathways. Cromolyn is an inhaled powder that is now available in a metered dose inhaler as well as in other less convenient preparations: dry powder (spinhaler) and wet aerosal (nebulizer). Cromolyn as well as drugs with similar pharmacologic activities such as nedocromil effectively protect most asthmatics from postexertional asthma. This prophylactic drug should be inhaled 30 to 60 minutes prior to exercise: the dose can be increased from two puffs to higher doses of four to six puffs if indicated. Its efficacy may be improved by use on a regular basis. Atlhough less potent than beta-sympathomimetics such as albuterol, cromolyn is often employed as a first line drug for the treatment of individuals with symptomatic exercise induced bronchospasm. This is especially true in situations in which an asthmatic is receiving regular therapy with inhaled beta agonists and increasing the dosage of this drug may be undesirable. In addition, combination therapy with cromolyn and a beta sympathomimetic drug appears to be more effective than either drug administered alone.

Although other bronchodilators such as theophylline and sympathomimetics administered orally can provide protection for exercise induced asthma, they are less potent than inhaled beta agonists. In addition, they can produce unwanted systemic side effects such as tachycardia, skeletal muscle tremor, gastrointestinal complaints, and anxiety. It also may be difficult to synchronize their peak effects with the onset of exercise. Thus, these drugs should be reserved for the treatment of underlying asthma or for use when an individual is unable to effectively use a metered dose inhaler. When there are difficulties with the administration of inhaled medications from a metered dose inhaler, a spacer should be tried before switching to medications administered orally. Ipratropium, an inhaled anticholinergic bronchodilator, can reduce exercise induced bronchospasm in some asthmatics. In this disorder it should be reserved for use as an adjunct to other medications rather than as a first line therapeutic agent. Inhaled or oral corticosteroid therapy does not effect exercise induced asthma when administered immediately before exercise. However, inhaled corticosteroids and perhaps cromolyn as part of long-term maintenance therapy may decrease asthmatic airway hyperreactivity and thus reduce the bronchospastic response to exercise.

For the prevention of exercise induced asthma in competitive athletes, an adequate range of bronchodilators is permitted by organizations such as the Olympic Committee. Albuterol, terbutaline, fenoterol, cromolyn, theophylline, and corticosteroids can be used, but nonselective beta$_2$-sympathomimetic drugs (epinephrine, ephedrine, isoproterenol, metaproterenol) are banned from use in competition. Specific rules should be checked, but usually the team physician and the sponsoring organization may need to be notified about the use of these medications by an athlete.

Since exercise induced asthma is a manifestation of asthmatic airway hyperreactivity, its management must be modified by changes that occur in the natural course of the underlying disease. For example, increases in bronchial reactivity may occur during an upper respiratory infection or after exposure to an allergen or environmental pollutants. These changes make asthmatics transiently more sensitive to exercise. Thus, individuals with asthma may have to avoid some forms of exercise in these situations, and the treatment of exercise induced bronchospasm must be integrated with the overall management of the underlying asthmatic condition.

EXERCISE INDUCED ANAPHYLAXIS

The rare syndrome of exercise induced anaphylaxis appears to be distinct from exercise induced asthma and exercise induced cholinergic urticaria. It occurs during or after strenuous exercise and often can be reproduced in the experimental laboratory. Exercise induced anaphylaxis is characterized by prodromal symptoms, which include the development of fatigue, itching, and erythema, which often precede urticaria, angioedema, choking, and upper airway obstruction as well as vas-

cular collapse and shock. This anaphylactic syndrome resembles mild systemic anaphylaxis produced by antigen exposure in a susceptible individual. Frequently there is either a personal allergy history or a family history of allergic disorders. It differs from cholinergic urticaria by the failure to develop an attack when there is an increase in body temperature and by the presence of circulatory shock. During these episodes increased serum levels of histamine have been found in individuals with positive exercise challenges; nonresponders do not exhibit elevations of plasma histamine levels. These attacks usually occur only after exercise and not in response to other physical stimuli. One or several episodes may recur yearly in an individual. The fact that this syndrome is not always associated with every episode of exercise indicates that other factors, including temperature and the relationship to ingestion of specific foods, may influence its development.

When exercise induced anaphylaxis occurs, management is directed toward the treatment of symptoms and is in general similar to the therapy of systemic anaphylaxis. Vascular collapse may require intensive therapy in a hospital or similar environment. Shock should be treated initially with epinephrine and fluid replacement, and urticaria, pruritus, and edema may be relieved by the administration of antihistamines. Bronchospasm should be reversed by the administration of bronchodilators, including inhaled beta sympathomimetic agonists and theophylline. Upper airway obstruction is almost never life threatening, but if significant occlusion of the upper airway occurs, emergency intubation or tracheostomy might be necessary. Since this rare syndrome occurs sporadically in the same individual, adequate prophylactic treatment is not well established, but strenuous activities may need to be limited and exercise should be stopped with the onset of prodromal symptoms. In addition, exercise should not be performed in hot, humid conditions or within 2 to 4 hours after food ingestion. Whenever an individual at risk for this disorder continues to exercise, he should be accompanied by someone with knowledge of its emergency management. Commercially available self-treatment kits are manufactured for the treatment of systemic anaphylaxis. These kits, which contain syringes preloaded with epinephrine (ANA-KIT, Hollister-Steir, or EpiPen, Center Laboratories), may be helpful in the emergency management of exercise induced anaphylaxis.

EXERCISE INDUCED URTICARIA

Cholinergic urticaria may develop after exercise, especially in warm or hot environmental conditions. In susceptible individuals exercise produces a pruritic erythematous rash consisting of small wheals, which may become confluent and edematous. This rash initially appears on the neck and thorax but may spread and become generalized over the entire body. Occasionally it is accompanied by other signs of cholinergic stimulation and by bronchospasm that resembles exercise induced asthma. It can be reproduced in some susceptible individuals by the intradermal injection of methacholine and in most by exercise challenge in a warm environment. Exercise induced urticaria may be initiated by the systemic release of histamine, and it appears to be associated with increased or hyperreactive cholinergic receptors in the skin that reflexly produce hives. Management consists of therapy with an antihistamine. For example, hydroxyzine (50 to 100 mg), taken four times daily or 30 to 60 minutes prior to exercise, usually prevents the development of exercise urticaria. Occasionally combinations of H_1 and H_2 antihistamines may be necessary. Associated bronchospasm can be prevented or treated with inhaled sympathomimetic drugs similar to the management of exercise induced asthma.

SUGGESTED READING

Anderson SD. Exercise-induced asthma. Chest 1985; 87S:191S–195S.
Anderson S, Seale JP, Ferris L, Schoeffel R, Lindsay DA. An evaluation of pharmacotherapy for exercise-induced asthma. J Allergy Clin Immunol 1979; 64:612–624.
Bleecker ER. Exercise-induced asthma—physiologic and clinical considerations. Clin Chest Med 1984; 5:109–119.
Kaplan AP. Exercise-induced hives. J Allergy Clin Immunol 1984; 73:704–707.
McFadden ER Jr. Respiratory heat and water exchange: physiological and clinical implications. J Appl Physiol 1983; 54:331–336.
Sheffer AL, Soter NA, McFadden ER, Austen KF. Exercise-induced anaphylaxis: a distinct form of physical allergy. J Allergy Clin Immunol 1983; 71:311–316.

SULFITE INDUCED ASTHMA

DAVID H. ALLEN, M.B., Ph.D, F.R.A.C.P.

For centuries sulfites have been used as preservatives in food and beverage processing and more recently as antioxidants in pharmaceutical solutions. Sulfites are added to foods or beverages as sodium or potassium metabisulfite or bisulfite or as gaseous sulfur dioxide. These preserved products are acidic, and the equilibrium reached in solution tends toward the formation of bisulfite and the liberation of gaseous sulfur dioxide. Up to 5 ppm of sulfur dioxide is present in the headspace gas above sulfited foods and beverages. When inhaled, sulfur dioxide gas is a potent bronchoconstrictor in asthmatic individuals.

Asthmatic reactions to the ingestion of sulfite containing foods and beverages are usually rapid, frequently occurring within 1 to 2 minutes after ingestion. The reactions can be best reproduced in the laboratory by ingestion of an acidified solution of metabisulfite. Extensive studies in our laboratory indicate that inhalation of sulfur dioxide during ingestion of a sulfite containing food or beverage is the most likely mechanism causing sulfite induced asthma. A number of factors, including the concentration of sulfite as well as the temperature and pH of the food or beverage, will modify the amount of sulfur dioxide liberated. The amount of sulfur dioxide inhaled by an asthmatic individual is further influenced by the route of inhalation, the nose removing more from inhaled air than the mouth. In addition the adequacy of asthma control at the time of sulfite ingestion affects the response. The mechanism of sulfite capsule induced asthma is probably eructation and inhalation of sulfur dioxide gas generated in the acid stomach. Absorbed sulfite is rapidly metabolized in the body to sulfate. There is no circulating sulfite level.

The diagnosis of sulfite induced asthma is best made by obtaining a detailed history of the event, attempting to identify a sulfited food or beverage provoking the rapid onset of asthma. This clinical diagnosis should be confirmed by a challenge with an acidified sulfite solution. Our challenge protocol is shown in Table 1. Asthmatic reactions to sulfite containing medications have been reported. Nonasthmatic reactions such as angioedema and anaphylaxis occur rarely.

THERAPEUTIC ALTERNATIVES

Optimal therapy of sulfite induced asthma requires a unique mixture of improved public health measures, declaration and decreased use of sulfites by industry together with comprehensive dietary chemical information for patients, as well as rapid treatment of acute attacks with appropriate sulfite free medications.

Public Health Aspects

Sulfite induced asthma is a significant public health problem. It was first reported in 1981 in North America. At that time sulfites were on the Food and Drug Administration's (FDA) generally regarded as safe (GRAS) list

TABLE 1 Sulfite Challenge Protocol

Preliminaries

1. No inhaled bronchodilators for 4 hours before test
2. Procedure explained to patient
3. Determine potential patient reactivity as follows:

Potential Reactivity

	Mild	Moderate	Severe	Very Severe
Sulfite history	Negative	Mild reaction	Severe reaction Hospital admission	Life threatening reaction

4. Challenges are not performed when FEV_1 is 70% of predicted value or below
5. Challenge doses are administered at 10 minute intervals with FEV_1 measured every 2 minutes; a positive response is a greater than 20% fall from the baseline level
6. Sulfite dissolved freshly in 30 ml of 0.5% W/V citric acid

	Mild	Moderate	Severe	Very Severe
Dose 1	Citric acid	Citric acid	Citric acid	Citric acid
2	25 mg	20	5	5
3	50 mg	25	25	10
4	—	50	50	25

Reverse challenge with nebulized sulfite-free beta agonist. A positive open challenge may be repeated after 24 hours.

and were widely used with minimal restriction in food and beverage processing. When the medical profession became aware of sulfite induced asthmatic reactions and advised patients to avoid sulfited foods, patients encountered problems in identifying sulfite containing foods because manufacturers were not required to indicate on labels the presence of sulfites. Furthermore sulfites were frequently used in restaurants on fresh foods, such as salads, to prevent browning. Thus, although it was possible to identify sulfite sensitive individuals, it was difficult to avoid sulfited foods.

Responding to evidence of the adverse effects of sulfites in some asthmatic individuals, the FDA recently has altered its regulations on sulfites. The use of sulfites is now forbidden on fruits and vegetables intended to be served raw or sold raw to customers or on those to be presented as fresh. In addition the FDA requires that all packaged foods and alcoholic beverages containing 10 ppm or more of sulfite be labeled to disclose the presence of the sulfiting agent. Similarly industry has responded to consumer and professional demands by using less sulfite. For example, the fruit juice industry has turned from sulfites to pasteurization and aseptic packaging, and some wine makers are now producing special sulfite free wines. A physician's management of sulfite induced asthma includes seeking out sulfite free products for his patients and pressuring both manufac-

turers to minimize the use of sulfite and local regulatory bodies to properly control its use.

Educating Patients to Identify Foods Likely to Contain Sulfite

In order to minimize reactions to sulfite containing foods, patients who have experienced sulfite induced asthmatic reactions should be given detailed lists of sulfite containing foods and beverages. Foods likely to provoke asthma are listed in Table 2. Physicians should develop a list appropriate to their locality.

Test strips are available to detect the presence of sulfites on fresh foods such as salads. Wines are a special problem because of the variable amount of sulfite present and the large number of factors that can influence the provoking dose of sulfur dioxide at the point of ingestion. For example, sweet white wines tend to contain more sulfite than dry whites or red wines, and if the wine is opened just before drinking, and particularly if the glass is warmed in the hand, the amount of sulfur dioxide generated will tend to be greater. Patients can prevent sulfite induced reactions to the ingestion of sulfited wines by allowing the wine to stand for at least 1 hour after opening and by minimizing the amount of sipping and thus inhalation of sulfur dioxide at the time of ingestion. The amount of sulfite in beer is low and unlikely to provoke asthma.

Medications

Preventative Medications

Blocking studies in sulfite sensitive asthma indicate that a variety of medications, including cromolyn, atro-

TABLE 2 Sulfited Foods and Beverages Likely to Provoke Asthmatic Reactions

In food purchased in grocery store

    Dried tree fruits
    Pickles, especially pickled onions
    Wines, especially sweet white wine and cider
    Dried vegetables
    Potato products—mashed potato, french fries, chips (at times)
    Chilled fruit juices
    Sausages (and other meats; check local regulations)

In restaurants*

    Fresh green salad
    Fresh fruit salad
    Seafood—fresh prawns
    Wine
    Guacamole

*The FDA has recommended a ban on the addition of sulfites to fresh foods in the United States.

pine, and zaditen (Ketotifen), effectively block sulfite induced asthma. In addition a beta-agonist inhaled immediately prior to a sulfite challenge will block. Premedication with an inhaled beta-agonist should be recommended for sulfite sensitive individuals when the concentration of sulfite in a particular food or beverage is unknown.

Treatment of Sulfite Induced Reactions

Immediate inhalation of a beta-agonist bronchodilator from a metered dose inhaler usually reverses a mild sulfite induced reaction. However, if the reaction is severe, with a marked reduction in expiratory flow rates, inhaled medications will be less effective. Parenteral beta-agonist therapy therefore may be required. Epinephrine injection, which may contain sulfite, is an inappropriate form of therapy.

Sulfite Containing Medications

Some bronchodilator solutions, including Bronkosol, isoetharine, and Isuprel, contain sulfites. Sulfite containing preparations for parenteral use include Decadron, hydrocortone injection, and epinephrine. Comprehensive lists of sulfite containing medications have recently been published. It should be noted that manufacturers are responding to demands for the removal of sulfites from medications used to treat asthma. For example, Metaprel nebulizer solution no longer contains sulfites, even in the multidose vial.

The Preferred Approach

Diagnosis requires a high degree of awareness on the part of the physician. Once diagnosed, the patient needs to be informed by the physician or dietitian about the sulfited foods and medications to avoid. Instruction should be given about the prevention of acute attacks in high risk situations by pretreatment with inhaled beta-agonists and the treatment of acute attacks with similar medications.

THE PROS AND CONS OF TREATMENT

Sulfites can induce severe life threatening attacks of asthma. Treatment is aimed primarily at preventing these severe reactions. However, it is inappropriate for a patient to commence a sulfite free diet in the expectation that sulfite avoidance will cure chronic asthma.

SUGGESTED READING

Dalton-Bunnow MF. Sulfite content of drug products. Am J Hosp Pharmacy 1985; 42:2196–2201.
Settipane GA. Sulfites in drugs: a new comprehensive list. NER Allergy Proc 1986; 6:543–545.

STATUS ASTHMATICUS

HOMER A. BOUSHEY Jr., M.D.

Status asthmaticus is defined as severe asthmatic bronchospasm that is unresponsive to acute bronchodilator therapy. It is not a distinct variant of asthma but rather a form in which the physiologic and pathologic changes of asthma are unusually severe. The treatment of status asthmaticus thus involves largely the vigorous, intensive application of therapies effective in relieving mild asthmatic bronchospasm, the use of measures to protect the patient against the consequences of severe obstruction to air flow, and the avoidance of injudicious therapies.

The clinical signs and symptoms of asthma are logical expressions of the underlying disease. In postmortem studies of patients dying of asthma the most impressive abnormality is the gross overinflation of the lungs due to widespread air trapping from diffuse obstruction of airways throughout the tracheobronchial tree. The airways themselves are filled with mucus, desquamated epithelial cells, and inflammatory cells, sometimes forming casts of small bronchi and their branches. The airway wall is thickened by an intense eosinophilic inflammatory infiltrate, and both airway smooth muscle and airway submucosal glands are hypertrophied and hyperplastic. These findings are not unique to patients dying of asthma, for similar but less pronounced changes are found in the lungs of people with asthma who die of other causes, as from accidents.

The physiologic consequences of diffuse airway narrowing include a reduction in maximal expiratory flow, an increase in the resistance to air flow, and an increase in lung volume. The increase in lung volume is due in part to the premature closure of narrowed peripheral airways (increasing residual volume) and is in part a compensatory mechanism, for the greater lung elastic recoil at high lung volumes tends to increase both the size of the airways and the driving force for expiration. Thus, the work that must be done to overcome both resistive and elastic forces is increased by diffuse airway narrowing, and hypoventilation occurs unless this increase in the work of breathing is matched by increases in respiratory drive and in the performance of the respiratory musculature.

The shift in functional residual capacity to a greater lung volume and the increased resistance to air flow result in a marked increase in the variation in pleural pressure from inspiration to expiration and thus to an exaggeration of the normal respiratory changes in arterial blood pressure (pulsus paradoxus). Alveolar pressure is markedly increased during the prolonged expiratory phase of breathing, and alveolar rupture with dissection of air within the pleural space or mediastinum sometimes occurs. Because small pulmonary vessels are exposed to this increased alveolar pressure, and because pulmonary arterial pressure must be greater than alveolar pressure to make possible pulmonary blood flow, pulmonary arterial pressure is increased and overload of the right ventricle may occur. Tests of the distribution of ventilation show that airway narrowing during an acute severe asthmatic attack is very uneven. This unevenness of ventilation inevitably leads to a mismatching of ventilation and perfusion, producing an increase in the alveolar-arterial oxygen difference, an increase in wasted ventilation, and compensatory vasoconstriction in poorly ventilated areas, further increasing pulmonary vascular resistance and pulmonary hypertension.

Despite the increases in the work of breathing and in wasted ventilation, alveolar and arterial Pco_2 values are characteristically below normal, indicating that the drive to maintain breathing is considerably increased. The increase in total ventilation helps to offset the fall in the Po_2 level caused by widening of the alveolar-arterial oxygen difference. The mechanisms responsible for alveolar hyperventilation are not precisely defined, but studies of animal models of asthma suggest that they depend on afferent innervation of the airways. Whatever the underlying mechanism, alveolar hyperventilation is typical in acute asthmatic attacks and means that carbon dioxide retention, or even a "normal" value for the Pco_2, indicates extremely severe air flow obstruction, fatigue of respiratory muscles, or exhaustion of the patient and is thus an indication for urgent aggressive therapy. These physiologic disturbances have a characteristic clinical expression, and certain clinical manifestations are now recognized as hallmarks of severe life-threatening asthma.

Rebuck and Read, reasoning that death results from suffocation, suggested that the risk of death could be estimated from assessments of the degree of air flow limitation (the "load"), the arterial oxygen and carbon dioxide tensions (the "outcome"), and the physical costs of producing a given outcome in the face of a given load. In brief, they demonstrated that the clinical features of severe life-threatening asthmatic attacks are consequences of airway narrowing and include an FEV_1

of less than 0.5 liter, an FVC of less than 1.0 liter, alveolar hypoventilation, pulmonary hypertension and right heart strain, pulsus paradoxus greater than 18 mm Hg, hypoxemia (Po_2 less than 65 mm), exhaustion or any disturbance in consciousness, and pneumomediastinum or pneumothorax. Later studies have added tachycardia (pulse rate greater than 120 per minute), tachypnea (respiratory rate greater than 30 per minute), accessory muscle use, orthopnea, diaphoresis, and a history of severe attacks requiring intubation as other indices of severe, potentially lethal asthmatic attacks.

THERAPY

The intensity of initial therapy for asthmatic bronchospasm is adjusted according to the severity of the attack. For patients without the features of life-threatening asthma, the administration of a selective beta$_2$ adrenergic agonist by aerosol (e.g., 0.3 ml of 5 percent metaproterenol solution in 1.5 to 2.5 ml of normal saline) is effective as is the subcutaneous injection of 0.3 ml of a 1:1000 dilution of epinephrine, and both are more effective than the intravenous administration of aminophylline. The response should be assessed clinically and by repeat spirometry and the treatment repeated if no improvement is noted at 30 minutes. Those who respond to this initial treatment generally continue to improve and may be discharged if they have minimal symptoms at rest, an FEV_1 of more than 40 percent predicted, the ability to use outpatient medications (most often a selective beta$_2$ agonist given by metered dose inhaler and an orally administered theophylline compound), and a follow-up appointment.

For patients who present with two or more of the features of life-threatening asthma or who fail to respond to the initial bronchodilator therapy just described, a more aggressive approach must be taken. For these patients it is useful to record the key features of the severity of disease on a flow sheet. Serial recording of the general state of consciousness, heart rate, respiratory rate, pulsus paradoxus, FEV_1 and FVC (or peak expiratory flow) values, and arterial blood gas levels provides a useful, quickly comprehensible profile of the patient's condition and response to therapy. When the initial assessment has been completed, supplemental oxygen should be given by nasal prongs at a rate of 4 liters per minute. In acute severe asthma there is no need for concern about inducing hypercapnia by giving excessive oxygen as there is in patients with exacerbations of chronic obstructive lung disease. Aerosol treatment with an inhaled beta$_2$ selective adrenergic agonist should be given initially, 1 hour later, and at 1 to 2 hour intervals for the first 8 hours or until a response is seen. An intravenous line should be secured for the administration of aminophylline and a corticosteroid. The initial or loading dose of aminophylline is 5.6 mg per kg given over 20 to 30 minutes in 100 to 250 ml of

0.5 normal saline, followed by a maintenance dose of 0.6 mg per kg per hour given by continuous infusion.

Care must be taken with both the loading dose and the maintenance dose. Many different bronchodilator compounds (e.g., Tedral, Quibron, Uniphyllin, Theodur, and Marax) contain theophylline, and if a full loading dose is given to a patient who already has a nearly therapeutic blood level (10 to 20 μg per ml), toxic effects may occur (nausea, vomiting, diarrhea, tachycardia, cardiac arrhythmias, grand mal seizures) and complicate an already difficult clinical situation. When in doubt, it is wisest simply to start the maintenance dose by continuous infusion and await the result of a stat analysis of a baseline blood sample of theophylline. The maintenance dose must also be adjusted in some patients. Since an age over 50 years, congestive heart failure, and liver disease impair metabolism, the rate of infusion should be lowered to 0.4 mg per kg per hour in patients with those conditions. Children and current cigarette smokers metabolize theophylline more rapidly and may require 0.8 mg per kg per hour. Because the rates of metabolism vary widely even in healthy individuals, the blood level of theophylline should be checked in all patients 12 to 24 hours after therapy is started and the dose adjusted to achieve a therapeutic level.

Corticosteroids are effective in acute severe asthma and are credited by some experts for the fall in the mortality of hospitalized asthmatic patients since they were introduced in the 1950s. Their efficacy has been demonstrated in several prospective placebo controlled, double blind studies, but these studies also show that the greater improvement in the steroid treated group becomes apparent only 6 to 12 hours after steroids are given. The studies do not show clear dose dependency, but it is common practice to give 0.5 to 1.0 mg per kg (0.5 to 1.0 mg per kg) of methylprednisolone intravenously initially and every 6 hours thereafter for the first 24 to 48 hours or until clinical improvement is seen. Because one of the actions of corticosteroids is to potentiate beta-adrenergic responsiveness of airway smooth muscle, their effect may first be apparent as an increase in the change in FEV_1 provoked by aerosolized metaproterenol.

The pathologic abnormalities responsible for airway narrowing in asthma are not confined to smooth muscle contraction, of course, and corticosteroids have other important actions in relieving air flow obstruction. The inhibition of phospholipase A_2, for example, may prevent the metabolism of arachidonic acid in inflammatory cells and inhibit the production of the prostaglandins and leukotrienes that may be responsible for attracting and activating other inflammatory cells, for altering water transport across the epithelium, and for altering mucus secretion from submucosal glands and goblet cells. Only limited means are available for increasing the clearance of airway secretions more directly. Beta-adrenergic drugs may increase mucociliary clearance but are already being given to relax airway smooth muscle. Adequate hydration is probably important, and many patients may be dehydrated as a result of the increase in insensible water loss from the respiratory tract, but overhydration has not been shown to be helpful in mobilizing airway secretions.

Thus the standard initial therapy for acute severe asthma or for asthma unresponsive to two or three treatments with an injected or inhaled adrenergic drug is administration of supplemental oxygen, repeated administration of an adrenergic aerosol, intravenous administration of aminophylline and corticosteroids, and generous intravenous and oral replacement of fluids.

TOXIC REACTIONS

The regimen we have discussed is usually effective and well tolerated but carries some risk of toxicity. Most severe is the risk of cardiac arrhythmias. Myocardial irritability is directly increased by aminophylline and by adrenergic drugs and may be potentiated, especially in patients taking digitalis, by the hypokalemia sometimes produced by adrenergic drugs. Electrocardiographic monitoring therefore should be maintained in patients with premature beats on initial examination, in patients over 40, and in all patients with a history of heart disease or arrhythmias, and the serum potassium level should be measured at 4 and 24 hours to rule out hypokalemia.

A more common but less severe form of toxicity is skeletal muscle tremor, an additive effect of theophylline and adrenergic drugs. This may be minimized by substituting inhaled ipratropium bromide aerosol (Atrovent, 40 to 60 μg from a metered dose inhaler) for every other aerosol treatment with an adrenergic drug. Ipratropium is a derivative of atropine that is poorly absorbed and that also crosses the blood-brain barrier poorly. It does not appear to be a more effective bronchodilator than adrenergic drugs in asthmatic subjects, but it may have an additive effect on airway caliber and at the least offers a means of maintaining the bronchodilation achieved with adrenergic drugs without adding to their cardiac or muscular toxicity.

Another common side effect of the standard initial therapy for severe asthma, but one that is rarely of great clinical importance, is modest worsening of hypoxemia due to reversal of the compensatory vasoconstriction of pulmonary vessels supplying poorly ventilated lung regions. The resulting fall in the arterial Po_2 level is usually small and requires no intervention. It is simply important to recognize that a fall in the PaO_2 level in the absence of a rise in the $PaCO_2$ level does not indicate that bronchodilator therapy is ineffective or that the patient's condition is worsening.

Although viral respiratory infections are common precipitants of acute severe asthmatic attacks, bacterial infections are not, and antibiotics should be given only for specific indications. Sputum purulence is not itself sufficient, for it may simply reflect the airway mucosal inflammation associated with viral infections or possibly with late reactions to intense antigen exposure. Similarly a localized perihilar infiltrate revealed on the chest radiograph may reflect large mucus plugs in central airways. Moderate leukocytosis is common in uncomplicated asthmatic attacks, especially in patients treated with parenteral doses of epinephrine or high doses of corticosteroids. Fever is not typical of acute asthma, however, and requires explanation (fever may be overlooked if the rectal temperature is not obtained because oral breathing is invariable with severe bronchospasm). In patients with clinical or laboratory signs of infection, sputum and blood cultures should be done and treatment started with a broad spectrum antibiotic, such as erythromycin trimethoprim-sulfamethoxazole, or ampicillin. Care must be taken to ensure the absence of a history of allergy to the antibiotic chosen, for asthmatic patients are apt to develop immediate hypersensitivity reactions.

The use of oxygen, an adrenergic aerosol, and aminophylline and methylprednisolone intravenously is effective in the majority of patients, and serial measurements of the respiratory rate, pulsus paradoxus, spirometry, and blood gas levels show steady improvement. Controversies over treatment are most likely to arise in the care of patients who do not improve over the first few hours. In such patients it is useful to distinguish failure to improve from clinical deterioration. In general, the more abrupt the onset of bronchospasm, the more promptly it is reversed with therapy. The acute severe attack provoked by aspirin or sulfites in a sensitive asthmatic patient often starts to reverse within a few hours after the beginning of therapy, and pulmonary function test results may be nearly normal on the following day. In contrast, the attack provoked by a viral illness is typically more gradual in onset and less quickly reversible with therapy, perhaps because smooth muscle contraction is relatively less important, and inflammation and mucus plugging are relatively more important as causes of airway narrowing. This may be the reason that improvement is not seen in some patients until the third to fifth day of therapy.

It is sometimes the case, however, that the condition worsens despite therapy. The patient appears to be fatiguing, the $PaCO_2$ has increased to 40 mm or higher, and pulsus paradoxus has increased. In this event the patient must be under constant surveillance, and preparations must be made for intubation and mechanical ventilation, for deterioration can be abrupt and absolute when the patient is exhausted. It is at this point that other therapeutic measures are sometimes tried. Giving beta-adrenergic agonists intravenously (e.g., isoproterenol) is sometimes effective, perhaps because intravenous administration increases delivery of the drug to severely obstructed airways not reached by inhaled aerosols. Another measure that has been attempted but that is best avoided is intermittent positive pressure breathing, because it further increases intrathoracic pressure and thus further compromises cardiac output and increases the risk of pneumothorax. Chest physiotherapy is poorly tolerated by acutely dyspneic patients; delivery of an ultrasonic mist of distilled water aerosol achieves little hydration of airway mucus and increases bronchoconstriction (distilled water aerosol is used to provoke bronchoconstriction in research studies). Sedatives, which are sometimes given in the expectation that they will reduce motor activity and thus oxygen consumption and ventilatory demands, are contraindicated. Sedatives depress the respiratory center and increase fatigue; they frequently have been implicated as the cause of death in severe asthma.

Intubation and mechanical ventilation are indicated for worsening hypercapnia, exhaustion, confusion, or impaired consciousness. Mechanical ventilation is hazardous in asthmatic patients, however, principally because of the high pressures needed to deliver an adequate tidal volume through narrowed airways into overdistended lungs. Pneumothorax, alveolar hypoventilation, and malfunction of the endotracheal tube or ventilator itself occur commonly. The risk of these complications can be reduced by using a volume cycled ventilator to ensure delivery of an adequate tidal volume and by taking measures to minimize inflation pressure: a large endotracheal tube, low inspiratory flow, and sedative and paralyzing drugs. Additional measures include using ketamine as a sedating, analgesic, and anesthetic drug with bronchodilating properties, and giving sodium bicarbonate to protect against respiratory acidosis if normal alveolar ventilation cannot be maintained except with dangerously high peak inspiratory pressures (60 cm H_2O and above). Cases have been reported in which bronchoscopy and lavage to remove mucus plugs from the airways were associated with clinical improvement, but they have yet to be shown to be effective in a prospective controlled study. The very low mortality in hospitalized asthmatic patients (estimated as 1 percent or less even for severe asthma) testifies to the effectiveness of current standard therapy. The reported recent increase in mortality from asthma seems not to be due to an increase in in-hospital deaths but to an increase in deaths in the hours before hospitalization.

The risk of sudden death appears to be increased in patients who have been hospitalized for asthma, especially if they have had attacks severe enough to require intubation, and especially in the first few weeks after discharge. Treatment therefore should be tapered slowly after discharge from the hospital and the severity of the disease should be monitored. It is our practice in hospitalized patients to switch from intravenous to oral therapy when objective signs show clear improvement, and not to discharge the patient until the response to oral and inhalation therapy has been observed for 24 hours. Oral doses of theophylline and the regular use of an inhaled beta-adrenergic drug are maintained, and the oral prednisone dosage is tapered over 7 to 10 days to 15 to 20 mg per day. The patient is then re-evaluated to determine the rate of further tapering. To permit this re-evaluation, tests of air flow obstruction must be carried out immediately prior to discharge and on return for outpatient evaluation. For patients with a history of abrupt attacks of severe bronchospasm without fore-warning, twice daily measurements with a portable peak flow meter may show increased variability or progressive deterioration as the prednisone dosage is tapered, indicating the need for resumption of higher dosages or the institution of inhalation therapy with corticosteroids.

SUGGESTED READING

Fanta CH, Rossing TH, et al. Glucocorticoids in acute asthma—a critical controlled trial. Am J Med 1983; 74:845–851.

Haskell RJ, Wong BM, et al. A double-blind, randomized clinical trial of methylprednisolone in status asthmaticus. Arch Intern Med 1983; 143:1324–1327.

Huber HL, Koessler KK. The pathology of bronchial asthma. Arch Intern Med 1922; 30:689–760.

Minitove SM, Goldring RM. Combined ventilator and bicarbonate strategy in the management of status asthmaticus. Am J Med 1983; 74:898–901.

Rebuck AS, Read J. Assessment and management of severe asthma. Am J Med 1971; 51:788–798.

Rock MJ, De La Rocha S, et al. Use of ketamine in asthmatic children to treat respiratory failure refractory to conventional therapy. Crit Care Med 1986; 14:514–516.

Scoggin CH, Sahn SA, et al. Status asthmaticus: a nine-year experience. JAMA 1977; 238:1158–1162.

CHEMICAL SENSITIVITY

JOHN C. SELNER, M.D.

The most perplexing questions raised in addressing the treatment of chemical sensitivities are immediately obvious to the clinician:

1. Who really has an intolerance to a suspect chemical exposure (disease)?
2. Who has signs and symptoms of disease even though the clinical course is dictated by other imperatives, i.e., social or marital advantage, personal injury potential, workman's compensation (illness)?
3. How should the clinician approach the environmentally ill patient when a specific disease is established but the absence of a recognized mechanism explaining observed physiologic events (e.g., sulfur dioxide) confounds efforts to offer the patient a meaningful intervention strategy?

The issue of pollution might be approached more effectively by recognizing the social, political, and economic considerations that tend to separate chemical exposures into four distinct categories: ambient (outdoor pollution), occupational (indoor pollution, workplace), domiciliary (indoor pollution, home), and universal reactors (allergic to the twentieth century). Each category has peculiar interactions involving prescribed and proscribed rules. A successful outcome for the patient and society demands recognition of the legal and social orders involved.

Entire texts have been devoted to air pollution, and many of the allergy literature citations relating to chemical sensitivity have addressed occupational investigations. Cutaneous eruptions are obvious examples of chemical sensitivity; contact dermatitis has been extensively reviewed elsewhere. Therefore, these subjects are not included in this treatment of chemical sensitivity. Our discussion here addresses domiciliary chemical considerations and the patient who is "allergic to the twentieth century."

The working position for most physicians regarding the treatment of chemical sensitivity can be reduced to avoidance strategies (e.g., respirators, masks, protective apparel, changes in job location). In some situations prophylactic drug strategies have been employed (e.g., cromolyn sodium with sulfur dioxide and platinum salt exposure). The protective effects of some drugs used prior to exposure are well established. However, a nagging uncertainty whether these exposure consequences (inflammation) masked by drug therapy are in the long term interest of the subjects involved raises certain ethical questions. It seems possible that one's genetic repertoire for detoxification of chemicals (e.g., cytochrome P-450) may determine the patient tolerance susceptibility potential. It is my opinion that patients should be advised of potential long term effects of chronic, even low dose, chemical exposure once specific sensitivity is established (e.g., toluene diisocyanate).

Although some physicians claim that sublingual drops and subcutaneous injection of chemicals can alter specific chemical intolerance, there is no body of scientifically derived information that supports such a contention. In our experience patients claiming relief of symptoms as a result of these unproven and controversial therapies have not demonstrated objective evidence of specific chemical sensitivity when evaluated under double blind, sham controlled conditions.

An extensive amount of literature on environmental chemicals (e.g., trimellitic anhydride, toluene diisocyanate, sulfur dioxide, formaldehyde) testifies to the continuing interest of allergists in chemical "sensitivities" as differentiated from the traditional aeroallergens (dust mite, pollens, animal antigens, organic dusts, mold spores), which have always been the special interest of the allergist. For instance, four distinct clinical syndromes have been identified with trimellitic anhydride. Symptoms associated with these syndromes appear to be the result of immunologic and toxicologic mechanisms and suggest that genetically determined host defense potentials are of primary importance in the expression of disease versus tolerance. Toluene diisocyanate is associated with the development of antibodies against a protein conjugated chemical. However, existing evidence does not relate the presence of this antibody to specific intolerance, and the suggestion has been made that disease may be the result of pharmacologic effects of diisocyanate metabolites.

Antibodies associated with sulfur dioxide have been suggested by the presence of wheal and flare reactions to the subcutaneous injection of small doses by sulfite material in a small number of patients demonstrating intolerance to metabisulfites. Asthma, urticaria, gastrointestinal symptoms, rhinitis, and even vasculitis-like symptoms have been described with exposures to this chemical. At the present state of our understanding, the inhalation of sulfur dioxide produced as a result of mastication of metabisulfite containing foods in a fluid acid medium results in bronchospasm. We may have little authoritative insight into other mechanisms operative in reactions to this chemical.

Chemical irritation of mucous membranes has been used to explain irritant mucous membrane symptoms resulting from exposure to formaldehyde gas. Whether formaldehyde specifically sensitizes given individuals continues to be a matter of debate. The extensive treatment of these disorders and those related to other chemicals (e.g., plicatic acid, ethylene diamine, colophony, monoethanolamines, pesticides) and their relation to immunologic phenomenology and host defense lay the foundation for a more aggressive assessment of chemical intolerance by allergists.

Until recently our knowledge of chemical disease was primarily restricted to industrial experience (occupational chemical illness). The oil crisis of the 1970s redefined architectural priorities and led to implementation of more energy efficient strategies for maintaining building interior thermostability (heating-cooling relationships). Almost immediately air quality questions arose, distinct from ambient air considerations that had previously dominated the air pollution question. Indoor air contains virtually all the toxins found in outdoor (ambient) pollution in addition to those produced and subsequently entrapped by building materials, decorative materials, and indoor fuel combustion sources (furnaces, appliances). Systematic investigation of indoor chemical sources has led to a humbling appreciation of the complexity of gas production and interaction and to a recognition of the limitations of existing standards for indoor air quality (Tables 1, 2).

"SICK BUILDING SYNDROME"

The allergist is confronted with questions regarding what can be called the "sick building syndrome," as

TABLE 1 The 10 Most Frequently Identified Chemicals Emanating from 42 Modern Building Materials*

Compound	Average Concentration (μg/cu m)	Frequency
Toluene	39.7	22
n-Decane	1.49	20
1,2,4-Trimethyl benzene	0.56	18
n-Undecane	1.00	17
3-Xylene	23.0	16
2-Xylene	3.81	14
n-Propyl benzene	0.20	13
Ethyl benzene	1.79	12
n-Nonane	1.05	11
1,3,5-Trimethyl benzene	0.36	11

* From Molhave L. In: Moghissi A, Moghissi B, eds. Environmental International. New York: Pergamon Press, Vol. 8. 1982: 117–127.

distinct from occupational illness, which is usually limited to industrial experience (e.g., trimellitic anhydride, toluene diisocyanate, platinum salts). Air entrapment at work and home in these instances often resulted in the following symptoms: irritation of mucous membranes of the eye and upper airway, a sensation of dryness of mucosa and skin, erythema and pruritus of the skin, mental fatigue (confusion and memory variations), and persistent awareness of an odor when this odor is not appreciated by others.

Because a large percentage of affected patients have coexisting signs of classic allergy, these patients are frequently referred to the allergist for definition of the source of these complaints and treatment. Many allergists no longer limit their assessment of these patients to IgE mediated factors readily assessed by skin testing or in vitro assessment of "sensitizing antibodies." Allergists are utilizing chemical provocation challenges and

TABLE 2 The 10 Compounds in the Highest Average Equilibrium Concentration from 42 Modern Building Materials*

Compound	Average Concentration (μg/cu m)	Frequency
Toluene	39.7	22
3-Xylene	23.0	16
$C_{10}H_{16}$ (Terpene)	20.8	6
n-Butylacetate	15.2	1
n-Butanol	9.4	5
n-Hexane	8.8	5
4-Xylene	7.3	8
Ethoxyethylacetate	5.9	1
n-Heptane	5.0	2
2-Xylene	3.8	14

* From Molhave L. In: Moghissi A, Moghissi B, eds. Environmental International. New York: Pergamon Press, Vol. 8. 1982: 117–127.

employing the same disciplines that were brought to bronchoprovocation challenges with pollens, molds, and mite antigen, as well as chemical provocation in the assessment of nonspecific airway reactivity (histamine, methacholine).

THE CHEMICAL CHALLENGE

Many chemical challenges can be safely and satisfactorily carried out on an outpatient basis without the need for sophisticated generation and monitoring equipment (e.g., the Pepys technique of painting isocyanate containing materials in a closed room). More complex questions, especially those with legal dimensions, frequently require expertise beyond that usually existing in a typical allergist's office. However, incorporating such expertise into allergy practice is not beyond the capabilities of many allergists willing to expend the investigative energies and financial requirements to develop these methods.

To do this in our office practice we have identified a need for close professional working relationships with several scientific disciplines. These include a psychiatrist or psychologist interested in sensory response modeling and psychophysiologic understanding of the dose response; a chemist with access to laboratory facilities, or an industrial hygienist; a ventilation engineer; and a toxicologist, preferably with a forensic background, who demonstrates a willingness to defend appropriately formulated conclusions. The allergist-immunologist who has assembled such a team is in a position to evaluate complaints of chemical sensitivity within the state of the art limitations of the science of environmental chemistry.

Facilities required for in-office evaluations have been previously described and include a challenge chamber with real time chemical measurement capabilities and access to laboratory facilities for measuring physiologic changes (cardiovascular, pulmonary, nasal, neuromuscular, and electroencephalographic).

A PROTOCOL APPROACH

The physician who evaluates chemical sensitivity must subscribe to a defined protocol in order to avoid the legal entrapments that presently surround the disability and injury compensation mentality, which some view as a kind of national entitlement scandal. This mentality seems to have its own agenda without regard for any impact on private or public interests. Further, it may have no regard for the prevailing scientific consensus or the accepted principles of the scientific method. To ignore the limitations imposed by these societal norms is to invite unproductive discord, which inhibits the progress of science in an area of intense national interest—environmental disease.

Without attempting to provide specific detail, clin-

ical investigations of chemical sensitivity require the discipline usually encountered in any successful research laboratory:
1. The development of an incident log detailing all activity associated with the case, from the initial contact to the conclusion, which may be long after the patient is actually seen (months to years).
2. Disciplined research relating to any chemical considered for challenge to determine its potential toxicity (thus ensuring safe challenge parameters).
3. Determination of the physical and chemical properties peculiar to a given chemical that determine the possibility of delivering this chemical under chamber conditions in a safe fashion.
4. Identification of the availability of instrumentation to measure the actual exposures involved.

CHEMICALS AND BODY LOADS

A sophisticated data base is emerging that allows clinicians to recognize the presence of environmental chemicals in serum, fat, and other body tissues. The presence of these chemicals can give an indication of prior exposure and, depending on the analyses carried out, can indicate day to day or week to week variations in exposure to specific chemicals (e.g., assessment of body chemical burden by analysis of expired air). The analysis of target compounds has led to designations of the frequency with which a chemical is detected in personal monitoring of some exposed populations. This has led to the following chemical designations:
1. Ubiquitous (60 to 98 percent of the time). Examples: trichloroethane, tetrachloroethylene, benzene, xylene isomers, ethyl benzene.
2. Often encountered (70 to 80 percent). Examples: carbon tetrachloride, trichloroethylene, chloroform (source: chlorinated water, dry cleaning), styrene (insulation, plastics), p-dichlorobenzine (moth crystals, room deodorizers).
3. Occasional (less than 10 percent). Example: ethylene dichloride.
4. Not found. Examples: tetrahalomethane, dibromochlorpropane.

These examples are offered not to confuse the reader but to emphasize that there are reliable data in the scientific literature that address these issues. Exposure analysis may allow the investigator insight into potential toxins that may influence clinical presentations, such as previous exposure to DDT and the existence of significant body loads for metabolites of DDT (e.g., DDE) some 30 years later. Although this is a fledgling science and controls for various clinical presentations confronting the clinician are not as yet satisfactorily established, the allergist has the unique opportunity to contribute to and become an integral part of a rapidly expanding medical science that eventually will encompass psycho-neuro-immuno-endocrinologic considerations. The foundation for such an expansion on the part of the allergist has already been laid by the extensive treatment in the allergy literature of environmental chemical exposures.

UNIVERSAL REACTOR

In the past 10 years we have encountered over 100 patients who would fill the generic description of the universal reactor—allergic to the twentieth century. These patients characteristically have no objective signs or symptoms of disease related to a specific chemical. Terr has reviewed a large number of these patients and demonstrated that laboratory data are normal except for those that can be related to objective disease. Our effort has gone beyond the limited goal of discrediting a bogus diagnosis based on unconventional and unproven techniques and has focused on the attempt to deprogram patients from a belief system necessitated by unresolved psychologic conflict.

In work with Dr. Herman Staudenmayer, we compared 36 patients with chemical intolerance to groups of patients with well characterized psychologic illness (71) and with well characterized chronic somatic disease (diabetes, arthritis, asthma; 37) and to normal subjects (11). Psychologic tests often do not differentiate among these patient groups. However, psychophysiologic parameters, especially low frequency electroencephalographic patterning, identify universal reactors with those patients experiencing well characterized psychologic impairment. We have found that patients receptive to an explanation for a disease other than environmental illness can be deprogramed from ecologic belief and return

to functional status 50 to 75 percent of the time. Success depends on the extent to which this belief is rooted in essential primary gain that requires the belief in order to avoid confrontation with painful life experiences. To date this work has involved too few cases to warrant speculation as to the long term outcome. Psychologic interaction has tended to reveal a disturbing incidence of life threatening physical abuse and sexual abuse in early childhood among these patients.

OLFACTION AND THE UNIVERSAL REACTOR

It is impossible to avoid recognition of the importance of the intriguing adaptive physiology of the sense of smell in chemical intolerance. Few clinicians and researchers appreciate the importance of this primitive survival potential, which affects psychosocial processing. Work done in the past 10 years has begun to reveal the directive nature of odor in human behavior. Our experience suggests that the organ of olfaction is in reality highly integrated into neuroendocrine processing and plays a determinant role in the body's efforts to maintain homeostasis. We have observed dramatic symptoms (pseudoconvulsions, paradoxical vocal cord dysfunction) and subtle symptoms (nausea, pruritus in the absence of cutaneous lesions) as the immediate result of odor detection. Frequently these dysfunctions are traceable to identifiable psychotrauma frequently experienced in childhood, but often continuing into adult life. The frequency with which coping mechanisms related to this phenomenon seem to deteriorate from age

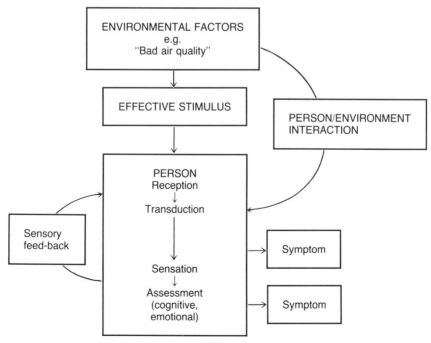

Figure 1 Factors controlling the response to chemical stimuli. (From Berglund B, Lindvall T. Environment International. New York: Pergamon Press, Vol. 12. 1986:147.)

30 through 50 is striking. Women seem to be affected more often than men. It has become clear that physician reinforcement of inappropriate phobic ideation regarding chemical intolerance must be avoided, because it can lead to disastrous psychologic and physical consequences.

SENSORY TOLERANCE

When considering challenges, a determination of "sensory tolerance" must be established. Many patients react with vague neuromuscular-cognitive-social symptoms simply as the result of an extraordinary impact of environmental chemicals on stimulus response. Such factors are only now revealing to researchers their importance in the qualitative and quantitative responses of specific individuals to chemical stimuli.

The model represented in Figure 1 might be described as an exercise in psychosocial reductionism that attempts to alert the clinician to the complexities of adaptive chemical-human interaction. It also underscores

the critical requirement for double blind, sham controlled challenge procedures, eliminating both observer and patient bias.

Our experience with "chemical sensitivity" suggests that a unique practice enhancing opportunity is available to both the allergist and other clinicians who encounter patients with "environmental illness." We believe that the price paid for the humanistic expansion required to work with these patients is well worth the investment when compared to the consequences of abandoning these patients to pseudoscientists.

SUGGESTED READING

Cullen M, ed. Occupational medicine: state of the art reviews. Workers with multiple chemical sensitivities. Philadelphia: Hanley & Belfus, 1987.
Selner JC, Staudenmeyer H. The relationship of environment and food to allergies and psychologic illness. In: Young SH, Rubin JM, Daman HR, eds. Psychobiological aspects of allergic disorders. New York: Praeger Publishing, 1986:102.
Whelan E. Toxic terror: the truth about the cancer scare. Ottawa: Jameson Books, 1985.

FOOD SENSITIVITY IN CHILDREN

HUGH A. SAMPSON, M.D.

"Food sensitivity" (an adverse reaction to food) is a general term used to denote any clinically abnormal response attributed to the ingestion of a food or food additive. Food sensitivity reactions are divided into two major categories: food intolerance (nonimmunologic) and food hypersensitivity or food allergy (immunologic). Four basic types of intolerance are recognized: toxicity or poisoning, pharmacologic reactions (caffeine), metabolic responses (lactase deficiency), and idiosyncratic reactions. Although an IgE mediated mechanism is the most well established hypersensitivity response, other less well defined immunologic mechanisms are believed to be responsible for such disorders as celiac disease, milk and soy induced enteropathies, and enterocolitis syndromes.

The often uncritical acceptance of published reports on food allergy has led to considerable confusion regarding the prevalence, diagnosis, and treatment of food sensitivity. Two prospective studies in children less than

6 years of age suggest that 4 to 6 percent of young children experience some adverse reaction to food. The majority of these reactions occur in young infants, consist of a "food intolerance," and generally are short lived. The most critical factor in treating food sensitivity is making an accurate diagnosis. Consequently the "diagnostic approach" will be emphasized in this discussion.

GENERAL COMMENTS ABOUT DIAGNOSIS

Although reports of food sensitivity can be verified by blinded challenge in only 30 to 40 percent of the cases, the history is an important component of the evaluation. Factors to be stressed in the history include the types of symptoms elicited, the timing of symptoms following ingestion, the severity of symptoms, and whether they have occurred on more than one occasion. In general, symptoms occurring soon after ingestion are more likely to be due to food hypersensitivity than those that take hours or days to develop.

A variety of symptoms secondary to food hypersensitivity have been confirmed by appropriate controlled studies and are listed in Table 1. Other symptoms have been attributed to "food allergy" but have never been substantiated in controlled trials. Some of these symptoms may be due to pharmacologic properties of

TABLE 1   Symptoms Substantiated by Blinded Food Challenges

1. Generalized anaphylaxis with cardiovascular collapse (sometimes associated with exercise)
2. Respiratory
   a. Upper airway: rhinoconjunctivitis, laryngeal edema
   b. Lower airway: wheezing (asthma)
3. Cutaneous
   a. Urticaria or angioedema, atopic dermatitis
   b. Urticaria associated with exercise
4. Gastrointestinal
   a. IgE mediated: lip swelling, palatal itching, tongue swelling, nausea, abdominal pain, cramps, emesis, diarrhea
      1. Oral syndrome—associated with birch pollen and apples, hazel nut, and carrots; and ragweed and watermelon, cantaloupe, and honeydew melon
   b. Celiac disease and dermatitis herpetiformis (IgA?)
   c. Malabsorption syndrome (steatorrhea, gross or occult blood loss, and eosinophilia) → enterocolitis (diarrhea, gross or occult blood loss, and failure to thrive), especially in response to soy and milk
   d. Heiner's syndrome—pulmonary infiltrates, iron deficiency anemia, emesis, diarrhea, failure to thrive
   e. Colic—cow's milk antigen in breast milk
5. Neurologic
   a. Migraine

certain foods, such as the high caffeine content of soft drinks.

The differential diagnosis of food sensitivity is broad, as indicated in Table 2, but a careful history often suggests the appropriate diagnostic category to pursue. Physical examination often is useful in excluding some disorders in the differential diagnosis. Various diagnostic studies (e.g., x-ray examination, biopsy) exclude many anatomic and metabolic abnormalities. Laboratory studies such as skin prick tests and IgE specific food antibody tests (e.g., RAST, FAST, MAST) are of some value in discriminating the foods responsible for

TABLE 2   Differential Diagnosis of Adverse Food Reactions

Gastrointestinal disorders
   Structural abnormalities (pyloric stenosis, hiatal hernia)
   Enzyme deficiencies—primary vs. secondary (lactase deficiency)
   Malignant disease (lymphoma)
   Other (cystic fibrosis, gallbladder disease)

Pharmacologic agents
   Caffeine (coffee, tea, soft drinks, cocoa)
   Theobromine (chocolate, tea)
   Tyramine (cheese, banana, tomato)
   Tryptamine (tomato, blue plum)
   Histamine (fish, beer, wine)
   Phenylethylamine (chocolate)

Contaminants and additives
   Flavorings and preservatives
   Dyes
   Toxins (bacterial, sea food associated)
   Infectious organisms

Psychologic reactions

immediate hypersensitivity reactions. There is no evidence to support the use of IgG specific food antibodies in the diagnosis of food sensitivity.

In order to establish whether a patient has food sensitivity, a provocative oral food challenge is necessary. The patient should abstain from eating a suspected food for 10 to 14 days prior to the challenge. Food challenges may be performed "openly" or as "single blind" or "double blind" procedures. Only the double blind procedure is free of psychologic factors and interpretational bias.

Freeze dried foods are most convenient for use in challenges and can be broken up into a fine powder using a blender. These foods can be purchased from grocery stores, health food stores, and camping outlets or in capsular form from Dura Pharmaceuticals (San Diego, California). Grape juice, cranberry juice, and tapioca-fruit mix provide good vehicles for administering food antigens. Freezing the challenge doses into small cubes often eliminates the smell and taste of particularly aromatic foods. For placebo controlled challenges, cornstarch or powdered lamb may be used to mimic the appearance and taste of various grain flours and meats.

Food challenges are initiated with small amounts of a test food antigen (less than 500 mg). Progressively larger doses of the test food are given over a 1 hour period until 10 to 15 g has been given or symptoms develop. Smaller initial doses, larger or smaller increments in the test doses, or a larger total dose may be given, depending upon the suspected sensitivity of the patient. A negative blinded challenge should be followed by an open feeding to insure that a food is tolerated in usual and customary portions. A single unequivocally positive objective reaction to a food tested in a double blind, placebo controlled manner may be taken as evidence of an acute reaction to food. However, in chronic disorders in which symptoms occur several times a week, two to three sets of positive challenges along with an equivalent number of negative placebo challenges are necessary to confirm a food sensitivity. If several placebo challenges are positive, the association with a food is unlikely. No patient with a convincing history of a recent life threatening reaction to a specific food should be subjected to an oral food challenge. When an immediate hypersensitivity reaction is considered, the patient should be observed for 2 to 4 hours following the challenge, since major reactions are likely to occur within this period.

PROTOCOL FOR DIAGNOSING FOOD HYPERSENSITIVITY

Table 3 outlines a protocol for evaluating food sensitivity. The initial evaluation should consist of a careful history, physical examination, and laboratory studies, which are suggested by the history and physical

TABLE 3 Evaluating Food Sensitivity

1. History and physical examination
   History: stress type of symptoms, timing, severity, and reproducibility
   Physical examination: exclude many possibilities in differential diagnosis

2. Laboratory tests
   Studies suggested by history and physical examination (e.g., x-ray study, breath hydrogen test, sweat test)
   Skin tests: prick technique with commercial extract or fresh food
      If negative (wheal <3 mm), immediate hypersensitivity very unlikely; further work-up probably unnecessary
      If positive (wheal > 3 mm), go to step 3

3. Strict allergen avoidance diet for 2 weeks
   Include foods suggested by history for most sensitivities; also foods suggested by skin prick tests for immediate hypersensitivity
      If unequivocal improvement and only one "major" or one or two "minor" foods are involved, continue restricted diet
      If improvement is equivocal or more than two foods are involved, go to step 4
   Elemental diet may be used in some cases

4. Single blind challenge in office
   Depending on the character and attitude of the patient, this may be done "openly" in circumstances in which blinding is very difficult
      If negative, discontinue restricted diet
      If positive to only one "major" food or less than four "minor" foods total, institute appropriate restricted diet
      If positive to more than one "major" food or more than four foods total, go to step 5

5. Double blind, placebo controlled oral food challenge

examination. If immediate hypersensitivity is suspected, skin prick testing should be performed with a battery of six to eight food extracts (egg, milk, peanut, fish, tree nuts, soy, and wheat) or foods suggested by the history. Negative skin prick test results in children 2 years of age and older (i.e., a wheal 3 mm larger than the negative control) make immediate hypersensitivity reactions extremely unlikely and preclude the need for further evaluation, unless the history is highly suggestive to the contrary. Foods eliciting a positive response should be eliminated from the patient's diet for 2 weeks.

When non-IgE mediated reactions are considered (e.g., cow's milk or soy protein enteropathy), foods suspected on the basis of the history should be eliminated from the diet for 2 to 3 weeks. If symptoms unequivocally improve, the diet should be continued unless it requires elimination of more than one "major" food (egg, milk, soy, wheat) or two or more "minor" foods (any food other than a major food). If symptoms persist unabated and food sensitivity is still contemplated, a brief trial (no longer than 2 weeks) of a severely restricted diet may be warranted. The following diets may be used: infants less than 4 months—milk substitute (Nutramigen, Pregestimil, or Vivonex); infants 4 to 8 months—milk substitute, rice cereal (many infant cereals contain more than one grain), and pears; 9 to 24 months—same as that for 4 to 8 months in addition to rice,

carrots, squash, and lamb; older than 2 years—same as that for 9 to 24 months in addition to fresh lettuce, potato, safflower oil, tea, and sugar. If symptoms fail to improve, food sensitivity can be considered ruled out.

When improvement is not clear-cut or several foods appear to be incriminated, an "open," or preferably a "single blind," challenge should be performed in the office setting under observation. Since food challenges, like immunotherapy administration, occasionally may result in severe anaphylaxis, appropriate equipment and personnel should be available in the office to deal with an emergency situation. If the office challenges reveal positive responses to only one major food or less than four foods total, an appropriate elimination diet may be instituted. Such a diet would not be overly restrictive and the results of such challenges would be acceptable. Positive challenges to more than one major food or more than four foods total should raise concern about the accuracy of the challenges and suggest the need for undertaking double blind, placebo controlled oral food challenges in an outpatient or inpatient setting. Restricting large numbers of foods without sound documentation subjects the patient to a diet that may be nutritionally deficient and that generally leads to noncompliance.

If the clinician follows the protocol outlined in Table 3, it is likely that a double blind, placebo controlled oral food challenge will be necessary in only a minority of patients. However, the need for sound documentation of food sensitivity by challenge procedures cannot be overemphasized. Overly restrictive diets in young children can lead to various eating disorders and create a great deal of family conflict, especially around mealtime. When various subjective complaints are being ruled out (e.g., vague abdominal complaints, behavioral problems) or when symptoms are reported to take several hours to days to develop, test challenges may be conducted at home. However, extreme caution should be exercised when recommending that parents administer a food suspected of eliciting an allergic reaction since life threatening anaphylaxis may occur.

TREATMENT OF FOOD SENSITIVITY REACTIONS

Strict avoidance of the offending food allergen is the only proven therapy for food sensitivity. Drugs may modify symptoms in some cases, but such measures should be considered only palliative. For example, corticosteroids alleviate symptoms in some protein enteropathy syndromes and may be life saving in some cases of fulminant secretory diarrhea, but the side effects of long term therapy are generally unacceptable. Antihistamines may modify symptoms of immediate hypersensitivity but rarely, if ever, block them completely. Oral doses of cromolyn sodium have been advocated by some, but carefully controlled trials in patients with challenge-confirmed food sensitivity failed to demonstrate efficacy. Preliminary studies with ketotifin suggest a potential therapeutic role in food hypersensitivity, but conclusions must await further confirmation. Rotational diets, immunotherapy, and sublingual or subcutaneous neutralization have never been shown to be efficacious in controlled trials.

Young infants who are sensitive to cow's milk generally can be managed adequately with elemental formulas, such as Pregestimil or Nutramigen. Infants with cow's milk protein enteropathy syndrome frequently develop sensitivity to soy. Although soy protein is immunogenic, it may be an acceptable alternative in other cow's milk sensitivities because its allergenic properties appear to be less marked. Many infants develop diarrhea and localized skin rashes following the ingestion of various fruits and fruit juices (citrus, apple, grapes, tomato). These reactions appear to represent ''intolerance'' and are generally short lived. In most infants with food sensitivity the diets can be expanded appropriately (i.e., addition of fruits, vegetables, and meats) without difficulty. However, the practice of adding only one new food every 3 to 5 days is probably a useful practice.

Children older than 2 years of age rarely (if ever) require an elemental diet for the treatment of food sensitivity. Appropriate oral challenge studies reveal only one or two specific food sensitivities in over 90 percent of the cases. The most practical method for implementing strict antigen avoidance diets is to teach parents (and older patients) to read food labels. Long lists of foods that patients ''may'' or ''may not'' eat are difficult to follow and are frequently outdated. Educating patients to recognize ''key words,'' ingredient listings that indicate the presence of a specific food, allows the formulation of the least restrictive diet possible and results in good dietary compliance. For example, the presence of milk may be indicated by any of the following ''key words'': milk, dried milk solids, whey, casein, lactalbumin, caseinates, cheese, butter, and curds. The assistance of a dietician in suggesting alternative food preparation techniques and insuring a nutritionally sufficient diet is invaluable.

Implementation of strict allergen avoidance frequently leads to the development of clinical tolerance to foods eliciting adverse responses. Virtually all young infants experiencing diarrhea in response to cow's milk or soy protein lose their sensitivity in 1 to 2 years. Several studies have demonstrated the loss of immediate hypersensitivity reactions in about one third of the patients after 1 year of antigen avoidance. Although young infants more consistently lose their food sensitivity, loss of hypersensitivity is by no means confined to the younger child. In addition, the clinical severity of the initial adverse reaction does not necessarily influence the longevity of the hypersensitivity. Infants less than 2 years of age with mild reactions may be rechallenged every 3 to 4 months to see whether symptoms persist. Older patients may be rechallenged every 1 to 2 years, depending upon how difficult it is to avoid the food in question. However, loss of sensitivity varies with the antigen in question. Clinically apparent sensitivity to peanut, tree nuts, and fish appears to be quite persistent, and rechallenging children with these foods at intervals less than every 4 to 5 years is probably unwarranted. In certain disorders, as in patients with celiac disease or dermatitis herpetiformis, restricted diets should be continued indefinitely.

Clinical reactivity to a food appears to be highly specific, and rarely are children sensitive to more than one or two foods. Although results of skin tests and in vitro tests of specific IgE commonly demonstrate cross reactivity among members of a botanical family or animal species, evaluation of over 180 children has revealed only one case of intrabotanical cross reactivity and no evidence of intraspecies cross reactivity, as determined by double blind, placebo controlled oral food challenges. Consequently the practice of avoiding all foods within a botanical family when one of its members is suspected of provoking allergic symptoms appears to be unwarranted. Elimination of this practice should improve patient compliance with elimination diets and reduce the likelihood of implementing a nutritionally deficient diet.

There are several contradictory reports in the literature regarding the role of breast feeding in the prevention of food allergy. Recent prospective studies from Scandinavia suggest that exclusive breast feeding for 6 months can reduce the number of infants developing food hypersensitivity at 1 year of age but may simply postpone the development of allergy to a later age in the majority. Avoidance of highly allergenic foods (peanut, egg, milk) by the lactating mother may be of further benefit, but dietary manipulation in the third trimester of pregnancy appears to offer no advantage and may compromise the pregnant mother's nutritional status.

Food intolerance reactions probably represent the majority of cases of food sensitivity in children, are most common in young infants, and are short lived. Both food intolerance and food hypersensitivity should be treated by strict avoidance of the inciting food. Repeated challenges should be conducted at varying intervals, depending upon the age of the child, the type of reaction provoked, and the food involved to ascertain whether the sensitivity persists. Appropriate studies to accurately document the presence of food sensitivity simplify the management of this disorder by reducing the number of foods that need to be eliminated from the patient's diet and the length of time they need to be avoided.

SUGGESTED READING

Bock SA. A critical evaluation of clinical trials in adverse reactions to foods in children. J Allergy Clin Immunol 1986; 78:165–173.

Leinhas JL, McCaskill CC, Sampson HA. Food allergy challenges: guidelines and implications. J Am Diet Assoc 1987; 87:604–608.

Sampson HA. Comparison of results of prick skin tests, RAST, and double-blind placebo-controlled food challenges. J Allergy Clin Immunol 1984; 74:26–33.

Sampson HA. Differential diagnosis in adverse reactions to foods. J Allergy Clin Immunol 1986; 78:212–219.

Walker-Smith JA, Ford RPK, Phillips AD. The spectrum of gastrointestinal allergies to food. Ann Allergy 1984; 53:629–636.

FOOD ALLERGY IN ADULTS

BRETT V. KETTELHUT, M.D.
DEAN D. METCALFE, M.D.

Food allergy is an immunologically mediated reaction to an ingested food antigen. In adults food allergy is uncommon and may present with a wide variety of symptoms. Although gastrointestinal symptoms (nausea, vomiting, and diarrhea) and cutaneous symptoms (urticaria, hives, and angioedema) predominate, respiratory symptoms (bronchospasm and rhinitis) and anaphylaxis may be observed in allergic individuals. When entertaining the diagnosis of food allergy, non-immunologically mediated adverse reactions to food must be excluded (Table 1). Corroboration of the patient's history may be obtained by positive prick skin test reactions to food extracts demonstrating mast cell bound IgE to a food antigen, the elimination of symptoms on exclusion of the suspected food(s) from the diet, and in selected patients, the reproduction of the symptoms on double blinded oral food challenge. Because skin testing and diagnostic oral food challenges pose a potential risk to the patient, only physicians skilled in these procedures, with support facilities to manage severe allergic reactions, should perform these diagnostic tests.

THERAPY

Once a food allergy has been identified and confirmed, the management consists of dietary avoidance to prevent the allergic reaction and pharmacologic therapy of symptoms resulting from inadvertent ingestion. A treatment plan must be individualized to account for the number and types of food involved, the degree of sensitivity, and the nature and severity of the symptoms.

TABLE 1 Examples of Adverse Food Reactions Due to Nonimmunologic Mechanisms

Enzyme deficiencies
  Lactase deficiency
  Sucrase deficiency
  Phenylketonuria

Gastrointestinal disease
  Hiatal hernia
  Peptic ulcer
  Gallbladder disease
  Postsurgical dumping syndrome
  Neoplasia
  Inflammatory bowel disease
  Pancreatic insufficiency

Additives and contaminants
  Dyes
    Tartrazine
  Exogenous chemicals
    Nitrates and nitrites
    Monosodium glutamate
    Sulfiting agents
    Antibiotics
  Endogenous chemicals
    Caffeine
    Tyramine
    Phenylethylamine
    Alcohol
    Theobromine
    Tryptamine
    Histamine

Toxins
  Bacterial toxins
    Botulism
    Staphylococcal toxin
  Endogenous toxins
    Certain mushrooms—α-amanitine
    "Shellfish"—saxitoxin
    Ichthyotoxin
  Fungi
    Aflatoxin
    Ergot

Other disorders
  Collagen vascular disease
  Endocrine disorders
Psychologic reactions
  Bulimia
  Anorexia nervosa

Diet

The treatment of choice in food allergy is elimination of the offending food(s) from the patient's diet. Care must be taken to provide optimal nutrition while completely eliminating the food(s) provoking adverse reactions. Palatability is an important consideration, because the success of the diet depends upon patient compliance. Diets that eliminate one or two foods are generally easy to design, but may become difficult to employ when common foodstuffs are to be avoided. For example, the dietary sources of milk and egg are numerous because of their widespread use in common foodstuffs. Elimination of these two foods alone results in a major loss of common commercially prepared foods from the diet. Hidden sources of these foods and others must be identified by the patient to reduce unexpected exposure to an offending food. The patient should be instructed to be wary of meals prepared by others who may include foods to which the patient may be sensitive. Cases have been reported in which patients with extreme sensitivities have experienced anaphylaxis, with subsequent death after such inadvertent exposures. Knowledge of the botanical families, as well as the classification of foods from animal sources, is necessary, for cross reacting antigens sometimes may be found among foods in the same group. For example, patients sensitive to shrimp often exhibit symptoms after ingestion of other crustaceans, such as crab, lobster, and crayfish. Cross reactivity in other food groups is not uniform, and diets should be planned in accordance with the patient's history of tolerance to these foods. Examples of these classifications of food groups are listed in Tables 2 and 3.

The preparation of a diet for a food sensitive patient should involve the skill of a dietician who is experienced in the treatment of these patients. One approach to the design of a diet for a patient with multiple food sensitivities is the institution of a well defined, limited diet as presented in Table 4. Foods that are not suspected of causing a reaction are then added one at a time every 2 days. Foods that provoke symptoms should be withheld from the diet, whereas foods not leading to a recurrence of symptoms may remain in the diet. This process is continued until enough foods have been reintroduced to provide a nutritious diet. Rarely a patient may be sensitive to numerous common foods. In these cases supplemental nutrition can be delivered by prescribing an elemental diet (e.g., Vivonex, Vital).

When treatment is first instituted, strict avoidance of all sources of the offending food should be observed. If the initial diagnosis is correct and compliance is maintained, improvement in the patient's condition should result. Eventually, in the absence of anaphylactic sensitivity, small amounts of the offending food may be tolerated upon cautious reintroduction into the diet. For example, small amounts of egg may be tolerated when used as an ingredient in the preparation of other foods.

In addition, certain foods not tolerated raw or partially cooked may be ingested without difficulty when completely cooked. Usually by practical experience most patients learn the method of preparation and the volume of a particular food that may be ingested without inducing symptoms, thereby making the diet more manageable.

Drugs

Even the most careful patient may inadvertently ingest the food to which he is sensitive. When the resulting symptoms of this exposure involve sites distant from the gastrointestinal tract, the treatment for each specific symptom is the same as that for similar allergic reactions. For example, the treatment of food induced urticaria is the same as the treatment of idiopathic urticaria, and asthma resulting from food ingestion is managed in the same way as asthma provoked by other allergens. The treatment for anaphylaxis due to a food ingestion differs only slightly from the treatment of other anaphylactic reactions. In addition to the standard therapy of anaphylaxis, gastric lavage may be necessary to reduce further antigen absorption and exposure. The patient with anaphylactic sensitivity should be taught how to self-administer epinephrine and should have an epinephrine-containing syringe and antihistamine available at all times. An identification tag stating the patient's sensitivity is also mandatory.

Gastrointestinal symptoms following inadvertent food ingestion are usually treated with antihistamines. An H_1 antihistamine, such as diphenhydramine hydrochloride in 25 to 50 mg doses three to four times daily, may be administered. As with other members of the ethanolamine series, diphenhydramine has marked sedative properties that may be undesirable in certain patients. Chlorpheniramine, an alkylamine, has a distinctly less sedative effect in most patients and may be given initially in doses of 4 mg three to four times daily.

Antihistamines, in addition to sedative effects, occasionally cause other central nervous system side effects, such as ataxia, dizziness, and difficulty in concentration. The anticholinergic properties of these drugs may lead to manifestations of atropine poisoning in susceptible patients or when given in large doses. Recently the nonsedating antihistamine terfenadine has been licensed for use in the treatment of allergic disease in the United States. This antihistamine may be useful in patients who are unable to tolerate other H_1 antihistamines because of sedation. The role of H_2 antihistamines such as cimetidine in the treatment of gastrointestinal food reactions has not been determined.

Corticosteroids are rarely used in the treatment of food allergy. Eosinophilic gastroenteritis and protein-losing gastroenteropathy associated with food allergy are two conditions in which steroid use may be instituted and the dosage tapered as symptoms resolve. Prednisone in oral dosages up to 60 mg a day may be required

TABLE 2   Classification of Foods from Plant Sources

Grain family	*Poppy family*	*Spurge family*	*Heath family*	*Composite family*	*Grape family*
Wheat	Poppy seed	Tapioca	Cranberry	Leaf lettuce	Grape
Graham flour			Blueberry	Head lettuce	Raisin
Gluten flour	*Plum family*	*Arrowroot family*		Endive	
Bran	Plum	Arrowroot	*Gooseberry family*	Escarole	*Myrtle family*
Wheat germ	Prune		Gooseberry	Artichoke	Allspice
Rye	Cherry	*Arum family*	Currant	Dandelion	Cloves
Barley	Peach	Taro		Oyster plant	Pimento
Malt	Apricot		*Honeysuckle family*	Chicory	Paprika
Corn	Nectarine	*Buckwheat family*	Elderberry		Guava
Oats	Almond	Buckwheat		*Legume family*	
Rice		Rhubarb	*Citrus family*	Navy bean	*Mint family*
Wild rice	*Laurel family*		Orange	Kidney bean	Mint
Sorghum	Avocado	*Potato family*	Grapefruit	Lima bean	Peppermint
Cane	Cinnamon	Potato	Lemon	String bean	Spearmint
	Bay leaf	Tomato	Lime	Soybean	Thyme
Mustard family		Eggplant	Tangerine	Lentil	Sage
Mustard	*Olive family*	Red pepper	Kumquat	Black-eyed pea	Marjoram
Cabbage	Green olive	Green pepper		Pea	Savory
Cauliflower	Ripe olive	Bell pepper	*Pineapple family*	Peanut	
Broccoli		Chili	Pineapple	Licorice	*Pepper family*
Brussel sprouts	*Ginger family*	Tabasco		Acacia	Black pepper
Turnip	Ginger	Pimento	*Papaw family*	Senna	
Rutabaga	Turmeric		Papaya		*Nutmeg family*
Kale	Cardamon	*Lily family*		*Morning glory family*	Nutmeg
Collard		Asparagus	*Birch family*	Sweet potato	
Celery cabbage	*Pine family*	Onion	Filbert	Yam	*Walnut family*
Kohlrabi	Juniper	Garlic	Hazelnut		English walnut
Radish		Leek		*Sunflower family*	Black walnut
Horseradish	*Orchid family*	Chive	*Mulberry family*	Jerusalem artichoke	Butternut
Watercress	Vanilla	Aloes	Mulberry	Sunflower seed	Hickory nut
			Fig		Pecan
Gourd family	*Madder family*	*Goosefoot family*	Hop	*Pomegranate family*	
Pumpkin	Coffee	Beet	Breadfruit	Pomegranate	*Cashew family*
Squash		Spinach			Cashew
Cucumber	*Tea family*	Swiss chard	*Maple family*	*Ebony family*	Pistachio
Cantaloupe	Tea		Maple syrup	Persimmon	Mango
Muskmelon		*Parsley family*			
Honeydew	*Pedalium family*	Parsley	*Palm family*	*Rose family*	*Beech family*
melon	Sesame seed	Parsnip	Coconut	Raspberry	Beechnut
Persian melon		Carrot	Date	Blackberry	Chestnut
Casaba	*Mallow family*	Celery	Sago	Loganberry	
Watermelon	Okra	Celeriac		Boysenberry	*Fungi family*
	Cottonseed	Caraway	*Legythis family*	Dewberry	Mushroom
Apple family		Anise	Brazil nut	Strawberry	Yeast
Apple		Dill			
Pear		Coriander		*Banana family*	*Sterculia family*
Quince		Fennel		Banana	Cocoa
				Plantain	Chocolate

initially to ameliorate symptoms. When prolonged steroid therapy is required, alternate day therapy with the minimal dosage required to control symptoms should be used. In these instances 5 to 10 mg of prednisone every other day is usually sufficient. Prolonged steroid therapy should be reserved for severe cases owing to the numerous side effects of this drug.

CONTROVERSIES IN FOOD ALLERGY

Controversy has arisen over the possible association of food allergy with poorly defined neurologic and behavioral complaints. It has been hypothesized for many years that symptoms such as depression, tension, and fatigue are associated with immunologically mediated reactions to foods. In spite of the long-standing nature of such claims, as yet no firm evidence has been presented to establish such an association. Thus, these problems should not be considered to be secondary to immunologically mediated food reactions.

Other areas of controversy center around two additional modes of treatment of food allergy. The first is either the parenteral or oral administration of dilute concentrations of food extract. No reasonable evidence exists to support this form of therapy. The second area of controversy concerns the prophylactic oral adminis-

TABLE 3 Classification of Foods from Animal Sources

Mollusks	Crustaceans	Fish
Abalone	Crab	Sturgeon
Mussel	Crayfish	Hake
Oyster	Lobster	Anchovy
Scallop	Shrimp	Sardine
Clam		Herring
Squid	*Reptiles*	Haddock
	Turtle	Bass
Amphibians		Trout
Frog	*Birds*	Salmon
	Chicken	Whitefish
Mammals	Duck	Scrod
Beef	Goose	Shad
Pork	Turkey	Eel
Goat	Guinea hen	Carp
Mutton	Squab	Codfish
Venison	Pheasant	Halibut
Horsemeat	Partridge	Catfish
Rabbit	Grouse	Sole
Squirrel		Pike
		Flounder
		Drum
		Mullet
		Weakfish
		Mackerel
		Tuna
		Pompano
		Bluefish
		Snapper
		Sunfish
		Swordfish

TABLE 4 Lamb and Rice Diet

Foods Allowed

Brown rice—natural long grain, short grain; parboiled

White rice—enriched, converted; cook without added fat

Brown or white rice, rice flour

Brown rice cakes—containing only brown rice and salt (if desired)

Puffed rice cereal—containing only brown rice

Lamb

Water

Salt

All food must be prepared without added fat. Rice, lamb, salt, and water are the only allowable foods. No food containing any other ingredients is to be eaten. Check labels. Salt or baking soda should be used to brush the teeth.

Eliminate

All foods not listed above, especially coffee, tea, soft drinks, and juices. Vitamins, aspirin, and any medication not ordered by a doctor must be eliminated.

Possible Menu

Breakfast	Lunch	Dinner	Snack
Rice mush	Rice patties	Rice and lamb sauté	Rice cakes
	Pan-fried lamb chops		

Instructions

Stay on basic diet for ____ days.

Then, on ____ add _____ all by itself, first thing in AM

Then, on ____ add _____ all by itself, first thing in AM

Then, on ____ add _____ all by itself, first thing in AM

Next, on ____ add _____ all by itself, first thing in AM

Next, on ____ add _____ all by itself, first thing in AM

Continue food additions one at a time at ____ day intervals until most or all other foods in the diet have been tested. Keep a diet diary as indicated. Add foods in large amounts, and eat them several times a day during addition period.

tration of cromolyn sodium or ketotifen. Insufficient clinical evidence exists to support use of cromolyn sodium use in food allergy, and it is not currently approved by the FDA for use in the disorder. Ketotifen, an antihistamine with mast cell stabilizing properties, has been suggested as being useful in the treatment of food allergy, although verification of this claim remains to be shown by careful clinical trials.

SUGGESTED READING

Atkins FM, Steinberg SS, et al. Evaluation of immediate adverse reactions to foods in adults. I. Correlation of demographic, laboratory, and prick skin test data with response to controlled oral challenge. J Allergy Clin Immunol 1985; 75:348–355.

Crawford LV. Allergy diets. In: Bierman CW, Pearlman DC, eds. Allergic diseases of infants, childhood and adolescence. Philadelphia: WB Saunders, 1980: 394.

Pearson DJ, Rix KJB. Allergy mimetic reactions to food and pseudo-food allergy. In: Dokor P, et al., eds. Pseudoallergic reactions. Vol. 4. Basel: Kargev, 1985: 59.

Reisman RE. American Academy of Allergy position statement—controversial techniques. J Allergy Clin Immunol 1981; 67:333–338

Sogn D. Medications and their use in the treatment of adverse reaction to foods. J Allergy Clin Immunol 1986; 78:238–243.

Terrill EE, Hill SR, et al. A checklist of names for 3,000 vascular plants of economic importance. Agriculture handbook 505. Washington, D.C.: United States Department of Agriculture, Agricultural Research Service, October 1986.

CHRONIC URTICARIA

NICHOLAS A. SOTER, M.D.

Urticaria occurs as circumscribed, raised, erythematous, usually pruritic, evanescent areas of edema that involve the superficial portions of the dermis. When the edematous process extends into the deep dermis and subcutaneous tissue, it is known as angioedema. About 50 percent of the patients experience both urticaria and angioedema, 10 percent angioedema alone, and 40 percent only urticaria. Episodes of urticaria lasting longer than 6 to 8 weeks are termed chronic. In addition to the skin, sites of clinical expression include the respiratory and gastrointestinal tracts and the cardiovascular system. Involvement of the upper respiratory tract may be fatal.

PREFERRED THERAPEUTIC APPROACH

The evaluation of a patient with recurrent (chronic) episodes of urticaria begins with a thorough history and physical examination. Although the ideal treatment for chronic urticaria is identification and removal of its cause, in the majority of instances no underlying cause can be discerned. The major clinical problem is the treatment of chronic idiopathic urticaria, and therapy focuses on measures to provide symptomatic relief.

In some instances it is important to avoid aspirin and other nonsteroidal anti-inflammatory drugs as well as nonspecific factors, such as alcohol, excessive heat, and exertion that may aggravate the episodes of urticaria. Antipruritic lotions containing menthol may provide temporary relief. Many patients respond to the administration of placebos.

Use of Antihistamines

H_1 antihistamines are the major class of therapeutic agents used in the management of chronic idiopathic urticaria. In addition to their antihistaminic actions, they possess a number of additional effects, including sedation, anticholinergic activity, local anesthesia, and antiemetic and antimotion sickness activities. The H_1 antagonists have been divided into subgroups based on their chemical structure (Table 1). Although the therapeutic superiority of individual drugs has not been substantiated, the effects just mentioned may be important in deciding which drug works best for an individual patient.

The H_1 antihistamines are absorbed from the stomach and small intestine, beginning within 20 minutes and reaching peak blood levels within 1 hour. The

TABLE 1   Antihistaminic Drugs

Chemical Class	Generic Name*
H_1 Receptor Antagonists	
Alkylamine	Chlorpheniramine maleate
Ethanolamine	Diphenhydramine hydrochloride
Ethylenediamine	Tripelennamine hydrochloride
Phenothiazine	Promethazine hydrochloride
Piperidine	Cyproheptadine hydrochloride
Piperazine	Hydroxyzine hydrochloride
Butyrophenone	Terfenadine
H_2 Receptor Antagonists	
Thioguanidine	Cimetidine hydrochloride
Ethenediamine	Ranitidine hydrochloride
H_1 and H_2 Receptor Antagonists	
Tricyclic antidepressant	Doxepin hydrochloride

* Commonly used representative examples.

duration of action ranges from 2 to 6 hours. Thus, for prolonged uniform therapeutic drug levels to be achieved, it is necessary to administer H_1 antihistamines in divided doses on a daily basis. The new nonsedative H_1 antihistamines have a much longer plasma half-life and can be administered in a twice or once daily regimen. Biotransformation of the H_1 antihistamines occurs in the liver, and the conjugated metabolites are cleared through the kidneys with complete excretion by 24 hours.

About 25 percent of individuals receiving H_1 antihistamines experience an adverse reaction, sedation being the most common problem. The sedative effect is pronounced in the ethanolamine and phenothiazine groups. The drugs of the ethylamine class have a less pronounced sedative side effect. Some tolerance to this sedative effect occurs in most individuals within a few days of continual administration of H_1 antihistamines. If tolerance does not occur, a trial of another subgroup can be undertaken. Patients should be warned about the accentuation of central depressive effects that H_1 antihistamines can cause when consumed in combination with alcohol.

New nonsedative antihistamines of the H_1 type, such as terfenadine and astemizole, are available in some countries, but only terfenadine has been approved for use in the United States. These therapeutic agents are particularly advantageous for individuals who must remain alert during their occupations or daily lives. Each drug achieves its nonsedative effect through a different mechanism. Terfenadine prevents sedation by not penetrating the blood-brain barrier. Although astemizole does pass into the brain, the drug has an affinity for peripheral H_1 receptors in the skin and elsewhere but not for central nervous system H_1 receptors. In addition, neither drug interacts with alcohol or other central nervous system depressants. Although no major side effects are known, there are no data regarding long term side effects.

Other central nervous system effects that may be experienced include dizziness, tinnitus, incoordination, blurred vision, and diplopia. At times the central nervous system effects can be stimulatory and include nervousness, insomnia, tremor, and irritability. Gastrointestinal manifestations include anorexia, nausea, vomiting, diarrhea, and epigastric distress. Some H_1 antihistamines also have anticholinergic properties that may result in dry mucous membranes, difficulty in micturition, urinary retention, dysuria, urinary frequency, and impotence. The cardiovascular effects of H_1 antihistamines usually are not experienced after oral administration.

The administration of H_1 antihistamines should be initiated at a low dosage level at defined regular intervals and increased to tolerance. For example, chlorpheniramine maleate, 4 mg, can be administered every 4 to 6 hours with a 4 mg increase in dosage every 48 to 72 hours to a maximal level of 16 mg at each time point. Moreover, some of the preparations, including chlorpheniramine maleate, are available in long acting forms that can be administered every 12 hours. If the H_1 antihistamine chosen is not effective or tolerated, therapy with another H_1 drug from a different chemical class should be instituted. Empiric trials of drugs from different classes may be carried out, and combinations of H_1 antihistamines also can be used. Once control of urticaria has been achieved antihistamine dosage should be tapered rather than stopped abruptly, inasmuch as flares may occur.

Topical preparations of antihistamines should not be used, owing to potential sensitization and resulting allergic contact dermatitis.

The combination of an H_1 and an H_2 antagonist may be used in cases of severe refractory idiopathic urticaria. Cimetidine hydrochloride, which is the H_2 antihistamine most frequently used, is absorbed from the small intestine, maximal blood concentrations being achieved within 80 to 90 minutes. Effective concentrations are present for 4 to 6 hours after an oral dose. The drug is eliminated unchanged in the urine with complete clearance by 24 hours. Both absorption of the drug and the duration of the therapeutic effect may be prolonged by administering it with meals.

Side effects occurring after the administration of cimetidine hydrochloride include occasional instances of headache, dizziness, and gastrointestinal symptoms. Cimetidine hydrochloride binds to androgen receptors, and this feature presumably is responsible for the occasional instances of gynecomastia and azoospermia in young male patients. An important side effect of cimetidine hydrochloride is its interference with the action of hepatic microsomal enzymes that metabolize drugs. This interaction may lead to potentiation of the effects of numerous other drugs, including warfarin, diphenylhydantoin, phenobarbital, diazepam, and propranolol. Although cimetidine hydrochloride was initially thought to have no effect on the bone marrow, a reversible granulocytopenia rarely may occur. The presence of an H_2 histamine receptor on T suppressor cells may in part explain the augmentation of delayed type hypersensitivity responses to intradermal antigens noted in some patients. Although cimetidine hydrochloride binds to nitrites in the gastrointestinal tract and may yield potential carcinogens in the form of nitroso compounds, prolonged administration has failed to result in gastric neoplasms.

The H_2 antihistamine ranitidine hydrochloride does not bind to androgen receptors, and it does not interfere with hepatic microsomal enzymes.

Other Therapeutic Approaches

The tricyclic antidepressant doxepin hydrochloride, which has activity against both H_1 and H_2 histamine receptors, may be of value. Terbutaline, a beta-adrenergic agonist, is of occasional benefit as an adjunct in combination with an H_1 antihistamine. The oral administration of disodium cromoglycate is ineffective in patients with chronic idiopathic urticaria, although a few individuals with urticaria secondary to food allergy may respond to administration of this drug.

Systemic corticosteroid therapy has no place in the routine management of chronic idiopathic urticaria. The side effects of corticosteroids are out of proportion to the therapeutic benefits in most patients. If corticosteroids are required in severe refractory urticaria, an alternate day regimen should be tried.

Epinephrine injections are widely employed, particularly in hospital emergency units, but their use is rarely required or indicated unless laryngeal edema or respiratory tract compromise complicates attacks.

Some forms of urticaria are elicited by physical stimuli, such as mechanical trauma, heat, cold, light, and water. The major therapeutic approach in these disorders is avoidance of the inciting stimulus. The administration of antihistamines may be helpful, and the induction of tolerance by repeated exposure to the appropriate physical stimulus has been achieved in some patients (see article on physical urticaria).

The role of dietary manipulation in chronic idiopathic urticaria is difficult to assess and is of limited value. In addition to foods, preservatives and food colorings are responsible for episodes of chronic urticaria in some instances. Removal of these agents from the diet is difficult but has been associated with therapeutic benefit in some individuals.

PROS AND CONS OF TREATMENT

The decision to treat chronic idiopathic urticaria depends on the frequency and severity of the symptoms and signs and focuses on empiric trials of H_1 antihistamines. In severe refractory urticaria, combinations of H_1 and H_2 antihistamines may be used. It is desirable to avoid repeated injections of epinephrine and the systemic administration of corticosteroids. Urticaria has a capricious course, may respond to the administration of placebos, and may resolve spontaneously. About 50 percent of the patients with urticaria are free of lesions within 1 year, but 20 percent continue to experience episodes for more than 20 years.

SUGGESTED READING

Champion RH, et al, eds. The urticarias. Edinburgh: Churchill Livingstone, 1985.

Coutts A, Greaves MW. Evaluation of six antihistamines *in vitro* and in patients with urticaria. Clin Exp Dermatol 1982; 7:529–535.
Czarnetzki BM. Urticaria. Berlin: Springer-Verlag, 1986.
Juhlin L. Recurrent urticaria: clinical investigation of 330 patients. Br J Dermatol 1981; 104:369–381.
Kerdel FA, Soter NA. Antihistamines in dermatology. In: Rook AJ, Maibach HI, eds. Recent advances in dermatology. Number 6. Edinburgh: Churchill Livingstone, 1983: 265.
Soter NA. Physical urticaria/angioedema as an experimental model of acute and chronic inflammation in human skin. Springer Semin Immunopathol 1981; 4:73–81.

PHYSICAL URTICARIA AND ANGIOEDEMA

ANTHONY D. ORMEROD, M.B., Ch.B., M.R.C.P
MALCOLM W. GREAVES, M.D., Ph.D., F.R.C.P.

The physical urticarias account for about 17 percent of the chronic cases of urticaria. The physical cause may be apparent from the patient's history or may be reproduced by physical testing with friction, pressure, heat, cold, water, vibration, or light. The response may be localized to the site of stimulation or generalized and commonly occurs within 10 minutes after stimulation, although in some types there is a delay of 2 to 12 hours. If the stimulus is sufficiently great, systemic symptoms of headache, flushing, dizziness, or syncope can occur in response to the systemic release of mediators. These urticarias tend to occur in young adults and begin spontaneously, remitting after a chronic course. Treatment is palliative and does not affect the course of the sensitivity. The coexistence of more than one type of physical urticaria is not uncommon.

In all common types of acquired physical urticaria, histamine release has been identified and mast cell degeneration is of undoubted importance (Table 1). This may be mediated by IgE as suggested by passive transfer of dermographism, cold urticaria, and some cases of solar urticaria. Nerve pathways may also be involved, as substance P released from sensory neurons participates in the flare response in dermographism, and depletion of substance P by the repeated topical application of capsaicin can render the area unresponsive to cold and heat in cold and heat contact urticaria. The low levels of certain protease inhibitors in physical urticaria (alpha$_1$-antichymotrypsin in cold and cholinergic urti-

TABLE 1 Classification of the Physical Urticarias

Dermographism*
Cholinergic urticaria*
Cold urticaria
Cold contact*
Reflex cold induced cholinergic
Cold dependent dermographism
Familial
Delayed
Delayed pressure urticaria*
Solar urticaria*
Local heat urticaria*
Delayed familial type
Vibratory angioedema
Familial
Sporadic*
Aquagenic
Urticaria*
Pruritus

*Histamine release demonstrated.

caria; alpha$_1$-antitrypsin in dermographism) may be a consumptive effect consequent upon widespread mast cell activation and whealing or may be primary, allowing unrestrained activity of mast cell derived enzymes.

There are few comparative studies of different antihistamines in physical urticaria, and most precede the recent introduction of the minimally sedating antihistamines, terfenadine and astemizole. These antihistamines have widely different pharmacokinetics, terfenadine having a rapid onset of activity and a half-life of 6 to 8 hours while astemizole has a slower onset, its maximal effect requiring 2 to 4 days' treatment. This delayed effect can be reduced by giving a loading dose. Astemizole has a long half-life (20 hours) and an active metabolite an even longer one (half-life 12 days), such that patients taking regular therapy demonstrate inhibition of histamine wheals and provocation tests for 4 to 6 weeks after stopping treatment. Side effects are few, but with terfenadine headaches, dysphoria, and rarely urticaria are reported. With astemizole, weight gain is sometimes seen and with overdosage ventricular arrhythmias are a serious complication. Neither of these drugs is considered safe in pregnancy. Studies in chronic idiopathic urticaria suggest that astemizole's effect increases in the first 3 weeks of therapy whereas tolerance occurs with terfenadine.

Individual responses to different antihistamines are widely variable and can be assessed by the patient using a self-assessment questionnaire while taking a series of antihistamines. Recent evidence that ketotifen prevents the release of histamine suggests that this may also have advantages in blocking the release of other important mediators. Oxatomide has been claimed to show similar properties in vitro, although this could not be confirmed in our own studies. Doxepin is a tricyclic antidepressant with potent antihistaminic activity and is useful in cold urticaria, perhaps by preventing the release of platelet activating factor. The use of hydroxyzine is a well established treatment in physical urticaria, and a single dose suppresses histamine wheals for 36 hours. Thus daily dosing at night is adequate. Other effects of hydroxyzine, including anticholinergic, antiserotonin, sedative, and anxiolytic effects, may account for its usefulness. Patients who are unwilling to take antihistamines or who have a poor response to therapy sometimes can be rendered tolerant by a graded repetitive stimulus given under supervision. Repeated restimulation is necessary during the refractory phase to maintain tolerance.

DERMOGRAPHISM

Dermographism is the commonest type of urticaria, accounting for 50 percent of the cases of physical urticaria. Firm stroking of the skin, which can be accurately reproduced using a spring loaded dermographometer, evokes a wheal and flare reaction within 10 minutes, which fades within the next 10 minutes. Whealing occurs in response to rubbing from clothing or bed sheets and minor trauma or pressure and is exacerbated by scratching. Less common variants include red dermographism, which occurs predominantly in dry skin of the elderly, and cold dependant dermographism in which rubbing followed by the application of cold water or ice is required to produce whealing. Dermographism has also been reported as a side effect of the anticancer drug bleomycin.

Terfenadine has been shown to potently reduce itching and whealing and is first line treatment, but because patients with dermographism may induce wheals by restlessness and scratching, a more sedative antihistamine such as brompheniramine may prove more effective. If the patient is not helped by an H_1 antagonist alone, an H_2 antagonist should be added: Hydroxyzine

and cimetidine are effective in combination, but in view of concern for possible antiandrogenic effects or, rarely, bone marrow depression from cimetidine, this treatment should be limited to the more symptomatic patients. Ketotifen may also be useful.

CHOLINERGIC URTICARIA

Cholinergic urticaria is a morphologically distinct reaction in which small 1 to 5 mm wheals develop with a variable degree of flare around lesions following exercise, heat, or emotional stimuli. The upper trunk and upper limbs are characteristically involved and palms and soles are spared. The diagnosis is best made by exercise or hot bath provocation testing. The stimulus for this type of urticaria is thought to be the release of acetylcholine and perhaps associated neuropeptides from cholinergic afferent fibers in response to activation of the autonomic cholinergic pathway for sweating. Lesions fade in 20 minutes to 1 hour.

In severely affected individuals cholinergic urticaria can produce facial angioedema and bronchospasm. Exercise induced anaphylaxis is often accompanied by cholinergic urticaria. Other uncommon variants include stress angioedema in which the typical rash of cholinergic urticaria is complicated by larger plaques of edema, and cholinergic dermographism in which stroking of the skin causes a rash resembling cholinergic urticaria. In a rare variant called persistent cholinergic erythema, small itchy macules of erythema appear continuously in response to the same stimuli. A rash closely resembling cholinergic urticaria can arise in aquagenic urticaria in which the reaction occurs following contact with water at any temperature.

Cholinergic urticaria is difficult to treat effectively. Hydroxyzine has been successful, but high dosages of 100 to 200 mg daily are often required. Anticholinergic drugs such as poldine methylsulfate are generally ineffective, because anticholinergic side effects appear at dosages too small to have a significant effect on the skin lesions. Desensitization has been reported but is possible in only a minority of patients. Up to 50 percent of the cases are exacerbated by aspirin, which should be avoided.

In severe intractable cholinergic urticaria, danazol is helpful, improvement being accompanied by an increase in the depressed levels of alpha$_1$-antichymotrypsin. Beneficial effects last for 2 to 3 months after cessation of therapy. This treatment is preferentially given to males because of androgenic side effects and the potential for fetal virilization when treating females.

COLD URTICARIA

Cold induced urticarias are a heterogeneous group of disorders in which the precipitating factor is cold.

Rarely it is secondary to systemic disorders giving rise to cryoglobulins, cold agglutinins, or cryofibrinogen secondary to underlying connective tissue disease, myeloma, viral infection, or syphilis. Cold urticaria may also follow viral illness or insect stings or may occur as a rare autosomally dominant familial type for which antihistamines are not effective. A recently recognized variant occurs in which generalized cooling in a cold room, especially if associated with exercise, gives rise to a rash indistinguishable from cholinergic urticaria. Ice cube tests in this type of reaction are negative. Other types include delayed and vasculitic variants and the cold induced dermographism already discussed.

In the common cold contact type the diagnosis can be confirmed by the application of ice to the skin for 10 to 20 minutes, and in other types generalized cooling in a cold room or cold wind is necessary. Patients with cold urticaria often describe severe systemic reactions when bathing in cold water, and because fatalities have occurred, unsupervised aquatic activities should be discouraged.

Cyproheptadine has produced favorable results in two trials. Four to 8 mg taken at night often prevents urticaria the following day. Side effects include drowsiness or weight gain, and some patients have an equivalent result using terfenadine. Ketotifen and hydroxyzine are frequently effective, and a recent study showed a preference for doxepin. The use of a mast cell stabilizing drug—tiaramide—has recently been proposed but it is not readily available. Combined H_1 and H_2 antihistamines also have been found to yield favorable responses in some instances.

Supervised desensitization with the induction of physical tolerance is frequently possible in cold urticaria and to some extent may occur naturally in exposed skin in winter. The problem of maintaining tolerance with once or twice daily cold baths or showers precludes a lasting effect in all but the strongly motivated.

DELAYED PRESSURE URTICARIA

In delayed pressure urticaria deep painful swellings occur 2 to 4 hours after the application of pressure to the skin. Lesions on the palms, soles, buttocks, and upper back are characteristic, and because of the delay their relationship to pressure may be overlooked. Systemic symptoms may accompany the swellings, with fever, malaise, headache, and leukocytosis. There is a marked association with chronic idiopathic urticaria, with different series showing an incidence of 27 to 82 percent. Histologically the lesions are characterized by a dense, deep, perivascular leukocyte infiltrate containing numerous eosinophils, and biopsy is useful in confirming the diagnosis. Also to confirm the diagnosis, weights of up to 10 kg can be placed in a sling strapped

over the shoulder or thighs for 20 to 30 minutes and read at 4 and 8 hours, but pressure testing gives variable results because refractory periods occur. Spring loaded devices have been used for quantitative studies, and a spring loaded dermographometer delivering firm pressure (200 g per sq mm) to the back for 1 to 2 minutes can be used as a screening test. Patients may also show delayed dermographic responses to rubbing and may develop lesions from the pressure effect of intradermal injections. Thus the results of intradermal tests require careful interpretation.

Antihistamines do not affect the pressure induced lesions but should help any concomitant chronic idiopathic urticaria. Nonsteroidal anti-inflammatory drugs were advantageous in a single study, but these findings have not been substantiated in subsequent investigations. Avoidance diets are also ineffective. Many patients respond to prednisolone, 20 to 30 mg, given on alternate days to minimize side effects. The decision to treat with prednisolone depends on the severity of the patient's disability and the dosage of steroid required.

SOLAR URTICARIA

Solar urticaria is a rare disorder in which pruritus and whealing develop within minutes after exposure to visible or ultraviolet light and resolve within 1 hour. It has been classified into subtypes depending on the action spectrum (Table 2), but the subdivision is arbitrary and some patients react to a wide spectrum. Dependent upon the action spectrum, patients may be troubled by light passing through window glass or light clothing or by fluorescent lights. In some patients light sensitivity is passively transferable, but the globulin fraction responsible has been only incompletely characterized.

In the action spectrum of 400 to 500 nm, erythropoietic protoporphyria needs to be excluded, especially in children. Systemic lupus erythematosus and drug reactions (sulfonamides and chlorpromazine) also need to be considered as possible etiologic factors in solar urticaria.

Although determination of the action spectrum may be useful in planning treatment, sunscreens and light avoidance often give disappointing results and antihis-

TABLE 2   Types of Solar Urticaria*

Group	Wavelength (nm)
Group I	290–320 (UVB)
Group II	320–400 (UVA)
Group III	400–700 (visible)
Group IV	290–700

* Adapted from Ramsey CA. Solar urticaria. Int J Dermatol 1980; 19:233–236.

tamines and beta-carotene are frequently unhelpful, although the latter may be useful in erythropoietic protoporphyria. Long term chloroquine therapy, successful in some instances, is potentially toxic. Cautious ultraviolet A therapy is most useful and achieves tolerance, which can be maintained by natural sunlight but which is quickly lost if there is a break in the treatment. PUVA is an effective alternative but may increase the risk of cutaneous malignant disease following long term treatment.

LOCALIZED HEAT URTICARIA

This very rare physical urticaria is induced by local heating of the skin in response to radiant heat, including sunlight or contact with warm surfaces or liquids. It is reproduced by the application of a beaker containing water at 45° C for 5 to 10 minutes. In some patients histamine is released during the reaction, but in others there is evidence of complement activation. Recently evidence of the corelease of histamine and prostaglandin D_2 has been described following heat challenge in heat urticaria. A distinct familial delayed form has been described that is responsive to antihistamines and atropine.

Desensitization is possible, and in one patient additional benefit was gained from indomethacin. H_1 antihistamines, such as hydroxyzine, used alone give variable results.

VIBRATORY ANGIOEDEMA

This rare type of urticaria was first described as an autosomally dominant inherited disorder and later in sporadic cases. Angioedema and flushing follow running, towelling, massage, or other vibratory stimuli. A laboratory vortex mixer has been used, secured to the arm for 5 minutes, to test for this disorder. Mast cell degranulation and histamine release occur. Induction of tolerance and avoidance of vibration have both been successful in treatment.

AQUAGENIC URTICARIA

The development, usually in young adults, of a cholinergic-like eruption mainly on the head, neck, and upper trunk, accompanied by intense itching, occurs in response to contact with water at any temperature. Sweat, sea water, and distilled water are equally effective, but organic solvents alone are ineffective. Although the rash resembles cholinergic urticaria, it is not provoked by heat, exercise, or emotional stimuli. The eruption, which is short lived and unaccompanied by systemic symptoms, is due to histamine release from degranulated mast cells. H_1 antihistamine treatment affords some relief from itching and ultraviolet B irradiation also may be helpful in some patients.

Aquagenic pruritus is a much more common reaction to contact with water in which intense itching without visible changes in the skin occurs in response to contact with water at any temperature. Although histamine release and mast cell degranulation have been observed in aquagenic pruritus, other mediators, possibly released as a result of increased fibrinolytic activity, may be involved. Polycythemia rubra vera causes water induced itching indistinguishable from aquagenic pruritus.

SUGGESTED READING

Breathnach SM, Allen R, et al. Symptomatic dermographism, natural history, clinical features, laboratory investigation and response to therapy. Clin Exper Dermatol 1983; 8:463–476.

Champion RH, Roberts SOB, et al. Urticaria and angio-oedema, a review of 554 patients. Br J Dermatol 1969; 81:588–597.

Greaves MW. Antihistamine treatment, a patient self assessment method in chronic urticaria. Br Med J 1981; 883:1435–1436.

Greaves MW, Sneddon IB, et al. Heat urticaria. Br J Dermatol 1974; 90:289–292.

Mayou SC, Black AK, et al. Cholinergic dermographism. Br J Dermatol 1986; 115:371–377.

Murphy GM, Black AK, et al. Persistant cholinergic erythema, a variant of cholinergic urticaria. Br J Dermatol 1983; 109:343–348.

Ramsay CA, Solar urticaria. Int J Dermatol 1980; 19:233–236.

Sibbald RG, Black AK, et al. Aquagenic urticaria, evidence of cholinergic and histaminergic basis. Br J Dermatol 1981; 105:297–300.

Steinmann HK, Greaves MW. Aquagenic pruritus. J Am Acad Dermatol 1985; 13:91–96.

HEREDITARY ANGIOEDEMA

ALLEN P. KAPLAN, M.D.

Hereditary angioedema is an autosomal dominant disorder associated with severe episodes of swelling of submucosal and subcutaneous tissues. Attacks may affect virtually any part of the body but most commonly involve the extremities or the face. Occasionally there may be edema of the submucosa of the small bowel that causes episodes of abdominal pain; the most severe of these may resemble an "acute abdomen." Episodes of swelling may also affect the upper respiratory tract to include the tongue, pharynx, and larynx. Laryngeal edema, in particular, can cause acute obstruction, stridor, and asphyxiation and therefore can present as a medical emergency. Attacks are sporadic and often occur in the absence of any precipitating event. However, in some patients there appears to be a preponderance of episodes in association with local trauma, concomitant illness, or emotional stress. The age of onset of episodes of angioedema can vary greatly; it most often occurs during childhood. However, episodes are seldom severe prior to puberty. The duration of attacks is typically 1 to 4 days; they are self-limited and most often require no therapy. However, attacks involving the upper airway or gastrointestinal tract require particular precautions, to be outlined.

Hereditary angioedema is caused by depressed function of the inhibitor of the activated first component of complement (C1 INH). Approximately 85 percent of the cases are attributable to diminished levels of the protein (typically less than 25 percent of normal), and 15 percent of the cases are attributable to synthesis of a dysfunctional protein and plasma levels may be normal or elevated. This protein is the only known physiologic inhibitor of the C1r and C1s components of the first component of complement. It is also the main plasma inhibitor of activated Hageman factor and kallikrein and is therefore the critical protein regulating the formation of the vasoactive peptide bradykinin. The swelling seen in hereditary angioedema is thought to be due to either a kinin-like molecule, which may be derived from one of the complement components, or to bradykinin (or both). Since the disease is transmitted as a dominant gene and patients are heterozygotes, one normal gene is present. The cause of C1 INH levels lower than 25 percent of normal (rather than the expected 50 percent) appears to be excessive catabolism. Similarly when an abnormal C1 INH is synthesized, small amounts of normal C1 INH are also present owing to transcription of the one normal gene.

In a patient presenting with angioedema, the diagnosis of hereditary angioedema is suspected if there is a positive family history. A low C4 level is suggestive regardless of the history, since sporadic cases or a new mutation occasionally may be found. A low C1 INH level is confirmatory. However, if the C1 INH level is normal or elevated in the presence of a low C4 level, a functional determination should be performed. During episodes of swelling the C4 level may approach zero and the C2 level also declines. Acquired angioedema with C1 INH deficiency is to be distinguished from the familial disorder. This is most often associated with B cell lymphomas or connective tissue diseases in which C1 INH levels are low as a result of unusual consumption. In these cases the C1q level is also often depressed; C1q levels are typically normal in hereditary angioedema. Therapy in acquired cases of C1 INH deficiency is directed to the underlying disease, but the modalities used to treat hereditary angioedema also can be utilized to prevent episodes of swelling.

Not all patients with hereditary angioedema require therapy. Some may have only mild attacks that do not have a major effect on life style. Others may have an attack frequency of less than one or two episodes per month. These do not require therapy unless severe episodes or life threatening situations are encountered. However, occasional patients such as these may be treated if the death of family members has created such anxiety that they prefer the risk of possible side effects associated with drug therapy. The clinical course of the patient should be the primary guide for therapy rather than the level of C4 or C1 INH.

TREATMENT OF ACUTE ATTACKS

Angioedema affecting the extremities requires no specific therapy, and the episode usually abates within a few days. Swelling affecting the face is more troublesome, and severe attacks can be aborted with repeated subcutaneous doses of epinephrine 1:1000. For example, 0.3 cc every 45 minutes for one to three doses would suffice for an otherwise healthy adult with prominent facial, lip, or tongue swelling. Abdominal attacks, although painful, require only supportive therapy. The main symptom is cramping abdominal pain, sometimes associated with nausea, vomiting, or diarrhea. These episodes are similarly self-limited, lasting for 1 to 4 days, but require careful observation if an episode is severe.

We admit patients with severe abdominal attacks, administer fluids intravenously (particularly if dehydration might result from fluid loss), and use mild analgesics. We generally avoid the use of narcotic analgesics; however, a single dose of Demerol administered early in an attack can be helpful. Repeated doses of epinephrine 1:1000 given every 1 to 2 hours sometimes can abort episodes after a few doses. An abdominal examination should be performed periodically with particular attention to the status of bowel sounds and evidence of rigidity. Typically a patient has areas of tenderness to palpation, or rebound may be elicited; bowel sounds are more often hyperactive than hypoactive. The areas of tenderness may vary over time as can rebound (likely the result of stretching of visceral but not parietal peritoneum). However, the abdominal wall remains soft. Fever, leukocytosis, an elevated sedimentation rate, and progressive rigidity of the abdominal wall are signs of an "acute abdomen" and alert one to the uncommon occurrence of another disease for which surgery might really be indicated.

Involvement of the airway is a true medical emergency, which is generally unresponsive to antihistamines or corticosteroids and may or may not respond to epinephrine. Early signs of laryngeal involvement include a change in voice, tone, or pitch or frank hoarseness. Pharyngeal involvement may cause a choking sensation and difficulty in swallowing food. This may not be an emergency, but careful observation is indicated because it can progress to difficulty in swallowing secretions, the risk of aspiration, or laryngeal symptoms. More severe laryngeal involvement can lead to inspiratory stridor and asphyxia. When angioedema of the airway appears likely, an otolaryngologic evaluation to examine the vocal cords and the laryngeal-pharyngeal area should be performed. Epinephrine should be administered (assuming that there are no contraindications)—about 0.3 ml of a 1:1000 dilution given repeatedly. Vital signs should be monitored to be sure that the cardiovascular effects of one dose have passed before another is given. Spacing can vary from every 45 to 120 minutes as indicated. Antihistamines or short acting corticosteroids may be given, but there is little rationale for their use and they are not likely to help.

The condition in a patient with airway involvement who is seen within hours after onset or during the first day may worsen during the ensuing 1 to 2 days before resolving by day 3 or 4. Such a patient should be observed, and if the attack appears to be progressive, admission to the hospital, the intravenous administration of fluids, and epinephrine are indicated. A patient seen at day 2 or 3 of an episode need not be admitted if the swelling is clearly nonprogressive after observation for many hours. Epsilon-aminocaproic acid can be used in an attempt to ameliorate the severity of edema of the airway. A dose of 8 g is given within the first 4 hours and then 16 g per day for the next 24 to 48 hours until the episode has ended. Thus a combination of subcutaneous doses of epinephrine administered periodically on day 1 with epsilon-aminocaproic acid for a few days is recommended. However, there is no truly reliable modality that one can count on and attacks may nevertheless progress in some patients.

In such a circumstance tracheostomy is indicated. An alternative is nasotracheal intubation in an operating room setting. The staff should be prepared to perform a tracheostomy if intubation is not successful. The tube remains in place until the episode abates.

The use of fresh frozen plasma in such circumstances is controversial. On the one hand C1 INH is being replenished and on the other hand substrate for circulating active enzyme is being given and generation of more permeability factor is possible. Fresh frozen plasma is best utilized as prophylactic therapy (to be discussed) and not administered during acute episodes.

SHORT TERM PROPHYLACTIC THERAPY

Patients with hereditary angioedema may require minor surgical or other invasive procedures, which could precipitate angioedema. Those involving the respiratory tract are of particular concern and include such circumstances as dental procedures (gingivectomy, extraction, root canal work, or even routine local anesthesia) and endoscopy. In such cases the use of fresh frozen plasma in a patient who is receiving no other therapy can prevent attacks. We recommend the infusion of 2 units of fresh frozen plasma the day prior to surgery and 2 units just before the procedure. One must be cautious because there is a finite risk of transmission of hepatitis or even AIDS, and all recommended precautions must be followed. Single doner volunteers who have been screened serologically may be used to allay patient anxiety. If such surgery is elective, the administration of androgens for 5 days prior to the procedure (e.g., 4 mg of stanozolol four times daily) should obviate the need for fresh frozen plasma and is a reasonable alternative. For major surgical procedures the approach is similar. In patients who are already taking maintenance dosages of androgens the dosage should be increased for the aforementioned 5 day period so that C4 and C1 INH levels rise.

MAINTENANCE THERAPY

The object of maintenance therapy is to prevent episodes of swelling by utilizing the least quantity of medication that is efficacious to minimize side effects and costs. The most effective drugs are androgens or androgen derivatives, such as methyltestosterone, danazol, and stanozolol. Methyltestosterone was the first androgenic compound shown to be effective in hereditary angioedema; its use is restricted to men but it is otherwise a satisfactory drug. It is efficacious, the cost is low, and the toxicity is minimal. One can start with 10 mg three times daily and, once the disease is quiescent, gradually decrease the dosage. The major danger in its use is cholestatic jaundice, and liver function should be assessed periodically—perhaps monthly at the start and then every few months.

For both women and men one can use attenuated androgens such as danazol or stanozolol. Both these drugs are capable of increasing synthesis of normal C1 INH and thereby correct the underlying biochemical defect. C4 levels also rise with therapy. In women taking birth control pills (estrogenic) there may be an increase in attacks, which can be reversed by discontinuing birth control tablets without further therapy. It has become clear that either drug can be effective for long term maintenance at dosages that produce little or no change in the plasma C4 or C1 INH level. It is not known whether the drug works by some other mechanism or whether small changes, perhaps within tissues, suffice in terms of protection. The main side effects of danazol use are weight gain (due in part to fluid retention and increased appetite), menometrorrhagia, headaches, muscle cramps, mild androgenic effects (voice deepening, hirsutism, alopecia, acne, altered libido), and a mild increase in the SGOT and SGPT levels.

The starting dosage is 600 mg per day and the dosage is then gradually decreased. As little as 50 mg every other day suffices for some patients, but this is highly variable. My experience with stanozolol is greater than that with danazol, and we utilize this as our first choice for long term therapy. Its efficacy is essentially the same as for danazol, the cost is less (about 10 to 20 percent), and the side effects, although similar in type, seem less prominent. An increase in SGOT, SGPT, or LDH levels can be seen but not frank jaundice or irreversible changes suggestive of chronic hepatitis or cirrhosis. Lowering the dosage or stopping therapy for a while leads to rapid reversal of the enzyme elevations. Stanozolol is marketed as a 2-mg tablet and most patients are controlled with 2 mg per day. For some, as little as 2 mg every other day is sufficient. One can proceed from 2 mg per day to 4 mg every other day and then to 2 mg every other day.

Epsilon-aminocaproic acid (7 to 8 g per day) also has been shown to control attacks of hereditary angioedema, although it has no effect on C4 or C1 INH levels, its mechanism of action is unclear. It is known to inhibit plasmin, plasminogen activation, and C1 activation even by immune complexes. Its effect is to decrease the severity of attacks of swelling rather than decreasing the frequency. It could be considered in severely ill patients who are unable to take any of the aforementioned androgens. It is clearly a "second line"

drug and particular caution is needed when there is a predisposition to thrombosis because it is antifibrinolytic. Thus it could be dangerous if a patient were to have a myocardial infarction or cerebrovascular accident. Epsilon-aminocaproic acid can also cause severe muscle toxicity, with pain and elevation of the aldolase and creatine phosphokinase levels. Therapy should be discontinued immediately if this occurs.

It is uncommon for therapy to be required in children prior to puberty, although episodes of swelling may occur. However, severe or life threatening episodes are rare in this age group and avoiding treatment is best. If therapy is needed, the minimal androgenic dosage should be used. This is perhaps less of a problem for males. Therapy of prepubescent girls should be carried out in conjunction with an endocrinologist. Epsilon-aminocaproic acid can be considered in this circumstance, since it does not affect gonadal development. We have successfully treated young females (age 10 to 14) with 2 mg of stanozolol every other day, with a normal onset of puberty, normal menses, and no evident side effects. We assess liver function every 3 months during the first year of therapy and every 6 months thereafter.

SUGGESTED READING

Frank MM, Sergeant JS, Kane MA, Alling DW. Epsilon aminocaproic acid therapy of hereditary angioneurotic edema: a double blind study. N Engl J Med 1972; 286:808–812.

Gelfand JA, Boss GR, Conley CL, Reinhart R, Frank MM. Acquired C1 esterase deficiency and angioedema: a review. Medicine 1979; 58:321–328.

Gelfand JA, Sherms RJ, Alling DW, Frank MM. Treatment of hereditary angioedema with danazol: reversal of clinical and biochemical abnormalities. N Engl J Med 1976; 295:1444–1448.

Kaplan AP. Urticaria and angioedema. In: Kaplan AP, ed. Allergy. New York: Churchill Livingstone, 1985:439–471.

Sheffer AL, Fearon DT, Austen KF. Clinical and biochemical effects of stanazolol therapy for hereditary angioedema. J Allergy Clin Immunol 1981; 68:181–187.

Sheffer AL, Fearon DT, Austen KF. Hereditary angioedema: a decade of management with stanozolol. J Allergy Clin Immunol; (In press).

PENICILLIN ALLERGY

JOHN A. ANDERSON, M.D.

Benzylpenicillin G and semisynthetic penicillin— the penicillins—as well as the cephalosporin drugs are all classified as beta-lactam antibiotics because of a

structural beta-lactam ring that all these drugs share. The penicillins, as a group, are among the most commonly prescribed drugs in the world today. The true incidence of allergic (immunologically mediated) reactions to the penicillin drugs in the world is not known. In continuing drug surveillance studies done in the United States among adult medical inpatients, however, the penicillin group of drugs is one of the most likely types of drugs to be involved in a significant adverse reaction.[1,2] IgE mediated systemic reactions complicate approximately 2 percent of the courses of penicillin therapy. In addition, since the prevalence of positive skin test reactions to penicillin drugs is estimated to be between 3 and 10 percent, a substantial proportion of the adult population is potentially at risk for anaphylactic reactions to these drugs. Anaphylaxis has been reported to occur with a frequency of 1 to 5 per 10,000 patient courses of penicillin treatment. Even if these incidence figures are inflated somewhat and even though the use of penicillins in the United States and other countries has declined in recent years because of the substitution of other less risky drugs in potentially susceptible patients, allergy to the penicillins and other beta-lactam antibiotics remains one of the most significant immunologically mediated adverse drug reactions.

Anaphylactic reactions to the penicillins occur most commonly in adults between the ages of 20 and 49, although anaphylaxis may occur at any age. Approximately 25 percent of these reactions occur within 48 hours after initial penicillin therapy. Seventy-five percent of the patients who have died of penicillin anaphylaxis had no history of allergy to these drugs. Sensitization to the penicillins can occur by any route, the topical route being most risky. Multiple short courses of administration of these drugs are most likely to result in sensitization. Once sensitization to the penicillins has occurred, the allergic reaction may occur following penicillin challenge by any route, but drug administration by the intramuscular route is most risky. The oral route is safest, since if reactions do occur, they tend to be mild, cutaneous in nature, and self-limited.[3]

The patient's sex, race, and HLA phenotype do not appear to affect the incidence of penicillin allergy. A personal or family history of allergy to other substances does not correlate with penicillin reactivity. Skin test reactions to penicillin drug products in atopic and nonatopic individuals have been shown to occur with equal frequency. Most reported deaths due to penicillin drugs have occurred in nonatopic patients. Patients who are allergic to the penicillin group of molds are not at an increased risk of developing sensitization to the penicillin drugs.

PENICILLIN ALLERGENS: PENICILLIN SKIN TESTING AND IN VITRO METHODS

Penicillin is a simple structure with a low molecular weight of 300 daltons.[1] As a hapten, it is itself not immunogenic, but it becomes so by combining with tissue proteins. The relative ease with which the parent drug, penicillin, and its drug metabolites combine with tissue proteins to become complete antigens (by forming stable covalent bonds) helps to explain the heightened "sensitivity" to this type of drug in humans compared with other drugs. The molecular nucleus of penicillin is 6-aminopenicillic acid, which contains a beta-lactam ring and a thiazolidine ring. Ninety-five percent of the parent penicillin drug is metabolized to the penicilloyl determinant (major penicillin determinant), and the rest of the drug is metabolized to minor haptenic determi-

nants. The exact structures of all minor penicillin haptenic determinants are unknown, but they include sodium benzylpenicilloate and penilloate (when benzylpenicillin is processed to form a "minor determinant mixture").

In vivo the amino or the hydroxyl terminal group on tissue proteins combines with the beta-lactam ring of the penicillins. For allergy skin testing, the penicilloyl "major" determinant is combined with polylysine to produce penicilloyl-polylysine.* This antigenic material is usually used in a prick-scratch-puncture skin test followed by intradermal skin testing according to the manufacturer's instructions. This test is usually combined with penicillin G or individually produced minor determinant mixtures.

Several protocols for allergy skin testing have been published. One common approach is to perform prick-scratch-puncture skin tests with penicilloyl-polylysine (6×10^{-5} molar), penicillin G (10,000 units per ml or 10^{-2} molar), or minor determinant mixture (10^{-2} molar) in addition to a histamine and saline control (Table 1).[4] It is clearly desirable to do skin testing with the minor determinant mixture; however, since a validated standardized commercial minor determinant mixture is not available, many clinicians simply use a fresh solution of penicillin G as a partial substitute for the penicillin minor determinants at the present time.[3] "Aging" penicillin has no advantage over freshly prepared penicillin allergens used for skin testing.

Prick-scratch-puncture skin tests are done with these reagents initially. If the results are negative, intradermal skin tests are then performed. A prick-scratch-puncture or intradermal skin test is considered to be positive when a wheal develops that is at least 2 mm larger than the diluent control skin test reaction read 10 to 20 minutes after the penicillin or other beta-lactam antibiotic antigen presentation. In vitro solid phase immunoassays for antigen specific IgE, such as the radioallergosorbent (RAST) or enzyme linked immune assay (ELISA), have been developed to detect antibodies to the penicilloyl determinant.[1,5] No similar in vitro assay exists for routine testing for IgE antigen specific antibodies to the minor penicillin haptenic determinants or to determinants to other beta-lactam antibiotics.

EVALUATION OF THE PATIENT PRESENTING WITH A HISTORY OF PENICILLIN ALLERGY

Penicillin skin testing is an extremely useful procedure in the evaluation of the patient who presents with a history of an adverse reaction to penicillin and in whom an IgE mediated immunologic mechanism for this reaction is suspected.[3] If the penicillin skin test is positive, the presence of IgE antigen against penicillin products can be considered confirmed and the patient is at risk for a clinical reaction if challenged with penicil-

---

*Produced commercially by the Kremer-Urban Company.

TABLE 1   Skin Testing for Beta-Lactam Antibiotic Allergy*

Skin Test Type	Skin Test Reagent	Drug Test Concentration	Skin Test Volume
Penicillin major determinant	Penicilloyl-polylysine †		
	1. Prick-scratch-puncture	Full skin test strength	One drop
	2. Intradermal	Full skin test strength	0.02 ml
Penicillin minor determinant	Fresh penicillin G‡		
	1. Prick-scratch-puncture	10,000 units/ml	One drop
	2. Intradermal	10,000 units/ml (serial skin testing optional e.g., 10 units/ml followed by 100 units/ml and 1,000 units/ml)§	0.02 ml (each)
and/or	Penicillin minor determinant mixture		
	1. Prick-scratch-puncture	10^{-2} molar	One drop
	2. Intradermal	10^{-2} molar (individual schedules for serial testing optional)§	0.02 ml
Semisynthetic penicillin or cephalosporin	Specific drug		
	1. Prick-scratch-puncture	0.25, 2.5, 25 mg/ml serial skin tests§	One drop (each)
	2. Intradermal	2.5, 25 mg/ml serial skin tests§	0.02 ml (each)
Histamine (positive control)	Histamine phosphate		
	1. Prick-scratch-puncture	1:1,000 w/vol	One drop
	2. Intradermal	1:10,000 w/vol (1:100,000 w/vol optional)	0.02 ml
Saline (negative control)	Buffered saline on appropriate dilution		
	1. Prick-scratch-puncture	N/A	One drop
	2. Intradermal	N/A	0.02 ml

* All skin tests are considered as immediate reacting in nature and can be read in 10 to 20 minutes. Prick, scratch, or puncture skin tests always should be done first. If negative, intradermal skin testing can then be done.
† Kremer Urban Co.—single skin test strength.
‡ Freshly prepared (1 week) benzyl potassium penicillin (1 million unit vial) mixed with 9.6 cc of sterile sodium chloride–penicillin stock solution (penn. stock on day of testing 0.5 ml of penn. stock + 4.5 ml of sodium chloride = 10,000 units per ml).
§ Serial skin testing: Although the usual patient can be safely skin tested with single strength reagents, sensitive patients should be serially tested with weaker strengths first before proceeding with stronger reagents.

lin. However, each patient who is history positive and penicillin skin test positive may not react clinically to a penicillin challenge on a given day (approximate risk, 60 to 70 percent).[4] The chance of finding a positive penicillin skin test reaction varies with the length of time from the time the patient had a clinical reaction to penicillin. Patients in whom the clinical reaction occurred between 2 weeks and 3 months after drug exposure have been shown to develop a positive penicillin skin test 70 to 100 percent of the time. On the other hand, positive penicillin skin test reactivity in patients shown to be allergic to penicillin decreases over time, approximately 50 percent being skin test negative 5 years following the allergic reaction and 70 to 80 percent being skin test negative 10 years or more after this allergic reaction.

In the majority of the studies involving patients who present to an allergist with a history of penicillin allergy at some time in the past, approximately 14 to 20 percent of the adults and no more than 10 percent of the children can be shown to be skin test positive to penicillin antigens.[4] A single group of investigators reported, however, that 63 percent of 740 patients presenting with a positive history of penicillin sensitivity were shown to be skin test positive on penicillin skin testing.[6]

If the penicillin skin test is negative, the patient generally can be considered to be not allergic to penicillin. The reliability of these tests has been reported to be as high as 96 percent in studies of patients who had a history of penicillin reactions, who were skin test negative, and who subsequently were challenged (4 percent reaction after penicillin challenge in 370 history positive patients who tested negative with penicilloyl-polylysine and penicillin G, and in 478 history positive patients who tested negative with penicilloyl-polylysine and minor determinant mixture).[4,7] Patients who have had a significant reaction to penicillin cannot be reliably tested to penicillin within the immediate 2 week period following the clinical reaction. Although a positive penicillin skin test reaction during this period of time may provide useful information, negative skin test reactions are considered as unreliable indices of the lack of penicillin sensitivity. The exact reason for the existence of this refractory period in some penicillin allergic patients is unknown.

In vitro penicilloyl RAST or ELISA assays may be helpful in the diagnosis of penicillin allergy only if they are positive. If negative, these assays do not rule out sensitivity, since they detect only 60 to 95 percent of the patients who react in a positive fashion to penicilloyl-polylysine skin tests, and these in vitro assays do not detect circulating IgE antibodies directed against penicillin minor determinant haptens.[1] A single investigator has reported a small number of patients who were shown to be clinically sensitive to penicillin and had circulating IgE antibodies directed against penicilloyl-polylysine by in vitro methods but who were also found to be skin test negative to penicilloyl-polylysine.[8]

These in vitro tests should be considered in situations in which reliable skin test reagents are not available, in which skin disease or conditions such as eczema or dermatographism preclude accurate determination of skin test reactivity, or in the presence of circulating drugs that affect the accuracy of skin test reactivity.

Some controversy surrounds the timing of the use of penicillin skin testing. Some allergists who deal primarily with adult patients recommend that skin testing with penicillin should be used only just before a therapeutic dose of penicillin is to be given. One of the reasons for this school of thought is that the penicillin skin test result is accurate only for that period of time or for that specific therapeutic endeavor. At any future time the patient may develop an initial penicillin sensitivity (or a renewed penicillin sensitivity). One investigator has recently shown that a select group of hospitalized patients who had a history of penicillin reactions but who were penicillin skin test negative following successful challenge with a full course of intravenous penicillin therapy had a high likelihood (60 percent) of developing subsequent positive penicillin skin test reactivity upon testing 2 to 3 months later.[9]

Many allergists who deal primarily with children as patients advocate elective penicillin skin testing. The reasoning behind this school of thought centers around the fact that only one of 10 children (versus one of five or more adults) who have a history of penicillin allergy is likely to be shown to have positive penicillin skin test reactivity. Many of these children developed urticaria or other rashes at a young age during the treatment of an "infection" with a penicillin product. Often the reaction in the child, in retrospect, was due to factors

other than an IgE immunologic reaction to penicillin (e.g., viral infection). One investigator has shown in a large number of patients (80 percent younger than 20 years of age) that elective skin testing can be done easily, is safe, and when followed by an oral challenge dose of penicillin is not likely to produce a clinical reaction in a skin test negative patient.[10,11] Finally, when these patients were given a full therapeutic course of oral penicillin therapy, only a few developed a rash, and no patient developed a systemic reaction to the antibiotic. Subsequently only 1 percent of the patients developed a positive skin test to penicillin when retested 4 weeks later. Thus elective skin testing, oral challenges in skin test negative patients, and oral penicillin therapy (in skin test negative, oral challenge negative patients) can help to "clear the air" for the physician who is in doubt about the patient who allegedly is sensitive to the drug. In the majority of the patients it is safe to give the penicillin again later without the necessity for retesting the patient for penicillin (before each treatment).

Some controversy also exists concerning the necessity for challenging a patient who has been found to be skin test negative. From the foregoing discussion it is evident that there is more risk of reaction in an adult who presents with a history of penicillin allergy than in a child. If the reaction is significant (e.g., life threatening), it is probably wise to challenge the patient with a single oral dose of penicillin following a negative penicillin skin test reaction. Following a full course of antibiotics, it is probably also wise to retest the patient at a future date. These recommendations are particularly important when the minor determinant mixture has not been used in the skin test protocol. However, in children who have had a questionable history of a penicillin allergic reaction at some time in the past, a negative penicillin skin test itself is a good index of the lack of penicillin sensitivity. In questionable cases, however, again an oral challenge under controlled conditions with a single dose of the penicillin product to be used is advised. It is wise also to advise the referring physician of the exact risk based on percentage of the reliability of the testing procedure for each given patient.

EVALUATION OF THE PATIENT SUSPECTED OF BEING ALLERGIC TO SEMISYNTHETIC PENICILLIN

Patients who are proven to be sensitive to any one type of penicillin by the demonstration of IgE antibodies against the parent penicillin drug or the metabolic by-product or by challenge with this drug should be considered allergic to all types of penicillins and semisynthetic penicillins.[3] 6-Aminopenicilloic acid is the nucleus of the penicillin G molecule. This nucleus is present in all semisynthetic penicillins, and thus it should not be surprising that cross allergenicity exists between these penicillins to some degree.

Routine skin testing procedures similar to those that have been recommended for the evaluation of the patient suspected of being allergic to penicillin G have not been perfected to the same degree for the evaluation of the patient suspected of being allergic to semisynthetic penicillins. Some investigators have shown that all reactors to the semisynthetic penicillins can be identified by skin testing with penicilloyl-polylysine, penicillin G, or minor determinant mixture.[3] These methods are the most studied and most validated. Other investigators contend that although defined cross reactivity exists between penicillin G and the semisynthetic penicillins, there may be unique antigens associated with the latter penicillins and, for this reason, additional skin testing with the specific semisynthetic penicillin is recommended. No commercially available major or minor individual semisynthetic hapten determinant skin test material is available; therefore, usually the parent (semisynthetic penicillin) drug is used.

One suggested routine involves serial prick-scratch-puncture skin testing utilizing concentrations of the semisynthetic penicillin of 0.25, 2.5 and 25 mg per ml (see Table 1). These tests are done serially with the weakest concentration first and then are read at 10 to 20 minute intervals. A positive test includes any in which the wheal is 2 mm or more larger than the control. If these prick-scratch-puncture tests are negative, serial intradermal skin testing is done with 2.5 mg per ml and then 25 mg per ml semisynthetic penicillin.

CEPHALOSPORIN SENSITIVITY AND CROSS SENSITIVITY TO CEPHALOSPORINS IN PATIENTS WHO ARE ALLERGIC TO PENICILLIN

The cephalosporins resemble the penicillins chemically; both drug nuclei contain a beta-lactam ring. However, in the case of the cephalosporins, the beta-lactam ring is attached to a six membered dihydrothiazine ring instead of a five membered thiazolidine ring as is the situation with the penicillins. Cephalosporin breakdown during body metabolism results in a major cephaloyl determinant or grouping and probably is associated with other "minor" antigenic determinants.

The skin testing procedures used by various investigators in an attempt to demonstrate IgE antibodies against cephalosporin drugs involve utilizing various concentrations of the parent cephalosporin drug and almost exclusively utilizing the prick-scratch-puncture method. These methods are at best crude and the experience of one investigator cannot be generalized.[12] If cephalosporin skin testing is done, care must be taken not to overinterpret a "positive" test, since nonspecific irritation is possible. Since so little clinical information exists about cephalosporins as skin test reagents, nega-

tive skin test reactions should be interpreted as "no information" rather than as a lack of cephalosporin allergy.

There are some clinical clues to the contention that each cephalosporin drug differs from another in the degree of risk of an allergic reaction. Thus skin testing with these general types of drugs may depend on the use of several cephalosporin antigens when these methods are perfected in the future.

Anaphylaxis to cephalosporin does occur but much less often than to the penicillins. Reactions have been reported both to cephalothin and to cephaloridine—the latter in two patients who had no evidence of penicillin allergy. The continuing Boston Collaborative Drug Surveillance Program studying cutaneous drug reactions has demonstrated that among adult medical inpatients cephalosporins account for only 1 percent of the cases of reactivity versus a 10 percent incidence with penicillin–semisynthetic penicillin.[2]

A recent study of children treated for otitis media with either amoxicillin or cefaclor demonstrated an allergy-like and nonallergy-like cutaneous reaction incidence with cefaclor of 5.4 percent versus 3.7 percent with amoxicillin.[12] The mechanism of reaction in this study was not investigated; however, it is possible that some cephalosporins will be shown to produce a toxic or idiopathic rash in a similar fashion to that shown for ampicillin. Although it is speculative, the incidence of such cutaneous allergy-like drug reactions may be increased by certain viral infections, as in the case of ampicillin rash with Epstein-Barr virus infection. If these speculations are true, many of the cutaneous reactions that are observed with the cephalosporins may be due to mechanisms other than IgE and therefore do not constitute a risk when penicillin is a substitute.

The true incidence of cross reactivity between penicillin–semisynthetic penicillin and the cephalosporin drugs is unknown. One investigator found in penicillin skin test positive patients that approximately half were allergic to ampicillin and half to cephalosporin utilizing prick-scratch-puncture and intradermal skin testing. None of the skin test positive (or negative) patients was challenged with these drugs, however. Another investigator challenged 27 patients known to be allergic to penicillin by history and skin testing (no cephalosporin skin testing), and none reacted. Furthermore, in the institution where the latter study was performed, it has become common practice to use cephalosporins in patients suspected of having penicillin allergy (without confirmation by either penicillin skin tests or challenges).

With all the published information as a base, it would seem that the risk of reaction using cephalosporins in patients suspected of being allergic to penicillin is approximately 2 percent.[12] Patients with a history of penicillin allergy should be skin tested with penicillin to define sensitivity. Most will be found to be nonallergic. In this group, cephalosporin administration is probably no more hazardous than it is in the general population. In confirmed penicillin allergic patients (history positive, penicillin skin test positive), up to half may have a positive cephalosporin skin test reaction. The latter group should be presumed to be allergic to both drugs unless challenged, and alternative drugs should be considered.

DESENSITIZATION OF PATIENTS WHO ARE ALLERGIC (IgE SENSITIVITY) TO BETA-LACTAM ANTIBIOTICS (PENICILLIN G, SEMISYNTHETIC PENICILLINS, OR CEPHALOSPORINS)

The principal preventive therapy of allergy to the beta-lactam drugs is to avoid use of these drugs if possible. When infection requires treatment in the face of allergy to these medications, a safe alternative drug is recommended. When this is not possible, and beta-lactam antibiotic therapy is required, desensitization should be attempted. This procedure is not recommended for non-IgE mediated reactions to the beta-lactam antibiotics, such as ampicillin rash, erythema multiforme, the Stevens-Johnson syndrome, toxic epidermal necrolysis or other exfoliative dermatitides, delayed (non-IgE mediated) eczema, drug fever, hemolytic anemia, or intestinal nephritis.

The basic process of the acute desensitization procedure involves the serial, fairly rapid administration of doses of a beta-lactam antibiotic in small increments of increasing strength over a short time course. In the usual situation the penicillin drug allergic patient is able to take a fixed amount of the medication to which he is allergic in this fashion without reaction or with minor controllable anaphylactic reactions.

The precise mechanism involved in the successful desensitization process to a drug like penicillin is not known. For many years it was assumed that mast cell–basophil preformed mediators (such as histamine) were being depleted. We now know that this does not completely explain the success of the desensitization procedure. Other hypotheses include antigen specific desensitization of tissue mast cells, hapten inhibition by the induction of circulating monovalent drug conjugates, the binding of circulating antipenicillin IgE antibodies by small amounts of drug haptens, and, finally, some induction of IgG antipenicillin "blocking antibodies."

It is recognized that a refractory period exists immediately following a penicillin anaphylactic reaction. Such a refractory period also occurs in the case of reactions to drugs not involving an IgE mechanism (e.g., aspirin). In some way the refractory period is induced by the desensitization procedure, allowing a "window of opportunity" to administer a necessary drug. Once

the cumulative drug dosage necessary to fight the infection process has been reached in the patient, this top dosage can be maintained in the allergic patient (chronic desensitization) as long as the interval between drug doses is not longer than 8 to 12 hours. If the interval of drug administration at this top dosage is prolonged beyond this narrow time frame, life threatening anaphylaxis may occur upon further drug administration as the refractory period or desensitized state dissolves.

DESENSITIZATION PROCEDURES: GENERAL PRINCIPLES

The desensitization procedure should be carried out with the appropriate informed consent of the patient, parent, or guardian. The procedure should be done under controlled conditions, such as in a hospital intensive care unit, so that not only can the patient be closely monitored but any adverse reaction to the drug administered during the procedure can be promptly recognized and appropriately treated. Whenever possible, the desensitization procedure should be performed on an elective basis instead of as an emergency—during the week and during regular hours so as to have the best chance of having available the optimal levels of support services and personnel for patient care. Any potential complicating factors should be corrected—if possible—before drug desensitization is started. This may include the control of urticaria, asthma, or shock and the discontinuation of beta-blocking drugs (and the control of disease by safer medications).

Premedication of the patient with antiallergic medications, such as those routinely used in patients with a history of adverse reactions to conventional radiocontrast media—such as antihistamines, cortisone, cimetidine, or ephedrine sulfate—is not recommended. It is important not to mask any early signs of anaphylaxis to the drug used in the desensitization process so that these reactions can be properly treated. The clinical status and vital signs should be monitored frequently throughout the procedure and throughout the first 12 hours of full dosage drug treatment. Finally, and most important, a knowledgeable physician should be present with the patient throughout the process.

DESENSITIZATION PROTOCOL: GUIDELINES

Individual protocols have been published by several authors over the years to help guide the less knowledgeable or less experienced physician through the desensitization procedure. The most widely published experience utilizing the desensitization procedure in patients who are allergic to penicillin involves the collective work of a single group of investigators.[5,13] Table 2

TABLE 2 Oral Desensitization Protocol*

Step†	Phenoxymethyl Penicillin (U/ml)	Amount (ml)	Dose (U)	Cumulative Dosage (U)
1	1,000	0.1	100	100
2	1,000	0.2	200	300
3	1,000	0.4	400	700
4	1,000	0.8	800	1,500
5	1,000	1.6	1,600	3,100
6	1,000	3.2	3,200	6,300
7	1,000	6.4	6,400	12,700
8	10,000	1.2	12,000	24,700
9	10,000	2.4	24,000	48,700
10	10,000	4.8	48,000	96,700
11	80,000	1.0	80,000	176,700
12	80,000	2.0	160,000	336,700
13	80,000	4.0	320,000	656,700
14	80,000	8.0	640,000	1,296,700

Observe patient for 30 minutes

Change to benzylpenicillin G — IV

15	500,000 U/ml	0.25	125,000	
16	500,000	0.50	250,000	
17	500,000	1.0	500,000	
18	500,000	2.25	1,125,000	

* From Sullivan TJ. Penicillin allergy. In: Lichtenstein LM, Fauci AS, eds. Current therapy in allergy, immunology and rheumatology. Toronto: BC Decker, 1985: 60.
† Interval between steps: 15 minutes.

represents an oral penicillin desensitization protocol devised by this group.*

Although the initial dose in the protocol (step 1) indicates 100 units, the author indicated that desensitization in patients who are very sensitive (e.g., penicillin prick rather than intradermal skin test positive) may be started at even more dilute antigen concentrations of 10 units, 1 unit, or 0.1 unit. The recommended interval between dosing is 15 minutes. This can be lengthened, however, in the patient who demonstrates reactions. Following stabilization of the patient who does react during the procedure, the next dose of desensitizing drug should be at a strength no greater than that two steps below the dose that precipitated the reaction.

As far as penicillin allergy is concerned, desensitization utilizing the oral route has been shown to be safer than any parenteral route (fewer reactions during the procedure).[5,13] In the case of allergy to the semisynthetic penicillins or cephalosporins, desensitization with oral penicillin therapy will not suffice. If oral drug forms of these other beta-lactam antibiotics are available, individual protocols should be made up, adapting to the general principles outlined in Table 2 for penicillin. On the other hand, when no oral beta-lactam antibiotic drug form exists, a parenteral desensitization protocol should be followed (Table 3). The experience of Stark et al,[5] utilizing the oral route of desensitization followed by beta-lactam antibiotic treatment in both adults and children for 1 to 40 days, shows a reaction incidence with the procedure of 38 percent. This incidence can be broken down further. Reactions during the acute desensitization process are as follows: pruritus, 4 percent; urticaria or angioedema, 5 percent; wheezing, 1 percent; total, 10 percent. Reactions during beta-lactam antibiotic therapy following attainment of the top dose during the desensitization process are as follows: pruritus, 3 percent; urticaria, 18 percent; large local reaction, 1 percent; serum sickness, 3 percent; hemolytic anemia, 1 percent; and glomerulonephritis, 1 percent. The total incidence of immunologic complications of the subsequent drug therapy was reported to be 27 percent. Stark and colleagues[5] also have shown that following the acute desensitization procedure, patients needing antibiotics for long periods may be maintained in the refractory or desensitized state for 3 weeks to more than 2 years (median duration, 10 weeks' therapy). In all cases the full dosage of therapy was given orally in divided doses daily, no longer than 12 hours apart.

Once therapy with the beta-lactam antibiotics has been completed, and antibiotics used in the desensiti-

*Lichtenstein LM, Fauci AS, eds. Current therapy in allergy, immunology and rheumatology. Toronto: BC Decker, 1985: 60–61.

TABLE 3 Parenteral Desensitization Protocol*

Step†	Concentration of β-Lactam Drug (mg/ml)	Amount (ml subcutaneously)	Dose (mg)	Cumulative Dosage (mg)
1	0.1	0.10	0.01	.01
2	0.1	0.20	0.02	.03
3	0.1	0.40	0.04	.07
4	0.1	0.80	0.08	.15
5	1	0.15	0.15	.30
6	1	0.30	0.3	.60
7	1	0.60	0.6	1.2
8	10	0.10	1	2.2
9	10	0.20	2	4.2
10	10	0.40	4	8.2
11	10	0.80	8	16.2
12	100	0.15	15	31.2
13	100	0.30	30	61.2
14	100	0.60	60	121.2
15	1,000	0.10	100	221.2
16	1,000	0.20	200	421.2
17	1,000	0.40	400	821.2
18	1,000	0.50	500	1,321.2
		Observe patient for 30 minutes		
19	1,000	IV	0.5 g	1,821.2
20	1,000	IV	1.5 g	3,321.2

* From Sullivan TJ. Penicillin allergy. In: Lichtenstein LM, Fauci AS, eds. Current therapy in allergy, immunology and rheumatology. Toronto: BC Decker, 1985: 61.

zation procedure or treatment have been stopped, the penicillin allergic patient is again at risk for reaction to a beta-lactam antibiotic. At a future date, if beta-lactam antibiotics are again needed, retesting and, if appropriate, desensitization are indicated.

Newer antibiotics, such as the newer penicillins, cephalosporins, or structurally unique monobactams, may be less reactive than the presently commercially available beta-lactam antibiotics. In the future these safer substitute antibiotics may become available for beta-lactam sensitive individuals.

NON-IgE MEDIATED IMMUNOLOGIC AND OTHER ADVERSE REACTIONS TO BETA-LACTAM ANTIBIOTICS

Other nonanaphylactic (but immunologic) reactions to the penicillins include hemolytic anemia, neutropenia and thrombocytopenia, serum sickness, glomerulonephritis, drug fever, and various cutaneous reactions. The antibody usually involved in the production of penicillin induced hemolytic anemia is IgG, although IgM and

IgA types of penicillin antibodies also have been implicated.[1] Positive direct antiglobulin (Coombs) tests can develop in 3 percent of the patients who receive large intravenous doses of penicillins. Only a small percentage of these patients, however, actively develop hemolytic anemia. Inhibition of factor VIII (blood coagulation factor) activity has been attributed to the presence of antipenicillin antibodies.

Penicillin is the most common cause of drug induced serum sickness-like reactions today. This syndrome of fever, rash, arthralgia, and arthritis results from circulating IgG and IgM drug-antibody complexes.[5] The local deposition of drug-antibody complexes is facilitated by IgE release of vasoactive amines. Antipenicillin IgE is involved in the urticarial rash associated with this condition. The reactions typically occur 7 to 14 days into therapy but may occur weeks following termination of the penicillin therapy. The majority of serum sickness-like reactions are mild and resolve spontaneously within a few days to weeks, although some may be treatable with cortisone.

Penicillin may induce drug fever. The penicillins, especially methacillin, have been associated with the induction of nephritis. One of the most common manifestations of an adverse reaction to a beta-lactam antibiotic is a maculopapular rash, which occurs with ampicillin therapy (approximately 5 percent risk). The risk of this rash has been reported to be higher in patients afflicted with Epstein-Barr virus (infectious mononucleosis) or cytomegalovirus infection than in chronic lymphocytic leukemia and hyperuricemia and patients receiving an allopurinol drug concomitantly. This rash is not associated with an IgE antibody; it has been shown to be safe to continue ampicillin in spite of this rash without adverse effects. However, since IgE drug antibody may involve a maculopapular rash, it may be impossible to definitively determine that the patient taking ampicillin who has a rash is not sensitive to penicillin. Therefore, in most cases ampicillin therapy, in such situations, should be discontinued. Two or more weeks following the episode involving the rash, and when the patient is stable, elective penicillin skin testing is recommended to determine the patient's allergic status. If penicillin skin testing is negative, reinstitution of any penicillin product should be considered safe for the immediate future.

Most serious cutaneous and mucocutaneous reactions to the beta-lactam antibiotics involve a rash such as erythema multiforme and either the Stevens-Johnson syndrome or toxic epidermal necrolysis or Lyell's syndrome. The latter types of febrile mucocutaneous syndromes are of particular importance in that they cannot be predicted, the prodrome is similar to an infectious disease, and in its severest form toxic epidermal necrolysis has been reported to be associated with up to a 30 percent mortality.[14] Although these reactions are allergy-like, IgE immune reactions have not been shown to be involved. Skin testing to penicillins is not helpful. In the few instances in which penicillin has been given on another occasion in patients who had such reactions, a repeated episode of the reaction has been documented. Penicillin desensitization has not been shown to be successful in such reactions and is not recommended.

It is well to point out that the desensitization process is applicable only in instances in which IgE immune reactions to penicillin are involved. Furthermore, the IgE desensitization procedure does not prevent the onset of serum sickness-like reactions, hemolytic anemia, or glomerulonephritis, as has been shown by the work of

Stark et al.[5] In all the cases of non-IgE adverse reactions to the beta-lactam antibiotics, data are insufficient to indicate that it is safe to readminister the beta-lactam antibiotics or to desensitize the patients, regardless of the specific mechanism of these reactions.

REFERENCES

1. DeSwarte RD. Special consideration of allergic drug problems: the beta-lactam antibiotics—penicillins and cephalosporins. In: Paterson R, ed. Allergic diseases: diagnosis and management. Philadelphia: JB Lippincott, 1985: 595.
2. Bigby M, Jick S, Jick H, Arndt K. Drug-induced cutaneous reactions—report from the Boston Collaborative Drug Surveillance Program on 15,438 consecutive inpatients, 1975–1982. JAMA 1986, 256:3358–3363.
3. Sogn DD. Penicillin allergy. J Allergy Clin Immunol 1984; 74:589–593.
4. Green G, Rosenblum A, Sweet L. Evaluation of penicillin hypersensitivity: value of clinical history and skin testing with penicilloyl-polylysine and penicillin G. J Allergy Clin Immunol 1977; 60:339–345.
5. Stark B, Earl H, Gross G, Lumry W, Goodman E, Sullivan T. Acute and chronic desensitization of penicillin-allergic patients using oral penicillin. J Allergy Clin Immunol 1987; 79:523–532.
6. Sullivan T, Wedner H, Shatz G, Yecies L, Parker G. Skin testing to detect penicillin allergy. J Allergy Clin Immunol 1981; 68:171–180.
7. Sogn D, Casale T, Condemi J, Evans R, Greenberger P, Kohler P, Saxon A, Shepherd G, Summers R, VanArsdel P, Levine B. Interim results of the NIAID collaborative clinical trial of skin testing with major and minor penicillin derivatives in hospitalized adults. J Allergy Clin Immunol 1983; 71 (Suppl):147 (abstract).
8. Sullivan T. Personal communication
9. Earl H, Stark B, Sullivan T. Penicillin induced IgE re-sensitization. J Allergy Clin Immunol 1987; 79:200 (abstract).
10. Mendelson L, Ressler C, Rosen J, Selcon J. Routine elective penicillin allergy skin testing in children and adolescents. J Allergy Clin Immunol 1984; 73:76–81.
11. Mendelson L, Ressler C, Page J, Selow J, Rosen J. Elective testing of penicillin allergic patients. J. Allergy Clin Immunol 1987; 79:200 (abstract).
12. Anderson J. Cross-sensitivity to cephalosporins in patients allergic to penicillin. Pediatr Infect Dis 1986; 5:557–561.
13. Sullivan T, Yecies L, Shatz G, Parker C, Wedner HJ. Desensitization of patients allergic to penicillin using orally administered beta-lactam antibiotics. J Allergy Clin Immunol 1982; 69:275–282.
14. Strom J. Aetiology of febrile mucocutaneous syndromes with special reference to the provocative role of infections and drugs. Acta Med Scan 1977; 201:131–136.

DRUG REACTIONS

DOROTHY D. SOGN, M.D.
PAUL P. VanARSDEL Jr., M.D.

The frequency of drug reactions is unknown. By estimate, in excess of 1 million American outpatients have drug reactions, necessitating 50,000 hospitalizations per annum. Additionally some believe that as many as 30 percent of all hospitalized patients (each receiving a mean of nine drugs) develop drug reactions. Most of these clinical events (approximately 75 percent) are nonimmunologic and are outlined in Table 1. According to the Coombs and Gell classification, there are four major types of immune mediated reactions.

CLASSIFICATION OF IMMUNE MEDIATED DRUG REACTIONS

The type I or immediate type of hypersensitivity reaction is responsible for common allergic reactions, including hay fever, some types of asthma, and hives as well as drug reactions leading to urticaria, angioedema, bronchospasm, hypotension, and anaphylactic shock. This type of reaction is mediated by immunoglobulin E (IgE). Drug reactions with clinical manifestations identical to type I reactions but not involving IgE are known as anaphylactoid reactions.

TABLE 1   Examples of Nonallergic Drug Reactions*

Overdosage

  May result from impaired handling of normal doses or excess intake

  Example: theophylline induced vomiting and headaches

Idiosyncratic reactions

  May result from unusual resistance to large doses or unexpected responses to ordinary or even low doses

  Example: Isoniazid induced polyneuritis

Side effects or unavoidable nontherapeutic effects

  Example: Tremulousness induced by metaproterenol (Alupent, Metaprel)

Paradoxical effects or effects opposite those expected

  Example: Sedative induced hyperactivity

Drug interactions

  Example: Deep sleep induced by simultaneous ingestion of tranquilizers and alcohol

*From Sogn D. How to avoid allergic reactions. Drug Therapy Clinical Therapeutics in the Hospital 1983; 73–81.

Type II reactions are dependent on complement and involve antibody directed against a cell membrane or cell membrane associated antigen, exemplified by certain drug induced anemias or thrombocytopenias.

Type III reactions are mediated by antigen-antibody complexes and are best illustrated by serum sickness reactions.

In the type IV reactions, sensitized thymus dependent lymphocytes are the mediators. Classic examples are contact dermatitides such as poison ivy, but can include contact type reactions to drugs such as neomycin and drug additives such as parabens and ethylenediamine.

An approach to drug allergy must comprise an understanding of the prevention, diagnosis, and treatment of these reactions. The focus in this article is the management of anaphylactic and anaphylactoid drug reactions.

PREVENTION AND DIAGNOSIS

As with other types of allergies, avoidance of the offending allergen is the best approach to management. Since avoiding a needed drug is not always an option, it is useful to screen patients at high risk for an allergic reaction to a given drug. For these reasons discussions of diagnosis and prevention are virtually inseparable when considering drug allergy.

In diagnosing drug allergy, as a first step a careful history of prior drug reactions must be obtained. Attention must be given to such factors as the nature and timing of the reaction, whether concurrent medications were being taken, and the nature of the underlying illness.

In the many cases when the history is ambiguous or multiple drugs are suspected, a confirmatory immunoassay would be of great help. Unfortunately such assays are few. The diagnostic value of skin testing with penicillin major and minor determinants has been discussed elsewhere, and as of this writing, a minor determinant mix is not commercially available. Prick and intradermal skin testing also should be employed prior to administration of protein or polypeptide agents such as heterologous antisera, including antithymocyte globulin and the increasingly used therapeutic monoclonal antibodies. Prick and, if negative, intradermal skin testing, read at 20 minutes, with dilutions $\frac{1}{10}$ and $\frac{1}{100}$, respectively, of these agents will reveal the presence or absence of reaginic antibody to these substances. Such testing is helpful only in predicting the risk of the immediate type of hypersensitivity.

When a convincing history of drug allergy with or without confirmatory immunoassay is obtained, reassessment of the need for the drug should be undertaken. This reassessment may include culture documentation of bacterial or viral infections or the ordering and review of other laboratory data. If the need for the drug is affirmed, consideration of an alternative drug should be pursued. Factors such as efficacy, side effects, and possible cross reactivity with the drug to which the patient is allergic must be weighed in making a decision.

Occasionally a drug can be administered even in the face of a convincing history of reaction to it. Such is the case with known anaphylactoid reactors to injection with radiographic contrast dye who are in need of a repeat procedure. The risk of a repeat reaction in such a patient ranges from 17 to 35 percent. A prophylactic regimen consisting of prednisone, 50 mg orally every 6 hours for three administrations and ending 1 hour prior to the procedure, and diphenhydramine, 50 mg intramuscularly 1 hour before the procedure, has been shown to reduce the risk of repeat reactions to 10.8 percent (usually minor skin reactions). The addition of ephedrine sulfate (25 mg) to this regimen was associated with a lessening of the reaction incidence to 5 percent. The addition of cimetidine hydrochloride was not useful; 14 reactions occurred during 100 procedures (14.0 percent).

A not infrequent clinical situation is that of the egg sensitive individual in need of immunization. Mumps, measles, influenza, typhus, and yellow fever vaccines are grown on materials originating from chickens, such that trace amounts of ovalbumin (0.5 to 1.0 ng) can be detected in these products. Reports of anaphylaxis in children with known egg allergy have occasioned a closer look at this population in which IgE directed against the ovalbumin in the vaccine could be detected. Results of these studies indicate that only patients with histories of anaphylactic reactions to egg are at high risk. These patients should undergo skin testing by the prick or scratch method with a $\frac{1}{10}$ dilution of the vaccine, followed by intradermal testing with a $\frac{1}{100}$ dilution if the result is negative. Negative responders have safely received the vaccine, but positive responders (with positive histories) should receive the vaccine only by slow incremental dosing.

A variation in the treatment of herniated lumbar disks came with the commercial availability of a papaya tree derived enzyme called chymopapain, which is capable of solubilizing the mucopolysaccharide of the human nucleus pulposus. Some 200,000 Americans are thought to be candidates for this procedure annually. A major drawback to this therapy is the development of anaphylaxis in an estimated 1 percent of the recipients. As a result of this observation, it has been appreciated that a large number of people outside the papain industry are exposed to and become sensitized to this substance through numerous exposures, including debriding ointments, digestive aids, some contact lens solutions, meat tenderizers, and beer. Thus, a careful history for papain hypersensitivity must be obtained. Since the procedure is performed with the aid of radiographic contrast dye, this hypersensitivity must also be ruled out. Premedication of the patient with antihistamines and steroids cannot be relied upon in the prevention of chymopapain

induced anaphylaxis. Patterson et al recommend the skin testing of candidates for these injections with chymopapain dilutions in saline with 0.1 percent human serum albumin as a stabilizer, proceeding with the medication only in skin test negative patients. Clinical trials to further study the efficacy of such screening techniques are about to commence.

Anaphylactoid reactions to aspirin affect about 1 million Americans. Reactions usually manifest as either wheezing or urticaria. About 4 percent of all asthmatics demonstrate aspirin sensitivity by exacerbations of wheezing. Another small group of asthmatics suffer from a triad of symptoms consisting of chronic sinusitis, nasal polyposis, and severe (usually late onset) asthma in addition to aspirin sensitivity. Because this reaction is not IgE mediated, patients can tolerate chemically similar compounds, including naturally occurring salicylates, but not certain nonsteroidal anti-inflammatory compounds such as mefenamic acid (Ponstel), ibuprofen (Motrin, Rufen), phenylbutazone, fenoprofen (Nalfon), naproxen (Anaprox, Naprosyn), and flufenamic acid. The diagnosis is usually made through the history; only occasionally is provocation testing needed. Acetaminophen is a useful aspirin substitute in these patients. The possible usefulness of aspirin desensitization for the treatment of asthma in certain aspirin sensitive asthmatics remains an intriguing therapeutic possibility.

DRUG ADDITIVES

Drug reactions may be induced by additives used to color or preserve drug preparations. Of particular concern are additives in medications used to treat allergic conditions, because they not only cause reactions but may confuse the diagnosis.

Certain stabilizing and bacteriostatic additives, such as ethylenediamine, thimerosol, and parabens, which are in some skin preparations, are associated with the induction of contact dermatitis (Coombs and Gell type IV). On re-exposure to these substances, even by another route, the patient may have a reaction.

Fisher described ethylenediamine allergic patients who experienced a hematogenous contact type of dermatitis upon receipt of theophylline ethylenediamine (aminophylline), or certain antihistamines. Patients receiving paraben containing medications can experience similar reactions. Thimerosal is a common contact sensitizer with widespread use, including some contact lens solutions and many vaccines. Very few data exist relating to challenging patients with clinical histories of thimerosal sensitivity or positive skin test results with this chemical.

Metabisulfites, antibrowning agents used in many foods and medications, are increasingly appreciated as

TABLE 2   Summary Outline of Anaphylaxis Treatment

General
    Epinephrine
    Tourniquet (when physically possible)
    Intravenous line, dextrose, in 0.5 normal saline
    Oxygen and emergency equipment on hand

Hypotension
    Epinephrine, slow intravenous; large volumes of dextrose in
        0.5 normal saline
    ECG monitor
    Monitor central venous pressure
    Vasopressor drug (?)

Upper airway obstruction
    Epinephrine
    Diphenhydramine
    Oxygen
    Endotrachial intubation or tracheostomy

Lower airway obstruction
    Epinephrine, isoproterenol
    Oxygen
    Aminophylline, intravenous
    Prepare for treatment of respiratory failure

Cardiac problems
    ECG monitor for dysrhythmias
    Monitor pulmonary artery wedge pressure
    Isoproterenol for cardiogenic shock

Late reactions
    Observe and monitor as necessary for 12 hours
    Glucocorticoid therapy

inducing asthmatic attacks. Steroid dependent asthmatics are considered at high risk for these reactions.

Desensitization, the administration of a drug by cautious incremental dosing, also can be undertaken when use of an allergy provoking drug is unavoidable. Although termed "desensitization," the exact mechanism(s) explaining this phenomenon is unknown; hypotheses include consumption of IgE in immune complexes, hapten inhibition, mast cell desensitization, and mediator depletion. This procedure is risky and should be undertaken in a controlled setting such as an intensive care unit where full capability for resuscitation is available. Guidelines for the treatment of anaphylaxis are shown in Table 2.

A general scheme for such drug administration consists of the subcutaneous administration of 0.1 ml of the concentration of the material giving the smallest positive skin reaction. The dose is progressively doubled every 15 to 30 minutes if tolerated until 1 ml of the undiluted medication has been administered. At this point the route is switched to intramuscular and then the full dose is given.

Allergic symptoms are treated as they occur and the timing of drug administration is adjusted accordingly, no further dosing being given until symptoms have resolved. Some allergists prefer to premedicate

patients undergoing desensitization, hoping to mitigate reactions; others do not premedicate, reasoning that early warning of major allergic reactions may be masked by such therapy.

Desensitization regimens have been tailored for insulin and penicillin allergy and are discussed elsewhere. Of particular interest because of its safety is the successful oral desensitization to penicillin associated with antigen specific desensitization of tissue mast cells.

Because performing a densensitization regimen is likely to be associated with provocation of symptoms, this is a logical point in the discussion to mention treatment modalities.

TREATMENT

Reactions that are thought to be allergic are listed in Table 3. Their clinical features are not discussed here except as they determine the type of treatment needed. In general, if a reaction develops, treatment with the suspected drug or drugs should be stopped unless, in the physician's judgment, the need for treatment is greater than the risk of the reaction and its symptoms

TABLE 3   Classification of Drug Reactions

Mast cell mediated reactions
    Systemic anaphylaxis
    Urticaria and angioedema
    Some pruritic maculopapular eruptions
    Serum sickness (in part)
    Anaphylactoid (nonimmunologic)

T-lymphocyte mediated reactions
    Allergic eczematous contact dermatitis

Photodermatitis

Other cutaneous reactions (mechanism uncertain)
    Maculopapular or exanthematous reactions
    Fixed eruptions
    Toxic epidermal necrolysis

Drug fever

Systemic lupus erythematosus and other autoimmune reactions

Organ systems reactions
    Blood: eosinophilia, hemolytic anemia, thrombocytopenia,
        granulocytopenia
    Lung
    Liver
    Kidney

Reactions with inconsistent drug associations
    Erythema multiforme
    Exfoliative dermatitis
    Vasculitis

can be controlled. Stopping treatment is a necessary step only for nonpruritic skin rashes, drug fever, and most reactions involving the major organ systems.

Pruritus

Urticaria and other pruritic skin rashes are treated with hydroxyzine, 25 to 100 mg by mouth (Atarax) or intramuscularly (Vistaril). Treatment can be repeated every 6 to 8 hours as needed until the eruption subsides. Alternative drugs are diphenhydramine (Benadryl), 25 to 100 mg and cyproheptadine (Periactin), 4 to 8 mg. The main side effect of treatment is drowsiness, not usually a problem with the hospitalized patient, but any ambulatory patient should be warned about the risk of operating a motor vehicle or other machinery while taking one of these drugs. Skin testing for IgE mediated sensitivity cannot be performed for at least 72 hours after the last dose of hydroxyzine and 48 hours after the last dose of the others. If the foregoing treatment is inadequate, one might consider adding an H_2 antihistamine, such as cimetidine or ranantidine, or substituting the tricyclic antihistamine doxepin, but the reaction is more likely to resolve if oral prednisone therapy, 40 mg daily, is given and rapidly tapered to zero when the reaction subsides.

Pain

Pain may be a prominent symptom with some reactions. The arthralgias of serum sickness and systemic lupus erythematosus and the cutaneous pain in vasculitis and some cases of urticaria can be treated with a nonsteroidal anti-inflammatory drug such as indomethacin (Indocin), 25 to 50 mg every 8 hours. If this is inadequate, prednisone treatment should be initiated (to be discussed).

Anaphylaxis

The treatment is summarized in Table 3 according to the usual sequence of events. Since shock and upper airway obstruction are the most likely causes of death, vital signs and the adequacy of respiration should be carefully followed from the onset of the reaction. As indicated in Table 3, epinephrine is effective in alleviating most of the features of anaphylaxis; 0.3 to 0.5 mg in a 1:1000 concentration should be given subcutaneously immediately. If the offending drug (an allergenic extract is a good example) was injected into an extremity, the injection site should be infiltrated with another 0.2 mg and a tourniquet placed above it. This usually is sufficient to prevent progression of the reaction.

Hypotension

If the patient is hypotensive (systolic pressure less than 60 mm), an intravenous line must be placed and a crystalloid solution such as 5 percent dextrose in 0.5 normal saline infused rapidly. Three to 4 liters of fluid may need to be infused to restore the plasma volume. Epinephrine is then infused through a side line at a dilution high enough (e.g., 1:100,000) to allow delivery of the drug at a rate of about 5 to 10 μg per minute, with continuous electrocardiographic monitoring for arrhythmias. Anaphylaxis may occur in a patient who has been taking a beta-adrenergic blocking drug. In such a patient epinephrine resistance may be overcome by increasing the dose, but this maneuver demands careful monitoring for side effects. Ancillary intravenous treatment with both the H_1 antihistamine diphenhydramine (Benadryl), 100 mg and the H_2 antihistamine cimetidine (Tagamet), 300 mg or ranitidine (Zantac), 50 mg, may be advisable. If the blood pressure remains low in the face of a rising central venous pressure, cardiogenic shock may have developed (to be discussed).

Upper Airway Obstruction

Hoarseness, stridor, or the use of accessory respiratory muscles should alert the observer to the possibility of obstructing angioedema. If this happens, diphenhydramine (Benadryl), 100 mg, should be given intravenously in addition to epinephrine, which can be given subcutaneously every 20 minutes. If a number 6 or 7 endotracheal tube cannot be inserted, one must be prepared to perform a tracheostomy or cricothyroid membrane puncture. Oxygen must be provided.

Lower Airway Obstruction

A few patients develop symptoms and signs of asthma as part of the anaphylactic reaction. Their treatment should be supplemented with the intravenous administration of aminophylline, 6 mg per kg over 20 minutes, followed by another 3 mg per kg if necessary. If the symptoms have not subsided, the drug should be continued in a constant infusion of 0.5 mg per kg per hour, adjusted to maintain the blood level at 10 to 20 g per ml. If toxic symptoms or signs appear (nausea, cardiac dysrhythmia), the infusion should be stopped until they subside. If the patient also is hypotensive, the aminophylline dose should be reduced by 50 percent.

Cardiac Problems

Dysrhymias may develop from a combination of factors such as drugs, anaphylactogenic mediators, and hypoxia. If a dysrhythmia develops, it is treated by conventional methods that need not be described here. If hypotension persists despite epinephrine infusion and fluid replacement, the patient is usually maximally vaso-constricted and adding treatment with an alpha-adren-ergic vasopressor drug serves no useful purpose. Usually pressure monitoring reveals a reduced cardiac output, which should be treated with isoproterenol (Isuprel), 1 to 5 μg per minute intravenously, with continuous elec-trocardiographic monitoring. Serving also as a broncho-dilator, this drug has a modest advantage over the alternative drugs dopamine and dobutamine.

Prevention of Late Reactions

The acute and potentially life threatening reactions usually resolve within 1 hour. A resurgence of the reaction, less serious but still uncomfortable, may appear 4 to 10 hours later. This may be prevented by giv-ing methylprednisolone (Solu-Medrol), 40 mg intrave-nously, after all other treatment has been started; this, or 40 mg of prednisone by mouth, can be given again 6 hours later. If no new symptoms develop within 12 hours after the onset, it is unlikely that any will appear later.

Glucocorticoid Treatment

Severe reactions should be treated with oral doses of prednisone or intravenous doses of methylpredniso-lone, 40 to 60 mg daily, from the start. In addition to the treatment of severe urticaria and serum sickness, and of the late phase of anaphylaxis already discussed, a glucocorticoid may be useful in the treatment of allergic contact dermatitis, erythema multiforme, and exfoliative dermatitis. Glucocorticoid treatment may also hasten recovery from pulmonary, hepatic, and hematologic re-actions. Toxic epidermal necrolysis, vasculitis, and in-terstitial nephritis do not usually respond to glucocorti-coids.

SUGGESTED READING

Drug allergy. NIH Publication 82–703, 1982, p. 1. Cited in: Sogn D. How to avoid allergic drug reactions. Drug Therapy Clinical Ther-apeutics in the Hospital 1983; 73–81.

Fisher AA. Allergic dermatitis medicamentosa: the systemic contact-type variety. Cutis 1976; 18: 637–641.

Greenberger PA, Patterson R, Tapio CM. Prophylaxis against repeated radiocontrast media reactions in 857 cases. Arch Intern Med 1985; 145:2197–2200.

Herman J, Radin R, et al. Allergic reactions to measles (rubeola) vaccine in patients hypersensitive to egg protein. J Pediatr 1983; 102:196–199.

Miller JR, Orgel HA, Meltzer EO. The safety of egg-containing vaccine for egg-allergic patients. J Allergy Clin Immunol 1983; 71:568–573.

Patterson R, Anderson J. Allergic reactions to drugs and biologic agents. In: Salvaggio JE, ed. Primer on allergic and immunologic diseases. JAMA 1982; 248:2643–2644.

Patterson R, DeSwarte RD, Greenberger PA, Grammer LC. Drug allergy and protocols for management of drug allergies. New En-gland and Regional Allergy Proceedings 1986; 325–342.

Stark BJ, Earl HS, Gross GN, et al. Acute and chronic desensitization of penicillin-allergic patients. J Allergy Clin Immunol 1987; 79:523–532.

Sullivan T. Antigen-specific desensitization of patients allergic to penicillin. J Allergy Clin Immunol 1982; 69:500–508.

VanArsdel PP Jr. Diagnosing drug allergy. JAMA 1982; 247:2576–2581.

INSECT STING ALLERGY IN ADULTS

LAWRENCE M. LICHTENSTEIN, M.D., Ph.D.

Sensitivity to the venoms of Hymenoptera species (honeybee, yellow hornet, white hornet, yellow jacket, and Polistes wasp) is far more common than generally supposed. An epidemiologic study carried out by Golden at Johns Hopkins demonstrated that fully 20 to 25 percent of the population is sensitive as judged by a

Study supported by grant A108270 from the National Institutes of Health, Bethesda, Maryland.

positive skin test result or a serum IgE antibody deter-mination. Usually these two indices of sensitivity co-exist. However, of this large group of sensitive individ-uals, only 3.3 percent have a history of systemic reactions, a larger number experiencing large local reactions. In a prospective study we found that approximately 20 per-cent of these skin test positive, history negative individ-uals have a systemic reaction when stung by the appro-priate insect.

It is, of course, necessary to become sensitized by a sting before one can have a reaction on being stung again. However, individuals may become sensitized by one sting or may be stung repeatedly for many years before suddenly becoming sensitive. As with other types of atopy, we have no information regarding what causes a sting to sensitize an individual.

The clinical manifestations of insect sting allergy are quite variable. A large local reaction is defined as a reaction at the site of the sting that is 8 cm or larger;

these evolve over 24 to 48 hours, resolving in the next 2 to 7 days. The majority of these large local reactions are IgE mediated and are accompanied by demonstrable IgE antibodies or positive skin test results to the appropriate venom. Individuals with large local reactions rarely (less than 5 percent) have a subsequent systemic reaction. Systemic reactions range from mild erythema to fatal shock. Although skin reactions are most common, the majority of adults also have respiratory symptoms, which may involve laryngeal edema or more diffuse bronchospasm, and approximately 30 percent have vascular symptoms, which may lead to hypotension and death. Individual patients may have many other manifestations, gastrointestinal symptoms of nausea, crampiness, or diarrhea probably being the next most common. In general, the pattern of the last reaction is repeated. That is, urticaria remains urticaria and bronchospasm remains bronchospasm. Although increases in severity can occur with successive stings, this is far rarer than is generally thought.

We have found in general that the patient's history in regard to the type of insect that caused the reaction is unreliable. It is also true that the common names for insects vary from country to country and perhaps from region to region. Many individuals have a characteristic prodrome, which is unique to the individual but repeats before each systemic reaction; the presence of this prodrome is a reliable diagnostic indicator.

DIAGNOSIS

The diagnosis of insect sting allergy is made by an appropriate history together with a positive skin test result. Skin test reagents in insect allergy are useful in a more narrow range than those in inhalant allergy, since the venoms are intrinsically irritating. With ragweed allergy, for example, 90 percent of clinically sensitive individuals have a positive skin test reaction with a concentration many orders of magnitude below that which causes irritation. With venoms this is not the case. Most individuals have a positive response only to 0.1 or 1 μg per ml, and the latter concentration is irritating in rare individuals. We have experimented with using 3 and 10 μg per ml concentrations in difficult patients, but this is not an established procedure. When a skin test result is equivocal or when for some reason this is not desirable, IgE antibody levels can be measured. These are found in about 85 percent of skin test positive individuals and often can be of real help when the skin test result is equivocal. We have seen virtually no individuals who have an appropriate and recent history in the absence of a positive skin test reaction or an increased IgE antibody level. Although others have reported this, it must be extremely rare.

In unusual circumstances individuals react to insect venoms that are not commercially available. Thus, for example, we have treated one individual who appears to be sensitive to sweat bee venom in addition to those of the other Hymenoptera species. A number of individuals are allergic to venom of the Polistes species, which have a very limited environmental niche.

One diagnostic test is of particular utility. In our area about 80 percent of the individuals who have a positive skin test reaction to yellow jacket venom are also sensitive to Polistes venom by skin testing. In most instances this is a cross reactivity and true Polistes sensitivity does not exist. This can be determined by doing a RAST inhibition test, a test that indicates whether a person has any antibodies to Polistes venom antigens, which do not cross react with yellow jacket antigens. Most patients tested are not truly sensitive to Polistes venom. Although this test is expensive, it can save the patient many thousands of dollars over the course of immunotherapy and eliminates immunization with an unneeded venom.

THERAPY

The treatment of an acute reaction to an insect sting is exactly the same as for anaphylaxis induced by any other cause; the treatment of this syndrome is covered in detail in another article in this volume. Epinephrine remains the treatment of choice. Although generalized cutaneous reactions do not necessarily require epinephrine, in the absence of a contraindication it may well stop a developing reaction. With mild reactions the patient must be observed for progression to more serious symptoms. Since most individuals, as noted, have a stereotypic response, epinephrine is used immediately in any individual who previously has had circulatory or respiratory distress. Individuals who are to be given immunotherapy (see following discussion) are supplied with an epinephrine injection kit, which they carry until their IgG antibody level has reached an adequate level. They are instructed to use this immediately and to report promptly to an emergency room. The dose of epinephrine initially is 0.3 to 0.5 cc subcutaneously. This is the only route of administration if the patient is conscious and has an obtainable blood pressure. This dose may be repeated every 10 to 15 minutes if it is not fully effective. Even with a good response to therapy, the patient with a severe reaction must be observed for at least 12 hours. In my opinion an individual who has had severe respiratory or circulatory distress should be hospitalized overnight, since a recurrence of symptoms 16 to 18 hours later may be life threatening.

As with any other sort of anaphylaxis, in addition to the use of epinephrine, the major therapeutic effort is designed to support airway function, applying artificial respiration or intubation if necessary. At times epinephrine does not restore the blood pressure, and in these instances it appears useful to provide large amounts of fluids using preparations that will maintain fluid in the vascular spaces, such as plasminate or albumin.

Most medical texts and emergency room manuals suggest that individuals suffering from anaphylaxis be treated with corticosteroids. There is no indication for corticosteroids during the acute reaction, since they are completely without efficacy. Some like to give these with the thought that they will abort a late phase relapse. Although this may be the case (and it has not been proven), I prefer observation, with prompt retreatment if a recurrence occurs.

Specific measures to prevent the occurrence of insect stings depend primarily on common sense. Patients should not walk barefoot and should avoid flowers, where honeybees may be active, or garbage cans, where yellow jackets are attracted. It is said that the wearing of bright clothes or perfumes can be dangerous.

Venom Immunotherapy

Patient Selection

Death from an insect sting is extremely rare. Literally millions of patients are sensitive, but the number of deaths that occur yearly probably does not exceed 100. However, to those of us who have seen a death or the far more common morbidity associated with the fear of insect stings, it is clear that venom immunotherapy plays a vital role in patient management. Since the therapy is not overly expensive (and should become much less expensive than it is), since it appears to be without serious toxicity, and particularly since it appears that it can be stopped after a number of years, I have no hesitation in recommending therapy to anyone with a serious systemic reaction. This recommendation is more or less forceful depending on the criteria to be discussed and summarized in Table 1. We recommend that all adults who have respiratory or vascular manifestations receive immunotherapy. However, in each case the possibilities and the risks are explored with each patient. Thus, for example, a 25 year old individual with minimal respiratory distress may wish not to undergo therapy, and we may respect this decision if we are sure that the pros and cons are understood.

TABLE 1   Patient Selection for Venom Immunotherapy*

Sting Reaction History	Skin Test, RAST	Venom Immunotherapy
Systemic (adult)	+	Yes
Systemic, life threatening (child)	+	Yes
Systemic, cutaneous (child)	+ or −	No
Systemic	−	No
Large local	+ or −	No
None	+ or −	No

* From Golden DBK. Insect sting allergy in adults. In: Lichtenstein LM, Fauci AS, eds. Current therapy in allergy and immunology 1983–1984. Toronto: BC Decker, 1983: 70–75.

We also recommend immunotherapy for most adults with merely cutaneous reactions. Age here is a major factor, since studies by our group have demonstrated that children with only cutaneous reactions do not require immunotherapy. We have been unable to study enough patients in the age range between 16 and 25 to determine whether they need therapy. However, in a young adult with only cutaneous reactions, we tend, after discussing the pros and cons, to be on the conservative side; whereas with an individual over 50, we tend to be more aggressive in suggesting immunotherapy.

In general, we do not recommend immunotherapy for large local reactions. However, I have offered such therapy to two kinds of individuals: those who are excessively fearful and the rare individual whose large local reaction is debilitating and in whom corticosteroid therapy may be contraindicated. We have not studied large local reactions specifically, but it seems likely from the data we have that immunotherapy is as effective in decreasing these reactions as it is in the systemic reaction.

Insect venom immunotherapy in children is discussed in chapter Sting Allergy in Children. For the sake of completeness I should like to point out that in general we do not treat children who have only cutaneous reactions, although in cases in which there is excessive fear on the part of the parents or the child, this may be done. It might be argued that many children with mild respiratory or vascular effects from stings need not be treated. Although this is probably true, we have been unable to accumulate a large enough group of these individuals to study the problem and we continue to advise immunotherapy in these patients.

Mechanism of Immunotherapy

Our group has been studying the mechanisms by which immunotherapy is effective in a variety of clinical conditions for the last two decades. Only in venom immunotherapy is there a clear-cut relationship between the IgG blocking antibody and clinical projection. A number of studies have demonstrated that patients who have more than 3 to 5 μg of IgG against a venom have a reaction incidence well under 2 percent, whereas individuals with half this much antibody have a significantly higher incidence of reactions. Therefore, as is to be elucidated, we decide on the eventual therapeutic dose of venom and the interval between venom injections by following the IgG antibody level. The significance and utility of IgG antibody measurements begin to disappear in the fourth and fifth years of venom immunotherapy. It can be demonstrated that immunotherapy can be stopped after 5 years (to be discussed) and that clinical protection then bears no relationship to the IgG level. The mechanism of clinical protection after 5 years of immunotherapy is not known.

Method of Immunotherapy

The regimen developed at Johns Hopkins for venom immunotherapy is outlined in Table 2 and contrasted with other recommended regimens. Although achieving maintenance levels of venom is critical to the success of this treatment, it is to be emphasized that the actual schedule by which this dose of venom is achieved may be quite variable. We have chosen a more rapid regimen than that used in most other centers because we have demonstrated that this regimen causes the least number of adverse side reactions. However, in our initial studies of this subject we treated many patients from abroad and in order to limit the duration of their stay in Baltimore often completed venom immunotherapy to maintenance levels in 2 or 3 weeks. Alternatively, in Europe some 1 to 2 day "rush" regimens are used. We see no purpose in these regimens because they require hospitalization and cause many systemic reactions, but in theory there is nothing wrong with this type of approach. From an immunologic point of view it is probably most effective to repeat injections every 10 to 14 days when the IgG response to the previous injection has maximized; however, this extends the time required to reach maintenance levels.

The venoms to be used depend entirely on the skin test response. A rare patient is found who responds only to yellow jacket venom and not to hornet venoms. For practical reasons we rarely treat such individuals with only yellow jacket venom. The dose then would have to be 200 μg rather than 100 μg in many patients, and this would be more expensive than using the mixed vespid therapy. As noted, in most areas outside of Texas, Louisiana, and neighboring areas, true sensitivity to Polistes venom is rare, and patients with positive skin test reactions to this insect venom should undergo RAST inhibition analysis, which in the majority of cases indicates that Polistes therapy is not needed.

As noted, the maintenance level of 100 μg of each

venom was arrived at by trial and error. It is, however, extremely important to reach this level, since, after the fact, we found that half the dose of venom (50 μg) is only 80 percent as effective as the full dose, which gives 98 percent protection. The reader will note that the patient who is sensitive to yellow jacket venom receives 300 μg of mixed vespid venoms as the maintenance dose, which in terms of cross reactivity is about the same as 200 μg of yellow jacket venom. The honeybee sensitive individual, however, receives only 100 μg. In 15 to 20 percent of the cases this 100 μg is not sufficient to avoid mild systemic reactions and has to be increased to 200 μg.

Once a maintenance level is achieved, the interval between injections is gradually increased from 1 week to 1 month. After several months an IgG level is obtained. Most individuals have a level well above 5 μg per ml at this point, and the interval between injections can be increased to every 6 weeks with, again, an IgG level being measured after several months. In at least 10 percent of the cases the immune response on a once monthly regimen is not adequate and the interval must be reduced to 2 weeks or in even rarer circumstances weekly injections to maintain the IgG level at about 3 to 5 μg. As noted, Dr. Golden at our institution has carried out sting challenge studies of individuals with less than 3 μg of antibody and has established clearly that they are at a greater risk of sustaining a systemic reaction than those with higher antibody levels. Although the systemic reactions are rarely serious, it should be the goal of therapy to completely obviate adverse reactions to a sting.

Adverse Reactions

In our experience adverse reactions to venom immunotherapy occur no more frequently than reactions to

TABLE 2   Regimens for Hymenoptera Venom Immunotherapy: Dose (μg)*

Week No.	Johns Hopkins Center for Allergic Diseases	Pharmalgen Package Insert	Albay Package Insert
1	0.1+1+3=4.1	0.001+0.01+0.1=0.111	0.05
2	10	0.1+0.5+1.0=1.6	0.10
3	20	1+5+10=16	0.20
4	40	10+20=30	0.40
5	60	20+30=50	0.50
6	80	30+30=60	1.0
7	100	40+40=80	2
8	100	50+50=100	4
9	—	100	5
10	100	100	10
11	—	—	20
12	—	100	40
13	100	—	60
14	(Repeat monthly)	—	80
15		100	100

* From Golden DBK. Insect sting allergy in adults. In: Lichtenstein LM, Fauci AS, eds. Current therapy in allergy and immunology 1983–1984. Toronto: BC Decker, 1983: 70–75.

injections of inhalant allergens. In that regard our experience apparently differs from that of other centers where the latter reactions are far less frequent. However, it is our opinion that the role of immunotherapy is to develop an adequate IgG antibody response, and if this is done with inhalant allergens, the dose of antigen required will lead to the same frequency of systemic and local reactions. The incidence of systemic reactions to venom immunotherapy is approximately 15 percent. These reactions usually occur at the initiation of venom immunotherapy when the dose is in the low microgram range. It is rare to see such a reaction once a dose above 25 to 50 μg of venom has been achieved. Most of these reactions are minor and, in experienced hands, do not require epinephrine therapy. There has been only one instance in the treatment of several thousand patients in which an injection induced a systemic response that appeared to be life threatening.

When an adverse reaction occurs, the dose is reduced to that (usually half) which caused no reaction and is then gradually increased. One important technique in getting past this point in the immunization regimen at which a systemic reaction occurs is to split the dose. That is, if a patient reacts to an injection of 5 μg of a venom, he will almost always not have an adverse reaction to 2.5 μg given twice at an interval of a half hour. In certain circumstances we have given individuals multiple injections at half hour intervals to expedite the immunization. We have never failed to get a patient to maintenance levels, and as mentioned elsewhere, it is critical to reach this level even in the patient who has severe and recurrent systemic reactions during therapy. In our worst case, reaching maintenance levels required 1 year's therapy with 30 or 40 significant systemic reactions. However, the dose was achieved and the patient has been taking this dose for many years without adverse reactions.

Large local reactions occur in approximately 50 percent of the individuals but rarely interfere with the progress of therapy. These reactions are much less common at doses under 15 μg or greater than 50 μg. In general, the presence of a large local reaction is not a contraindication to continuing the usual schedule of therapy, since it does not indicate that a more severe systemic reaction will occur at higher doses. We ask the patient to try to tolerate this reaction, and if it is overly bothersome, we may pretreat the patient with an antihistamine before the injection and continue this for 24 to 48 hours. In rare situations it has been necessary to pretreat a patient with prednisone to avoid a serious large local reaction. In this instance we would use 30 mg of prednisone 12 hours before the injection with a repeat dose 24 hours later.

Other adverse reactions to venom immunotherapy have not been observed. There are individuals who complain of malaise for a day after the injection, but it is not clear whether this incidence would be different following placebo injections. In a decade of administering venom immunotherapy to thousands of individuals, no long term toxic effect has been seen. Some years ago Yversinger studied beekeepers, who receive 100 to many thousands of times more venom over protracted periods of time, and found that the incidence of disease in this group was not different from that in control subjects. Thus, venom immunotherapy is quite safe.

Monitoring Immunotherapy

Table 3 indicates the way that we follow patients at Johns Hopkins. This is probably more intensive than is necessary in an office practice and is changing as we gain more experience. At the outset of our studies we carried out RAST IgE antivenom analyses in every patient. As noted, this is now necessary only if the skin test result is equivocal or if there is another reason to use a serologic test. We also followed IgE antibody levels over the years of venom immunotherapy with the thought that a decrease in this antibody level or its disappearance would give us an indication of when to stop therapy. The IgE level has not proved useful in this regard and this practice has been largely abandoned.

As already mentioned, however, we believe that

TABLE 3 Monitoring Venom Immunotherapy*

Test	Indication	Frequency
Skin test (venom)	Diagnosis	Pretreatment
	Loss of sensitivity	Every 2 to 3 years
IgE (venom)	Diagnosis	Pretreatment
	Loss of sensitivity	Every 2 to 3 years
IgG (venom)	Response to induction	Pretreatment, achievement of maintenance
	Maintenance efficacy	Maintenance
	Prolonged interval	Every 12 months for 5 years
	Problems during therapy	
Sting challenge	Efficacy of therapy	Maintenance
Leukocyte histamine release	Diagnosis	Pretreatment
RAST inhibition	Vespid venom cross-reactivity	Pretreatment

* From Golden DBK. Insect sting allergy in adults. In: Lichtenstein LM, Fauci AS, eds. Current therapy in allergy and immunology 1983–1984. Toronto: BC Decker, 1983: 70–75.

IgG antibody levels must be monitored closely. We generally draw blood for a baseline value and measure the IgG antibody level in this serum and in the serum obtained about 6 weeks after the maintenance dose of venom immunotherapy has been achieved. Earlier we emphasized the importance of a doubling or tripling of the baseline value. We now think that this is less important and focus on seeing that the patient has at least 5 μg of IgG venom antibody against each insect to which he is sensitive. This level is used to make the decision to increase the interval of venom immunotherapy injections to monthly and, later, every 6 weeks. It probably would be possible to spread injections to intervals of 8 to 10 weeks in a subset of patients who have a particularly good immune response. Since the duration of venom immunotherapy is limited, however, we have not pursued such studies. Once a maintenance regimen is established, IgG antibody levels should be obtained yearly for the first 4 or 5 years. As noted, they have little value after this period.

Cessation of Immunotherapy

To this point the diagnosis and treatment of venom hypersensitivity have been logical and based on firm immunologic principles. Information regarding the cessation of venom immunotherapy is based on clinical observations alone. To our surprise we found that after 5 years of immunotherapy, even in the face of continuing positive skin test results and elevated IgE antibody levels against venom, patients could tolerate a sting with no difficulty. The incidence of reactions is about 3 percent, which is not significantly different from what would be observed if the patient had continued with immunotherapy. These studies have just been completed. Dr. Golden has stung individuals after 1 year or 2 years without venom immunotherapy. He has also stung the first group at yearly intervals for 4 years and most recently repeated a sting 4 weeks after the first, trying to ascertain whether the first sting sensitized people. In all these studies the cited low incidence of reactions has been observed and no serious reactions have been encountered.

Our current position is to explain these data to the patients and advise them that in our opinion it is safe to stop immunotherapy after 5 years. It should be emphasized that this is new clinical information and that employing this strategy requires that both the patient and the physician feel comfortable. Certainly there are some individuals who do not wish to stop therapy (although well over 90 percent follow this course). Further, there are some individuals whose previous reactions have been of such a nature or whose physical condition is such that we would not feel comfortable taking the risk of even a mild systemic reaction. These patients, however, are rare.

The mechanism by which patients are protected after 5 years is not clear. I believe, however, that this protection is the result of the immunotherapy and not simply attributable to the passage of time. The only reliable data one can use to support this belief are derived from our study with children who had cutaneous manifestations. In those studies it was observed that patients taking venom immunotherapy had an incidence of systemic reactions of about 1 percent, whereas those given a placebo had a 10 percent reaction rate. This was highly significant, but since none of the placebo treated children had a reaction that was more serious than the initial reaction, we stopped this therapy after 5 to 7 years. What is of great interest, however, is that in following these two groups of children with field stings, we discovered that the treated group had maintained its 1 percent reaction rate, whereas the untreated group had maintained its 10 percent reaction rate. This strongly suggests that venom immunotherapy had an effect over and above that due to the passage of time.

SUGGESTED READING

Golden DBK, Johnson K, Addison BI, Valentine MD, Kagey-Sobotka A, Lichtenstein LM. Clinical and immunologic observations in patients who discontinue venom immunotherapy. J Allergy Clin Immunol 1986; 77:435–442.

Golden DBK, Kagey-Sobotka A, Valentine MD, Lichtenstein LM. Dose dependence of Hymenoptera venom immunotherapy. J Allergy Clin Immunol 1981; 67:370–374.

Golden DBK, Marsh DG, Kagey-Sobotka A, Addison BI, Friedhoff L, Szklo M, Valentine MD, Lichtenstein LM. Epidemiology of insect sting allergy. JAMA (in press).

Golden DBK, Meyers DA, Kagey-Sobotka A, Valentine MD, Lichtenstein LM. Clinical relevance of the venom-specific immunoglobulin G antibody level during immunotherapy. J Allergy Clin Immunol 1982; 69:489–493.

Golden DBK, Valentine MD, Kagey-Sobotka A, Lichtenstein LM. Regimens of Hymenoptera venom immunotherapy. Ann Intern Med 1980; 92:620.

INSECT STING ALLERGY IN CHILDREN

ROBERT E. REISMAN, M.D.

Allergic reactions due to insect stings are a major medical problem and occur with increased frequency in children. The reaction pattern varies from mild generalized urticaria to severe anaphylaxis, and even death. For individuals at potential risk, the fear of subsequent reactions significantly modifies daily activities and behavior.

The availability of purified venoms has provided a major diagnostic and therapeutic advance and in addition has led to a reinvestigation of the natural history of insect sting allergy. The general guidelines for diagnosis and treatment are applicable to both children and adults. Children may differ significantly in some aspects, including the severity of reactions and the natural history of the disease process.

TYPES OF REACTIONS

Reactions to stinging insects may be classified as follows:

1. Normal reaction. A normal reaction following an insect sting consists of transient pain, swelling, and erythema at the injection site. As a rule, the reaction subsides within 1 hour and requires no treatment.

2. Local reaction. Large local reactions consist of extensive swelling, extending from the sting site to adjacent tissue. Such reactions may peak at 24 to 48 hours and last for up to 1 week. For example, a sting on the back of the hand may extend to the elbow. These reactions are not accompanied by systemic symptoms.

3. Anaphylactic reaction. Anaphylactic reactions following insect stings have the same clinical features as those due to other etiologies. The usual symptoms include generalized urticaria, angioedema, generalized pruritus, nausea, vomiting, diarrhea, hypotension, shock, upper airway edema, and asthma. As a rule, the symptoms start within a few minutes after the insect sting, although some reactions may start as late as several hours following the sting.

4. Toxic reaction. Toxic reactions occur as the result of multiple stings and the symptoms mimic those seen in anaphylaxis.

5. Unusual reaction. A variety of unusual reactions have been described in a temporal relationship to the insect sting. These include neurologic reactions, such as encephalitis, the Guillain-Barré-syndrome, serum sickness, nephropathies, and vasculitis. These reactions may or may not be accompanied by immediate anaphylaxis.

CLINICAL FEATURES OF STING ANAPHYLAXIS

Retrospective population studies have suggested that anaphylactic reactions following insect stings occur in 0.4 to 0.8 percent of the population. More recent studies suggest that the incidence may be even higher. The majority of the reactions have occurred in individuals under age 20, with a 2:1 male to female ratio. This may be a reflection of exposure rather than a predisposition of males or younger individuals to develop anaphylactic reactions. The majority of reactions have occurred following stings about the face and neck, but stings on any part of the body may lead to anaphylaxis. The majority of fatalities have occurred in individuals over age 40, with an estimated 40 to 50 deaths per year in the United States. The increased incidence of fatality in adults compared to the increased incidence in children suggests that adults are unable to withstand the fairly profound biochemical and physiologic consequences of anaphylaxis. Autopsy examinations have shown a fairly high incidence of cardiovascular disease in individuals who have died following insect stings.

DIAGNOSIS

The diagnosis of insect sting allergy is made on the basis of a history of an acute allergic reaction following an insect sting and the presence of specific IgE antibodies detected by skin testing or in the serum by the RAST. For individuals suspected of being at risk, current recommendations are to test with the five available insect venoms (honeybee, yellow jacket, bald-faced hornet, white-faced hornet, and Polistes [wasp]). Initial prick tests are recommended using a solution of 1.0 μg per ml. If the prick test result is negative, intradermal tests are done with increasing concentrations of each of these venoms, usually starting at concentrations between 0.0001 and 0.001 μg per ml. If the test results are negative, the concentrations of venom are increased to a maximal concentration of 1.0 μg per ml. Dilutions are made in a special albumin diluent provided with the venoms. The albumin diluent control and histamine are used as negative and positive controls, respectively. A positive skin test result has been defined as a reaction to 1.0 μg per ml or less, with a negative diluent control. We have found that this 1.0 μg per ml concentration is often irritating, causing a high incidence of nonspecific reactions in noninsect allergic controls. For these reasons we recommend a maximal dose of 0.1 μg per ml.

Testing is usually done with 0.02 ml rather than the 0.05 ml recommended in the product brochure. The venom dilutions have recommended expiration dates, depending upon the concentration: less than 0.1 μg per ml—prepare fresh daily; 0.1 μg per ml—14 days; 1.0 μg per ml—1 month; 10 μg per ml—1 month; 100 μg per ml—5 months.

The RAST has been used as a diagnostic test. As in other systems, the RAST is less sensitive and more expensive than the skin test. It is a useful test for following the course of individuals over time or with therapy. As an initial diagnostic test, it usually is not necessary. On rare occasions a high RAST titer is found with low or even minimal skin test reactivity.

THERAPY

Principles of Avoidance

Simple precautions may decrease the risk of insect stings. Individuals at risk should be careful during outdoor activities. Food and odors attract insects and thus garbage should be well wrapped and covered. Allergic patients should be wary of outdoor cooking and eating. They should wear shoes and long pants or slacks when walking in the grass of fields, and gloves when gardening. Bright colors and perfumes should be avoided. The use of insect repellents has not been shown to prevent insect stings.

Medical Therapy

Acute allergic reactions due to insect stings are treated in the same manner as anaphylaxis of any cause. The drug of choice for the immediate treatment of acute allergic reactions is epinephrine hydrochloride, usually administered subcutaneously in doses ranging from 0.15 to 0.3 ml. On rare occasions intravenous injection may be necessary. Epinephrine should be given at the earliest sign of any systemic symptoms. Antihistamines, such as chlorpheniramine, 4 to 8 mg, or diphenhydramine, 50 mg, may be given orally or parenterally and may be helpful in the treatment of pruritus and urticaria.

The effectiveness of antihistamines in the treatment of more severe anaphylactic symptoms is difficult to document. Aminophylline, vasopressors, oxygen, and other medications may be needed for bronchospasm, shock, and hypoxemia with cyanosis. Careful attention must be given to maintenance of the airway, since upper airway edema has been identified as a common cause of death. The heart rhythm should be carefully monitored. Generally, acute reactions subside within a matter of minutes to hours, even without therapy. Rarely the reaction may continue for a long period of time and, if so, steroids and restoration of plasma volume may also be necessary.

Patients at risk of anaphylaxis are taught to self-inject epinephrine and are advised to have epinephrine and an orally administered antihistamine preparation available at all times. Kits containing these medications are available. The Ana-Kit (Hollister-Stier Laboratories) has a syringe that delivers two 0.3 doses of epinephrine (1:1000) and chewable, 2 mg, chlorpheniramine maleate tablets, alcohol wipes, and a tourniquet. The Epi-Pen unit (Center Laboratories) is a pressure sensitive, syringe loaded device that makes the needle puncture and injects the medication. It is more expensive than the Ana-Kit but more attractive to patients who are not accustomed to the use of a syringe and self-injection. The Epi-Pen, designed for older children and adults, delivers a single dose of 0.3 ml of aqueous epinephrine, 1:1000 (0.3 mg). The Epi-Pen Jr. delivers 0.3 ml of epinephrine, 1:2000 (0.15 mg). Aerosols of epinephrine may be helpful in alleviating upper airway edema but require excessive use in order to be absorbed in sufficient quantity for the treatment of systemic symptoms. Patients should wear an identification bracelet describing their insect allergy.

The treatment of local reactions generally consists of the application of cold and the use of oral doses of antihistamines and analgesics. When the reactions are extremely large and painful, steroids may be beneficial in reducing the swelling (e.g., prednisone, 20 to 40 mg daily in the morning for several days, as indicated).

As previously noted, the pathogenesis of the rare neurologic and vascular complications that have been described following insect stings is still unknown. In these situations steroid therapy may be helpful.

Venom Immunotherapy

Selection of Patients

Venom immunotherapy has been shown to provide protection for over 95 percent of the patients who have had prior anaphylaxis following an insect sting. The current recommendations are to administer venom immunotherapy to individuals who have a history of sting anaphylaxis and have venom specific IgE, detected by skin testing or in the serum by the RAST. It is important to emphasize that only approximately 50 percent of the patients meeting these criteria really require immunotherapy.

Studies of the natural history of insect sting sensitivity have shown that there is not a simplistic relationship between the presence of venom specific IgE and clinical anaphylaxis. In the initial study that established the efficacy of venom immunotherapy, about 40 percent of the patients who were thought to be allergic on the basis of history of sting anaphylaxis and positive skin test results failed to react to a sting challenge after placebo or whole body extract therapy. Further evaluation with deliberate sting challenges in other studies also demonstrated the variability of the sting response in presumably sensitive patients, leading one group of authors to conclude that "no in vitro or in vivo tests predicted with certainty the status of the sting-sensitive person."

Most intriguing have been the observations of Schuberth and colleagues, who studied children with dermal reactions as the only manifestation of anaphylaxis and were followed without venom immunotherapy. Subsequent re-stings in these children led to only a small number of recurrent reactions, and when reactions did occur, the symptoms were similar or less severe than the initial reaction. Children who received immunotherapy achieved almost 100 percent protection against subsequent re-sting reactions. These observations have led to the conclusion that children who have had only dermal reactions due to sting anaphylaxis could be treated with available symptomatic medication and do not require venom immunotherapy.

Our own studies, in adults who have had dermal reactions only, suggest that the reaction pattern may be similar, and that these individuals are far less likely to have re-sting reactions than are patients who have had initial cardiovascular or respiratory symptoms. Further observations are needed before extending the recommendations regarding the lack of need for immunotherapy to adults with dermal reactions only.

On rare occasions individuals have had negative skin test results when evaluated following sting anaphylaxis. Such individuals are not considered candidates for venom immunotherapy. It would be difficult to select the proper venom, and in the absence of a defined IgE pathogenesis the effectiveness of venom immunotherapy is unknown.

Patients with toxic reactions following multiple stings present an unresolved issue. When subsequently evaluated, these patients often have positive skin test results and may then be susceptible to single sting anaphylaxis. In such cases venom immunotherapy might be appropriate.

Patients who have had only local reactions do not require venom immunotherapy. In studies of both children and adults it has been shown that the majority of individuals continue to have local reactions if re-stung and are at very low risk for systemic anaphylaxis. For these reasons patients who have had only local reactions do not even require skin tests. Table 1 summarizes the recommendations for immunotherapy.

Selection of Venom

The recommendations established in 1979, when commercial venoms became available, are to give immunotherapy with each of the venoms to which a patient has had positive skin test results. For most individuals this has led to multiple venom injections, particularly with vespid (yellow jacket, hornet, wasp) venoms. Stud-

TABLE 1 Indications for Venom Immunotherapy

Sting Reaction	Skin Test	Venom Immunotherapy
Anaphylaxis, adult	+	+
Anaphylaxis, children		
Cardiovascular, respiratory symptoms	+	+
Dermal reaction only	+	−
Anaphylaxis, children or adults	−	−
Large local reaction	Not indicated	−
Toxic reaction	+	?

ies of cross reactivity of venoms have shown extensive cross reactivity between venoms of the two different hornet species (bald-faced hornet and white-faced hornet), and yellow jacket venom and hornet venom. For these reasons it should be anticipated that an individual who is allergic to a yellow jacket sting will have positive reactions to hornet venoms. The failure to find positive skin test results is the exception, not the rule.

The relationship of Polistes (wasp) venom is not so clear-cut. Approximately 50 percent of those who are allergic to Polistes react to other vespids, and vice versa. For these reasons we have attempted to treat with individual venoms, depending on the history and skin test findings. When the culprit insect clearly cannot be identified, the mixed vespid venoms or the Polistes venom may be necessary. Knowledge of the cross reactivity patterns, however, helps in interpretation of the skin test findings. Thus, we recommend the following:

1. If the insect causing the reaction is positively identified as a yellow jacket, yellow jacket venom alone is given.

2. If the insect cannot be positively identified and the skin test reaction to yellow jacket venom is stronger than that to hornet venom, yellow jacket venom is given.

3. If the insect cannot be identified and the patient reacts equally to the yellow jacket and hornet venoms, both venoms are given.

The honeybee and vespids belong to different families. Nevertheless there is some cross reaction between honeybee and yellow jacket venoms, but the relationship is fairly complex. Thus, if an individual reacts to both venoms, it may be necessary to use both for immunotherapy. However, careful attention to details of the sting history, differences in the degree of skin test reactivity, and knowledge of the cross reactions between venoms can lead to an educated decision for single venom immunotherapy.

Dosing

The basic concepts of venom immunotherapy are the same as with other types of allergen immunotherapy. Treatment is started with very small doses of venom

TABLE 2   Dose Schedules for Hymenoptera Venom Immunotherapy

Dose No.	Individual Venoms			Mixed Vespid Venom		
	Volume (ml)	Concentration (μg/ml)	Dose (μg)	Volume (ml)	Concentration (μg/ml)	Dose (μg)
1	0.10	1*	0.10	0.10	3	0.30
2	0.20	1	0.20	0.20	3	0.60
3	0.40	1	0.40	0.40	3	1.2
4	0.70	1	0.70	0.70	3	2.1
5	0.10	10	1.0	0.10	30	3.0
6	0.20	10	2.0	0.20	30	6.0
7	0.40	10	4.0	0.40	30	12
8	0.70	10	7.0	0.70	30	21
9	0.10	100	10	0.10	300	30
10	0.15	100	15	0.15	300	45
11	0.20	100	20	0.20	300	60
12	0.35	100	35	0.35	300	105
13	0.50	100	50†	0.50	300	150
14	0.65	100	65	0.65	300	195
15	0.80	100	80	0.80	300	240
16	1.00	100	100	1.00	300	300

*With this venom concentration the first two and second two doses are often given 20 minutes apart at one office visit. Subsequent incremental doses are given once or twice weekly. The maximal maintenance dose is administered every 4 weeks. After 1 year the interval between maintenance doses is extended to 6 to 8 weeks.
†The product brochure recommends a maximal dose of 100 μg of individual venoms. Our recommendation is 50 μg.

and gradually increased to the maximal maintenance dose. Dosing schedules have varied from the traditional one injection per week to rush immunotherapy utilizing multiple injections over several days, usually in a hospital setting. As a general rule initial venom doses usually range from 0.1 to 0.001 μg. This depends somewhat upon the patient's sensitivity, as judged clinically and by skin tests. Early venom doses may be rapidly increased; with higher doses the increase is effected more slowly. A typical dosing schedule is shown in Table 2.

Top Dose.   The initial studies of venom immunotherapy were done with maximal doses of 100 μg of single venoms and 300 μg of mixed vespid venom (bald-faced hornet, white-faced hornet, and yellow jacket). In our experience 50 μg of individual venoms has been found to be equally effective. This dose has provided clinical protection and stimulated a good immunologic response.

Maintenance Interval.   The usual interval between maintenance doses is 4 weeks. Recent studies have clearly shown that once individuals have been taking maintenance doses for about 1 year, the maintenance dose interval can be successfully extended to 6 to 8 weeks with no loss of efficacy.

Duration of Therapy.   A major problem is duration of therapy. Several criteria have been suggested as

guidelines for the cessation of therapy. If the venom skin test becomes negative, which occurs in a minority of patients, therapy can be stopped. Repeat skin tests should be performed every 2 to 3 years in patients taking therapy in order to monitor their sensitivity. A fall in the serum venom specific IgE to insignificant levels has been suggested as another reliable criterion for stopping treatment. Observations to date have shown a very low incidence of re-sting reactions in patients in whom therapy was stopped, on the basis of this criterion. Most recently it has been suggested that 5 years of venom immunotherapy might be sufficient, even though skin test results remain positive and the serum venom specific IgE level remains elevated. Further experience will be necessary before this guideline can be generally adopted.

Reactions to Venom Immunotherapy

Local and systemic reactions may occur following venom immunotherapy. Because it is important to reach maximal maintenance doses to ensure adequate protection, it is necessary to persist with attempts to develop patient tolerance to full doses. In the case of local reactions the dose may be split into several sites. On occasion the addition of a small amount of epinephrine may decrease the swelling. Following systemic reactions the venom dose must be decreased and then raised very slowly. Often this is a long term, tedious process, but most times it is successful. The utilization of single venoms rather than multiple venoms and a maximal maintenance dose of 50 μg often eliminates some of these reactions.

Treatment Failures

On rare occasions treated patients have continued to have re-sting reactions. It is important to identify the culprit re-sting insect and perhaps repeat skin testing to be sure that the patient is being treated with the appropriate venom. If the treatment venom is correct, the dose of venom immunotherapy should be increased, perhaps doubled. Measurement of the serum venom specific IgG level may be helpful in these situations. This antibody has been identified as the immunologic mediator of immunity to insect stings. If the IgG antibody titers are low, the protective effects of higher venom doses might be suggested by an increase in the titers. The routine measurement of serum venom specific

IgG is unnecessary in view of the extremely high incidence of success with venom immunotherapy and the observation that other factors are related to tolerance to re-stings in individuals with prior allergic reactions.

SUGGESTED READING

Graft DF, Schuberth KC. Hymenoptera allergy in children. Pediatr Clin North Am 1983; 30:873–886.
Graft DF, Schuberth KC, Kagey-Sobotka A, Kwiterovich KA, Niv Y, Lichtenstein LM, Valentine, MD. Assessment of prolonged venom immunotherapy in children. J Allergy Clin Immunol 1987.
Mauriello PM, Barde SH, Georgitis JW, Reisman RE. Natural history of large local reactions from stinging insects. J Allergy Clin Immunol 1984; 74:494–498.
Parker JL, Santrach PJ, Dahlberg JE, Yunginger JW. Evaluation of hymenoptera sting sensitivity with deliberate sting challenge: inadequacy of present diagnostic methods. J Allergy Clin Immunol 1982; 69:200–207.
Reisman RE, Dvorin DJ, Randolph CC, Georgitis JW. Stinging insect allergy: natural history and modification with venom immunotherapy. J Allergy Clin Immunol 1985; 75:735–740.
Valentine MD. Insect venom allergy: diagnosis and treatment. J Allergy Clin Immunol 1984; 73:299–304.

SYSTEMIC ANAPHYLAXIS

TIMOTHY J. SULLIVAN III, M.D.

Anaphylaxis is an acute, life endangering syndrome resulting from the sudden release of large amounts of diverse mediators from mast cells. The clinical manifestations include rapidly evolving respiratory tract obstruction or cardiovascular collapse. Anaphylaxis occurs in approximately one of every 2700 hospitalized patients, and the overall lifetime risk in the United States is approximately 1 percent.

The causes of anaphylaxis can be divided into four groups—antigens, direct mast cell activating agents, anaphylatoxin generating agents, and factors acting by mechanisms not currently understood (Table 1). IgE antibodies can initiate anaphylaxis by binding to complete antigens, such as insulin, or to determinants formed by covalent attachment of highly reactive drugs (e.g., penicillin) to large molecules, such as albumin or immunoglobulin. Some drugs can directly activate mast cell mediator release in the absence of specific IgE. Massive complement activation can generate formation

TABLE 1 Classification of Causes of Systemic Anaphylaxis*

IgE mediated anaphylaxis
  Haptens
    Antimicrobial drugs
      Penicillins and cephalosporins
      Tetracyclines
      Aminoglycosides
      Nitrofurantoin
      Amphotericin B
      Sulfonamides
    Other drugs
      Ethylene oxide
      Local anesthetics (some reactions)

  Complete antigens

    Proteins
      Hymenoptera venoms
      Chymopapain
      Insulin
      Streptokinase
      Heterologous immunoglobulins (some reactions)
      Allergen extracts
      Protamine
      Seminal fluid
      Foods
        Milk
        Egg
        Shellfish
        Fish
        Peanut
        Nuts
        Chocolate

TABLE 1 (Continued)   Classification of Causes of Systemic Anaphylaxis

Other agents
    Quarternary ammonium muscle relaxants (some reactions)

Direct activation of mast cell mediator release
    Opiates
    Radiocontrast media
    Vancomycin
    Polymyxin B
    Dextran
    Quarternary ammonium muscle relaxants (some reactions)

Anaphylatoxin mediated anaphylaxis
    Human plasma and blood products
    Homologous and heterologous immunoglobulins (some reactions)
    Dialysis membranes (some reactions)

Anaphylaxis initiated by unknown mechanisms
    Exercise
    Mastocytosis
    Nonsteroidal anti-inflammatory drugs, including aspirin
    Synthetic steroid hormones
    Recombinant immunoregulatory molecules
    Idiopathic anaphylaxis

* The substances, disease states, and activities noted are examples of common provocative factors. Numerous other agents are known or strongly suspected in each category.

of large amounts of the anaphylatoxins C3a and C5a. Anaphylatoxins bind to specific mast cell receptors and, as the name implies, can initiate marked mast cell mediator release. Several other causes of anaphylaxis are known, ranging from exercise to aspirin, that induce mast cell mediator release by unknown mechanisms.

These diverse stimuli induce similar pathophysiologic events. Activated mast cells secrete mediator containing granules and can form potent mediators from membrane lipids. Granule mediators include histamine, proteolytic enzymes such as mast cell tryptase, glycosidases, and granulocyte chemotactic factors. Newly formed lipid mediators include prostaglandin D_2, sulfidopeptide leukotrienes, and platelet activating factor. These mediators induce marked changes in the microenvironment and activate complex local reflex mechanisms. Histamine (acting through H_1 and H_2 receptors), PGD_2, the leukotrienes, and possibly platelet activating factor appear to be the principal mediators of anaphylaxis. These mediators can cause diminished arteriolar tone, increased permeability of postcapillary venules, increased venous capacitance, diminished force of ventricular contraction, cardiac rhythm disturbances, and ventricular conduction abnormalities, all of which can contribute to the hypotension occurring during anaphylaxis. Interstitial respiratory tract vessel engorgement, edema, contraction of respiratory tract smooth muscle, and increased bronchial gland secretion lead to the respiratory tract disorders noted during anaphylaxis.

CLINICAL MANIFESTATIONS OF ANAPHYLAXIS

As summarized in Table 2, characteristic clinical manifestations of anaphylaxis can appear in many organ systems. Anaphylaxis usually begins within minutes after exposure to the causative factor, although the onset may be delayed for several hours. Once under way, the reaction usually progresses in an explosive manner, reaching a peak intensity within 1 hour. Nonfatal reactions resolve over a period of up to 48 hours. Pruritic cutaneous reactions often are the first manifestations of anaphylaxis. Acute asthma, rhinitis, and conjunctivitis may occur. Acute perineal pruritus and a metallic taste in the mouth may be present.

Respiratory or cardiovascular dysfunction during anaphylaxis can be fatal. As noted in Table 3, respiratory failure may be the result of upper airway obstruction or severe acute asthma. Cardiovascular collapse may be the result of peripheral vascular dysfunction or cardiac dysfunction. The relative frequencies of these disorders on presentation to a medical facility have been estimated to be as follows: hypotension, 68 percent; bronchial obstruction, 52 percent; laryngeal obstruction, 36 percent; respiratory arrest, 12 percent; and cardiac arrest, 12 percent.

Several nonimmunologic factors appear to increase the risk that anaphylaxis will progress to a severe or

TABLE 2   Clinical Manifestations of Anaphylaxis

System	Manifestation
Skin	Generalized, perineal, or vaginal pruritus; angioedema; urticaria and other pruritic rashes
Eye	Pruritus, conjunctival suffusion, lacrimation
Nose	Pruritus, congestion, sneezing, rhinorrhea
Mouth	Metallic taste
Upper airway	Sensation of narrowing airway, hoarseness, stridor, oropharyngeal or laryngeal edema, complete obstruction
Lower airway	Dyspnea, tachypnea, wheezing, use of accessory muscles of respiration, cyanosis, respiratory arrest
Cardiovascular	Tachycardia, hypotension, ventricular and supraventricular rhythm disturbances, cardiac arrest
Gastrointestinal	Nausea, vomiting, cramping abdominal pain, diarrhea, bloody diarrhea
Neurologic	Fear of impending death, weakness, dizziness, syncope, seizure

TABLE 3   Causes of Death from Anaphylaxis*

Cardiovascular dysfunction
   Peripheral vessel dysfunction
      Loss of arteriolar tone
      Increased vascular permeability
      Increased capacitance of veins
   Cardiac dysfunction
      Diminished force of contraction
      Diminished coronary blood flow
      Rhythm disturbances
      Conduction abnormalities
Respiratory dysfunction
   Upper respiratory tract obstruction
      Angioedema
   Pulmonary dysfunction
      Airway narrowing from interstitial edema and smooth muscle contraction
      Increased bronchial secretions

* Ischemia and hypoxia during anaphylaxis can cause extensive injury to the heart, brain, kidneys, and liver.

TABLE 4   Nonimmunologic Risk Factors for Severe or Fatal Anaphylaxis

Beta-adrenergic blockade
Bronchial asthma
Cardiac disease

fatal outcome (Table 4). The presence of beta-adrenergic blocking drugs appears to increase the likelihood and severity of anaphylaxis and interferes with the use of beta-adrenergic agonists to treat anaphylaxis. Asthmatic patients appear to be twice as likely to die if anaphylaxis occurs. Anaphylaxis is more likely to be severe or fatal in patients with congestive heart failure or arteriosclerotic coronary artery disease.

DIAGNOSIS OF ANAPHYLAXIS

A diagnosis of anaphylaxis is based upon clinical and biochemical evidence of acute, life endangering secretion of mast cell mediators (Table 5). Essential to the diagnosis is the presence of acute upper airway obstruction, bronchial obstruction, or hypotension. The presence of other distinctive allergic symptoms and signs, evidence of allergy to the agent in question, and elevated serum mast cell tryptase levels should suggest or support the diagnosis of anaphylaxis. Exposure to stimuli known to cause anaphylaxis immediately before the onset of the syndrome supports the diagnosis of anaphylaxis as does evidence of the presence of IgE to this agent.

TABLE 5   Diagnosis of Anaphylaxis*

At least one of the following must be present: acute hypotension, bronchial obstruction, or upper airway obstruction (cardiac or respiratory arrest)

Presence of distinctive allergic symptoms and signs in other systems

Recent exposure to agents or activities known to be capable of inducing anaphylaxis

Evidence of IgE to an agent encountered just before onset of anaphylaxis

Absence of conditions that can mimic anaphylaxis

Elevated serum levels of mast cell tryptase

Elevated levels of other molecules associated with mast cell secretion: plasma and urinary histamine and metabolites, serum high molecular weight neutrophil chemotactic factor, and urinary PGD_2 metabolites

* Effective therapy of acute anaphylaxis requires accurate diagnosis based upon clinical criteria.

Serum levels of mast cell tryptase are unequivocally elevated during anaphylaxis, providing a useful biochemical dimension for the diagnosis of anaphylaxis. Tryptase blood levels peak approximately 1 hour after the onset of the reaction and have an approximately 3 hour half-clearance time. Other possible biochemical markers of mast cell secretion include histamine and metabolites of histamine, and PGD_2 and metabolites of PGD_2, but measurements of these molecules have not yet been proven useful for routine clinical assessment.

Several illnesses that can be mistaken for anaphylaxis must be excluded. The differential diagnosis of anaphylaxis includes myocardial infarction, primary cardiac dysrhythmias, vasovagal syncope, pulmonary embolism, hypovolemic shock, stroke, aspiration pneumonia, adverse pharmacologic reactions to drugs, hereditary angioedema, foreign body in the airway, epiglottitis, other causes of upper airway obstruction, hyperventilation, anxiety attack, and Munchausen syndrome.

MANAGEMENT OF ANAPHYLAXIS

Assessment

The initial evaluation of a patient experiencing anaphylaxis should establish the nature and intensity of the clinical manifestations (see Table 2), the rate of progression of the reaction, medications the patient has received recently and for prolonged periods, and concurrent illnesses (particularly asthma and cardiac disease). Knowledge of the presence or absence of therapy with beta-adrenergic blocking drugs is especially important. Administration of any drug suspected of having caused the reaction should be discontinued. High priority must be given to assessment of the respiratory and cardiovascular systems: upper airway patency, pulmonary function, cardiac rhythm, and blood pressure (see Table 3). These four factors should be monitored (when feasible) by direct visualization, spirometry, electrocardiography, and serial blood pressure measurements.

The initial assessment permits formulation of a plan of management that takes into consideration the severity and nature of the anaphylaxis and individual patient factors. If the patient is receiving beta-adrenergic receptor blocking drugs, immediate institution of management approaches not dependent on beta-receptor activation by epinephrine or isoproterenol is mandatory (Table 6). Severe pulmonary problems should be anticipated and pharmacologically pre-empted in asthmatic patients (see Table 6). Steps should be taken to prepare for intubation, cricothyrotomy, assisted ventilation, cardiac monitoring, or intra-aortic balloon pumping as indicated by the initial examination. Delay in preparation for the use of potentially essential sophisticated measures, while assessing

TABLE 6 Management of Anaphylaxis

General therapeutic measures
  Clinical assessment
  Epinephrine (subcutaneously or by infusion)

Specific interventions
  Hypotension
    Peripheral vascular defects
      Trendelenburg position
      Intravenous administration of isotonic sodium chloride
      Norepinephrine or other vasopressor infusion
      H_1 and H_2 blocking drugs
    Cardiac dysfunction
      Conventional therapy of dysrhythmias
      Isoproterenol infusion
      H_1 and H_2 blocking drugs
      Intra-aortic balloon pump
  Airway obstruction
    Upper airway obstruction
      Supplemental inspired oxygen
      Extension of neck
      Oropharyngeal airway
      Endotracheal intubation
      Cricothyrotomy
    Lower airway obstruction
      Supplemental inspired oxygen
      Intravenous administration of theophylline
      Aerosol bronchodilator therapy
      Endotracheal intubation
      Conventional treatment for status asthmaticus
      Assisted ventilation
Biphasic anaphylaxis
  Monitor by direct observation for at least 12 hours after onset of anaphylaxis
  Systemic corticosteroid therapy after acute reaction has been treated and again 6 hours later
  H_1 and H_2 blocking drugs initially and again 6 hours later
  Recurrent anaphylaxis treated according to guidelines for acute anaphylaxis

the effects of epinephrine or other initial medical therapy, can contribute to a fatal outcome.

Epinephrine

This adrenergic receptor agonist is the drug of choice for the initial management of anaphylaxis. The capacity of epinephrine to suppress mediator release from mast cells and basophils and to reverse many of the end organ effects of the mediators of anaphylaxis, while producing peripheral vasoconstriction, makes this a nearly ideal drug for initial therapy in most patients. Complete remission of the signs of anaphylaxis often occurs within minutes after the injection of epinephrine (Table 7).

Subcutaneous doses of 300 to 500 μg (0.3 to 0.5 ml of a 1:1000 solution) for an adult usually are effective. Asthmatic adults should receive 500 μg, since they often are relatively insensitive to beta-adrenergic receptor stimulation. This dose can be repeated after 10 minutes if the first dose has not induced improvement or untoward effects. If serious manifestations of the reaction persist, an intravenous infusion of epinephrine at an initial infusion rate of 2 μg per minute (for an adult) can be instituted. One milligram of epinephrine (e.g., 1 ml of a 1:1000 solution or 10 ml of a 1:10,000 solution) can be diluted in 500 ml of fluid for intravenous infusion at a rate of 1 ml per minute. Intravenous bolus injections of epinephrine, in the context of anaphylaxis, often induce serious cardiac rhythm disturbances that can cause or contribute to a fatal outcome. Intravenous bolus therapy should be avoided. Excessive subcutaneous doses of epinephrine can induce similar cardiac complications. Inappropriately high doses of epinephrine also can induce hypertension, acute catecholamine cardiac toxicity, or other serious side effects.

Failure to use epinephrine early in the management of anaphylaxis increases the probability of a fatal outcome. The likelihood of prompt marked benefit is high, and the risk of serious untoward effects from properly administered epinephrine is low. The proper use of epinephrine remains the initial treatment of choice in most patients.

TABLE 7 Epinephrine in Anaphylaxis

Drug of choice in most cases

Arrests mediator release and reverses many mediator actions

Intravenous bolus therapy dangerous because of cardiac rhythm disturbances

Subcutaneous therapy usually effective

Intravenous infusions of 2 μg/ml usually safe in adults

Failure to use epinephrine more dangerous than proper use of epinephrine

Hypotension

Peripheral Vascular Defects

Diminished arteriolar tone, increased postcapillary venule permeability with loss of intravascular volume, and vasodilation can contribute to hypotension during anaphylaxis. Epinephrine is the initial treatment of choice and usually is sufficient to restore vascular tone and normal permeability properties.

If epinephrine is not effective, or if the patient is being treated with beta-adrenergic blocking drugs, expansion of intravascular volume, vasopressor infusion, and combined H_1 and H_2 antihistamine therapy should be considered. A supine position with elevation of the legs (Trendelenburg position) may be helpful. Normal saline, or another salt containing fluid, can be administered rapidly to an adult at a rate of up to 100 ml per minute to a limit of 3 liters. Administration of fluid, especially amounts of more than 3 liters in an adult or the equivalent in a child, should be guided by the patient's response, cardiovascular status, age, and urine output.

If fluid administration and the Trendelenburg position are ineffective, or if hypotension is profound, a vasopressor may be needed. Norepinephrine appears to be the most consistently effective pressor in anaphylaxis, although success with other drugs has been reported. Norepinephrine should be diluted to a 4 μg per ml (4 ml of a 1 mg per ml solution in 1000 ml of 5 percent dextrose in water). The initial infusion rate for adults is 8 to 12 μg per minute (2 to 3 ml per minute). The rate of infusion should be adjusted to sustain a systolic blood pressure of 80 to 100 mm Hg. Previously hypertensive patients may require higher pressures, but the systolic pressure should be 40 mm Hg or more below the patient's usual systolic pressure. Conventional measures should be taken to avoid or treat extravasation of the drug.

Histamine, acting through both H_1 and H_2 receptors, appears to play a significant role in the peripheral vascular and cardiac disorders that contribute to hypotension. Concurrent blockage of H_1 and H_2 receptors appears to be necessary to block the hypotensive effects of histamine. Effective blockade can be achieved by using an H_1 antihistamine such as diphenhydramine (1 mg per kg of body weight in an adult, intravenously) and an H_2 antihistamine such as cimetidine (4 mg per kg infused intravenously over at least 5 minutes).

Cardiac Dysfunction

Dysrhythmias and diminished force of cardiac contraction can contribute to hypotension during anaphylaxis. Markedly decreased force of ventricular contraction may be the sole origin of hypotension in anaphylaxis.

Complex and life endangering rhythm disturbances may arise from the combined impact of intercardiac mast cell mediator release, intravascular mediators, hypoxia, hypotension, or excessive doses of epinephrine. Electrocardiographic monitoring is desirable during anaphylaxis, when possible.

Epinephrine is the initial treatment of choice and usually is sufficient to restore normal cardiac function. Hypoxia and hypotension should be corrected immediately. Conventional therapy for ventricular rhythm disturbances usually is successful.

Cardiac contractility disorders may respond to the infusion of a $beta_1$-adrenergic agonist. Epinephrine is the usual drug of choice, but if a concurrent alpha-adrenergic effect is not desired, isoproterenol can be infused. For an adult, 1 mg of isoproterenol is dissolved in 500 ml of 5 percent dextrose in water (2 μg per ml) and administered at a rate of 0.25 to 2.50 ml per minute (0.5 to 5 μg per minute). The speed of infusion is adjusted according to the clinical response and the effect on heart rate. Dopamine has complex effects that could have both beneficial and undesirable effects on anaphylaxis. This drug appears to be less effective than other drugs for pressor or inotropic effects. Potent nonadrenergic inotropic drugs are available, but they often induce peripheral vasodilation that can be severe and difficult to reverse. This property renders available nonadrenergic inotropic drugs dangerous to use in anaphylaxis.

Cardiac dysfunction during anaphylaxis in a patient receiving beta-adrenergic blocking drugs presents an especially challenging problem. Attempts to overcome the block with high doses of epinephrine can cause excessive alpha-adrenergic effects. High doses of either epinephrine or isoproterenol can induce acute cardiac catecholamine toxicity despite beta-receptor blockade. General measures addressing hypoxia, ventricular rhythm disturbances, and hypotension should be applied. Combined blockade of H_1 and H_2 receptors may be beneficial.

Refractory hypotension may reflect acute myocardial infarction caused by acute hypoxia or hypotension during anaphylaxis.

Upper Airway Obstruction

The effective management of laryngeal or oropharyngeal angioedema depends upon aggressive use of the steps outlined in Tables 6 and 8. Epinephrine can induce remission rapidly, but direct intervention should be undertaken if significant obstruction is present. An H_1 antihistamine (e.g., diphenhydramine, 1 mg per kg intravenously in an adult) can be given. Aerosolized epinephrine may be used topically to complement parenteral doses of epinephrine. Supplemental inspired oxygen, extension of the neck, and insertion of an oropharyngeal airway may be helpful.

TABLE 8 Cricothyrotomy Procedure

1. Extend neck to place cricothyroid membrane and overlying skin under tension and to make membrane immediately accessible.
2. Locate cricothyroid membrane below thyroid cartilage and above cricoid cartilage.
3. Make small transverse incision in skin in anterior third of cricothyroid space just above upper border of cricoid cartilage (use vertical incision if patient is combative).
4. Puncture cricothyroid membrane in midline.
5. Enlarge opening with scalpel handle or another form of blunt dissection.
6. Insert endotracheal tube with internal diameter of 4 to 5 mm (smaller in children).

When initial measures are not sufficient or when severe obstruction is present at the beginning of therapy, endotracheal intubation is indicated. An endotracheal tube with a 4 or 5 mm internal diameter is sufficient to ventilate an adult and is more likely to be placed successfully than a conventional larger endotracheal tube. Airway needles and similar small aperture devices are not sufficient for the management of severe obstruction. If intubation is not possible, a cricothyrotomy should be performed. This procedure is much faster, safer, and more feasible in an emergency than a tracheotomy. Details of this intervention are presented in Table 8.

Lower Airway Obstruction

Pulmonary dysfunction in anaphylaxis can be managed with a stepwise approach similar to that used for severe acute asthma (see Table 6). Measurements of FEV_1, peak expiratory flow rate, pulsus paradoxus, and blood gas levels are useful in assessing the severity of the disease and the impact of therapy. Systemic epinephrine therapy may be sufficient to suppress pulmonary reactions. If epinephrine fails to halt the pulmonary reaction, if the reaction is severe at initial evaluations ($FEV_1 \leq 1.0$ liter, peak flow ≤ 299 liters per minute, pulsus paradoxus ≥ 18 mm Hg, $PCO_2 \geq 42$ mm Hg), or if the patient is being treated with beta-adrenergic blocking drugs, other measures are used to control the pulmonary dysfunction. Supplemental inspired oxygen should be administered by nasal cannula (5 liters per minute) or face mask (40 to 60 percent oxygen) as needed to sustain a PO_2 above 60 mm Hg (preferably 80 to 100 mm Hg).

Theophylline can exert powerful beneficial effects on pulmonary disorders in anaphylaxis, but a loading dose must be administered over 20 minutes and the therapeutic range of the drug is quite narrow. Decisions about dosages must be made with attention to prior theophylline therapy, concurrent illnesses, concurrent drug therapy, and other factors. In patients who are not taking theophylline therapy, an intravenous loading dose of 6 mg of aminophylline (the ethylene diamine salt of theophylline) per kg of body weight can be given over 20 minutes. If the patient has been receiving theophylline therapy, the dosage is selected according to the maintenance dosage being given, the time since the last dose, and the serum theophylline level; usually no more than half the usual loading dose is given. Theophylline blood levels of 10 to 20 μg per ml are maintained by infusions of aminophylline, usually 0.3 to 0.9 mg per kg per hour intravenously.

Theophylline clearance rates can vary markedly from patient to patient and are influenced by several intercurrent factors. Theophylline metabolism can be slow in cases of hepatic dysfunction, congestive heart failure, or concurrent therapy with drugs such as cimetidine or erythromycin. Cigarette smokers tend to metabolize theophylline more rapidly. The appearance of nausea, vomiting, or cardiac rhythm disturbances during theophylline infusion indicates possible theophylline toxicity; infusion should be halted until the blood level is determined. Clearly serial serum theophylline levels can be useful in achieving therapeutic but nontoxic blood levels.

Biphasic Anaphylaxis

The initial therapy of severe anaphylaxis induces prompt, complete, sustained clinical remissions in approximately half the cases. Protracted anaphylaxis (respiratory or cardiovascular manifestations at least partially resistant to therapy for hours to more than 1 day) occurs in approximately one fourth of the severe cases. A particularly dangerous pattern, biphasic anaphylaxis, occurs in approximately one fourth of the severe cases. Biphasic anaphylaxis is characterized by complete remission of symptoms and signs of anaphylaxis in response to initial therapy, followed by recurrence of potentially life endangering disorders after an asymptomatic interval of up to 8 hours.

Since no methods are available to predict whether the remission will be temporary or sustained, the patient should be observed for at least 12 hours after the onset of anaphylaxis. Laryngeal obstruction, bronchial obstruction, or hypotension may recur, but these disorders have not been observed to occur for the first time during the second episode. Thus, clinical monitoring is focused on possible recurrence of the life endangering features present during the initial phase.

Once the initial manifestations of anaphylaxis are controlled, systemic corticosteroid therapy can be given. Biphasic anaphylaxis can occur despite this intervention, but the use of corticosteroids is based upon studies of biphasic immediate hypersensitivity reactions in the lung, skin, and nose that demonstrate corticosteroid suppression of late reactions. The initial dose, equivalent to 60 mg of prednisone, should be given intravenously to permit a rapid onset of action. This dose should be repeated with oral medication 6 hours later.

Combined H_1 and H_2 blockade also should be considered. Although pruritus, wheal and flare reactions, and angioedema reactions are primarily H_1 receptor mediated, histamine induced hypotension is mediated by both H_1 and H_2 receptors. An H_1 antihistamine (e.g., diphenhydramine, 1 mg per kg intravenously in an adult) and an H_2 antihistamine (e.g., cimetidine, 4 mg per kg intravenously in an adult) should be given initially and again 6 hours later (a longer interval for long acting H_2 antihistamines).

Most of the reported instances of biphasic anaphylaxis have occurred in patients who received corticosteroids and H_1 antihistamine therapy, indicating that current prophylactic measures are not ideal. These reactions often are mild to moderate in severity, but immediately life endangering reactions do occur. Recurrent anaphylaxis is treated according to the same principles used to treat acute anaphylaxis.

Urticaria and Angioedema

Acute urticaria and angioedema associated with anaphylaxis usually remit with epinephrine therapy. Conventional therapy with an H_1 antihistamine or combined therapy with H_1 and H_2 antihistamines also exerts powerful suppressive effects. Corticosteroids suppress most continuing urticaria and angioedema reactions associated with anaphylaxis, but the onset of action is 4 to 6 hours after the first dose.

AVOIDANCE OF ANAPHYLAXIS

The incidence and severity of anaphylaxis can be reduced to a very low level by utilizing the approaches summarized in Table 9. Expanded precautions are indicated for patients who are at increased risk for severe anaphylaxis—those with a history of anaphylaxis, asthmatic patients, patients receiving beta-adrenergic blocking drugs, and those with cardiac disease. Patients with a history of multiple drug allergies may be at increased risk of anaphylaxis from other drugs. Immunologic tests are available to assist in the detection of IgE sensitivity to beta-lactam antibiotics, chymopapain, and a variety of other agents.

Immunization with specific Hymenoptera venoms can induce effective protection for approximately 98

TABLE 9   Approaches to Avoidance of Anaphylaxis

General precautions
  Control exposure to factors known to have caused immediate hypersensitivity reactions in past (e.g., drugs, stinging insects, foods, exercise)
  Administer drugs by oral route when possible
  Observe for at least 30 minutes after first dose of drugs that are common causes of anaphylaxis
  Special precautions for patients at increased risk of severe anaphylaxis:
    Discontinuation of beta-adrenergic blocking drugs during periods of risk (e.g., hospitalization, radiocontrast studies, stinging insect season)
    Optimization of therapy of asthma before surgery; radiocontrast studies; new, high risk drug therapy
    Immunologic screening for allergy before drug therapy when tests are available
    Introduction of beta-lactam drug therapy with an oral dose when possible
    Premedication before radiocontrast studies, general anesthesia, mediator releasing drugs

Immunologic screening for specific IgE before drug therapy

Immunization
  Hymenoptera venom sensitive patients

Premedication
  Before radiocontrast medium injections
    Prednisone: 50 mg oral doses 13, 7, and 1 hour before procedure in adults
    Diphenhydramine: 1 mg/kg 1 hour before procedure in adults

Acute desensitization of allergic patients
  Oral desensitization (e.g., penicillin, sulfonamides)
  Parenteral desensitization (e.g., insulin, aminoglycosides, heteroantisera)

Self-administered epinephrine

percent of the patients who have had anaphylactic reactions to stings by bees, wasps, yellow jackets, or hornets. The efficacy and safety of similar therapy with fire ant materials are under investigation.

Premedication with corticosteroids and H_1 antihistamines has been proven effective in reducing the frequency and severity of anaphylactic reactions to radiocontrast media. This approach is ineffective against penicillin and other antigen induced anaphylaxis and should not be considered effective outside the context of radiocontrast reactions.

When strong indications for use of a drug are present in patients with anaphylactic sensitivity to that drug, acute desensitization can be considered. Acceptably safe oral desensitization protocols have been reported for beta-lactam drugs and sulfonamides. Similar approaches could be considered for other drugs available in an oral form. Parenteral desensitization, although associated with more frequent and more severe complications, has been successful for drugs such as insulin, aminoglycosides, and heteroantisera. Similar protocols could be considered for other drugs. In nearly all instances anaphylactic sensitivity can be bypassed by these procedures.

Self-administered epinephrine should be provided for patients who are likely to experience anaphylaxis outside a medical facility. The patient should be taught the indications and details of self-administration. These procedures should be reviewed with the patient and the patient's family on a regular basis. Speed and simplicity of administration favor the use of Epi-Pens for this purpose.

The patient and physicians involved in the patient's care should be thoroughly integrated into plans for avoidance and future therapy. These diverse strategies, carefully applied, can reduce the morbidity and mortality from episodes of recurrent anaphylaxis to a very low level.

SUGGESTED READING

Goldenberg IF, Cohn JN. New inotropic drugs for heart failure. JAMA 1987; 258:493–496.
Kravis TC, Warner CG, eds. Emergency medicine. Rockville: Aspen Publishers, 1987: 69, 1061–1063.
Patterson R, DeSwarte RD, Greenberger PA, Grammer LC. Drug allergy and protocols for management of drug allergies. N Engl Reg Allergy Proc 1986; 7:325–342.
Porter J, Jick H. Drug-induced anaphylaxis, convulsions, deafness, and extrapyramidal symptoms. Lancet 1977; 1:587–588.
Schwartz LB, Metcalfe DD, Sullivan TJ. Tryptase levels as an indicator of mast-cell activation in systemic anaphylaxis and mastocytosis. N Engl J Med 1987; 316:1622–1626.
Sheffer AL. Anaphylaxis. J Allergy Clin Immunol 1985; 75:227–233.
Stark BJ, Earl HS, Gross GN, Lumry WR, Goodman EL, Sullivan TJ. Acute and chronic desensitization of penicillin-allergic patients using oral penicillin. J Allergy Clin Immunol 1987; 79:523–532.
Stark BJ, Sullivan TJ. Biphasic and protracted anaphylaxis. J Allergy Clin Immunol 1986; 78:76–83.

RECURRENT IDIOPATHIC AND CRYPTOGENIC ANAPHYLAXIS

PAUL T. McBRIDE, M.S., M.D.
MICHAEL A. KALINER, M.D.

Anaphylaxis is a term used to describe symptoms ranging from isolated cutaneous flushing to life threatening vasomotor or respiratory collapse. The etiology ranges from classic IgE related mast cell mediated hypersensitivity reactions to anaphylactoid reactions, which, although identical in presentation, result from mast cell activation that is not IgE mediated. The commonest signs and symptoms of anaphylaxis are summarized in Table 1. They include flushing, tachycardia, pruritus, urticaria, and angioedema and often progress to asthma, airway edema, gastrointestinal dysfunction, and even death. The most common causes of true anaphylactic or IgE mediated hypersensitivity reactions are allergic reactions to penicillin and Hymenoptera stings; additional causes are listed in Table 2. Iodinated radiocontrast media are the most common cause of anaphylactoid reactions.

The sudden development of such distinctive multisystem symptoms usually makes the diagnosis of anaphylaxis obvious, but the differential diagnosis of similar reactions is often necessary (Table 3). Vasovagal reactions usually present with acute collapse, but bradycar-

TABLE 1 Clinical Findings in Anaphylaxis

System	Signs	Symptoms
Cutaneous	Flushing, urticaria, angioedema	Flushing, pruritus
Cardiovascular	Tachycardia, shock, hypotension, syncope, arrhythmias	Faintness, weakness, palpitations
Gastrointestinal	Abdominal distention, vomiting, diarrhea	Bloating, nausea, cramps, pain
Respiratory	Rhinorrhea, laryngeal edema, wheezing, bronchorrhea, asphyxiation	Nasal congestion, shortness of breath, difficult breathing, choking, cough, hoarseness, lump in throat
Others	Diaphoresis, fecal or urinary incontinence	Feeling of impending doom, conjunctival pruritus and edema, sneezing, headache, disorientation, hallucinations, genital burning, metallic taste

dia, diaphoresis, and abdominal symptoms in the absence of flushing, urticaria, and pruritus are diagnostic. Other medical emergencies such as cardiac arrhythmias, myocardial infarction, pulmonary embolism, seizure, cerebrovascular accident, asphyxiation, and hypoglycemia have distinctive presentations without urticaria, flushing, and pruritus. The prolonged time course and lack of associated symptoms, including pruritus, differentiate hereditary angioedema and serum sickness from anaphylaxis. Systemic mastocytosis with mast cell degranulation can mimic anaphylaxis because of mediator release, but the lesions of urticaria pigmentosa usually can be found. Unappreciated drug or chemical ingestion,

TABLE 2   Causes of Anaphylaxis and Anaphylactoid Reactions

1. IgE mediated reactions
   Antibiotics and other drugs
   Foreign proteins (horse serum, chymopapain)
   Food
   Immunotherapy
   Hymenoptera stings
   Seminal plasma
2. Complement mediated reactions
   Blood, blood products
3. Nonimmunologic mast cell activators
   Opiates (narcotics)
   Muscle depolarizing drugs
   Radiocontrast media
4. Modulators of arachidonic acid metabolism
   Nonsteroidal anti-inflammatory drugs (aspirin)
   Tartrazine (possible)
5. Idiopathic recurrent anaphylaxis
6. Other causes, as yet unclassified
   Exercise
   Cholinergic urticaria with anaphylaxis
   Cold induced urticaria with anaphylaxis
   Hormonally related reactions
   Sulfiting drugs
   Many drugs and chemicals

carcinoid syndrome, and pheochromocytoma must be ruled out.

Episodes of recurrent anaphylaxis present a diagnostic dilemma, and if no etiology can be identified are termed idiopathic anaphylaxis. The medical work-up consists mainly of obtaining a careful history concerning possible cryptogenic causes of anaphylaxis, the time course or pattern of symptoms, drug or food ingestion,

TABLE 3   Differential Diagnosis of Anaphylaxis

Vasovagal

Syncope

Arrhythmia	Hypoglycemia
Cardiac arrest	Asphyxiation
Myocardial infarct	Hyperventilation
Seizure	Cerebrovascular
Pulmonary embolus	accident

Laryngeal edema

Hereditary angioedema

Serum sickness

Cold urticaria

Mastocytosis (with or without urticaria pigmentosa)

Medication overdose

Endocrine—pheochromocytoma, carcinoid

Sulfite, monosodium glutamate exposure

Idiopathic urticaria and asthma

Foreign body in trachea

Damage to larynx

Idiosyncratic reaction to medication

activity level, and environmental conditions. This is followed by appropriate skin testing for aeroallergens and food allergens and then laboratory studies to rule out other possible diagnoses. A careful detailed review of each recurrent event is necessary to identify the inciting agent.

Multiple causes of "cryptogenic" anaphylaxis have been identified. Probably the most common cause is unrecognized drug or chemical sensitivity. A newly recognized syndrome is exercise induced anaphylaxis. This diagnosis must be distinguished from cholinergic or heat induced anaphylaxis by provocation testing. Cold induced urticaria with anaphylaxis is diagnosed by the history of cold exposure prior to the event. Specific foods and food additives may be implicated as possible causes but often remain unconfirmed. Idiopathic recurrent anaphylaxis, which is the diagnosis once other causes have been ruled out, recently has been linked to ovarian hormone sensitization in women with recurrent anaphylactic syndromes.

Hormonally related anaphylaxis is a distinct form of recurring anaphylaxis seen in women of childbearing age. The symptoms vary from mild to profound anaphylaxis, differ markedly in severity from patient to patient, and often (but not always) increase at the time of menses. There is no correlation with food or other allergens. The mechanism or trigger for the attacks remains unidentified, but anaphylactic attacks may be provoked after skin tests or subcutaneous provocations with 0.2 to 1.0 mg of progesterone. Reactions in these hormonally sensitive subjects may be provoked by infusion with luteinizing hormone releasing hormone, which stimulates ovarian secretion of gonadal hormones. In a continuing study at the NIH a synthetic luteinizing hormone releasing hormone analogue that blocks gonadal function and suppresses menses has shown promise in a limited number of subjects with hormonally mediated anaphylaxis but remains investigational. In these hormonally sensitive patients, oophorectomy has been curative.

Exercise induced anaphylaxis is one of the most common causes of anaphylaxis recognized today. Most of these patients are conditioned athletes, and symptoms can occur at any level of exercise. The disease is rare in children and unpredictable in occurrence. Positive skin test results to foods ingested prior to exercise related anaphylaxis are found in about 50 percent of the patients, and often ingestion of a particular food near the time of exercising is required for an attack to occur. Celery and shellfish are the foods most commonly implicated. In many instances isolated exercise or food ingestion does not provoke a reaction, but the combination of food and exercise invariably does. This pattern suggests the necessity for multiple triggers. The differential diagnosis is narrowed by the association with exercise, but food associated and cholinergic anaphylaxis must be investigated.

Acute exercise related anaphylactic attacks are treated as outlined in Table 4. Prophylactic therapy with H_1 and

TABLE 4   Treatment of Acute Anaphylaxis (Adult)

1. When possible, apply a tourniquet to halt blood flow from source of antigen or inciting medication; remove stinger if an insect sting; remove tourniquet every 15 minutes
2. Place patient in recumbent position; elevate legs; keep warm; provide oxygen
3. Epinephrine aqueous 1:1000, 0.3–0.5 ml subcutaneously; from this amount inject epinephrine 1:1000, 0.1–0.2 ml directly into source of antigen to reduce blood flow
4. Diphenhydramine, 25–50 mg intramuscularly or intravenously over 3 minutes
5. Ranitidine, 50 mg, or cimetidine, 300 mg, intravenously over 3 to 5 minutes
6. Establish and maintain airway; administer racemic epinephrine via metered dose inhaler or epinephrine (1:1000) by nebulizer to closed airway if laryngeal edema is present; if ineffective, tracheal intubation may be required
7. Maintain blood pressure with fluids, volume expanders, or pressors: dopamine hydrochloride, 2–10 μg/kg/min, or norepinephrine bitartrate, 2–4 μg/min
8. If wheezing is a problem that does not respond to H_1 antihistamines, administer aminophylline, 5.6 mg/kg intravenously over 20 minutes followed by a maintenance dose of 0.9 mg/kg/hr intravenously thereafter
9. For prolonged reactions, repeat epinephrine every 20 minutes x 3; provide hydrocortisone, 100 mg intravenously every 6 hours

H_2 antihistamines, cromolyn sodium, theophylline, corticosteroids, and beta-agonists has met with mixed success. Anecdotal reports of success with ketotifen therapy (Zaditen, Sandoz) have been published, and this regimen is currently under study. Modification or reduction of exercise, avoidance of incriminated foods before and after exercise, exercising with a companion, and immediate access to an anaphylaxis emergency kit are advised.

The term cholinergic anaphylaxis defines a syndrome of recurrent anaphylaxis associated with elevations of the core body temperature. The history often reveals attacks following exertion, hot baths or showers, anxiety, and an increased frequency during the hot summer months. Fever associated with an infectious agent is not associated with similar events. Typically there is no involvement of the face or hands, and characteristic 1 to 3 mm "cholinergic" wheals surrounded by extensive erythema are observed on the trunk. Skin testing with methacholine is positive in about half the subjects, who develop satellite wheals in the area of flare, which support the diagnosis.

The etiology of this syndrome is unclear, but attacks are always associated with sweating and involvement of the cutaneous cholinergic nervous system is postulated. Preventive therapy is aimed at maintaining the normal body core temperature, but once an attack has begun, standard therapy for acute anaphylaxis is usually effective.

Therapy for nonhormonally mediated idiopathic anaphylaxis is symptomatic and often ineffective because the cause remains unknown. Standard therapy for acute anaphylactic events—epinephrine, 0.3 to 0.5 mg subcutaneously; diphenhydramine, 25 to 50 mg intravenously; ranitidine (or other H_2 antihistamines); 50 mg given slowly intravenously; and fluids, oxygen, and theophylline-bronchodilator therapy (as needed)—is necessary and is summarized in Table 4. Specific therapy for laryngeal edema is often required, since maintenance of an open airway is essential. Administration of racemic epinephrine via a metered dose inhaler or epinephrine (1:1000) by nebulizer is usually effective early in the course, but tracheal intubation is sometimes required and tracheal fenestration may be necessary for recurrent laryngeal edema. Trials of nonsteroidal anti-inflammatory drugs and orally administered contraceptives are almost always ineffective. Prolonged prophylactic therapy with H_1 and H_2 antihistamines and trials of daily or alternate day prednisone therapy should be instituted with expectations of occasional success.

SUGGESTED READING

Broom BC, Fitzharris P. Life-threatening inhalent allergy: typical anaphylaxis induced by inhalational allergen challenge in patients with idiopathic recurrent anaphylaxis. Clin Allergy 1983; 13:169–179.
Casale TB, Keahey TM, et al. Exercise-induced anaphylactic syndromes: insights into diagnostic and pathophysiologic features. JAMA 1986; 255:2049–2053.
Kaliner MA. Anaphylaxis. NER Allergy Proc 1984; 4:324–328.
Slater JE, Raphael G, et al. Recurrent anaphylaxis in menstruating women: treatment with a luteinizing hormone releasing agonist, a preliminary report. Obstet Gynecol 1987; 70:542–546.
Sonin L, Grammer LC, et al. Idiopathic anaphylaxis—a clinical summary. Ann Int Med 1983; 99:634–635.
Stricker WE, Anawe-Lopez E, et al. Food skin testing in patients with idiopathic anaphylaxis. J Allergy Clin Immol 1986; 77:516–519.

SYSTEMIC LUPUS ERYTHEMATOSUS

JOHN H. KLIPPEL, M.D.

Systemic lupus erythematosus is a chronic, relapsing, and remitting inflammatory disease with multiple potential target organs. Although the cause, or perhaps more likely causes, of the disease are unknown, there is sufficient knowledge of the clinical course and pathologic processes to allow for the development of effective patient management. These include patient education, careful attention to the general internal medicine needs of the patient, regular monitoring to detect early evidence of disease exacerbations, and finally a limited number of drugs and other medical therapies used in treatment. Medical therapies are directed primarily at suppression of inflammation or dysfunction of the immune system thought to be of basic importance in pathogenesis. The success of the management of patients has been a major factor in the progressive improvements in prognosis of the disease over the past several decades.

EDUCATION

Patient education is an essential part of lupus management that is far too often neglected. The need for education is perhaps most evident during the early months of disease, although this need clearly persists throughout the course. The newly diagnosed patient often focuses only on the worst of all possibilities and becomes overwhelmed to learn that the disease may be fatal, involve vital organs, complicate pregnancy, and require drug treatment with serious possible side effects. These in fact may be major issues in the seriously ill patient that need to be addressed promptly from the onset. However, in the majority of patients emphasis on the marked variability of the disease, information about the specific details of the patient's illness, and reassurance that most patients respond well to management serve to minimize anxiety. Patient support groups as well as the distribution of appropriate patient literature concerning lupus are often very effective. Two of the better sources of patient information that can be highly recommended are *Living with S.L.E. A Handbook for Patients with Systemic Lupus Erythematosus* (W.V. Epstein and G. Clewley, Millberry Union Bookstore, 500 Parnassus Avenue, San Francisco, CA 94143) and *Lupus Erythematosus: A Handbook for Physicians, Patients and Their Families* (Lupus Foundation of America, Inc., Suite 203, 1717 Massachusetts Avenue, N.W., Washington, D.C. 20036).

GENERAL MEDICAL MANAGEMENT

The physician caring for a patient with systemic lupus erythematosus must be prepared to deal with many problems that fall within the category of general internal medicine. The care and well-being of the patient are as much, if not even more, dependent on attention to these aspects of management as those few therapies directed at the disease per se. Among the more common needs of the patient with lupus in addition to supportive care is the treatment of infections, hypertension, seizures, and minor psychiatric illness. In addition, there are several principles of preventive medical care that apply to essentially all such patients (Table 1).

DISEASE ACTIVITY

Therapy is guided by the concept of lupus disease activity. Although somewhat difficult to define precisely, disease activity is a composite of clinical and laboratory features suggesting the presence of uncontrolled lupus (Table 2). On the basis of the potential for these features to cause serious morbidity or mortality, the individual clinical manifestations or laboratory abnormalities can be categorized as to minor or major disease activity. These may reflect direct evidence of continuing lupus organ disease (e.g., nephritis, cardiopulmonary disease, dermatitis, serositis), indirect nonspecific manifestations of systemic inflammation (e.g., fever, fatigue, elevated erythrocyte sedimentation rate), or simply evidence of a deranged immune system (antinuclear antibody, anti-DNA antibodies, or hypocomplementemia).

TABLE 1   Important Preventive Measures in the Medical Management of Systemic Lupus Erythematosus

1. Regular monitoring	Patient should be evaluated every 6 months at a minimum to assess disease activity and review therapy; minimal standard laboratory studies should include BUN and creatinine, CBC, platelet count, urinalysis
2. Immunizations	Influenza vaccine should be given yearly Pneumoccocal vaccine should be given to splenectomized patients
3. Antibiotic prophylaxis	Antibiotic prophylaxis should be used for all dental or genitourinary procedures
4. Photoprotection	Patients with photosensitivity should be reminded to avoid intense sun exposure and to use sun screens
5. Birth control	Pregnancy should be avoided at times when the disease is active and uncontrolled or the patient is under treatment with major therapies

TABLE 2 Disease Activity in Systemic Lupus Erythematosus

	Clinical Features	Laboratory Features
Minor disease activity	Fatigue	Elevated ESR
	Fever	Leukopenia
	Rash	Proteinuria
	Oral and nasal ulcers	Hematuria
	Arthritis	Red cell casts
	Alopecia	Antinuclear antibodies
		Anti DNA antibodies
		Hypocomplementemia
Major disease activity	Serositis	Thrombocytopenia
	Myocarditis	Hemolytic anemia
	Pneumonitis	Rising BUN and
	Nephrotic syndrome	creatinine levels
	Vasculitis	
	Myositis	
	Psychosis	
	Status epilepticus	
	Cranial neuropathy	
	Transverse myelopathy	

The assessment of lupus disease activity is used to plan appropriate therapy as well as to gauge the success or failure of the therapy. In general, major disease activity warrants more intensive, aggressive approaches to management, whereas minor disease activity typically can be controlled with more conservative, less toxic forms of treatment. Changes in disease activity over time are useful in determining the effectiveness of therapy and whether more, less, or even another form of therapy is indicated. In most instances objective measures of disease activity, such as urine sediment examination, renal function tests, or the detection of proteinuria in nephritis or the hemoglobin level, white blood cell count, or platelet count for hematologic involvement, make the task of assessing disease activity for any given organ system affected by lupus relatively straightforward and easy.

Far more complicated is the patient with multisystem disease. A patient may have multiple minor abnormalities that when combined clearly constitute a major serious illness. Moreover, in the course of therapy certain features of the disease often decrease and others worsen. Thus, it may be difficult to assess the extent of disease activity and plan appropriate changes in therapy.

To address this clinical problem, a number of different methods to quantify overall lupus disease activity have been proposed. These range from relatively simple, four tier disease activity schemes (none, mild, moderate, severe) to more complex systems, which assign scores to individual measures, which are then summed to give a global disease activity index score. Although the latter type of scheme would be valuable in the clinical management of patients, in particular, in clinical trials involving therapy, none of the systems that have been developed have yet been properly validated.

Finally, it is important to note that measures of abnormal immunity are not by themselves markers of disease activity. However, they may be useful as adjunctive supportive evidence of disease activity in conjunction with clinical findings or other laboratory abnormalities. The patient with high titer antinuclear antibody, anti-DNA antibody, or depressed serum complement levels who is otherwise completely well should not be judged to have active lupus or be treated for these abnormalities.

DRUG THERAPY

The drug management of systemic lupus erythematosus is simplified by the limited number of drugs used in treatment. The pathologic changes seen in lupus as well as findings of abnormal immune function imply that drugs that suppress inflammation or immunity are likely to be of benefit. However, for the most part, detailed understanding of the exact mechanisms of action of drugs possessing either of these properties is lacking. Moreover, clinical use of these drugs is mostly empirical. With perhaps the single exception of lupus nephritis, there are no controlled trials upon which decisions can be based. Drug treatment thus comes to be based more on clinical experience and opinion than on scientific facts.

Nonsteroidal Anti-inflammatory Drugs

Nonsteroidal anti-inflammatory drugs are commonly used for the treatment of minor clinical manifestations of lupus. In addition to various salicylate compounds, there are now a number of prescription drugs of this type available. There is no reason to believe that one such drug is preferable to another. In fact, the only comparative study that has been done to evaluate this class of drugs in lupus found aspirin and ibuprofen to be equally effective. The selection among these drugs thus is based on such factors as physician or patient preference, cost, patient tolerance, or, in individual patients, the apparent capacity of one particular drug to best control the disease. The latter finding accounts for a good deal of changing from one drug to another until a nearly optimal drug is found. For unexplained reasons, certain patients appear to respond better to one drug, whereas others seem to experience no beneficial effect from that drug. The combining of nonsteroidal anti-inflammatory drugs is to be discouraged.

Several complications induced by nonsteroidal anti-inflammatory drugs may be mistaken for lupus activity. Since appropriate therapy is to discontinue the use of such a drug as opposed to intensifying drug therapy for lupus, these become important clinical considerations.

Although a spectrum of rare clinical manifestations such as fever, anaphylaxis, and pulmonary and cutaneous vasculitis has been described with these drugs, their effects on the kidneys and the central nervous system are of particular relevance in patients with lupus.

The inhibitory effect of these drugs on prostaglandins may produce a reduction in renal function with an elevation of the serum creatinine level or depression of creatinine clearance. These influences are particularly pronounced in the kidney with pre-existent active or chronic lupus nephritis in which prostaglandins become an important adjunct to maintain renal function. In this setting these drugs serve almost as a stress test to evaluate kidney involvement. In order to accurately determine renal function, it is therefore essential that all nonsteroidal drug therapy be discontinued for several days prior to the study. This is of particular importance if the recent loss of renal function prompts consideration of further evaluation by renal biopsy or the need for major changes in therapy. If these drugs are contributing to the impairment of renal function, their discontinuation will result in a rapid improvement in function.

Several nonsteroidal anti-inflammatory drugs have been associated with aseptic meningitis. Although these drugs appear to be capable of producing this reaction in patients without autoimmune disease, the majority of cases reported have involved patients with lupus or a lupus-like illness, thus suggesting a heightened predisposition to this drug complication in this patient population. The typical clinical presentation involves headaches, meningismus, and fever and rarely pruritus, facial edema, and conjunctivitis. Study of the cerebrospinal fluid reveals lymphocytosis, an elevated protein level, and a sterile culture. Azathioprine has also been incriminated in the production of aseptic meningitis in patients with lupus.

Corticosteroids

Corticosteroids are the single most important class of drugs used in lupus treatment. They are used topically for cutaneous manifestations, in low doses for minor disease activity, and in high doses for major disease activity (Table 3). The oral doses of prednisone recommended are arbitrary but generally are adequate to control most disease manifestations that might be categorized under minor or major activity. Ideally oral corticosteroid therapy should be given as a single daily morning dose. In the event that this is inadequate, the same total daily dosage should be divided into a two or three times a day schedule before the total dosage of corticosteroid is increased.

The reduction in the corticosteroid dosage (tapering) once the disease process is under control is of particular importance for high dose corticosteroid programs. There are few agreed upon rules as to how best

TABLE 3   The Multiple Uses of Corticosteroids in Systemic Lupus Erythematosus

Indication	
Rashes	Topical corticosteroid ointments and creams
	Short acting Hydrocortisone (0.125–1.0%)
	Intermediate acting Methylprednisolone (0.025–1.0%) Triamcinolone
	Long acting Betamethasone (0.025–0.2%) Dexamethasone
Minor disease activity	Prednisone (equivalent) at a dose of <0.5 mg/kg in single or divided daily dose
Major disease activity	Prednisone (equivalent) at a dose of 1 mg/kg in single or divided daily dose
	Intravenous bolus megadose (1 g or 15 mg/kg) of methylprednisolone given over 30 minutes; often repeated for three consecutive days

to go about dosage reduction. An attempt to change to an alternate day schedule after 4 to 6 weeks of therapy is common practice. The rate of dose reduction should approximate 5 mg of prednisone (or equivalent) on alternate days weekly until the patient is on a pure alternate day schedule. Some patients do not tolerate alternate day corticosteroids and begin to show evidence of disease activity starting in the afternoon or evening of the off-corticosteroid day. Nonsteroidal anti-inflammatory drugs are frequently used as a substitute; if these fail, efforts should be made to maintain the patient on the lowest possible daily corticosteroid dosage that controls the disease.

Many, or perhaps even most, lupus specialists reason that the risks of disease relapse when corticosteroids are discontinued far outweigh the potential long term toxic effects of chronic low dose corticosteroid therapy. Thus, the institution of corticosteroid therapy represents a lifelong treatment for many patients. There is, however, no evidence that low dose corticosteroid therapy prevents lupus flares or is associated with a high incidence of relapse once discontinued in certain clinical settings. Thus, in patients with prolonged periods of disease remission, slow reduction of the corticosteroid dosage with an aim toward eventual discontinuation of corticosteroid therapy should be a goal of patient management.

Megadose bolus intravenous methylprednisolone therapy should be regarded as an alternative to traditional high dose oral drug use in the treatment of major lupus activity. Several small randomized trials evaluating the efficacy of bolus methylprednisolone therapy appear to confirm at least the short term benefits of this approach.

A number of side effects of bolus megadose methyl-prednisolone not evident with high dose oral corticosteroid therapy have been reported. Common minor events noted have included facial flushing, a metallic taste, hypertension, hyperglycemia, and noninflammatory arthritis. Of considerable concern, however, are several presumably rare serious toxic effects such as intractable hiccups, anaphylaxis, seizures and other neurologic complications, and cardiac arrhythmias.

Antimalarial Drugs

Antimalarial drugs are effective in the management of mild systemic, cutaneous, and musculoskeletal features of lupus. The clinical efficacy of these drugs in systemic lupus erythematosus has never been subjected to rigorous randomized testing, although many years of clinical experience leave little doubt as to their importance. The mechanism of action of these drugs relevant to lupus is unknown; anti-inflammatory, immunosuppressive, photoprotective, and nucleoprotein stabilizing properties of antimalarial drugs have been described.

The antimalarial drugs commonly used in lupus include hydroxychloroquine or chloroquine (4-amino-quinolines) and less frequently mepacrine (a 9-aminoacridine compound; Table 4). Many advocate starting antimalarial therapy with a loading dose regimen (400 mg of hydroxychloroquine or 500 mg of chloroquine) for 4 weeks and then switching to a lower dosage maintenance schedule once the disease process is under control. The response to antimalarial drugs, particularly

in terms of cutaneous manifestations, can be remarkably rapid, with improvement often evident in a matter of days after starting the drug. Patients taking long term antimalarial therapy in complete clinical remission pose a minor dilemma. As with corticosteroids, many believe that discontinuation of therapy often results in disease relapse. Thus there is, in general, a reluctance to discontinue therapy completely. Reduction of the dosage of antimalarial drugs to one or two tablets a week in these patients is worthwhile.

There are a number of potential toxic effects of antimalarial therapy (see Table 4). However, with the small drug doses used in the treatment of lupus, the risks of most of these adverse effects are exceedingly small. The major concern is ocular toxicity of which there are two types. Deposition of antimalarial drugs in the cornea is relatively common. This may be responsible for visual disturbances such as complaints of a halo effect around lights often within several weeks after starting the drug. Corneal deposits can be detected by slit lamp examination and are not a contraindication to continued antimalarial therapy. In addition, corneal deposits are not in any way related to retinopathy, the other form of antimalarial eye toxicity. Clearly antimalarial retinopathy has been the major concern regarding the long term use of these drugs in lupus. The frequency with which antimalarial retinopathy occurs in the disease and whether daily drug doses or cumulative drug doses are the major important factors are not known. An ophthalmologic examination should be performed prior to therapy and then annually to detect any evidence of retinal toxicity early. Since antimalarial retinopathy has been reported to be exacerbated by light, patients treated with antimalarial drugs should be advised to wear sunglasses in bright sunlight.

TABLE 4 Doses and Toxic Effects of Antimalarial Drugs in Systemic Lupus Erythematosus

	Tablet Size	Daily Dosage
Drugs and dose		
Hydroxychloroquine (Plaquenil)	200 mg	200–400 mg
Chloroquine phosphate (Aralen)	500 mg	250–500 mg
Mepacrine (Atabrine)	100 mg	100 mg
Toxic effects		
Gastrointestinal	Anorexia, cramps, nausea, diarrhea	
Cutaneous	Erythematous rashes, bleaching of hair, yellow staining (mepacrine)	
Neurologic	Headaches, dizziness, irritability, peripheral myopathy and neuropathy	
Ophthalmologic	Corneal deposits, retinopathy	
Hematologic	Leukopenia, toxic granulations, thrombocytopenia, aplastic anemia	
Cardiac	Cardiomyopathy	

Immunosuppressive Drugs, Plasmapheresis, and Other Experimental Therapies

Cytotoxic and antimetabolite (immunosuppressive) drugs, plasmapheresis, as well as newer more experimental therapies such as total lymphoid irradiation are discussed in the chapter on *Lupus Nephritis*. The indications for these forms of therapy in systemic lupus erythematosus are serious major disease activity that is unresponsive to acceptable doses of corticosteroids and cases in which high doses of corticosteroids are contraindicated. With the exception of lupus nephritis, experimental therapies have not been rigorously evaluated in serious forms of lupus, and evidence that they are effective in this setting is derived mostly from case reports. It is not clear that any of these therapies allow lower dosages of corticosteroids to be given. Finally, it is important to recognize that these experimental forms of therapy are associated with significant risks and require careful assessment of potential benefits versus risks on a case by case basis.

SPECIAL THERAPEUTIC CONSIDERATIONS

Lupus Pregnancy

Potential complications in the mother and developing fetus require special considerations in managing the pregnant lupus patient. The increased risk of spontaneous abortion as well as rare manifestations of lupus in the newborn, such as skin, cardiac, and hematologic involvement, requires that obstetrical care be provided by a specialist in the management of high risk pregnancies. Recurrent abortion in a patient with systemic lupus appears to be associated with antibody to cardiolipin. The treatment of these patients with high doses of prednisone combined with low dose aspirin or anticoagulation therapy has been reported to be effective in the prevention of abortion.

For the expectant mother there is a definite increased risk of worsening lupus throughout the pregnancy as well as in the postpartum period. Patients need to be followed more closely than usual during this period to monitor disease activity. The major treatment approach for increased lupus activity involves the use of prednisone. Although prednisone crosses the placenta, there is little evidence that the fetus is harmed even by high doses of prednisone. Stress doses of corticosteroids are often given to the mother for several days at the time of delivery to prevent a postpartum relapse of lupus. In general, other drugs used in the treatment of lupus are discontinued during pregnancy. Although it is common practice to discontinue antimalarial and immunosuppressive drugs for fear of damage to the fetus, the evidence that these drugs are teratogenic is meager.

Lupus Thrombocytopenia

Thrombocytopenia in systemic lupus represents a unique manifestation in which there are several alternatives to the general approaches to drug treatments already described. Chemotherapy with vinca alkyloids such as vinblastine and vincristine is an effective means of drug therapy. These drugs bind avidly to tubulin contained in platelets, and upon phagocytosis of the platelet the drug is selectively delivered to cells of the reticuloendothelial system (chemical splenectomy). Danazol, a synthetic analogue of androgenic steroids and progesterone, appears to have a potentially important role in the treatment of refractory lupus thrombocytopenia. Finally high dose intravenous therapy with monomeric gamma globulin has been used effectively to treat lupus thrombocytopenia. Although the effects on the platelet count are typically of short duration, prolonged responses have been observed.

The role of splenectomy in lupus thrombocytopenia has long been the subject of controversy, including at one time an allegation that splenectomy might actually promote dissemination of the disease. The recent literature regarding the effects of splenectomy in lupus thrombocytopenia is divided between studies advocating and those emphasizing the failure of the procedure to significantly affect the short or long term outcome. In selected patients splenectomy has proved to be the only modality capable of managing lupus thrombocytopenia. However, it clearly should be reserved for patients who have failed to benefit from conventional medical approaches.

SUGGESTED READING

Decker JL. The management of systemic lupus erythematosus. Arthritis Rheum 1982; 25S: 891–895.

Kimberly RP. Steroid use in systemic lupus erythematosus. In: Lahita RG, ed. Systemic lupus erythematosus. New York: John Wiley, 1987: 889.

Klippel JH, Decker JL. Systemic lupus erythematosus. In: Zvaifler NJ, sect. ed. Internal medicine. Boston: Little, Brown, 1987: 1270.

Klippel JH. Immunosuppressive therapy. In: Lahita RG, ed. Systemic lupus erythematosus. New York: John Wiley, 1987: 923.

Lanham JG, Hughes GRV. Antimalarial therapy in SLE. In: Hughes GRV, ed. Clinics in rheumatic diseases. East Sussex: WB Saunders, 1982: 279.

Rothfield NF, Parke A. Pregnancy in SLE: risks to mother and fetus and current methods of management. In: Pinals R, ed. Post-graduate advances in rheumatology. Princeton: Forum Medicus, 1986: I–IV; 1–16.

RHEUMATOID ARTHRITIS

SHAUN RUDDY, M.D.
W. NEAL ROBERTS, M.D.

PROBLEMS IN PLANNING RHEUMATOID ARTHRITIS THERAPY

Rheumatoid arthritis is a chronic systemic inflammatory disease of unclear etiology, the sine qua non of which is joint inflammation. Other prominent characteristics are symmetry of joint involvement over time (although not necessarily at presentation), variability of presentation, and volatility of clinical course. Spontaneous partial remissions and exacerbations during the course characterize the course in three quarters of the patients with rheumatoid arthritis; another 10 percent progress relentlessly to debilitating deformity and 15 percent have monocyclic disease with no recurrence after the first episode (Fig. 1). The joints involved during the first year or two tend to be the most troublesome joints throughout the course. Admixtures of inflammatory joint symptoms, secondary mechanical joint symptoms, non-articular pain (fibrositis, bursitis, tendonitis), the psychologic impact of chronic disease, an increased incidence of septic joints, and extra-articular features (including Sjögren syndrome, scleritis, vasculitic skin ulcers, and Felty syndrome) can all contribute to the variability of the clinical course, precluding a linear approach to the therapeutic choices.

The mainstays of long term treatment are appropriate control of exercise and rest, including splinting, and the use of a relatively safe salicylate or nonsteroidal anti-inflammatory drug. Most patients have mild rheumatoid disease with only moderate threat of permanent structural damage to articular cartilage surfaces and respond satisfactorily to these two categories of treatment. Excessive pain and especially continued rapid loss of function or progression of deformity justify the use of more toxic, slow acting antirheumatic drugs. The latter include primarily gold salts, penicillamine, and hydroxychloroquine. Hydroxychloroquine has special value in the control of moderately severe synovitis as an intermediate step between nonsteroidal anti-inflammatory drugs and other slow acting antirheumatic drugs. Following the latter are the cytotoxic drugs methotrexate, azathioprine, and cyclophosphamide. Methotrexate now has become nearly coequal with the slow acting antirheumatic drugs owing to its relatively low toxicity; cyclophosphamide is generally withheld because of its recognized long term risk of inducing cancer.

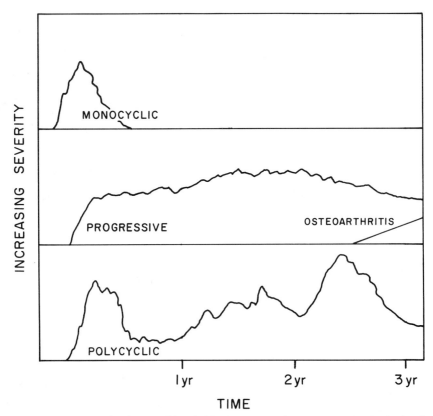

Figure 1 Clinical courses common in rheumatoid arthritis. Note secondary osteoarthritis beginning in the second panel.

Of the patients who require a slow acting antirheumatic drug for rheumatoid arthritis, most will have ceased taking the medication within several years. The extensive dropout from this second line antirheumatic therapy is attributable partially to side effects and partially to a lack of efficacy, but in any case the overall impact of these drugs on the course of the disease probably is not as great as initial responses to therapy would lead one to suspect.

Treatments for which the efficacy in the usual clinical situation, the benefit-toxicity ratio, or the role relative to other established therapies is as yet poorly defined include low dose daily oral therapy with prednisone, supplemental eicosopentanoic acid, sulfasalazine, thalidomide, therafectin, cyclosporine, total nodal irradiation, and low dose combinations of cytotoxic drugs such as cyclophosphamide and methotrexate. Nontraditional remedies, many with little or no apparent efficacy, add additional complexity.

Finally, surgical replacement of worn-out joints with extensive cartilage loss remarkably improves the function of hips and knees. The threshold for invoking this therapy continues to decrease every few years as technical improvements in joint replacement, particularly at the prosthesis-cement-bone interfaces, lengthen the half-lives of these implants. Therefore, in the face of slow acting antirheumatic drug toxicity or lack of efficacy, a strategy of last resort for severe rheumatoid arthritis is to abandon the latter therapy, using only salicylates (or nonsteroidal anti-inflammatory drugs) and replacing joints as they fail.

SPECIFIC THERAPIES AND MANAGEMENT APPROACHES IN RHEUMATOID ARTHRITIS

Physical Measures

The goal of physical management—including formal physiotherapy as well as specific prescriptions for rest, exercise, and splinting of involved joints—is to steer a course between overuse of a joint leading to an increase in inflammatory symptoms and underuse permitting contractures of the surrounding joint capsule with loss of range of motion. The more actively involved a joint, the more immobilization it requires, sometimes requiring splinting accompanied by local steroid injection. With lessening inflammation, range of motion exercise should be intensified in order to recover range lost during the exacerbation.

The most frequent error in general physical management is failure to withdraw a prescription for rest after an exacerbation subsides. After several exacerbations and admonitions to rest, the patient forms the impression that activity should be restricted even when inflammation is minimal. The resulting generalized deconditioning and excessive fatigue may be difficult to distinguish from that of systemic disease activity.

The most frequent error in physical treatment of specific joints is failure to splint involved wrists in order to prevent excessive flexion while the patient is sleeping. Also important is the liberal use of metatarsal bars, orthotics, or metatarsal pads to decrease the load on the most involved metatarsophalangeal joints.

In two randomized trials comparing inpatient multidisciplinary treatment of flares of rheumatoid arthritis with vigorous outpatient team treatment with home visits, hospitalization proved to be more expensive and more effective, with benefits lasting for up to 1 year. The low priority accorded patients with rheumatoid arthritis by health planners and cost control schemes obviates this approach in most settings. In contrast to acute care hospitals, rehabilitation units are exempt from diagnosis related group regulations and may provide a setting for more prolonged care of patients with rheumatoid arthritis.

Family and Social Considerations

Support groups of patients with rheumatoid arthritis as well as other social services serve at least two important functions. First, they may define functional thresholds such as the appropriate degree of social activity in adolescents, the ability to remain on a job, and the ability to move around the house and carry out the activities of daily living sufficiently well to remain independent of the family. These thresholds should be vigorously defended with a multidisciplinary approach involving social services at the same time that toxic drugs are introduced for disease control. Even when the patient's course of deterioration has slowed and is not approaching one of these functional thresholds, a social support group can combat the unfavorable psychologic aspects of chronic illness.

Second, social services, hospital admissions, and interviews with the family regarding drug toxicity serve to certify the patient in the sick role. Without this certification, the family may see no obvious deformity in the early stages, and may conclude that the patient's fatigue and complaints are out of proportion to physical changes.

Salicylates and Nonsteroidal Anti-inflammatory Drugs

Of all the medications effective for rheumatoid arthritis, aspirin and nonsteroidal anti-inflammatory drugs are the safest and the ones with which physicians generally have the most experience. The traditional argument in favor of aspirin as an initial drug has been its lower cost. However, if costs of work-ups and treatment for peptic ulceration and gastrointestinal hemorrhage are counted, the cost advantage of aspirin over the nonsteroidal anti-inflammatory drugs may disappear. The availability of salicylate levels to monitor compliance constitutes another advantage of aspirin over nonsteroidal anti-inflammatory drugs. The toxic consequences of full anti-inflammatory dosages of aspirin include one death from gastrointestinal hemorrhage in every 100 patients every 5 years. The major advantage of the nonsteroidal anti-inflammatory drugs is their longer pharmacologic half-lives, which lengthen the dosing interval, thereby increasing compliance. For example, piroxicam can be given once a day, although the incidence of significant gastrointestinal bleeding may be high in older patients. In addition, once or twice a day dosing limits dosage flexibility. For example, stiffness may be much worse in the morning, suggesting weighting the major portion of the day's dosage toward the previous night. Indomethacin seems to cause a higher incidence of central nervous system side effects such as headache and dysphoria in older patients. Consequently the first choice of many rheumatologists is a nonsteroidal anti-inflammatory drug, avoiding piroxicam and indomethacin in older patients. Sulindac may be particularly valuable in patients with mild renal insufficiency when a minimal effect on renal prostaglandins is desired, and when the patient is taking other medications that are renally excreted and whose toxicity may be augmented by any decrease in glomerular filtration rate.

How long should therapy with an ineffective nonsteroidal anti-inflammatory drug be continued before one switches to another medication? The only prospective trial that specifically sought an answer to this question suggested that new responses still occurred 4 weeks into the therapy. The usual recommendation is for 2 weeks of full dosages of nonsteroidal anti-inflammatory drug before concluding that there is a lack of efficacy. When patient noncompliance is factored in, the probable average trial is 7 to 10 days, however. This discrepancy between data and practice probably arises from differences between the patient's and the doctor's concerns, the former being more interested in the analgesia and the latter in the anti-inflammatory effect. Combinations of nonsteroidal drugs with salicylates or other nonsteroidal drugs appear to increase the risk of toxic effects with no increase in efficacy. Most patients decide for themselves to use some additional medication for analgesia. In the majority of cases this is acetaminophen, but sometimes it is an aspirin containing medication or over the counter ibuprofen.

When the first nonsteroidal anti-inflammatory drug employed proves ineffective after at least 2 weeks, what drug should replace it? Most rheumatologists would pick second and third choice nonsteroidal anti-inflammatory drugs on the basis of the principle of switching from one chemical class to another. There are five chemically distinct groups of nonsteroidal anti-inflammatory drugs, all of which inhibit cyclo-oxygenase activity. The major classes other than salicylates are propionic acids (ibuprofen, naproxyn), indole related compounds (indomethacin, sulindac, tolmetin), which are structurally closest to phenylbutazone, fenamates (meclofenamate), and oxicams (piroxicam). Data supporting the switching of classes over random choice of subsequent nonsteroidal anti-inflammatory drugs or their complete omission are lacking.

The main toxic effects of salicylates and nonsteroidal anti-inflammatory drugs are peptic gastritis, erosions, and ulcers. These lesions correlate imperfectly both with symptoms of upper gastrointestinal upset and with detectable gastrointestinal blood loss. For example, ulcers can occur, bleed, and heal while the patient continues to take nonsteroidal anti-inflammatory drug without symptoms. By default most clinicians merely monitor symptoms to detect erosions and ulcers, although a case could be made for periodic monitoring of the hematocrit. Periodic testing of the stool for occult blood is of no value because positive test results occur in most patients taking these drugs for long periods. A strategy for handling gastrointestinal upset is to discontinue all nonsteroidal and salicylate medications until 5 days after all symptoms have subsided. Therapy with the same or a different drug then can be restarted. Extra meals, over the counter antacids, H_2 blockers, sucralfate, and, when available, prostaglandin congeners may permit continued nonsteroidal anti-inflammatory drug therapy. Nonacetylated salicylates (magnesium choline salicylate or salicyl salicylate) have the least effect on the gastric mucosa but may be less effective in moderate to severe inflammation.

Additional nonsteroidal anti-inflammatory drug effects for which there is no agreed upon detection strategy include drug induced hepatitis and agranulocytosis. A complete blood count including a differential count and a chemistry battery should be carried out within the first 2 weeks after initiating nonsteroidal anti-inflammatory drug treatment.

A difficult-to-control feature of nonsteroidal anti-inflammatory drug prescribing is the patient's expectation for relief, which often exceeds what the medication can accomplish. The total effect of these drugs on the pain and inflammation of moderate rheumatoid arthritis may be in the range of 15 percent on a visual analogue scale, so that the medication may be of benefit but be seen by the patient as "only taking the edge off." The effect of the nonsteroidal drug may be evident only when it is discontinued. If pain is due to cartilage loss and secondary osteoarthritis, the patient almost certainly will be disappointed with the effect of the drug.

General Considerations in Therapy with Slow Acting Anti-inflammatory Drugs

The therapy of rheumatoid arthritis with slow acting anti-inflammatory drugs is one of the most unusual areas in modern medicine: the doctor gives the drug and then waits for 1 to 6 months for a clinical response. This delay in response makes the clinical effect of the drug difficult to differentiate from the natural history of a variable disease. Careful follow-up of certain clinical parameters is therefore imperative. Probably the easiest measurements to follow are the patient's global assessment, measured grip strength, length of the period of early morning stiffness, and the erythrocyte sedimentation rate. In general, slow acting antirheumatic drugs have minimal immediate anti-inflammatory effects but in the long run are several-fold more effective against moderate rheumatoid inflammation than are nonsteroidal anti-inflammatory drugs. True remissions are rare, but approximately two thirds of the patients who are able to take a full course of a given slow acting antirheumatic drug improve and about half of these do so to a great degree. Adverse drug reactions requiring discontinuation of therapy occur in about one third of the patients. Long term benefit from these drugs is reduced because of the continuing occurrence of side effects throughout the period of drug use and the tendency of the disease to relapse when the drugs are withdrawn. It is possible but not certain that a patient who initially responds to a slow acting antirheumatic drug can be "recaptured" with the same medication later. Failure to respond to one such drug does not predict a failure to respond to another; neither does toxicity with one accurately predict a recurrence of similar toxicity with another.

Some side effects of slow acting antirheumatic drugs, particularly oral ulcers and mild skin rashes from gold, can be circumvented by discontinuing the medication long enough for the side effect to resolve and then reinstituting the same drug, perhaps by a different route of administration (e.g., oral instead of injectable doses of gold), at a low dosage, and slowly advancing the dosage over a period of weeks to months. Methotrexate hepatotoxicity can be "treated through" if it is manifested only by hepatocellular enzyme increases of two and a half-fold or less. Toxic effects for which this strategy definitely should not be tried include agranulocytosis, hydroxychloroquine retinopathy, proteinuria with a change in renal function (in contrast to mild proteinuria with a normal creatinine level), and gold colitis.

The choice of timing for beginning slow acting antirheumatic drug therapy is complex (Table 1). The choice of such a drug is influenced by additional factors shown in Table 2. Hydroxychloroquine is clearly the least toxic, but is also less effective than gold, penicillamine, and cytotoxic drugs. Of all the medications other than nonsteroidal anti-inflammatory drugs and aspirin, methotrexate and steroids in low oral doses act most rapidly. Penicillamine is the slowest. Despite the multiple in vitro mechanisms of action ascribed to each of the slow acting antirheumatic drugs, it appears likely that gold and hydroxychloroquine operate by affecting monocyte function and that penicillamine interferes with T lymphocyte function.

TABLE 1 The Decision to Begin Therapy with Slow Acting Antirheumatic Drugs

In favor
  Progressive deformity or loss of function
  Persistent active inflammation despite nonsteroidal anti-inflammatory drug therapy
  Radiographic evidence of erosions
  Steroid dependency

Against
  No evidence of active synovitis on physical examination
  Questionable diagnosis
  Less than 6 months of disease
  Child bearing potential, off birth control therapy
  Lack of compliance or laboratory follow-up

Hydroxychloroquine

Although the beneficial effects of hydroxychloroquine are not marked, this drug is the easiest of the slow acting antirheumatic drugs to administer. It only rarely leads to gastrointestinal upset and otherwise causes a vanishingly small incidence of nuisance side effects. Skeletal muscle and myocardial toxic effects have been reported rarely. The abrupt onset of new heart failure in a patient taking hydroxychloroquine is reason to discontinue the drug. Unfortunately, rare instances of pigmentary macular degeneration in the retina occur with hydroxychloroquine. Most reported cases have occurred at high dosages; it is recommended that the dosage not exceed 6.5 mg per kg per day. Dosage schedules that vary every other day may have to be used because the tablets come in only a 200 mg size. With this low dosage of one or two tablets per day the incidence of pigmentary macular degeneration appears to be less than 1 percent and is related to the daily dosage rather than the total cumulative dosage. Unfortunately the prospect of visual loss, no matter how small statistically, often frightens patients. Nevertheless informed consent about visual loss is mandatory.

Appropriate monitoring of hydroxychloroquine includes a full retinal examination initially to exclude senile macular degeneration, which may be difficult to differentiate from pigmentary macular degeneration, along with an ophthalmologic follow-up every 6 months. It may take 3 months for the drug to have a beneficial effect. Patients who are in need of a rapid decrease in inflammatory symptoms are often given a more rapidly acting drug such as methotrexate. For those who need therapy in addition to nonsteroidal drugs but who can be expected to maintain function for a number of months, hydroxychloroquine is the slow acting antirheumatic drug of choice.

TABLE 2   Slow Acting Antirheumatic and Cytotoxic Drugs for the Treatment of Rheumatoid Arthritis

	Hydroxychloroquine	Auranofin	Injectable Gold Salts
Indications	Mild to moderate synovitis Symptoms unresponsive to nonsteroidal anti-inflammatory drugs, splinting, physiotherapy, local steroid injections	Persistent or progressive disease despite hydroxychloroquine therapy	Persistent or progressive disease with hydroxychloroquine, diarrhea with auranofin
Relative contraindications	Pre-existing macular disease	Proteinuria, renal disease Expected poor compliance with monitoring	Proteinuria, renal disease; history of gold rash, oral lesions
Usual dosage	200 mg q.d. or b.i.d.	3 mg b.i.d.	10 mg test dose, week 1 50 mg per wk × 20 wk Taper to 50 mg per mo
Maximal dosage	200 mg b.i.d.	3 mg t.i.d.	50 mg per wk
Major toxic effects	Pigmented macular degeneration (1%) Gastrointestinal upset (11%)	Mucocutaneous lesions (23%), rare exfoliation, diarrhea (25%), membranous nephropathy (2%), hematologic complication (1%)	Mucocutaneous lesions (48%), rare exfoliation, membranous nephropathy (6%), hematologic complication (7%)
Recommended monitoring	Baseline and q 6 mo retinal examinations with photographs and Ishikawa dot and Amsler grid tests	CBC, differential and platelet counts, urine dipstick for protein q 2 wk; may lengthen interval to q 3 wk at 2 mo	Same as oral gold, but check laboratory test results prior to each injection
Length of usual trial	3 mo	6–8 mo	4–6 mo

Gold

Adverse drug reactions to gold include extensive skin eruptions, oral ulcers, and a membranous glomerulopathy, the latter manifested by proteinuria. There may be about a 0.5 percent incidence of mortality from agranulocytosis, aplastic anemia, or uncontrollable secretory diarrhea due to gold induced colitis. Patients with HLA-DR3 disease may be more susceptible to gold induced thrombocytopenia. Rarely intramuscular doses of gold result in a "nitrotoid" reaction of acute vasodilation and hypotension when the rapidly absorbed aqueous solution (thiomalate salt) is used.

Most toxic reactions to gold occur during the first 4 months of treatment, but they may occur at any time during treatment, making complete blood counts with differential counts and urine tests for protein every 2 to 4 weeks the standard of monitoring for gold therapy, whether given by injection or orally. Hematuria without proteinuria probably is not gold membranous nephropathy and should be studied diagnostically as would any other hematuria.

Laboratory monitoring is the major expense in gold therapy. On the other hand, all the slow acting antirheumatic drugs (with the exception of hydroxychloroquine) require similar monitoring. Monthly laboratory monitoring can be decreased in frequency to every 2 months in patients who are stable with gold therapy for years. Gold is the slow acting antirheumatic drug for which the best case for protection of the patient from bone erosions can be made. High dose prednisone, cyclophosphamide, or methotrexate may also prevent erosions, but the first two of these drugs are much more toxic than gold. Oral gold therapy may not be the equivalent of injectable therapy; the disease in patients who are stable with injectable gold therapy often flares when they are switched to the oral preparation.

D-penicillamine

D-penicillamine is a difficult drug to manage. In addition to the membranous nephropathy and bone marrow toxicity characteristic of gold, penicillamine produces the nuisance side effect of loss of taste in 20 percent of patients and rarely the more serious autoimmune side effects of a myasthenia gravis-like syndrome and pemphigus. If the dosage is accelerated rapidly (e.g., over 2 months rather than 6 months), the incidence of thrombocytopenia, gastrointestinal intolerance, and other adverse reactions increases significantly. On the "go low, go slow" regimen (125 mg as a starting dosage with 125 mg monthly increments to a daily dosage of 750 mg), it takes 6 months to reach the full dosage and another month to decide that the full dosage has been of no value. Patients who seem likely to tolerate the 6

Methotrexate	Penicillamine	Azathioprine
Failure of gold; need (often social or psychologic) for rapid reliable response	Failure of gold and methotrexate	Failure of gold, methotrexate, and penicillamine
Liver disease; alcohol consumption 4 oz per wk Renal disease Trimethoprim sulfa	Proteinuria, renal disease History of drug rash, oral lesions	Renal disease, liver disease
2.5 or 5.0 mg q 12 h × 3 doses weekly	125 mg daily, raising dose by 125 mg per mo	50 mg daily, raising dose by 25 mg per 2 wk, guided by CBC
15 mg per wk	750 mg daily	200 mg daily
Hepatic fibrosis, rarely cirrhosis (irreversible)	Mucocutaneous lesions (30%), membranous nephropathy (15–20%), hematologic complications (5%), autoimmune syndromes (1%)	Bone marrow suppression, hepatitis (1%)
CBC, differential and platelet counts, liver chemistries, creatinine q 2 wk May lengthen interval to q 3 wk at 2 mo	CBC, differential and platelet counts, urine dipstick for protein q 2 wk; may lengthen interval to monthly at 6 mo	CBC, differential and platelet counts prior to adjusting dose; liver chemistries monthly
3 mo (many respond in first month)	7–9 mo	3 mo

to 9 months with no response are the best candidates for penicillamine. Penicillamine may be ineffective in seronegative rheumatoid arthritis.

Cytotoxic Drugs

Methotrexate

Cytotoxic drugs are probably as effective or more effective, and also faster acting (see Table 2), than the slow acting antirheumatic drugs against moderate to severe rheumatoid inflammation. However, the uncertain frequency and the known severity of adverse effects, including liver and lung toxicity in the case of methotrexate, make their exact role relative to the slow acting antirheumatic drugs debatable. Methotrexate is a reasonable drug to try if hydroxychloroquine and gold have been of no value. For many therapists methotrexate is preferable to penicillamine. In two large continuing trials methotrexate is being compared directly to oral therapy with gold. Responses to methotrexate tend to occur at 2 to 12 weeks of treatment in contrast to a longer period that may be needed for gold "loading" and the up to 9 months necessary for the evaluation of penicillamine treatment.

Experience with methotrexate in the treatment of psoriasis shows that it is not associated with any increase in malignant disease, but in animal models methotrexate breaks chromosomes at their fragile sites. The main clinical complications of methotrexate treatment are hepatic fibrosis and an interstitial-alveolar pulmonary infiltrate. These complications may occur in 1 to 2 percent of the patients, and there is no reliable way to predict when they will occur or to treat them when they do. Detection of hepatic toxicity is only marginally facilitated by carrying out the recommended liver chemistry panel every 2 to 4 weeks. The enzyme measurements should be made several days after the methotrexate dose. A decrease in the serum albumin level may also signify liver fibrosis due to methotrexate.

The role of liver biopsy in detecting hepatic toxicity is still unclear. Baseline liver biopsies are unnecessary, but rheumatologists still use needle biopsies of the liver as part of the routine monitoring when the total dosage reaches 1 to 2 g. Bone marrow suppression is usually not a problem with the low dosages of methotrexate used in the treatment of rheumatoid arthritis. However, renal insufficiency, seriously impaired pulmonary function, folate deficiency, severe infections, alcohol consumption greater than 4 ounces per week, and obesity great enough to preclude liver biopsy are contraindications to the use of methotrexate. Shortness of breath, a nonproductive cough, and fever are characteristics of methotrexate pulmonary toxicity. The clinical picture is one of a cold without rhinorrhea. A chest cold without a runny nose should be a red flag prompting physician evaluation for a patient taking methotrexate.

Other Cytotoxic Drugs

Anecdotal evidence indicates that azathioprine may be somewhat less effective than methotrexate and more apt to produce bone marrow suppression in the dosages commonly used. The one controlled comparison between methotrexate and azathioprine showed only a trend toward greater efficacy of methotrexate. Rarely idiosyncratic hepatotoxicity from azathioprine occurs in the first few weeks of the course. An excess of lymphoreticular malignant disease has been observed among allograft recipients treated with azathioprine but not among patients with rheumatic diseases treated with this drug. Severe effects of rheumatoid vasculitis such as nonhealing lower extremity ulcers may require brief pulse treatment with cyclophosphamide for which there is an established protocol. Despite its efficacy, continuous use of cyclophosphamide for rheumatoid arthritis without vasculitis is precluded by an increased incidence of the development of neoplasia.

Oral Steroid Therapy

There is general agreement that the risks of osteoporosis and other adverse effects from pharmacologic doses of prednisone are great enough to counterbalance their beneficial effect in rheumatoid arthritis. Using steroids for rheumatoid arthritis is like buying an automobile on time: all the benefits occur in the first 2 years and payment continues almost indefinitely. Nevertheless as many as 15 or 20 percent of the patients with moderately severe rheumatoid arthritis take steroids. There may be some role for low dosages of 5.0 to 7.5 mg a day. Every other day regimens usually fail owing to an exacerbation of symptoms on the "off" day ("every other day arthritis"). The role of steroid therapy hinges on the critical unanswered question of how much treatment with low dosages adds to the risk of osteoporosis. The risk-benefit ratio for low dose prednisone treatment of rheumatoid arthritis therefore may be affected profoundly by increases in the use of estrogen for the prevention of postmenopausal osteoporosis or coronary artery disease. Prednisone given at a dosage of 7.5 mg daily is probably a reasonable addition to slow acting antirheumatic drug treatment for patients with a lower baseline risk of osteoporosis, including those with high bone density determined by densitometry, large framed individuals, men, and blacks.

Injectable Steroids

Steroid injections are most useful when one or a few joints dominate the clinical picture. Almost any joint or surrounding periarticular structure can be injected successfully by an experienced operator. Intra-articular injections should be limited to three or four per joint per year because animal evidence indicates that repeated intra-articular injections accelerate cartilage degeneration. Serious complications from steroid injections are rare, although "postinjection flares" from steroid crystal deposition can occur 2 to 8 hours following the injection and the vitiligo that occurs when some of the injectable steroid infiltrates the dermis in black patients is cosmetically undesirable. Local steroid injection is one of the most effective treatments for geographically limited rheumatoid arthritis.

Surgery in Rheumatoid Arthritis

Secondary osteoarthritis and "bone on bone" pain are indications for joint replacement. Open surgical synovectomy is no longer performed, but arthroscopic synovectomy of the knee may provide relief of symptoms if the knee dominates the clinical picture or is the remaining troublesome joint after successful slow acting antirheumatic or cytotoxic drug therapy. Total joint replacement of the hips and the knees has a 95 percent certainty of affording pain relief, a 1 percent per year chance of resulting in loosening, and a 1 percent chance of resulting in postoperative infection.

Prosthetic replacements of other joints are less satisfactory. There is still no widely available prosthesis that withstands the stress put on an ankle. If the ankle joints or joints of the midfoot are destroyed by rheumatoid arthritis but remain painful, arthrodesis is the best option; the same is generally true of the wrist and elbow. Shoulder replacement eliminates pain as effectively as lower extremity joint replacements but adds little to function because the rotator cuff is usually destroyed and cannot be reconstructed. Silastic joint replacements in the small joints of the hands improve the hands cosmetically but often fracture and fail to increase strength even though they restore mechanical relationships. It is wise not to use hand surgery as a patient's first joint replacement surgery in order to avoid leaving the patient with an unrealistically pessimistic view of the functional value of joint replacement. Dorsal synovectomy to prevent rupture of the extensor tendons of the hands with consequent loss of function is an effective prophylactic surgical measure.

Experimental Treatments

There are a number of apparently effective treatments with major limitations imposed by side effects or inconvenience. Among these are radiation synovectomy with injected yttrium or dysprosium, which can be performed only in centers adjacent to a cyclotron or linear accelerator capable of creating these short lived isotopes.

Radiation synovectomy is 90 percent effective and may be superior to surgical synovectomy. Cyclosporine A produces a partially reversible loss of renal function and is ineffective at doses that minimize this effect. Total nodal irradiation (2000 to 3000 rads) has produced remissions lasting 2 years but also deaths due to infection. Lower doses of total nodal irradiation (200 to 750 rads) are currently being investigated. Plasmapheresis is ineffective. Pulse methylprednisone offers no advantage over low dose steroid therapy. Needed advances include: more dosing information in regard to radiation, risk to benefit information delineating the role of low dose prednisone therapy, and a clearer definition of the risk to benefit ratio inherent in the strategy of using cytotoxic and slow acting antirheumatic drugs earlier in the course of the disease.

SPECIAL PROBLEMATIC SITUATIONS

Early Aggressive Disease

The patient who has severe synovitis during the first year of disease with considerable functional loss poses a major question. Does early aggressive treatment have a better chance of succeeding than late aggressive treatment? One point of view holds that as soon as one is certain of the diagnosis, one should use the drug most likely to suppress synovitis before the disease gets a foothold. The contrasting point of view suggests that slow acting antirheumatic or cytotoxic drugs are rarely continued for many years consecutively and ultimately have little impact on the final outcome. One therefore should withhold them as long as possible in order to avoid unnecessary exposure to toxic drugs in patients in whom spontaneous remission might occur. Most rheumatologists have become increasingly aggressive in the early use of slow acting antirheumatic drugs. Previous recommendations centered on the caution that one should avoid such drugs during the first year when the likelihood of spontaneous remission was the greatest. Most rheumatologists now place this limit at 6 months. Many use oral gold therapy even earlier. Hydroxychloroquine has always been available for early use.

The Discouraged Patient

The patient who adopts a therapeutically nihilistic attitude and gives up trying to maintain joint mobility is in a precarious situation. Flexion contractures may become permanent, and often function lost in this way cannot be regained even surgically. Two approaches greatly encourage the patient at almost zero cost. The first is to allow the patient as much control over the therapy as possible. Creating options of more or less equal value and presenting them to the patient as choices

generate a sense of control on the part of the patient. Second, steroids can be injected into the two or three most actively inflamed joints. A long lasting (e.g., 3 month) benefit from injection may occur, and the systemic spillover during the initial week after injection may also help psychologically. The contrast between the response to intra-articular steroid therapy, even if it is short-lived, and the baseline to which the patient returns demonstrates that effective treatment is at least possible and that the situation is not hopeless.

Night Pain

Pain that awakens the patient at night usually leads to a specific treatment. The three most likely causes of night pain in patients with rheumatoid arthritis are: (1) bursitis-tendonitis in the shoulder, hip, or anserine bursa, which responds to local steroid injections (patients use the medial surface of the knees to push off against the mattress when turning over and may experience patellar and anserine bursa pain from this seemingly innocuous action); (2) compression neuropathy, which can be treated with steroid injection or decompression of the nerve (e.g., median nerve release); and (3) structurally diseased joints with bone on bone pain from cartilage loss (these patients may benefit from surgery).

The Patient Who Has Failed to Improve

The diagnosis should be reviewed (Table 3). In the patient who has experienced failure with multiple slow acting antirheumatic drugs as a result of toxicity, a detailed re-examination of the history should be made in order to determine whether the "toxicities" that led to discontinuing such a drug, particularly gold, are toxicities that definitely warrant abandoning the drug. These include nephrotoxicity with rising creatinine levels, cytopenias, and gold colitis. Mild (trace to 1^+) proteinuria, stomatitis, or a mild skin rash sometimes can be "treated through" by restarting at a lower dosage

TABLE 3 Rheumatic Diseases That May Resemble Rheumatoid Arthritis

Consider the following in seronegative rheumatoid arthritis failing to respond to treatment:

Erosive interphalangeal osteoarthritis	Reiter's syndrome (especially if metacarpophalangeal involvement is asymmetric)
Calcium pyrophosphate deposition disease	
Chronic tophaceous gout (especially steroid treated)	Psoriatic arthritis
Ankylosing spondylitis (especially if metacarpophalangeal involvement is asymmetric)	Systemic lupus erythematosus

and advancing the dosage more slowly. The probability of success using this strategy may be augmented by switching the route or form of administration of gold. Thus, if the toxic effect was minor and occurred with aurothioglucose, the patient is switched to gold sodium thiomalate, or auranofin. As an alternative to restarting slow acting antirheumatic drug therapy, local steroid injections and nonsteroidal anti-inflammatory drugs may be used for the control of symptoms, using surgical replacements for joints as they fail. A patient with advanced widespread disease is sometimes paradoxically a very good candidate for multiple joint replacements, since the level of physical activity is so low that it puts little stress on the bone-cement interface. This conservative strategy of aspirin combined with replacement of joints as they fail from cumulative cartilage loss is often superior to repeated excursions into obscure areas of therapeutics such as plasmapheresis and long term cyclophosphamide therapy.

The "Burnt Out" Patient

There is some debate about whether rheumatoid arthritis "burns" itself out. Fibrotic pannus may both insulate the examining hand from signs of inflammation in the joint and physically limit the volume of effusion. Some patients appear to have very limited inflammation on examination and yet have malaise and easy fatigability accompanied by laboratory evidence of disease activity, such as decreased albumin and hematocrit levels with increased erythrocyte sedimentation rate. These patients sometimes benefit from aggressive treatment even though they have long-standing rheumatoid arthritis with little apparent evidence of active synovitis on examination.

Generalized Fatigue and Aching Without Physical Signs

A patient who has had rheumatoid arthritis for a short period of time may not have the deformity and scarred pannus of the "burnt out" patient but still may not be doing well. Such a person may have a mild synovitis or synovitis in a few joints but complain of generalized aching, which may turn out to be secondary fibrositis or depression (treatable with amitriptyline). Comorbidity such as hypothyroidism is common. When symptoms of aching are disproportionate to physical findings or laboratory test results, special attention to the patient's home, family, or other social situation is indicated.

A Single Inflamed Joint or a Dominant Joint

This is the most important special situation in the treatment of patients with rheumatoid arthritis. A single dominant joint in a patient with rheumatoid arthritis should be aspirated the first time it is seen to effect symptomatic relief, diagnosis by culture, and drainage of a potentially infected joint space. Shoulders in particular require prompt aspiration. Unlike joints in the lower extremities, shoulders usually can be spared physical stress and are voluntarily and involuntarily splinted by the patient when a small effusion stretches the joint capsule. Therefore, a large palpable effusion makes the shoulder more likely to be infected even if not warm. In patients with rheumatoid arthritis there may be several reasons why there is not so much warmth over a septic joint as in other patients. Nonsteroidal anti-inflammatory drugs, steroids, and generalized debility may contribute to decreasing the signs of inflammation.

In a particularly stubborn, culture negative joint, especially one that is as anatomically complex as the shoulder, the failure of one local steroid injection to produce relief should prompt more careful examination of all the tendon and bursal structures around the joint. Injections directed at the structure that seems by physical examination to be most involved are more successful than steroid injections given intra-articularly by the anterior approach regardless of physical findings.

SUGGESTED READING

Furst DE, et al. A controlled study of concurrent therapy with nonacetylated salicylate and naproxen in rheumatoid arthritis. Arthritis Rheum 1987; 30: 146–154.

Hamdy H, McKendry RJ, Mierins E, Liver JA. Low-dose methotrexate compared with azathioprine in the treatment of rheumatoid arthritis. Arthritis Rheum 1987; 30: 361–368.

Healey LA. The current status of methotrexate use in rheumatic diseases. Bull Rheum Dis 1986; 36: (4).

Helewa A, et al. A cost-effectiveness analysis of in-patient and intensive out-patient therapy for patients with rheumatoid arthritis: a randomized controlled trial. Arthritis Rheum 1987; 30: S31 (abstract).

Panush RS. Controversial arthritis remedies. Bull Rheum Dis 1985; 34 (5).

Scott DGI, Bacon PA. Intravenous cyclophosphamide plus methylprednisolone in the treatment of systemic rheumatoid vasculitis. Am J Med 1984; 76: 377–384.

JUVENILE RHEUMATOID ARTHRITIS

SUZANNE L. BOWYER, M.D.

Juvenile rheumatoid arthritis is an inflammatory disease of unknown etiology. In some patients systemic features may be present in addition to the arthritis. Pain at rest is extremely rare; moving a joint through its full range of motion seems to cause the most discomfort. Stiffness affecting the joints and adjacent soft tissues is usually a prominent symptom, and without constant attention to range of motion, contractures can and will result. The disease remains active for several years, but in the majority of children remission eventually occurs. Because of the chronic yet self-limited nature of this disease, which affects young children, safe, well tested medications having no long term side effects should be used. The patient and parents should have a good understanding of the disease process and work with the medical team in therapeutic planning.

The goals of treatment are to control the inflammation and stiffness, to prevent and correct any musculoskeletal deformities, and to ensure that the child reaches adulthood as functional as possible despite the illness. Throughout the treatment period the child's normal social, emotional, and intellectual development must continue. The problems encountered during the course of the illness are multidisciplinary in nature, and ideally these children should be cared for by a team of individuals familiar with the medical and psychologic issues created by the disease. Such a team usually includes a pediatric rheumatologist, a nurse-clinician, a social worker, and physical and occupational therapists. A general approach to the treatment of juvenile rheumatoid arthritis is outlined in Table 1.

Juvenile rheumatoid arthritis has three distinct types of onset. The patients in each group differ in presentation, disease course, and prognosis (Table 2). The general approach to treating arthritis is the same regardless of the subgroup into which the patient best fits. The severity and extent of joint involvement, which may vary between subtypes, determine the exact nature of the treatment regimen needed for any individual patient. Aggressive arthritis accompanied by early bone erosions implies the need for equally aggressive treatment. Drugs with the potential for causing side effects can be justified when the alternative is irreversible joint damage in a young patient. On the other hand, a more conservative regimen would be appropriate for a child with mild monoarticular arthritis, little functional disability, and no evidence of erosions on x-ray examination of the involved joints.

TABLE 1   Approach to Treatment in Juvenile Rheumatoid Arthritis

1. The patient and family should be educated regarding the nature of the disease, the expected disease course, and its prognosis
2. Adequate nutrition, rest, and exercise should be encouraged
3. Medications are prescribed to decrease inflammation and associated pain and stiffness
4. Exercises are prescribed to:
   a. Preserve range of motion in involved joints
   b. Increase the strength of muscles crossing involved joints
   c. Prevent deformity
5. Splints may be prescribed to decrease stiffness and prevent contractures
6. The patient's ability to perform activities of daily living must be maximized
7. Potential complications should be screened for, dealt with, and prevented if possible
8. Emotional support must be provided to the patient and family

GENERAL MEASURES

Like children with any chronic inflammatory disease, patients with juvenile rheumatoid arthritis tend to be more tired than other children their own age. An after-school rest period can make a major difference in their disposition and ability to function in the evening.

Good nutrition is important for these children. No form of dietary manipulation has consistently been shown by rigorous scientific testing to significantly alter the course of arthritis. We recommend a regular balanced diet appropriate for the child's age. Because many children tend to have a poor appetite when the disease is active, administration of a multivitamin preparation is probably a good idea as well.

Children with juvenile rheumatoid arthritis stiffen up when they remain in one position for a long time. This process is called "gelling." It is most common in the morning, and a warm bath can be helpful in getting the child moving. When at school, the child should be allowed to get up, walk around, and stretch from time to time.

PHYSIOTHERAPY AND OCCUPATIONAL THERAPY

Pain and stiffness in joints and surrounding soft tissues keep children with juvenile rheumatoid arthritis from moving normally during the day, putting them at risk for contractures. Thus, physiotherapy becomes important as a means for maintaining joint range of motion. The type of therapy prescribed differs according to the level of disease activity present. Acutely inflamed joints should not be subjected to vigorous or weight bearing exercise, for example. Therefore, during a flare only range of motion exercises are prescribed. Later stretching and strengthening are added in order to preserve or

TABLE 2   Classification of Juvenile Rheumatoid Arthritis

Type of Onset	Age at Onset	Males/Females	Clinical Characteristics	Laboratory Findings	Prognosis
Systemic	Any	Equal	Rash, fever, lymphade-nopathy, hepatosple-nomegaly, pericarditis; may have a few or many joints involved	↑ ↑ ESR ↑ WBC ↓ Hb Negative ANA, RF	All mortality (1–2%) in this group. 50% develop persistent arthritis and more than half of these have severe arthritis
Polyarticular Rheumatoid factor negative	Usually under 5 years old	Majority are female	More than five joints, symmetrical, few systemic features	↑ ESR ↑ WBC ↓ Hb May have positive ANA	10–15% develop severe arthritis
Rheumatoid factor positive	Usually older (teenage)	Majority are female	Symmetrical polyarthritis, small joint involvement similar to adult rheumatoid arthritis, nodules	↑ ESR ↑ WBC ↓ Hb RF positive ANA negative	Prolonged course, rare remission, more than 50% with severe joint disease
Pauciarticular Type I	Usually under 5 years old	Majority are female	Fewer than five joints involved, usually lower extremity; uveitis in 20%	ESR slightly ↑ ANA frequently positive RF negative	Arthritis frequently goes into full remission. 10–20% have residual eye damage, some become polyarticular.
Type II	Usually older (teenage)	Majority are male	Lower extremity involvement; hip commonly involved; enthesopathy; symptomatic acute iritis	HLAB27 positive	Some may develop ankylosing spondylitis as adults

increase the strength of the muscles surrounding the affected joints. Heat, provided as a warm bath, hot packs, paraffin, or ultrasound, can be helpful for increasing range of motion. Exercises such as swimming and pedaling a bicycle are excellent for preserving range of motion in a nonweight bearing fashion.

Occupational therapists can assess a child's ability to carry out the activities of daily living. In order to maintain and improve their self-image, children with juvenile rheumatoid arthritis should be encouraged to do as much as possible for themselves. If functional deficits exist, an occupational therapist can provide assistive devices to help the child perform particularly difficult tasks.

Splints are used when a child is steadily losing range of motion in a particular joint. These devices are pieces of plastic molded to the areas of interest, padded, and held in place with Velcro straps. A resting splint temporarily immobilizes a joint in a comfortable but functional position. Splints often are worn at night during periods of active disease so that even though joint stiffening occurs, the joint will still be in a usable position.

COMPLICATIONS

Part of the physician's role in treating a child with juvenile rheumatoid arthritis is to anticipate and treat complications. The most common are joint contractures, leg length discrepancies, and chronic uveitis.

Prevention of contractures has been discussed in the previous section. If a contracture does occur, a vigorous program of stretching is indicated. Serial splinting and casting procedures have been successful in patients with contractures that have been unresponsive to more conservative measures. Rarely a patient requires soft tissue release or balanced traction to relieve the contracture.

Children with pauciarticular arthritis affecting only one knee may develop overgrowth of the affected leg. If the leg becomes more than 1 inch longer than the other leg, a compensatory hip tilt and associated back problems may result. If this problem is identified, it can be easily treated by placing a small lift on the shoe on the unaffected side. In most patients the magnitude of the difference in leg lengths tends to diminish with time. Rarely, however, differences of as much as 3 to 4 cm may result. In these cases epiphyseal stapling procedures may be necessary.

Chronic uveitis occurs primarily in patients with antinuclear antibody positive pauciarticular juvenile rheumatoid arthritis. It can be seen, however, in antinuclear antibody negative patients as well. Because the condition is asymptomatic, screening must be performed at regular intervals in order to start treatment before permanent damage is done to the eye. A slit lamp examination done by an ophthalmologist will identify the earliest signs of inflammation. Treatment consisting of topical steroid therapy, mydriatics, and occasionally low dose systemic steroid therapy should be supervised by an ophthalmologist.

DRUG THERAPY

Nonsteroidal Anti-inflammatory Drugs

Many nonsteroidal anti-inflammatory drugs are available for the treatment of arthritis (Table 3). Aspirin remains the drug of first choice in the treatment of juvenile rheumatoid arthritis. It has a long history of use, and its good and bad points are well characterized. This drug is given four times a day with a meal or snack. It is not necessary to awaken the child for a nighttime dose, however, because a steady level is reached within the first week of therapy. Levels of 20 to 30 mg per dl are therapeutic.

In 50 percent of the children taking aspirin the liver enzyme levels temporarily are increased to two to three times normal values. If the levels rise to five to ten times normal or if the child has abdominal pain, aspirin should be stopped and Tolectin or Naprosyn substituted. True hepatotoxicity occurs primarily in patients with systemic disease and in those with aspirin levels greater than 30 mg per dl. In some patients with systemic disease it is difficult to obtain a therapeutic aspirin level despite dosages in excess of 100 mg per kg per day. When the disease is brought under control, however, salicylate levels may rise into the toxic range. This phenomenon may be secondary to gastrointestinal absorption problems during the acute phase of the illness or to a corticosteroid effect on aspirin metabolism. In these patients salicylate levels may rise as the steroid dosages are tapered.

Because of recent concern about the relationship between the use of salicylates and the development of Reye's syndrome, it is suggested that aspirin be stopped temporarily if the child develops chickenpox or influ-

TABLE 3 Nonsteroidal Anti-inflammatory Drugs Useful in Children Less Than 12 Years Old

Drug	How Supplied	Dose	Dosing Interval	Side Effects
I. Salicylates				
A. Aspirin	325 mg tablet	75–100 mg/kg/d	q.i.d.	Tinnitus, bruising, gastrointestinal irritation, hepatotoxicity, allergic reactions, papillary necrosis, decreased renal blood flow
1. Enteric coated				
Ecotrin	325 and 500 mg tabs 325 and 500 mg caps			
Encaprin	325 and 500 mg caps			
2. Baby aspirin	80 mg tabs (chewable)			
B. Choline salicylate (Arthropan)	600 mg/tsp liquid			
C. Choline-magnesium salicylate (Trilisate)	Scored 500, 750, 1000 mg tabs 500 mg/tsp liquid			
II. Indomethacin group				
A. Indomethacin (Indocin)	25 and 50 mg caps (25 mg/tsp liquid available from manufacturer)	1.5–3.0 mg/kg/d	t.i.d.	Side effects common to all nonsteroidal anti-inflammatory drugs: gastrointestinal irritation, allergic reactions, papillary necrosis, fluid retention, headache, dizziness
B. Tolmetin sodium (Tolectin)	Scored 200 mg tabs (can be chewed or dissolved in 1 tsp milk) 400 mg caps	15–30 mg/kg/d	t.i.d.	
III. Propionic acid derivatives				
* A. Ibuprofen				
Motrin	400, 600, 800 mg tabs	Preliminary data suggest 1200–1600 mg/sq m	q.i.d.	As above
Rufen	400, 600 mg tabs			
Nuprin, Advil, Medipren	200 mg tabs available over the counter			
* B. Naproxen (Naprosyn)	250, 375, 500 mg tabs 125 mg/tsp liquid	10–16 mg/kg/d	b.i.d.	

*Not yet approved by the FDA for use in children under 12 years.

enza. It is not necessary to stop the drug for a mild upper respiratory infection. The Public Health Service recommends influenza vaccine for children taking long term aspirin therapy.

Nonsteroidal anti-inflammatory drugs decrease the symptoms of inflammation via several mechanisms, among them suppression of prostaglandin synthesis. These drugs do not change the values of the laboratory tests measuring disease activity (sedimentation rate, rheumatoid factor titer, platelet count) nor do they alter the eventual course of the disease. They do provide relief of pain, swelling, warmth, and morning stiffness, however, and their effects are seen within days to weeks after starting the medications. The decrease in pain and stiffness allows the patient to do more effective range of motion exercises, thus preserving the ultimate functional state of the affected joints. The side effects of nonsteroidal anti-inflammatory drugs are listed in Table 3 as well.

In some cases it may be helpful to give two nonsteroidal anti-inflammatory drugs—each from a different drug class—for a short period. Although children do not seem to be as susceptible as adults to the adverse renal effects of nonsteroidal anti-inflammatory drugs, it is wise to monitor the blood urea nitrogen and creatinine levels and serial urinalyses if two drugs are going to be used for longer than 1 week.

Slow Acting Antirheumatic Drugs

If arthritis remains active after 6 months of treatment with nonsteroidal anti-inflammatory drugs or if periarticular bone erosions are evident on x-ray examination, more aggressive treatment is indicated. This course is most common in patients with polyarticular juvenile rheumatoid arthritis. Slow acting antirheumatic drugs are rarely indicated in patients with pauciarticular or systemic disease. They actually modify the course of the arthritis, decreasing the incidence of erosions and causing changes in laboratory values such as the erythrocyte sedimentation rate and the rheumatoid factor titer. These medications are given along with, not in place of, nonsteroidal anti-inflammatory drugs. No obvious improvement should be expected for about 2 to 4 months after starting therapy with one of these drugs—hence the name. If the patient is significantly disabled by the degree of disease activity, low dose corticosteroid therapy can be used to allow the child to function while waiting for the slow acting antirheumatic drugs to take effect.

Gold

Gold is the oldest and best studied drug in this group. Intramuscular gold therapy has been used for years to treat adult and pediatric rheumatoid arthritis. It

TABLE 4 Guidelines for Gold Administration

1. Check CBC, urinalysis, and liver function tests
2. Baseline x-ray views of involved joints should be obtained
3. Give test dose of 5 mg intramuscularly
4. If test dose is tolerated, increase weekly dose gradually to a maximum of 0.75–1.0 mg/kg/dose (maximal dose, 50 mg) per week
5. Prior to each injection, CBC and urinalysis should be checked and results obtained
6. Injection should not be given if:
   a. WBC is less than 4500
   b. Platelet count is less than 150,000
   c. Urine is positive for blood or protein
   d. Patient develops mouth sores, rash, or eosinophilia
7. If response is favorable after 20 weeks, interval between injections may be lengthened to 2 weeks for next 3 months, 3 weeks for following 3 months, and eventually 4 weeks

probably modifies disease activity by interfering with monocyte and macrophage function. Fifty to 60 percent of treated patients improve significantly, but some 25 percent are unable to tolerate the drug because of side effects. Guidelines for the administration of gold are given in Table 4.

Two gold salts are available for injection—gold sodium aurothiomalate (Myochrysine) and aurothioglucose (Solganol). Myochrysine tends to cause more pain on injection and causes a higher incidence of nitritoid reactions (flushing and dizziness) after injection than does Solganol.

The most common sites of gold toxicity are the skin and mucous membranes, bone marrow, and kidneys. If the disease develops a rash, mouth sores, eosinophilia, neutropenia, thrombocytopenia, hematuria, or proteinuria, the drug should be stopped. When the abnormality has completely resolved, the medication can be cautiously started again at a lower dosage. The reappearance of gold toxicity should prompt the change to another drug. Extreme cytopenia and the development of exfoliative dermatitis are contraindications to restarting the drug.

An oral form of gold is now available (Auranofin). Although it has not yet been approved by the FDA for use in children under 12 years of age, it has been studied in juvenile rheumatoid arthritis. The dosage is 0.1 to 0.2 mg per kg per day. Auranofin appears to be less effective than injectable gold in controlling the disease. The blood count and urinalysis should be monitored weekly in patients taking the drug.

Hydroxychloroquine (Plaquenil)

Although the exact mechanism of action of hydroxychloroquine is currently unknown, in vitro the drug has a stabilizing effect on the lysosomal membranes of inflammatory cells. The dosage is 7 mg per kg per day for 8 weeks and then 5 mg per kg per day. A recent multicenter collaborative study suggested that Plaquenil was not effective for the treatment of childhood arthritis. Although the drug is not as effective as gold, it still has a role in the treatment of selected patients. It is given in pill form and thus spares the child the pain of an intramuscular injection. Plaquenil's side effects are completely different from those associated with gold, and the drug thus can be used in patients who are intolerant to gold. The main toxic effect of this drug is retinopathy. A baseline eye examination should be obtained and ophthalmologic screening should be done every 4 to 6 months. Although complications are rare in this dosage range, the drug should be stopped if signs of toxicity occur because the damage is cumulative. The total duration of therapy probably should not exceed 2 years.

Penicillamine

Although penicillamine has many demonstrable effects on the immune system, the mechanism of its beneficial effect in the treatment of arthritis remains a mystery. Guidelines for the use of this drug are given in Table 5. The most common side effects of penicillamine are similar to those caused by gold. With both drugs, side effects are most often seen in patients who carry the HLA marker DR3. The penicillamine dosage should be lowered at the first sign of bone marrow or renal toxicity. Autoimmune phenomena such as lupus, polymyositis, myasthenia gravis, Goodpasture's syndrome, and pemphigoid are seen occasionally in patients treated with this drug. The spectrum of rare but serious side effects as well as a recent multicenter study that questions the usefulness of the drug in juvenile rheumatoid arthritis has resulted in fewer patients being given this drug.

Corticosteroids

The indications for steroid use in juvenile rheumatoid arthritis are given in Table 6. These drugs should

TABLE 5   Guidelines for Treatment with Penicillamine

1. Baseline CBC and urinalysis should be obtained
2. Dosage: Begin at 125 mg/day; increase in increments of 125 mg every 2–3 months to a maximal dose of 10 mg/kg/day or 750 mg/day total (whichever value is less)
3. Monitor CBC and urinalysis weekly for 2 months, every other week for 6 months, then monthly
4. Dosage should be lowered if patient develops a decrease in WBC, mild proteinuria, or rash
5. Drug should be discontinued if patient develops marked decrease in WBC or platelets, nephrotic range proteinuria, or autoimmune disease, or if mild changes listed above do not clear on lower dosage
6. Drug ideally should be taken on an empty stomach

TABLE 6   Indications for Corticosteroid Use in Juvenile Rheumatoid Arthritis

1. Severe systemic symptoms unresponsive to nonsteroidal anti-inflammatory drugs
2. Symptomatic pericarditis unresponsive to nonsteroidal anti-inflammatory drugs
3. Symptomatic relief while starting slow acting antirheumatic drug therapy
4. Intra-articular injection into a single troublesome joint
5. Topically for uveitis
6. Orally in low doses for patients with uveitis unresponsive to topical therapy

be used in the lowest dosage possible for the shortest reasonable period of time. Steroids are not disease modifying drugs. They do not prevent erosions or alter the disease course. However, they do mask the symptoms of the disease and give the patient a sense of well-being. Consequently they are useful in mobilizing a patient who would otherwise be confined to bed because of pain and stiffness.

When treating the pericarditis of systemic disease, dosages in the range of 1 mg per kg per day of prednisone are needed. Fever, arthritis, and uveitis, on the other hand, frequently respond to very low dosages, on the order of 5 to 10 mg per day. For intra-articular injection, 10 to 30 mg of prednisone tebutate or 20 to 40 mg of triamcinolone acetonide is appropriate. A joint should not be injected more than three times. In patients troubled by severe debilitating morning stiffness, giving all or most of the steroid dosage at night, rather than in the morning, can be helpful. With the low dosages used, giving the drug at night does not seem to increase the side effects. However, the arthritis associated with HLA-B27 positivity does not respond to steroids.

Once corticosteroids have been started, they are extremely difficult to taper. The decrease in dosage must be very slow—1 mg per day each week, for example, in order to avoid a flare of the underlying disease. The side effects of prolonged corticosteroid treatment are well known and are listed in Table 7.

Methotrexate

Methotrexate has been used by dermatologists since the 1950s for the treatment of psoriasis. The same dosing regimen was adopted for the treatment of adult rheu-

TABLE 7   Side Effects of Corticosteroid Treatment

1. Growth suppression	6. Cataracts
2. Cushingoid body habitus	7. Osteoporosis
3. Weight gain and fluid retention	8. Gastric irritation
4. Striae	9. Myopathy
5. Hirsutism	

matoid arthritis during the 1970s. Methotrexate is now being tried in selected pediatric patients who have progressive erosive disease unresponsive to nonsteroidal anti-inflammatory and slow acting antirheumatic drugs. It is also useful in patients with HLA-B27 positive arthritis. The drug is a folate antagonist and probably interferes with the immune phenomena associated with juvenile rheumatoid arthritis through its effect on DNA synthesis. It seems to have a direct anti-inflammatory effect as well.

The drug is given in a low dosage oral regimen, beginning with three doses of 2.5 mg every 12 hours once a week (example: 8 AM Friday, 8 PM Friday, 8 AM Saturday). The dosage may be increased to a maximum of 15 mg per week. In adult studies symptomatic relief has been noted within 2 to 4 weeks after starting the drug. Methotrexate's effect on the disease course will be clarified by continuing long term studies; a multicenter pediatric study is currently in progress as well.

Although occasionally methotrexate causes gastrointestinal irritation, liver toxicity has not been a major problem with this dosing regimen in the pediatric age group. Pulmonary toxicity also has not been a problem in children, but again experience is limited. In patients taking this drug the complete blood count should be checked every other week and liver function tests monthly. If persistent elevation of liver enzyme levels is noted, the drug should be temporarily stopped. It is probably a good rule of thumb not to use the drug in patients with pre-existing lung disease.

OTHER FORMS OF TREATMENT

Several forms of treatment that initially showed promise for patients with juvenile rheumatoid arthritis have fallen into disuse in recent years. Examples include pulse steroid therapy, plasmapheresis, leukapheresis, and cytotoxic drug therapy. The small additional therapeutic effects these modes of therapy offered did not seem to justify their increased toxicity except in very rare patients. Total lymphoid irradiation, which has been used in some adults with rheumatoid arthritis, is considered too toxic for use in juvenile rheumatoid arthritis.

Surgery

Soft tissue release can be helpful in severe contractures. Synovectomy is performed occasionally in cases of chronically active disease confined to a single joint (usually the knee). We have used the procedure in patients with severe pauciarticular disease unresponsive over a period of at least 1 year to therapeutic doses of nonsteroidal anti-inflammatory drugs and intra-articular corticosteroid injection. The ability to perform synovectomy via arthroscopy has shortened the recovery time significantly.

The availability of hip replacement for children with severe juvenile rheumatoid arthritis has made a vast difference in their ability to function as adults. Joint replacement should be delayed as long as possible in order to allow the child to reach maximal growth. Until the replacement is done, vigorous physiotherapy must be continued. Strengthening and range of motion exercises are necessary to maintain muscle tone and strength and to prevent contractures around the joint. If the supporting structures are maintained, a return to good function is possible after joint replacement. If the muscles are allowed to become weak and contracted, however, even a new joint will not restore lost function to the limb.

In summary, the treatment of juvenile rheumatoid arthritis is vigorous, intense, and multidisciplinary in scope. It must include education of the patient and parent regarding the nature of the illness and the purpose of treatment. Medications are used to decrease pain and inflammation and to prevent long term joint damage. Physiotherapy and occupational therapy are essential to keep the patient moving and functional. Screening for and treatment of complications are also important. Last but not least, normal social, emotional, and intellectual development should be encouraged.

SUGGESTED READING

Baum J. Aspirin in the treatment of juvenile arthritis. Am J Med 1983; 10–16.
Baum J. Treatment of juvenile arthritis. Hosp Prac 1983; 121–136.
Brewer EJ, Giannini EH, et al. Gold therapy in the management of juvenile rheumatoid arthritis. Arthritis Rheum 1983; 23:404–410.
Brewer EJ, Nickeson RW. Diagnosis and management of juvenile rheumatoid arthritis. Part II. Drug treatment. Hosp Phys 1983; 30–35.
Howard-Lock HE, Lock CJL, et al. d-Penicillamine: chemistry and clinical use in rheumatic disease. Semin Arthritis Rheum 1986; 15:261–281.
Truckenbrodt H, Hafner R. Methotrexate therapy in juvenile rheumatoid arthritis: a retrospective study. Arthritis Rheum 1986; 29:801–807.

REITER'S SYNDROME

PAUL KATZ, M.D.

Historically the diagnosis of Reiter's syndrome was applied to patients with the clinical tetrad of arthritis, nongonococcal urethritis, conjunctivitis, and typical mucocutaneous lesions. However, it is now apparent that it may not only affect young males. It is recognized that "incomplete" forms of the disease exist in which not all these manifestations are present. Some females with oligoarthritis primarily involving the lower extremities who originally were misdiagnosed as having seronegative rheumatoid arthritis are afflicted with Reiter's syndrome. Furthermore, the disease may have manifestations other than those in the classic tetrad (Table 1).

Reiter's syndrome most frequently occurs in genetically susceptible individuals exposed to specific microorganisms. Thus, 60 to 80 percent of the patients have the HLA-B27 antigen. Infectious agents known to "trigger" Reiter's syndrome generally fall into two classes: postvenereal (or endemic) secondary to Chlamydia or Ureaplasma, and postdysenteric (or epidemic) related to Salmonella, *Shigella flexneri*, Yersinia, and Campylobacter. Nonetheless patients frequently have no history that suggests infection with either group of organisms. Perhaps 25 percent of HLA-B27 positive individuals exposed to these agents develop Reiter's syndrome. The manifestations of Reiter's syndrome are not secondary to persistence of the offending bacterium, but rather constitute an aberrant "reactive" host response to the infection, which can develop and recur despite absence of the organism.

Although many patients have an initial acute illness that does not reappear, most patients have chronic or recurrent symptoms. Five years after the onset approximately 80 percent of the patients with Reiter's syndrome are still symptomatic. Apart from an increased incidence of chronic uveitis and sacroiliitis in HLA-B27 positive individuals after 5 years, there is no difference in outcome between HLA-B27 positive and HLA-B27 negative patients or between males and females.

APPROACH TO THE PATIENT

Diagnosis

A primary problem in the approach to the patient with Reiter's syndrome is establishing the correct diagnosis. Unfortunately there may be significant delays in patients with atypical presentations or those lacking the clinical tetrad. As already noted and shown in Table 1, there may be confusion in the diagnosis or even a misdiagnosis because of the rarity of the disease and its protean manifestations. Additionally some patients with Reiter's syndrome have an acute and self-limited course; these patients are disserved by long term treatment with potentially toxic drugs.

Patient Education

The importance of patient education cannot be overemphasized. Because of the perceived stigma of a disease that may be sexually acquired, the inability to predict the natural history and outcome, the periods of remission and exacerbation, and the lack of a "cure," it is incumbent upon the physician treating patients with Reiter's syndrome to inform them of these potential problems. The concept of a disease initiated by an infection but not responsive to antibiotics is often difficult for patients to grasp. Affected individuals may benefit from a comparison of Reiter's syndrome to an "allergy" in which environmental agents "cause" the symptoms. It is probably imprudent to speak of the potential long term problems of the disease with patients who have been ill for less than 2 to 3 months, since some of these subjects will never have a recurrence.

Given the genetic predisposition to Reiter's syndrome, patients may express concern about the possibility of the disease in offspring. It should be emphasized that even if the affected individual is HLA-B27 positive, there is only a 50 percent chance that any child will carry this haplotype. Should the child have this antigen, there is only a 20 to 25 percent chance that he will develop Reiter's syndrome, and the likelihood of this is

TABLE 1 Clinical Manifestations of Reiter's Syndrome During the Initial Attack

Signs or Symptoms	Frequency (%)
Musculoskeletal	100
Tendinitis	25
Back pain	50
Heel pain	40
Polyarthritis	80
Monarthritis	15
Sausage digits	20
Genitourinary	90
Urethritis	85
Cervicitis	70
Conjunctivitis	60
Skin lesions	50
Keratodermia blennorrhagica	15
Balanitis	40
Nail changes	10
Fever	35
Weight loss	40

dependent upon contact with the offending agent. Therefore, patients should be told that the chance of ''passing'' the disease to a son or daughter is relatively low and that there is no reason to avoid childbearing.

Physical and Local Therapy

Articular and Periarticular Disorders

The importance of physical and local treatment in the management of Reiter's syndrome cannot be overemphasized. As is the case with any acute arthritis, inflamed joints initially should be rested and even splinted if necessary. Once the inflammation has begun to subside, range of motion exercises and maintenance of muscle strength should be instituted under the supervision of a physical therapist. Individuals afflicted with chronic arthritis and joint dysfunction should receive maintenance therapy and instruction in ways to carry out the activities of daily living.

Since Reiter's syndrome often involves the lower extremities, patients with foot symptoms may benefit from orthotics, shoe inserts, or custom shoes; this treatment often can be facilitated through consultation with an experienced podiatrist.

Patients with localized enthesopathies, tendinitis, or monarticular arthritis despite systemic therapy often can be aided by local corticosteroid injections. Tendon injection with corticosteroids should be performed carefully because of the danger of tendon rupture induced by overzealous infiltration. The use of a mixture of a local anesthetic and a depot corticosteroid preparation often can produce prompt and long lasting relief from tendinitis. Intra-articular corticosteroid injections in patients with one or two disproportionately ''active'' joints may be useful and may avoid changes in treatment in a patient who is otherwise doing well. My experience with corticosteroid injections in Reiter's syndrome is similar to that of others: although many patients respond, the results are usually not as dramatic or as lasting as those in rheumatoid arthritis or gout.

Ocular Disorders

The mild conjunctivitis that may accompany Reiter's syndrome usually does not require therapy; however, this determination should be made by an opthalmologist, who should also look for anterior uveitis. Symptomatic conjunctivitis or uveitis usually remits with topical or intralesional corticosteroid therapy. Some patients may report a response to systemic treatment with anti-inflammatory drugs; nonetheless topical treatment of the eye symptoms of Reiter's syndrome is preferable.

Mucocutaneous Lesions

The circinate balanitis, keratodermia blennorrhagica, and nail lesions of Reiter's syndrome are usually asymptomatic or mildly symptomatic and require no therapy. Because of the risk of corticosteroid induced skin atrophy, these compounds generally should be avoided except when lesions on the soles or palms are so severe as to limit function.

Pulmonary Disease

A late complication of Reiter's syndrome may be the development of apical fibrosis and cavitary disease similar to that in ankylosing spondylitis. This unusual condition needs to be recognized in order to avoid needless diagnostic intervention. The complication of a secondary mycetoma, or fungus ball, and the possible need for surgical resection should be appreciated.

Cardiac Disease

Pericarditis, conduction abnormalities, and aortic regurgitation are recognized complications of Reiter's syndrome. Pericarditis and conduction abnormalities are most common early in the disease and require systemic anti-inflammatory therapy such as the nonsteroidal drugs (see next section) or corticosteroids. Fewer patients develop chronic conduction disturbances or aortic regurgitation, and these problems and the need for invasive therapy should be guided by a cardiologist.

Systemic Therapy

Anti-inflammatory Therapy

The nonsteroidal anti-inflammatory drugs are the primary therapeutic modalities in Reiter's syndrome, and most patients require these drugs at some time during the course of the illness. Numerous drugs are available (Table 2), and a logical scheme is dependent upon the physician's familiarity with the drugs, side effects, efficacy, and cost. These drugs are not approved for use in Reiter's syndrome, yet their proven effectiveness is established. Unlike therapy in rheumatoid arthritis or osteoarthritis, salicylates are generally not useful in Reiter's syndrome. Historically indomethacin has been the drug used initially by most rheumatologists, since phenylbutazone has fallen into disfavor (to be discussed). It may be that indomethacin is considered the first drug of choice because it has been available longer than any of the ''modern'' nonsteroidal anti-inflammatory drugs. Nonetheless there are many rheumatologists,

TABLE 2 Commonly Used Nonsteroidal Anti-inflammatory Drugs for Reiter's Syndrome

Chemical Group	Dosage Interval	Maximal Daily Dosage (mg)
Propionic acid		
Ibuprofen	tid–qid	3,200
Naproxen	bid	1,500
Fenoprofen	tid–qid	2,400
Ketoprofen	tid–qid	300
Indole derivatives		
Indomethacin	tid–qid	200
Sulindac	bid	400
Tolectin	tid–qid	1,600
Pyrazolones		
Phenylbutazone	tid–qid	400
Fenamates		
Meclofenamate	tid–qid	400
Oxicams		
Piroxicam	qd	20

TABLE 3 Side Effects of Nonsteroidal Anti-inflammatory Drugs

Gastrointestinal	Dyspepsia, nausea, vomiting, abdominal pain, constipation, diarrhea, ulcers, gastric erosions, hemorrhage
Renal	Edema, azotemia, proteinuria, nephrotic syndrome, allergic interstitial nephritis, renal tubular acidosis
Hematologic	Platelet dysfunction, agranulocytosis, aplasia, potentiation of anticoagulant action
Hepatic	Liver function abnormalities, jaundice
Cardiac	Congestive failure, hypertension
Central nervous system	Headache, cognitive dysfunction, depression, lethargy
Pulmonary	Asthma in aspirin sensitive individuals, hypersensitivity pneumonitis
Allergic	Hypersensitivity reactions, asthma in aspirin sensitive individuals

including myself, who generally begin treatment with indomethacin with the doses listed in Table 2. Therapy, if tolerated, is continued for at least 2 to 3 weeks, the time that may be required for a maximal response to be observed. If the patient has not responded to maximal doses of indomethacin, or if unacceptable side effects have occurred, I switch to another nonsteroidal anti-inflammatory drug, usually in a different chemical class (Table 2). Again a 2 to 3 week trial is mandatory with any of these drugs before considering the trial a "failure." It may be necessary to try multiple nonsteroidal anti-inflammatory drugs until one is found that is efficacious and well tolerated. Patients should be told that all these drugs are effective but that there is great variability in the response from patient to patient.

Although originally it was a first line drug for the treatment of Reiter's syndrome, the toxicity of phenylbutazone (to be discussed) as well as the availability of other nonsteroidal anti-inflammatory drugs has made it a second line choice. Nevertheless, I occasionally utilize this drug for a 1 to 2 week period in patients with severe Reiter's syndrome that has been unresponsive to other drugs. In this group, phenylbutazone may reduce the activity of a "flare" and permit the institution of therapy with another nonsteroidal anti-inflammatory drug.

Nonsteroidal anti-inflammatory drug therapy should be continued as long as the patient is symptomatic. It is desirable to utilize as low a dosage as possible to reduce the likelihood of complications. Some patients may be capable of achieving many "drug free" periods when the disease is quiescent.

Unfortunately the beneficial effects of the nonsteroidal anti-inflammatory drugs are often limited by their side effects, which in some instances may be life threatening. A partial list of the toxic effects of these drugs is contained in Table 3. Nonsteroidal anti-inflammatory

drugs exert their effects on the inflammatory and immune responses through inhibition of the enzyme cyclooxygenase, which catalyzes an early step in the synthesis of prostaglandins. Thus, many (but not all) of the adverse effects of these drugs are secondary to local decreases in prostaglandin production.

Gastrointestinal symptoms are the most common side effects of this class of drugs and can include dyspepsia, nausea, vomiting, abdominal pain, constipation, diarrhea, erosions, ulcers, and hemorrhage. There is often poor correlation between abdominal symptoms and the severity of nonsteroidal anti-inflammatory drug induced lesions; thus patients with significant mucosal ulceration and massive hemorrhage may have no preceding symptoms, whereas patients with significant abdominal pain may have normal endoscopically visualized mucosa. Elderly patients or those with renal, liver, or cardiac disease may have significant reductions in glomerular filtration due to inhibition of prostaglandin dependent renal blood flow; in this group particular caution should be exercised when using a nonsteroidal anti-inflammatory drug. I generally avoid using longer acting drugs (e.g., piroxicam) in these individuals. There are data that suggest that sulindac may have less effect on renal blood flow, and this drug may be tried cautiously in patients at risk. The reduction in the glomerular filtration rate is generally reversible upon discontinuation of the nonsteroidal anti-inflammatory drug. Other renal side effects such as the nephrotic syndrome, allergic interstitial nephritis, and renal tubular acidosis can occur with any of these drugs.

Platelet dysfunction related to prostaglandin inhibition is observed in the presence of active drug; this is reversible upon discontinuation of therapy with the offending drug. Hepatic toxicity with increased serum transaminase levels is not uncommon, but two- to three-fold increases do not necessitate discontinuation of the drug. These elevations are reversible, however. Hyperbilirubinemia is more serious and calls for cessation of drug use.

Central nervous system symptoms are also observed, headache being the most common complaint. This is a particular problem with indomethacin. Cognitive dysfunction, depression, and lethargy are also reported, especially in older age groups. As is the case with most drugs, true allergic reactions can occur with nonsteroidal anti-inflammatory drugs; in such cases it may be relatively safe to switch to a drug in another chemical class.

As noted, the idiosyncratic and dose dependent toxic effects of phenylbutazone have limited its present day utility. The aplastic anemia originally reported was most commonly observed with long term use in the elderly. However, the unpredictable agranulocytosis that occurs within weeks after beginning therapy with the drug is of grave concern, and patients should be monitored with frequent white cell counts while receiving this drug.

Antibiotics

Despite the infectious "trigger" in most cases of Reiter's syndrome, there are no data indicating that persistent infection is responsible for symptoms. However, some patients with urethritis may respond to treatment with doxycycline or tetracycline.

Corticosteroids

Apart from topical, intra-articular, and periarticular treatment, corticosteroids are rarely indicated in patients with Reiter's syndrome. However, selected individuals with severe systemic symptoms may respond to short courses of low dose prednisone therapy (5 to 10 mg per day). This drug may be useful while awaiting the hoped-for beneficial effects of conventional drugs.

Cytotoxic Drugs

Although most patients with Reiter's syndrome respond to the foregoing therapies, there are a few whose arthritis and mucocutaneous disease mandate more aggressive treatment. In general, the remittive drugs used in rheumatoid arthritis are of no proven efficacy in Reiter's syndrome. Although there are few data regarding the controlled use of cytotoxic drugs, it appears that methotrexate and azathioprine may be useful in selected patients.

Because of similarities between the cutaneous lesions of psoriasis and those of Reiter's syndrome, there are reports of the successful use of methotrexate in Reiter's syndrome. I have used this drug in long term, low dose therapy (similar to the protocols for psoriasis and rheumatoid arthritis) and have found it to be efficacious in many patients. The drug can be given parenterally or orally as a single weekly dose. Treatment is usually begun with 5 mg per week, and the dosage is gradually increased in 2.5 to 5.0 mg increments; the usual maintenance dosage is approximately 15 to 20 mg per week. Joint symptoms usually decrease after the skin disease is controlled.

A number of side effects of methotrexate may curtail therapy. Included among these are mucositis, leukopenia, and pneumonitis. Liver fibrosis with prolonged methotrexate treatment has been reported in psoriasis, and this may not be detectable with liver function tests. Patients with pre-existing liver disease, hepatitis B antigenemia, or alcohol abuse should undergo a pre-methotrexate liver biopsy with a subsequent biopsy after a cumulative dosage of 1.5 g has been given. Liver biopsy in patients who are not at risk for liver disease is controversial; in general, I have not obtained tissue in these subjects.

Another cytotoxic drug that has been employed less frequently in Reiter's syndrome is azathioprine. Limited experience suggests that 1 to 2 mg per kg per day of this drug as a single oral dose may be effective in some patients with Reiter's syndrome. The major side effect of this drug, namely, leukopenia, may limit its use in this disease.

SUGGESTED READING

Fox R, Calin A, Gerber RC, Gibson D. The chronicity of symptoms and disability in Reiter's syndrome. An analysis of 131 consecutive cases. Ann Intern Med 1979; 91:190–193.

Keat A. Reiter's syndrome and reactive arthritis in perspective. N Engl J Med 1983; 309:1606–1615.

Lally EV, Ho G Jr. A review of methotrexate therapy in Reiter's syndrome. Sem Arthritis Rheum 1985; 15:139–145.

Willkens RF, Arnett FC, Bitter T, Calin A, Fisher L, Ford DK, Good AE, Masi AT. Reiter's syndrome. Evaluation of preliminary criteria for definite diagnosis. Bull Rheum Dis 1982; 32:31–34.

Wright V. Seronegative polyarthritis, a unified concept. Arthritis Rheum 1978; 21:619–633.

SJÖGREN'S SYNDROME

ELAINE L. ALEXANDER, M.D., Ph.D.

Sjögren's syndrome is a common autoimmune connective tissue disorder, which conservatively affects 2 percent of the adult population (more than 4 million Americans), the majority of whom are women (9:1). The disorder is often unrecognized or misdiagnosed by unsuspecting patients and physicians because of the characteristic insidious, slowly progressive, and subtle symptoms. The term autoimmune exocrinopathy has been used to describe the sicca (dryness) manifestations caused by progressive infiltration and destruction of salivary, lacrimal, and other glands by mononuclear inflammatory cells (predominantly lymphocytes and plasma cells). The syndrome has not only glandular (nonsystemic) but also extraglandular (systemic) manifestations. The disorder can occur alone (primary Sjögren's syndrome) or may be associated with another connective tissue disorder (secondary Sjögren's syndrome). Secondary Sjögren's syndrome most commonly is associated with rheumatoid arthritis and less commonly with systemic lupus erythematosus, progressive systemic sclerosis, or overlap syndromes or a lymphoproliferative disorder (benign [pseudolymphoma or angioblastic lymphadenopathy with dysproteinemia] or malignant [lymphoma or lymphosarcoma]). The management of the glandular and extraglandular manifestations is the same in primary and secondary Sjögren's syndrome.

The major clinical manifestations of the sicca complex are xerophthalmia (keratoconjunctivitis sicca [dry eyes]), xerostomia (dry mouth), and recurrent or chronic episodes of major salivary gland enlargement. Other glands may be affected, giving rise to dryness of mucous membranes in the nasopharynx and upper respiratory tract, dry skin (xerosis or cutaneous sicca), and vaginal dryness (vaginitis sicca). Extraglandular complications essentially can involve any organ in the body with associated mononuclear cell infiltrates, focal tissue damage, and organ dysfunction. Musculoskeletal symptoms including polyarthralgias-polyarthritis (nondeforming, nonerosive, often transient and migratory, and usually asymmetric) and myalgias are common. Their presence is not necessarily associated with more serious manifestations of systemic disease. Inflammation of blood vessels by either neutrophils or mononuclear cells also can cause cutaneous or systemic vasculitis. Basically the approach to the therapy of Sjögren's syndrome can be divided into the treatment of glandular and extraglandular manifestations.

GENERAL CONCEPTS

The management of the patient with Sjögren's syndrome requires a multidisciplinary approach. Successful treatment requires a working partnership between the patient and the physician. Patient education is of utmost importance. In patients with glandular manifestations alone, the rheumatologist, ophthalmologist, otolaryngologist, and dentist provide the basic support system. The rheumatologist is perhaps best qualified to monitor the patient for the potential emergence of extraglandular (systemic) disease and to coordinate diagnostic workups and therapeutic intervention. Because Sjögren's syndrome potentially may affect every organ in the body, additional consultation with appropriate specialists may be required for appropriate diagnosis and therapy. Ideally in complicated cases an internist should coordinate the multidimensional care recommended by specialists. Because of the diversity of symptoms, the patient with Sjögren's syndrome is often subject to the phenomena of "polydoctors" and "polypharmacy," which actually may impair optimal management.

There are several important general principles in the management of Sjögren's syndrome. First, most patients with Sjögren's syndrome can be treated successfully for sicca symptoms and other manifestations, such as musculoskeletal symptoms. Second, only a minority of patients require potent anti-inflammatory or immunosuppressive therapy. In fact, immunosuppressive therapy should be reserved for very specific indications (to be discussed). In particular, we do not recommend the use of these drugs for the treatment of sicca or musculoskeletal symptoms alone.

Sjögren's syndrome is a chronic disease. Because of the insidious and fluctuating pattern of sicca and musculoskeletal symptoms, the efficacy of a given therapeutic modality may be difficult to assess. Therefore, controlled blinded trials with serial assessment of objective parameters are required to verify the therapeutic efficacy of any given modality before it is incorporated into the therapeutic regimen. In some instances the patient's complaints may seem out of proportion to objective or pathologically defined documented abnormalities. In such cases physicians under pressure by patients for treatment should not resort to the use of immunosuppressive drugs but rather provide patient education and the appropriate utilization of conservative measures.

As with all chronic diseases, the symptoms of Sjögren's syndrome clearly are affected by stress. There may be important immunologic control mechanisms operative in the exacerbation of connective tissue disease by stress. The removal of stressful life situations is an important adjunct in the care of the patient with Sjögren's syndrome. Conversely, all the patient's symptoms and problems cannot be attributed to Sjögren's syndrome. Patient support groups appear to be an effective means for patient education and dissemination of information as well as serving as an important psychologic and emotional support system. Some patients, however, are uncomfortable with these groups and actually may react adversely with an increase in symptomatology and a decrease in subjective well-being and functional status. The physician may be helpful in assisting a patient in deciding whether a support group may be beneficial.

Most important in terms of therapy, there are numerous "common sense" alterations in the patient's behavior and life style that may result in a significant decrease in the symptom complex. Furthermore, there are a number of relatively minor therapeutic modalities that also may result in significant improvement. The patient may resist such a basic approach, searching instead for a "magic pill or remedy" to cure all symptoms.

TREATMENT OF GLANDULAR DISEASE

The management of glandular disease in Sjögren's syndrome is directed primarily at the treatment of ophthalmologic, oral, nasopharyngeal–upper respiratory tract, cutaneous, and vaginal sicca symptoms (Table 1).

Ophthalmologic Disease

The treatment of "dry eyes" is aimed primarily at alleviating symptoms, avoiding the development of superficial erosions of the corneal epithelium, preventing conjunctivitis and blepharitis, and appropriately treating complications as they develop.

The correction of environmental or extrinsic factors that may aggregate ocular sicca symptoms is important. The patient should be maintained in a high humidity environment year round. Air conditioning, forced heat, windy and dry environments, and high altitudes (including airplanes) worsen symptoms. Environmental toxins (tobacco smoke, fixatives, solvents) and other chemical agents also aggravate ocular dryness. Drugs, particularly those with anticholinergic side effects (phenothiazines, tricyclic antidepressants, antispasmodics, antiparkinsonian drugs, decongestants, and antihistamines), should be avoided.

TABLE 1 Glandular Manifestations (Symptomatic or Conservative Treatment): Sicca Manifestations

Ocular
Oral
Nasopharynx and upper respiratory tract
Skin
Vagina
Musculoskeletal syndrome

The primary treatment for dry eyes is lubrication with artificial tears, which can be used as often as necessary. These preparations vary in viscosity and preservative content. The selection of an artificial tear product is usually an empiric choice by the patient. Eye irritation from these preparations may reflect the preservatives they contain, such as benzalkonium chloride, thimerosal, or chlorobutanol. Lubricating ointments can be used at night to provide protection over a longer period of time but may cause significant blurring of vision. Slow release capsules (Lacrisent, Merk, Sharp and Dohme) containing a polymer of hydroxypropyl cellulose can be inserted every 6 to 12 hours beneath the inferior tarsal margin. The capsule absorbs tears, dissolves slowly, and releases polymer. These capsules are particularly useful for patients who use artificial tears frequently. In some patients with extremely dry eyes, however, the capsule adheres to the conjunctiva and sclera and may not dissolve. Some investigators have suggested using the patient's own serum as an artificial tear. Data at present are insufficient to determine whether this approach is effective.

Drugs have had limited and inconsistent effects in the treatment of ocular sicca symptoms. Parasympathomimetics, especially the muscarines, serve to stimulate tear flow. The efficacy of pilocarpine in the treatment of ocular sicca is still under experimental investigation (see discussion of oral disease). Bromhexine (see discussion of oral disease) and acetylcysteine, a mucolytic drug, have not been documented to be effective consistently in controlled trials. The topical application of vitamin A has not proven effective in controlled trials. The topical use of corticosteroids in the treatment of corneal ulcers may actually worsen the condition and is not recommended. Uveitis can occur in Sjögren's syndrome and is treated with topical, or if necessary systemic, corticosteroid therapy.

The use of contact lenses in the treatment of ocular sicca symptoms is controversial. Some patients with emerging Sjögren's syndrome actually develop an intolerance to the use of contact lenses, which may be a subtle clue to the presence of the disorder. In others soft contact lenses actually may protect the cornea and prevent or treat corneal erosion or ulcers. Patients using contact lenses must observe meticulous hygienic standards and be followed very carefully, particularly since there is an increased risk of infection.

Surgical intervention is reserved for severe cases of keratoconjunctivitis sicca with progressive disease. Punctal occlusion of lacrimal canaliculi can be performed by electrolysis or diathermy but is irreversible. Less effective, but reversible, methods include strangling sutures of the canaliculi, laser photocoagulation of the lacrimal points, or the use of gelatine or silicone plugs. Recently diversion of the lacrimal canaliculus by surgical displacement of the punctum lacrimale onto the anterior edge of the lid, where it cannot collect tears, has been used and is reversible; the small quantity of residual tears is maintained in the lacrimal basin. Autografting of salivary glands to the lacrimal basin is an experimental procedure.

Oral Disease

The treatment of xerostomia in documented Sjögren's syndrome can be a difficult management problem. At the present time most treatment modalities are palliative. Identification of contributing factors that may aggravate xerostomia by further reducing salivary flow is important (sleep disorders, mouth breathing, cigarette and alcohol consumption, and drugs with anticholinergic side effects). Patients may consume increased quantities of liquids and may keep water at the bedside. The consumption of large quantities of fluid during the day may produce nocturia and disrupt normal sleep patterns. Unless fluid consumption is pushed to pathologic extremes, resulting in iatrogenic diabetes insipidus, however, there is no contraindication to liberal fluid intake. The majority of patients have residual salivary function and can stimulate salivary flow by using sugarless, highly flavored lozenges, chewing gum, candy, or beverages. The use of these agents prior to meals may enhance lubrication and the digestion of food. Dietary counseling to avoid dry food and the use of foods known to stimulate saliva production may be helpful. The slow ingestion of small pieces or portions of food, with complete chewing and wetting prior to swallowing, is an important practical aid.

Artificial saliva preparations are useful in some patients. The effects are transient, however, and the preparations are relatively expensive. Several preparations are available from different manufacturers, but essentially they are the same, containing sorbitol, sodium carboxymethylcellulose, and methylparaben in either liquid or spray form. Saliva substitutes should be used sparingly (approximately 2 ml) before and after meals, at bedtime, and following oral hygiene.

Dental care is an important cornerstone of the management of Sjögren's syndrome because of associated dental caries and periodontal disease with gum recession. Oral hygiene should be performed after meals and at bedtime with daily flossing. Dental check-ups and removal of dental plaque should be scheduled at least every 6 months and in some cases more frequently. When gingivitis is present, aggressive and persistent treatment is required to prevent the loss of teeth. Every attempt to maintain impeccable oral hygiene should be made because patients with Sjögren's syndrome have difficulty with the adequate fitting of dentures because of continuing problems with gum resorption. Single crystal aluminum oxide dental implants may be effective in preserving existing teeth. Topical or liquid treatment with stannous fluoride promotes mineralization and retards damage to tooth surfaces. The fluoride can be applied at night directly to the teeth from plastic trays, providing better coverage at the gingival margins.

Several preparations designed to stimulate the production of saliva have been used with variable success. Expectorants containing potassium iodide or iodinated glycerol may be useful. Parasympathomimetic drugs, such as pilocarpine (5 mg three to four times a day), recently have been shown in controlled trials to decrease xerostomia and increase salivary function. Pilocarpine may cause sweating approximately 30 minutes after ingestion and is contraindicated in patients taking beta-blockers or those with pulmonary or cardiac disease. Bromhexine, originally used as a mucolytic agent in cough syrups, and Efamol, derived from the evening primrose and containing gamma-linoleic acid, have been used in Scandinavia with reported success in decreasing xerostomia in some but not all patients. These drugs have not been studied in controlled trials in the United States. Efamol is available in the United States, but bromhexine is not. An electronic device for stimulating salivary flow has not undergone clinical research trials.

It is important to keep the mucous membranes of the mouth, nose, and upper tracheobronchial system moist. Normal saline nasal sprays used four to six times a day maintain moisture. Nasal irrigation with normal saline may prevent desiccation and crusting. Humidifiers should be attached to heating systems and a portable unit used within the bedroom at night. Adequate humidification decreases respiratory symptoms and decreases mouth breathing, which worsens xerostomia. Particular attention to increased fluid consumption and adequate humidification is needed in dry climates, with increased elevation, and during airplane flights.

Persistent or chronic salivary gland enlargement may occur. Infection, tumor, and obstruction are treatable causes. If these disorders are excluded and parotid gland enlargement is severe, a short course of moderate dose corticosteroid therapy may be effective.

Other Glandular Manifestations

Cutaneous sicca is a common and aggravating symptom in Sjögren's syndrome. Hot baths and showers should be avoided and the duration of exposure limited. Soaps containing a moisturizing cream are preferred. Moisturizing creams, particularly those that trap the body's natural moisture, should be applied while the skin is still wet. Avoidance of excessive sun exposure is important, and sun blocks should be used routinely to prevent premature aging of the skin. Hypoallergenic and nonscented cosmetics are preferred by some patients.

Vaginitis sicca is a serious symptom that may result in dyspareunia and impaired sexual performance and enjoyment. Standard lubricants are often effective in alleviating symptoms. Patients in whom symptoms are not controlled by this method should be evaluated by a gynecologist to assess the need for topical or systemic hormonal supplementation and to insure that there are no attendant infections (e.g., candidiasis).

TREATMENT OF EXTRAGLANDULAR DISEASE

There are two basic approaches to the treatment of the extraglandular manifestations of Sjögren's syndrome (Table 2). For extraglandular manifestations that result in end-organ damage and dysfunction, there is replacement therapy. For extraglandular manifestations secondary to an active destructive inflammatory process, immunosuppressive therapy is used. Both approaches may be required in certain instances.

Organ Specific Disease

Sjögren's syndrome can affect any organ in the body. Organ specific involvement may result in an autoimmune process indistinguishable from a disorder occurring as an isolated manifestation (e.g., Graves' disease, Hashimoto's thyroiditis, pancreatitis, pernicious anemia, chronic active hepatitis, primary biliary cirrhosis, pulmonary fibrosis, interstitial nephritis). Cytopenias such as autoimmune thrombocytopenia or neutropenia and Coomb's positive autoimmune hemolytic anemia may be severe and require therapy. These disorders in

Sjögren's syndrome are treated as if they occurred outside the setting of Sjögren's syndrome and with appropriate replacement therapy when indicated.

Two specific organ systems commonly involved in primary Sjögren's syndrome warrant special comment with respect to therapy. Interstitial pneumonitis resulting in pulmonary infiltrates, mild to moderate restrictive pulmonary disease, and decreased diffusing capacity usually does not require treatment. In some cases, however, the inflammatory process may be very aggressive and result in marked deterioration in pulmonary function. Obstructive lung disease secondary to inflammatory bronchioalveolitis may be severe and rapidly progressive. Lung biopsy should be performed in such cases to establish the presence of potentially treatable active inflammation or fibrosis, which is not treated.

Renal disease in Sjögren's syndrome is also common and usually does not require immunosuppressive therapy. The most common form of renal disease is interstitial nephritis, which results in overt or latent renal tubular acidosis and chronic sterile pyuria and hematuria. In rare instances this form of renal disease may be severe and associated with deteriorating renal function. Furthermore, patients with Sjögren's syndrome rarely can develop glomerulonephritis, particularly those with cryoglobulins. The latter two forms of aggressive renal disease need to be treated with immunosuppressive therapy.

TREATMENT OF SYSTEMIC DISEASE

Two other recently recognized systemic complications of Sjögren's syndrome may need to be treated with immunosuppressive therapy—inflammatory vascular disease (i.e., vasculitis) and neuromuscular disease (central and peripheral nervous system disease and inflammatory myopathies).

Cutaneous vasculitis, manifested most commonly by palpable purpura, petechiae, or chronic urticaria, is a common manifestation of Sjögren's syndrome. All patients with Sjögren's syndrome and cutaneous vasculitis should be carefully evaluated for systemic complications because of the potential for systemic or nervous system disease in such patients. Cutaneous vasculitis alone can be treated successfully with one or more drugs: hydroxychloroquine, dapsone, or low doses of corticosteroids. Patients should be monitored serially for the re-emergence of cutaneous lesions or the development of systemic complications.

Systemic vasculitis can occur in Sjögren's syndrome, often with nervous system involvement. Both histopathologic types of vasculitis (neutrophilic [leukocytoclastic] and mononuclear [lymphocytic]) can cause serious end-organ damage. Small to medium sized vessels are predominantly involved, but in some instances large vessels may be affected. Although vasculitis in the

**TABLE 2 Extraglandular Manifestations
(Immunosuppressive or Replacement Therapy)**

Organ Specific	
Thyroid	Graves' disease
	Hashimoto's thyroiditis
Pancreas	Pancreatitis, malabsorption
Stomach	Pernicious anemia
Liver	Chronic active hepatitis
	Primary biliary cirrhosis
Lung	Interstitial pulmonary fibrosis
	Bronchioalveolitis
Kidney	Interstitial nephritis
	Glomerulonephritis
Cytopenias	Neutropenia
	Thrombocytopenia
	Hemolytic anemia
Systemic	
Vasculitis, vasculopathy	Spectrum of small to medium sized, rarely large vessels
Neuromuscular disease	
Central nervous system	"Central nervous system Sjögren's syndrome"
Peripheral nervous system	Neuropathy
Muscle disease	Myositis
Lymph node disease	Pseudolymphoma
	Lymphoma
	Lymphosarcoma

lungs, kidneys, gastrointestinal tract, heart, or nervous system (to be discussed) is most apt to result in clinically significant disease manifestations, vessels in any organ in the body can be affected. Patients with Sjögren's syndrome with systemic vasculitis require immunosuppressive therapy.

Recent investigations have indicated that central nervous system disease can occur in Sjögren's syndrome and may result in a multifocal neurologic disease affecting both the brain and the spinal cord, in addition to causing psychiatric or cognitive dysfunction. A spectrum of inflammatory insults are associated with neurologic disease in Sjögren's syndrome, ranging from frank vasculitis (predominantly small to medium sized vessels and rarely large vessels), to small vessel cerebral vasculopathy, to destructive lymphocytic infiltrates.

Currently we are recommending aggressive therapy only for patients with focal neurologic syndromes who have progressive disease documented by objective abnormalities by at least one of the following: magnetic resonance imaging study, multimodality evoked response testing, electroencephalography, cerebrospinal fluid analysis, or angiography. The abnormal parameter(s) can be followed serially to objectively assess the response to therapy. At present we do not recommend immunosuppressive therapy for patients with cognitive or psychiatric dysfunction alone. Inflammatory muscle disease (myositis) documented by biopsy associated with enzyme level elevation or electromyographic changes is another indication for immunosuppressive therapy.

The Musculoskeletal Syndrome

Many patients with Sjögren's syndrome have a recurrent transient symptom complex characterized by low grade fever, parotid gland enlargement, lymphadenopathy, malaise, fatigue, and musculoskeletal symptoms including arthralgias and myalgias. The syndrome may resemble a flu-like illness and can be very debilitating. The musculoskeletal symptoms and fatigue also may occur alone. Some patients have a soft tissue syndrome that resembles fibromyalgia or fibrositis. Nonsteroidal anti-inflammatory drugs, physical therapy, weight reduction (if indicated), an exercise program, and patient education are recommended for the management of these symptoms. Corticosteroids are not recommended for the management of these chronic recurrent musculoskeletal problems.

Frank arthritis is uncommon but does occur. Synovitis is usually transient, asymmetrical, migratory, and nondeforming. A transient symmetrical polyarthritis can occur. Nonsteroidal anti-inflammatory drugs usually are effective, but some patients may require a short course of low to moderate dose corticosteroid therapy. If rheumatoid arthritis coexists, the management of arthritis is the same as for rheumatoid arthritis alone.

Immunosuppressive Therapy

The approach to the treatment of systemic complications of Sjögren's syndrome is general and similar to that used in other autoimmune disorders, such as lupus erythematosus and multiple sclerosis. In general, Sjögren's syndrome appears to be a subtle, subacute, or insidious disease, but disease manifestations can be acute, devastating, and rapidly fatal.

There have been no controlled trials comparing the therapeutic efficacy of different approaches in treating the systemic complications of Sjögren's syndrome. Treatment is usually initiated with daily oral dosages of corticosteroids in the range of 0.5 to 1.0 mg per kg. More seriously ill patients initially may need intravenous therapy in divided doses. Treatment is continued for 3 to 6 months, and the dosage is tapered over several months to approximately half the starting dosage. Corticosteroids with little or no mineralocorticoid effects should be used at the lowest possible dosage and for the shortest possible duration; when possible, alternate day therapy should be used. Conversely, in patients with serious life threatening illness, adequate dosages of steroids should be given for appropriate periods of time without tapering too rapidly. Often such patients initially are not treated aggressively enough to control disease manifestations and dosages are tapered too quickly. There is no reported experience in the use and efficacy of pulse intravenous corticosteroid therapy in Sjögren's syndrome. Supplemental drugs that may permit lower corticosteroid dosages include salicylates, nonsteroidal anti-inflammatory drugs, hydroxychloroquine, and dapsone. Careful monitoring for potential steroid complications should be routine.

If corticosteroids are ineffective or toxic effects are unacceptable, there are several options. Antimetabolites, azathioprine, or an alkylating drug, cyclophosphamide, may be used in patients with potentially life threatening complications. Oral therapy with azathioprine or cyclophosphamide may be administered in the daily dosage of 1.0 to 3.0 mg per kg. To avoid corticosteroid side effects and the complications of daily immunosuppression, intravenous pulse cyclophosphamide therapy may be used for 6 to 12 months and every 3 to 4 months thereafter, depending on the severity of the disease and the therapeutic response. The starting dosage is 0.75 g per sq m, adjusting the dosage to maintain the white blood cell count nadir 10 days after administration at approximately 3000 cells per cubic mm. It appears to be important to induce leukopenia-lymphopenia for the successful treatment of the systemic complications of Sjögren's syndrome. This regimen should be accompanied by adequate hydration, intravenous corticosteroid therapy, and usually pretreatment with antiemetics. In very seriously ill patients therapy may be initiated with corticosteroids and cyclophosphamide concomitantly. Cyclosporine has been used in a small number of cases at low doses and is not recommended because of renal toxicity and the potential for the development of lymphoma.

Plasmapheresis is reserved for patients with systemic complications associated with hyperglobulinemia or cryoglobulinemia and is used in conjunction with corticosteroids and alkylating drugs, such as cyclophosphamide or chlorambucil, to prevent immunologic rebound. Newer experimental research approaches used in other autoimmune diseases, such as total body lymphoid radiation, monoclonal antibodies, and interferons, have not been studied in clinical trials in Sjögren's syndrome.

Lymphoma

Lymphoma is another systemic complication of Sjögren's syndrome requiring treatment. Patients with Sjögren's syndrome develop a spectrum of lymphoproliferative disease, from benign polyclonal gammopathy, to pseudolymphoma, to lymphoma (usually of the non-Hodgkin B cell type), to angioimmunoblastic lymphadenopathy with dysproteinemia. These disorders may be treated effectively with corticosteroids or cyclophosphamide. Patients with Sjögren's syndrome should be under constant surveillance for the development of lymphoma, for they have a 43-fold increased risk of developing

lymphoma compared to normal individuals. Patients with rheumatoid arthritis with Sjögren's syndrome have a similar risk. The treatment of lymphoma or lymphosarcoma with chemotherapy or radiation therapy should be directed by experienced oncologists.

SUGGESTED READING

Alexander EL. Inflammatory vascular disease in Sjögren's syndrome. In: Talal N, Moutsopoulos HM, Kassan SS, eds. Sjögren's syndrome: clinical and immunological aspects. Heidelberg: Springer-Verlag, 1987:102.
Alexander EL. Neuromuscular complications of primary Sjögren's syndrome. In: Talal N, Moutsopoulos HM, Kassan SS, eds. Sjögren's syndrome: clinical and immunological aspects. Heidelberg: Springer-Verlag, 1987:61.
Alexander EL, Lijewski JE, Jerdan MS, Alexander GE. Evidence of an immunopathogenic basis for central nervous system disease in primary Sjögren's syndrome. Arthritis Rheum 1986; 29:1223–1231.
Alexander EL, Malinow K, Lijewski JE, Jerdan MS, Provost TT, Alexander GE. Primary Sjögren's syndrome with central nervous system dysfunction mimicking multiple sclerosis. Ann Intern Med 1986; 104:323–330.
Proceedings of 1st International Seminar on Sjögren's Syndrome. Chapter 8. Treatment. Scand J Rheum Suppl 1986; 61:237–270.
Talal N, Moutsopoulos HM. Treatment of Sjögren's syndrome. In: Talal N, Moutsopoulos HM, Kassan SS, eds. Sjögren's syndrome: clinical and immunological aspects. Heidelberg: Springer-Verlag, 1987:291.

ANKYLOSING SPONDYLITIS

JOSEPH H. KORN, M.D.

Ankylosing spondylitis, or Marie-Strümpell arthritis, is the prototype of the group of disorders known as the seronegative spondyloarthropathies. It is both a true arthritis or synovitis of diarthrodial joints and an enthesopathy, an inflammatory and destructive process involving tendinous and ligamentous attachments to bone. It differs from the other polyarthritides such as rheumatoid arthritis in the pattern of joint involvement. Although peripheral joint disease does occur in ankylosing spondylitis, the hallmark of the disease is axial involvement—the spine and the pelvic and shoulder girdles. It is this pattern of involvement that both distinguishes the disease from most inflammatory arthritides and leads to confusion with degenerative and muscular conditions of the lower back. Thus, diagnostic accuracy is important in selecting an appropriate approach to therapy.

In making the correct diagnosis, historical and physical findings are paramount. Clinical studies have shown that the patient's history is reliable in distinguishing inflammatory (e.g., spondylitic) back pain from mechanical back pain. An early age of onset, such as the late teens and early twenties, is found more commonly in ankylosing spondylitis. In addition, the back pain is more diffuse than in mechanical disorders, involving the entire spine and not just the lower back; thus, the symptoms are concordant with the radiographic and pathologic findings. Like other inflammatory arthritides, spondylitic back pain improves with activity, is made worse by prolonged recumbency, and is characterized by stiffness after sitting or lying in a single position (gelling). Night pain is a common associated feature. Finally, the presence of inflammatory peripheral arthritis, inflammatory enthesopathy, and extra-articular disease manifestations (see later discussion) distinguishes the spondyloarthropathies, including ankylosing spondylitis, from mechanical back pain.

The distinction between ankylosing spondylitis and other spondyloarthropathies is made largely on the basis of associated clinical findings. Extra-articular features of ankylosing spondylitis include uveitis, aortitis, apical pulmonary fibrosis, and enthesopathic findings (e.g., heel pain). Both uveitis and aortitis may be found in

Reiter's syndrome, and the distinction between ankylosing spondylitis and Reiter's syndrome is often difficult. Such characteristic features of Reiter's syndrome as balanitis, keratodermia blennorrhagica, and urethritis, when present, differentiate the disorder from ankylosing spondylitis. Similarly, the presence of inflammatory bowel disease or psoriasis allows the distinction of spondyloarthropathy associated with these disorders from ankylosing spondylitis.

Early in the disease the symptom complex is a result of inflammatory processes in diarthrodial (synovial) joints, in synarthroses (nonsynovial joints), at cartilage-bone junctions, and at ligamentous and tendinous attachments to bone and cartilage. Thus, involvement of apophyseal and costovertebral joints leads to limited motion of the spine (at the intervertebral joints) and rib cage, respectively. Sacroiliac pain, often referred to the buttocks, is a result of involvement of both the true sacroiliac joints (approximately the lower two thirds of the sacroiliac articulation) and the synarthrosis of the upper articulation. Enthesopathy is common at ligamentous attachments to vertebrae, pelvic bones, ankles (Achilles tendon and plantar fascial attachment), and femurs. At the intervertebral discs, costochondral junctions, and symphysis pubis, inflammatory processes lead to pain, swelling, and erosive changes at the cartilage-bone interfaces. During the course of the disease there is both fusion of diarthrodial and synarthrodial joints and calcification of ligamentous structures leading to loss of mobility and function. These processes obviously are not amenable to medical therapy. The cauda equina syndrome with sphincter dysfunction secondary to root compression has been reported occasionally and may require surgery.

As noted earlier, the diagnosis of ankylosing spondylitis is best made on the basis of a characteristic symptom complex. In early disease both physical and radiographic findings may be normal. With progression, physical examination shows decreased chest expansion and decreased flexion of the lumbar spine. Physical maneuvers to elicit the pain of sacroiliitis, such as sacroiliac compression or hyperextension of the opposite hip, have not been of demonstrated value. With progressive disease there is often forward protrusion of the neck, kyphosis in the upper thoracic spine, and fixed flexion at the hips giving rise to a characteristic posture. Such features as iritis, aortic regurgitation, apical pulmonary fibrosis, and enthesopathic signs and symptoms (e.g., costochondral pain and tenderness) are unusual in mechanical back disease and in inflammatory arthritides other than the spondyloarthropathies, and their presence lends support to a diagnosis of ankylosing spondylitis. Laboratory tests show no consistent abnormalities that are diagnostically useful; the erythrocyte sedimentation rate, which is usually abnormal in other types of inflammatory arthritis, is often normal in ankylosing spondylitis.

Radiographic findings are helpful in the diagnosis. In the spine these include erosions at the vertebral corners and vertebral squaring, calcification in the outer border of the annulus fibrosus (syndesmophyte) followed by calcification of the anterior longitudinal ligament and other ligamentous structures giving the characteristic bamboo spine appearance, and erosion and fusion at apophyseal and costochondral joints. The sacroiliac joints may show definite erosions, which may be manifested as irregular widening of the joint, areas of narrowing and sclerosis, and, later, fusion. Calcification of ligamentous structures, heel spurs, and costochondral erosion are a few of the other radiographic changes that may be seen.

No discussion of ankylosing spondylitis would be complete without mention of the genetic associations of this disorder. In various studies, 90 to 95 percent of Caucasian patients with ankylosing spondylitis have the histocompatibility antigen HLA-B27; a similar association exists for B27 and Reiter's syndrome. In contrast, HLA-B27 is found in only 6 to 8 percent of the control population. Epidemiologic studies suggest that 1 to 2 percent of the population have symptoms attributable to ankylosing spondylitis; one may then calculate an attack incidence of approximately 20 percent for the B27 positive population. Interestingly, in epidemics of Reiter's syndrome associated with bacterial agents, susceptibility is largely limited to B27 positive individuals, and the attack incidence among these is approximately 20 percent.

Clinically overt ankylosing spondylitis is predominantly a male disease. Subclinical or undiagnosed disease occurs with considerable frequency in women; similarly, there is a reservoir of low grade disease—under the tip of the iceberg, so to speak—among B27 positive males. This is supported by the demonstration of radiographic evidence of sacroiliitis in B27 positive individuals who have not had symptoms of back pain requiring medical consultation. However, given the fact that approximately one of 14 individuals in the population is B27 positive, and given the high incidence of mechanical back pain in the population, a positive test for HLA-B27 does not sustain a diagnosis of ankylosing spondylitis. Indeed, in most instances testing for B27 is not diagnostically helpful.

Genetic linkage of a disorder raises questions in patients as to genetic transmission. Although half the children of B27 positive patients with ankylosing spondylitis are B27 positive, it is not clear that the risk of ankylosing spondylitis in these children is substantially greater than that in other B27 positive individuals. Although families with several cases of ankylosing spondylitis have been observed, it is clear that the disease is not transmitted in a typical mendelian dominant fashion.

THERAPY

In the treatment of the arthritis of ankylosing spondylitis the goals are to provide pain relief and to limit deformity, thus providing maximal function. It is not clear that any therapy, with the possible exception of axial irradiation (vide infra), halts the erosive, destructive, and ankylosing features of the disease. Nonetheless a program encompassing both anti-inflammatory therapy and physical therapy can prove of long term benefit to the patient. If ankylosis of the spine or other joints is to occur, these measures can help to insure that joint fusion will occur in the best functional position. The patient in whom the hips are fused in flexion and who has severe dorsal kyphosis and anterior protrusion at the neck represents a failure of medial management.

Physical Measures

Physical measures and physical therapy should be directed at mitigating the deformities just outlined and maintaining maximal mobility of the spine and hips. The physician's role in this regard is educating the patient as to possible long term consequences of the disease and the important role that the patient can play in treatment. Prolonged periods in any position are harmful, certainly in regard to immediate symptoms and probably long term outcome as well. Jobs requiring prolonged periods of sitting in one place, particularly while stooping forward, as over a desk or work bench, aggravate forward displacement of the head and dorsal kyphosis. The patient should make a point of arising from a sitting position at least hourly for a short walk. Standing jobs similarly require frequent changes of position and intermittent exercise. When possible, raising the work surface to obviate the need for leaning forward is helpful. Long drives, in the course of either work or leisure, should be interrupted hourly for brief periods of standing, stretching, or walking.

Furniture should be chosen for proper support of the spine rather than for apparent immediate comfort. Chairs should be straight-backed and not deeply cushioned; furthermore, the patient should be instructed to sit with appropriate posture, not curled up or slouched. The patient should sleep on his back and not in a fetal position with hips flexed. Pillows should be thin and compressible, if used at all. Firm back support is essential; because one rarely encounters a patient who admits to anything other than a "firm" mattress, the most prudent course is to use a ¼ inch thickness of plywood even under "firm" mattresses.

"Physical therapy" should combine a generous measure of general physical activity along with specific exercises. Swimming provides excellent range of motion for most joints, including the spine, and at the same time protects joints from weight bearing stress. In this respect it is perhaps the best form of general exercise for arthritis. Depending on the individual patient, the severity and activity of the disease, and pre-existing deformity, activities ranging from walking to vigorous competitive sports may be appropriate.

Specific exercises should be directed at maximizing the range of motion of the spine and other joints and counteracting the direction in which deformities tend to develop. In the latter regard, instruction should be provided in exercises to counter forward propulsion of the head, to extend the dorsal spine, and to extend the hips. Other exercises should be directed at improving motion of the spine in all planes: rotation, flexion-extension, and lateral flexion. Breathing exercises to maintain the capacity for full chest expansion are often overlooked. A commitment of time for training with a physical therapist who understands the disease and the goals of physical therapy in ankylosing spondylitis is a worthwhile investment for the patient.

Drug Management

The ability of the patient to function normally in day to day activities and to follow an outlined program of physical activity is dependent upon the control of the inflammatory process. To the extent that physical therapy protects from or limits spinal and joint deformity and disability, control of acute symptoms of pain and stiffness permits the execution of a physical program that, we hope, leads to better spine and joint function in the long term. Conversely there is no evidence to indicate that anti-inflammatory therapy retards the destructive joint disease, and it is unlikely that ankylosis that would otherwise occur can be more than partially ameliorated.

The basis of therapy is the group of drugs called nonsteroidal anti-inflammatory drugs. The list of these drugs grows longer each year, and a comprehensive review of the benefits, side effects, and dollar cost of each is both beyond the scope of this article and unnecessary. Several general statements may be made. To varying degrees, all are effective in the management of ankylosing spondylitis. Indomethacin and phenylbutazone, in my experience and that of most others, are considerably more efficacious than other nonsteroidal anti-inflammatory drugs in most patients. Aspirin, for reasons that are unclear, is least effective in this disorder; this is in contrast with rheumatoid arthritis in which aspirin is effective on a par with all the newer nonsteroidal anti-inflammatory drugs. In general, the newer nonsteroidal anti-inflammatory drugs are equivalent to each other in effectiveness, although individual patients appear to respond better to one or another drug. In addition to effectiveness, both side effects and relative costs of the various drugs must be considered.

My preference is to initiate therapy with one of the new nonsteroidal anti-inflammatory drugs rather than with indomethacin and phenylbutazone, which, though generally more effective, are associated with greater toxicity. It is important to use these drugs at an adequate dosage (Table 1); too commonly they are prescribed at the lowest recommended dosage and the erroneous con-

TABLE 1 Nonsteroidal Anti-inflammatory Drugs for Ankylosing Spondylitis*

Drug	Total Daily Dosage	Frequency of Administration
Ibuprofen	2400–3200 mg †	t.i.d.-q.i.d.
Indomethacin	100–200 mg	b.i.d.-t.i.d.
Meclofenemate	300–400 mg	t.i.d.-q.i.d.
Naproxen	750–1500 mg	b.i.d.
Phenylbutazone	300–400 mg ‡	t.i.d.-q.i.d.
Piroxicam	20 mg	q.d.
Sulindac	300–400 mg	b.i.d.
Tolectin	1200–1600 mg	t.i.d.-q.i.d.

*This is not an all encompassing list but rather those with which the author has had experience.
† Dosages of 3600 to 4200 mg daily have been used on rare occasion; 3200 mg represents upper limit of the officially recommended dosage.
‡ 400 mg only rarely required.

clusion is drawn that they are ineffective. Within the group of available drugs the choice is based on drug half-life and cost. Drugs with short half-lifes are less effective in the management of morning stiffness, and the requirement for more frequent daily administration decreases compliance. It is important that patients take the drug around the clock and not only when they hurt. I would thus initiate treatment with a drug that requires no more than a three times daily dosage. It is worth advising the patient to check several pharmacies for relative cost as this may vary considerably in a given geographic area.

In my experience at least half the patients do not achieve sustained relief of symptoms with the newer group of nonsteroidal anti-inflammatory drugs, even when taken at maximal therapeutic dosages. Most of these respond well to indomethacin. Taken at a dosage of 150 to 200 mg daily initially, indomethacin provides good relief from pain and stiffness. The patient should be cautioned to take the drug with meals to ameliorate headache, light-headedness, and other neurologic symptoms. After an initial response the dosage of the drug may be tapered. It is not clear that "sustained release" formulations of the drug greatly enhance its effectiveness, but the incidence and severity of side effects may be lower. In patients who do not respond to indomethacin, phenylbutazone is usually effective. Despite the potential for serious side effects (to be outlined), ankylosing spondylitis is one disorder in which use of this drug is clearly indicated.

Side Effects of Therapy

Many of the adverse effects of therapy are shared, to greater or lesser extent, by all the nonsteroidal anti-inflammatory drugs and are a direct result of the pharmacology of drug action. All these drugs inhibit pros-

taglandin synthesis, and PGE_2 prevents back-diffusion of hydrogen ion in the gastric mucosa; this effect may be related to the high frequency of gastric irritation and, in some patients, gastrointestinal ulceration or bleeding. Bleeding is promoted by the inhibitory effects of these drugs on platelet function via inhibition of thromboxane and PGE synthesis. In patients with pre-existent gastric or duodenal ulcers, exacerbation of symptoms, new ulceration, and gastrointestinal bleeding should be carefully watched for. Some patients cannot tolerate any of the nonsteroidal anti-inflammatory drugs without the concomitant use of antacids, H_2 antagonists, or cytoprotective drugs. These, however, should not be used as a routine adjunct of nonsteroidal anti-inflammatory drug therapy in most patients.

Like the gastrointestinal side effects, renal toxicity may result from pharmacologic effects of the drug. Inhibition of renal prostaglandin synthesis results in decreased renal blood flow, an effect that is most often of clinical consequence in the elderly and those with pre-existent renal disease. The pharmacologic decrease in renal blood flow, however, is reversible, and a mild stable increase in the serum creatinine level should not require drug discontinuation. Sulindac, which is administered as a prodrug and not metabolized efficiently to an active metabolite in the kidney, appears to be associated with a lower incidence of decreased renal function.

More serious is the infrequent development of irreversible and, in rare instances, fatal renal disease. This has been reported with the majority, if not all, of the nonsteroidal anti-inflammatory drugs, is apparently due to an idiosyncratic reaction, and is usually manifested histologically as interstitial nephritis. Elderly patients and those with pre-existent renal disease may be at greater risk for the development of this side effect as well. In addition to the shared side effects already noted, individual drugs have unique but generally not serious side effects.

Indomethacin and phenylbutazone, because of their unique role in the treatment of ankylosing spondylitis and because of their generally greater toxicity, should be discussed separately. As noted, indomethacin causes neurologic side effects that are more pronounced in the elderly but are seen in all age groups, particularly when the drug is taken on an empty stomach. Thrombocytopenia has been reported as a consequence of indomethacin treatment, and platelet counts should be checked every few months, at least initially. Indomethacin is generally more gastric irritative than other nonsteroidal anti-inflammatory drugs, and gastric bleeding may be seen. Despite these side effects, indomethacin is a singularly useful drug in the management of ankylosing spondylitis.

Phenylbutazone is also associated with a greater frequency and severity of gastric intolerance than other nonsteroidal anti-inflammatory drugs and in the author's experience is associated with a greater frequency of gastrointestinal bleeding. Phenylbutazone may cause sodium retention to an extent sufficient to precipitate cardiac failure. Most worrying to many are the reported instances of agranulocytosis and general bone marrow depression due to this drug. Estimates suggest that this complication occurs in one of 10,000 treated patients each year and that half the reactions are fatal. For many patients, however, phenylbutazone is the only drug that provides relief from symptoms and allows physical mobility and function; the physician and patient therefore must weigh these benefits against the potential risk. If therapy with phenylbutazone is instituted, hematologic parameters should be followed regularly. Once an initial response is achieved, the patient may be able to be managed with another drug.

Corticosteroids and Immunosuppressive Drugs

There is no demonstrated benefit from corticosteroids in the management of spinal disease in ankylosing spondylitis. Occasional patients with peripheral arthritis may benefit from brief courses of steroids in low dosages (5 to 15 mg of prednisone daily) to suppress disease activity. When single peripheral joints are a persistent problem, intra-articular steroid instillation may be beneficial. Immunosuppressive drugs have not been shown to have a place in the treatment of ankylosing spondylitis. One exception may be in the rare patient who has predominant peripheral disease in whom weekly low dosage methotrexate (5 to 15 mg) may be tried. This approach is directed by analogy to Reiter's syndrome and psoriatic arthritis, as there is no published experience with methotrexate in ankylosing spondylitis. Whether axial disease might also respond to methotrexate is unknown, and the author has had no experience in this regard.

Irradiation

Irradiation of the axial skeleton can ameliorate spinal arthritis. This modality of treatment has been largely abandoned after reports of leukemia in patients with ankylosing spondylitis who had received irradiation. Nonetheless, in the patient who cannot tolerate any of the nonsteroidal anti-inflammatory drugs (e.g., because of activation of peptic ulcer disease), irradiation may be the only therapeutic intervention that will enable the patient to function. Administration of 400 to 600 rads to the axial skeleton over two sessions may provide good relief while leading to lower risks than previously encountered with higher dosages of radiation.

Surgery

The most common surgical procedure required in patients with ankylosing spondylitis is total hip replace-

ment to correct or prevent hip ankylosis. These patients unfortunately have a tendency to develop periarticular calcium deposition and reankylosis following total hip replacement. The frequency of reankylosis has varied among different series, and the possibility of ankylosis should not preclude total hip replacement which is otherwise indicated. Surgery to correct spinal deformity is of limited utility and should not be attempted unless the deformity markedly limits function and the surgeon has had experience with these patients. There has been some experience with spinal osteotomy to correct severe kyphosis. Finally, it should be noted that many patients with ankylosing spondylitis, owing to a failure of diagnosis, have undergone surgical procedures for low back pain. The clinician should entertain the diagnosis of ankylosing spondylitis in young men with back disease and protect them from surgical procedures that will provide no therapeutic benefit.

Extra-articular Disease

Most extra-articular disease manifestations are not readily amenable to therapy. Thus the cardiac abnormalities of conduction disturbances and aortitis have not been treated medically except for control of arrhythmias; aortic valve replacement may be necessary, depending on the hemodynamic consequences of the lesion. There is little published experience about treatment of the pulmonary fibrotic lesion; although occasionally cavitary, it is more commonly a mild fibrosis. Acute iritis requires the use of topical corticosteroid therapy.

PATIENT EDUCATION

As with other disorders, taking the time to explain the disease to the patient—what we know about its course and its treatment, what the patient is free to do and what he should avoid, and how even if a disease is incurable, that does not mean that it is untreatable—is critically important. This is often best done over a period of several office visits rather than all at one time during the first encounter. Questions about the hereditary nature of the disease and the risk in offspring should be discussed frankly. Finally, in the course of a chronic disease it is a rare patient who does not seek second, third, or more opinions. This option should be discussed with the patient openly both so that care can be coherent and coordinated and so that the patient may be referred to knowledgeable specialists (lists are usually available from the local Arthritis Foundation). Otherwise many patients will find those who promise cures from diet, vitamins, enemas, or magic drugs, treatments that will have a great impact on the patient's wealth but no beneficial effect on his health.

SUGGESTED READING

Calin A, Fries JF. Striking prevalance of ankylosing spondylitis in healthy W27 positive males and females. N Engl J Med 1975; 293:835–839.

Calin A, Porta J, Fries JF. The clinical history as a screening test for ankylosing spondylitis. JAMA 1977; 237:2613–2617.

Carette S, Graham D, Little H, Rubenstein J, Rosen P. The natural disease course of ankylosing spondylitis. Arthritis Rheum 1983; 26:186–190.

Shanahan WR Jr, Kaprove RE, Major PA, Hunter T, Bargar FD. Assessment of longterm benefit of total hip replacement in patients with ankylosing spondylitis. J Rheumatol 1982; 9:101–114.

SYSTEMIC SCLEROSIS

ETHAN WEINER, M.D.
JOSEPH H. KORN, M.D.

Systemic sclerosis, or scleroderma, is a multisystem disease characterized by cutaneous and visceral fibrosis and obliteration of small vessels. Clinical expression of the disease is a reflection of these connective tissue and vascular processes. The skin is the most visible organ affected by this process, with thickening and induration usually beginning distally and extending proximally. Dermal fibrosis and atrophy of hair follicles and sweat glands are noted on histologic study of involved skin. A similar process in the gastrointestinal tract causes atrophy of the muscularis mucosae and of the longitudinal and circular layers of smooth muscle, resulting in loss of lower esophageal tone, motility disturbance, and malabsorption. In the lungs vascular obliteration or interstitial fibrosis can occur, leading to restrictive lung disease and cor pulmonale. Obliteration of the renal vascular bed can cause an abrupt hypertensive crisis, with the rapid onset of renal failure. The heart can be affected by pericarditis, restrictive cardiomyopathy, or conduction system disturbance. Obliteration of the vessels supplying peripheral nerves (vasa nervorum) can result in mononeuritis multiplex, often affecting the trigeminal nerve.

Almost all patients with scleroderma suffer from Raynaud's phenomenon, classically a triphasic vascular response to cold, emotion, or other stimuli manifested by pallor, cyanosis, and then reactive hyperemia of affected areas, most commonly the fingers. If no history of Raynaud's phenomenon is obtained, the diagnosis of scleroderma should be questioned. Likewise, if skin tightening proceeds from the trunk outward rather than from the extremities inward, other causes of skin tightening such as scleredema or eosinophilic fasciitis should be carefully ruled out before the diagnosis of scleroderma is made. Conversely, true scleroderma can present as a low grade myositis or arthritis, accompanied by

edematous "puffy" skin that has not yet become hidebound. The diagnosis of scleroderma can be elusive until more characteristic cutaneous and visceral manifestations ultimately develop.

Scleroderma can present with a wide spectrum of organ involvement. In a subgroup of patients with what is often labeled the CREST syndrome (an acronym for calcinosis, Raynaud's phenomenon, esophageal dysmotility, sclerodactyly, and telangiectasia), skin changes are limited primarily to the fingers. In this subgroup pulmonary hypertension without fibrosis often develops late in the course of the disease, but other visceral involvement (except for esophageal) is uncommon. At the opposite end of the spectrum are patients who, within several months after the onset of Raynaud's phenomenon and sclerodactyly, develop thickened skin in more proximal areas such as the upper arms, thighs, and chest with or without associated involvement of the lungs, heart, kidneys, and gastrointestinal tract. Finally, many patients defy easy classification—they may have prominent CREST features but may have proximal skin disease or more aggressive organ system disease as well. Alternatively patients have associated features of other connective tissue diseases, such as systemic lupus erythematosus or rheumatoid arthritis, that only after some years develop into a single classic connective tissue disease. From a therapeutic viewpoint this means that the clinical manifestations that require treatment vary greatly from patient to patient, as does the pace of the disease, which can be indolent or rapidly life-threatening.

The pathogenesis of scleroderma is poorly understood. Fibroblasts isolated from patients with scleroderma produce more collagen than do normal cells. There is also both morphologic and functional evidence of endothelial cell dysfunction in scleroderma and associated evidence of platelet activation and aggregation in patients with active disease. However, there is no single underlying abnormality yet known to explain both the vascular and fibrotic phenomena that are the hallmarks of the disease.

There is no characteristic laboratory abnormality in scleroderma. Most patients have antinuclear antibodies, often with a speckled or nucleolar pattern, and some patients (particularly those with the CREST syndrome) have anticentromere antibodies. None of these antibodies is absolutely specific for scleroderma, however. Antibodies to topoisomerase I, formerly called Scl-70, are largely restricted to scleroderma. They are present in only about one third of the patients and therefore lack sufficient sensitivity to be diagnostically useful. Absence of all detectable autoantibodies does not rule out the diagnosis of scleroderma, but should invite closer scrutiny and further efforts to rule out other diseases with similar cutaneous manifestations. The erythrocyte sedimentation rate is often normal in scleroderma. Mild anemia or a low serum albumin level can occur if the patient has significant gastrointestinal involvement and is in a poor nutritional state. As a rule, complement levels are not depressed, and there is little evidence for immune complex disease.

Owing to the lack of understanding of the pathogenesis of scleroderma, treatment has been most successful when used to palliate specific organ system manifestations. Remittive therapies, designed to modulate the course of the disease in general, have yielded much less success, and their role in disease management remains to be clarified.

THERAPY FOR SPECIFIC ORGAN INVOLVEMENT

Skin Care

The skin should be kept warm and moisturizers should be used liberally, especially in the winter. Dry skin fissures easily and because of the poor vascular supply in scleroderma heals slowly. Wearing thin cotton gloves or glove liners under mittens provides optimal warmth and hand protection when mittens must be removed. Areas of calcinosis cutis should be kept clean, and local infections around calcium deposits should be treated early with systemic antibiotic therapy. Calcium deposits, which form niduses for recurrent or severe infections, may require surgical removal. Warfarin, probenecid, colchicine, and diphosphonates have been used to try to reduce the size of cutaneous calcium deposits or prevent the development of new ones. Unfortunately none of these drugs has been clearly successful. Pruritus in areas of involved skin is a common problem; although no treatment has proved uniformly successful, some patients benefit greatly from colchicine.

Raynaud's Phenomenon and Vascular Phenomenona

One of the most troublesome problems for scleroderma patients, both those with the CREST variant and those with diffuse systemic sclerosis, is Raynaud's phenomenon. Although typically episodic, it often can be severe and persistent, leading to painful digital ulcerations and resorption of the distal finger pads. Locally infected digital ulcerations should be treated with oral doses of antibiotics active against penicillinase producing staphylococci (dicloxacillin, erythromycin, or orally administered cephalosporins). Slowly healing ulcerations may conceal occult infection under scabs or crusts and may also benefit from antibiotics. In addition to scrupulous attention to keeping core and peripheral body temperature warm and keeping the skin lubricated, the use of vasodilators may be of significant benefit. We prefer to start with either nifedipine or topical nitrate therapy. Nifedipine therapy is initiated at low dosages (10 mg twice or three times daily) and gradually increased. Nitroglycerine ointment applied to the forearm or chest (½ to 1 inch every 4 to 6 hours) has been successful in many patients. Long acting nitrate patches, in our experience, have been much less successful perhaps because of tachyphylaxis in response to constant circulating drug levels. Pentoxifylline, a drug which lowers blood viscosity, is very useful in some patients. Alternative drugs such as alpha-adrenergic blocking drugs (prazosin, dibenzyline) or centrally acting drugs (methyldopa, reserpine) tend to be associated with more side effects. Prazosin, in particular, may be associated with syncope after the initial dose, and the patient should be warned and started on the lowest dosage (1 mg). Beta-blockers and other potentially vasoconstricting drugs should be avoided if substitute drugs are available. Some clinicians advocate the long term use of antiplatelet drugs such as aspirin and persantine to impede the platelet aggregation, release of vasoactive substances, and microthrombus formation that take place at sites of microvasculature injury in scleroderma. Such therapy has not been of demonstrated value but is appealing on theoretic grounds and, at least for low dose aspirin, is of little risk.

Occasionally patients need more aggressive intervention to save a digit from impending gangrene. Our initial approach was the intra-arterial infusion of reserpine (0.75 to 1.0 mg slowly) into the brachial artery of the affected side. Unfortunately reserpine for parenteral administration is no longer readily available. Local sympathetic blockage by repeated daily anesthetic injection has helped break the cycle of vasospasm, leading to ischemia and further vasospasm. Systemic intravenous infusion of PGE_1 (given by continuous central venous catheter infusion at doses of 6 to 10 ng per kilogram per minute for 3 days) also can be helpful in this situation. Surgical sympathectomies, however, are not recommended because their benefit is usually transient, lasting for weeks to months, and the patient is left with an uncomfortable, sometimes edematous, extremity. In our experience surgical amputation of digits is rarely necessary if the aggressive medical approaches just outlined are undertaken.

TABLE 1 Therapy for End Organ Involvement in Scleroderma

Skin disease
  Keep skin warm, lubricated, and protected from injury
  Antibiotics (dicloxacillin, erythromycin, cephalexin) for infected or poorly healing digital ulcerations
  Colchicine for pruritus due to calcinosis

Raynaud's phenomenon
  Vasodilators
    Nifedipine, 10–20 mg b.i.d.-q.i.d.
    Nitroglycerin ointment, 1/4 to 1 inch q 4–6 hr
    Prazosin, 1 mg then 1 mg t.i.d. to start
    Pentoxifylline, 400 mg t.i.d.
  Persistent Raynaud's phenomenon or impending gangrene of a digit
    Intravenous PGE₁ infusion via central catheter (6–10 ng/kg/minute continued for 3 days)
    Sympathetic block repeated daily or every other day for several days

Gastrointestinal disorders
  Antireflux measures
    Elevate head of bed
    Antacids p.c. and h.s.
    H₂ antagonists (ranitidine, 150 mg h.s.; famotidine, 40 mg h.s.; cimetidine 200 mg h.s.)
    Metaclopramide, 5–10 mg before meals
  Malabsorption, diarrhea
    Trial of tetracycline, 500 mg q.i.d.
  Constipation
    Stool softeners

Arthritis
  Nonsteroidal anti-inflammatory drugs including aspirin and nonacetylated salicylates
  Low doses of steroids for early puffy scleroderma

Myositis (symptomatic)
  Prednisone, 20–60 mg/day initially, tapering according to clinical and laboratory response

Acute interstitial lung disease
  Corticosteroids, 40–60 mg daily initially, tapering according to response
  ? Cyclophosphamide for severe or steroid unresponsive disease

Pericarditis
  Prednisone, 20–60 mg/day for significant or symptomatic disease

Hypertension and renal crisis
  Enalapril, 5–20 mg b.i.d., or captopril, 25–150 mg t.i.d., increasing rapidly from starting dose until blood pressure control is achieved; after initial control, adjust dosage to maintain diastolic blood pressure ≤80 mm Hg

Sjögren's syndrome
  Artificial tears, t.i.d. to q.i.d.; lubricating ophthalmic ointment before bed

Specialized dental care may be needed

Psychologic and social support
  Physician time, patient support groups

Gastrointestinal Dysmotility

Esophageal stricture formation can occur in scleroderma after prolonged acid reflux. In many but not all of these patients there is an antecedent history of reflux symptoms. It is reasonable therefore to apply antireflux measures in all patients with scleroderma to prevent potential stricture formation. These measures should include elevating the head of the bed 4 to 6 inches and the liberal use of antacids, particularly before sleep. Symptomatic patients may also benefit from the use of an H₂ blocker (cimetidine, famotidine, or ranitidine) at bedtime. Patients complaining of dysphagia or severe reflux symptoms may also benefit from metaclopramide, 5 to 10 mg, given before meals to increase lower esophageal sphincter pressure.

In the small bowel a malabsorption state may develop because of poor bowel motility, leading to stasis and bacterial overgrowth. This often is manifested as diarrhea and weight loss clinically and hypoalbuminemia on laboratory evaluation. Many patients benefit from the administration of tetracycline during exacerbations of this condition. Excessive use of tetracycline should be avoided, however, since alteration of the bacterial flora for extended periods may allow the development of pseudomembranous colitis. Alternatively constipation can develop as a result of impaired bowel motility; it should be treated with stool softeners.

Musculoskeletal Disorders

Frank arthritis is an infrequent manifestation of scleroderma but may occur early in the disease. Management with aspirin or other nonsteroidal anti-inflammatory drugs often suffices, but small dosages of prednisone (5 to 10 mg per day) can be used on a short term basis if nonsteroidal drugs alone do not provide relief from pain and swelling. In patients with renal dysfunction nonsteroidal drugs generally should be avoided, except for the nonacetylated salycylates, which do not interfere with prostaglandin production. A common problem in patients with scleroderma is the development of flexion contractures at many joints due to the tightening of skin and ligaments around them. Regular physical therapy, with range of motion exercises at these joints, is vital both to prevent worsening of this condition and, it is hoped, to effect improvement.

Cardiac and Pulmonary Disease

Early aggressive therapy of the interstitial lung lesion of scleroderma with high dose steroid therapy (1 mg per kilogram per day of prednisone or the equivalent) or cytotoxic drugs may be beneficial in preventing or reducing the amount of pulmonary fibrosis. Such treatment should be undertaken only if there is ample evidence of active interstitial inflammation by gallium scan, bronchoalveolar lavage, and/or lung biopsy. Once established, however, pulmonary fibrosis is not reversible. In late disease supervening pulmonary hypertension may be treated by the use of pulmonary vasodilators, such as nifedipine or hydralazine, and by the use of supplemental oxygen if significant desaturation occurs with exercise.

Pleuritis or pericarditis frequently occurs during the course of the disease. These disorders respond well to moderate dosages of steroids (20 to 30 mg per day of prednisone), which are tapered when the patient is no longer symptomatic and pleural or pericardial fluid accumulation is resolving. All patients should be followed with periodic electrocardiograms, and if there is evidence of a conduction disturbance or the patient gives a history of palpitations or light-headedness, a 24 hour ambulatory electrocardiogram should be obtained. Some patients with scleroderma show evidence of a significant arrhythmia, which may be amenable to or require treatment by either drugs or pacemaker insertion.

Scleroderma Renal Crisis

Renal involvement in scleroderma is often abrupt in onset, manifesting as severe hypertension and progressing in days to weeks to renal failure. Rarely, progressive renal disease develops in the absence of associated hypertension. Associated proteinuria is common as is evidence of microangiopathy, including microangiopathic hemolysis resulting from fibrin thrombi occluding small vessels in the kidney and elsewhere. The pathophysiology involves marked narrowing or cortical renal vessels with associated areas of cortical infarction in severe cases.

Such renal involvement in scleroderma formerly (until 10 to 12 years ago) was almost uniformly and rapidly fatal. The advent of angiotensin converting enzyme inhibitors for the treatment of hypertension has dramatically reversed the previously poor prognosis in scleroderma renal disease. Thus, the currently available inhibitors enalapril and captopril are the initial drugs of choice in treating scleroderma associated hypertension. We also favor treating scleroderma renal failure without

hypertension with angiotensin converting enzyme inhibitors on the assumption that there is disordered microvascular flow, which may respond to such therapy. In such instances other causes of renal insufficiency must first be considered and the diagnosis of scleroderma renal disease substantiated by the finding of microangiopathic changes on the peripheral blood smear or compatible renal angiographic or biopsy findings.

Aggressive treatment with angiotensin converting enzyme inhibitors has usually resulted in normalization of renal function when therapy has been initiated before there has been a two- to three-fold increase in the serum creatinine level (i.e., a 50 to 75 percent loss of renal function). Even in some patients whose renal disease has progressed to the point of requiring dialysis for acute scleroderma renal crisis, continued aggressive treatment with such inhibitors has resulted in the return of renal function to reasonable levels. It is our practice to "push" therapy to diastolic blood pressures of 80 mm Hg or lower, particularly in patients already showing impairment of renal function. Our experience has been that at such blood pressures improvement of renal function is more likely to occur. In most cases no additional therapy besides angiotensin converting enzyme inhibitors is required. We would particularly avoid diuretics because they tend to further decrease renal perfusion pressure and may aggravate what is often already a hyperreninemic state. Glucocorticoids have not been shown to be of any value in treatment and indeed may aggravate the hypertension and renal disease.

Ideally one would like to institute treatment of scleroderma hypertension before it becomes symptomatic. For this reason it is wise to teach patients to take their own blood pressure weekly. A trend toward rising blood pressures (e.g., from 110/70 to 150/90) would warrant treatment even if the diastolic blood pressure remained technically within the normal range. Here also we would be inclined to treat with angiotensin converting enzyme inhibitors rather than with milder antihypertensive drugs.

Sjögren's Syndrome

About 25 percent of the patients with scleroderma also suffer from Sjögren's syndrome, a polyglandular exocrinopathy resulting in decreased tear and saliva production. Increased dental caries often result from decreased saliva flow, and patients complaining of dry mouth should undergo frequent dental check-ups and should observe scrupulous dental hygeine. The decreased oral aperture in patients with scleroderma makes dental work and dental hygiene more difficult. Patients complaining of dry gritty eyes should be given artifical tears during the day and lubricating ophthalmic ointments for use at night. There is no systemic pharmacologic agent to increase tear and saliva production.

THE ROLE OF DISEASE MODIFYING DRUGS

Many drugs have been tried to alter the course of scleroderma in a global way. These have included anti-inflammatory drugs, such as colchicine, immunosuppressive drugs, including corticosteroids and cytotoxic drugs, and p-aminobenzoate, which has been advocated as an antifibrosis drug. Unfortunately reports of success with these drugs have been largely anecdotal, and efficacy has not been reproducibly demonstrated. Recent reports of the successful use of plasmapheresis and lymphoplasmapheresis are encouraging but require further documentation.

Attention has focused recently on D-penicillamine, a chelating drug that can prevent extracellular collagen fibril cross linking by reversibly blocking aldehyde groups on the fibril surface. D-penicillamine also may decrease the rate of collagen synthesis and increase the rate of collagen degradation. In addition, it has suppressive effects on T lymphocytes in vitro and could mediate an effect based on suppression of synthesis of lymphokines, which stimulate collagen synthesis.

All the studies with penicillamine have been uncontrolled and have largely been retrospective. There is, however, a suggestion that progression of skin disease can be slowed by the drug. Data suggesting that the development of renal crisis or pulmonary fibrosis may be prevented in some patients by the early use of penicillamine are inconclusive at best. The patients who have the most to gain from D-penicillamine are those with rapidly progressive, diffuse skin disease, since these are the patients for whom slowing of the skin progression would be most beneficial. This subgroup may also be the patients at greatest risk of developing pulmonary or renal involvement. The natural history of scleroderma is often one of gradual spontaneous skin softening after several years, and therefore patients with long-standing stable skin disease would be less likely to benefit from penicillamine. Likewise patients with the CREST syndrome, who have little skin involvement and who rarely develop renal crises or pulmonary fibrosis, would be less likely to benefit from penicillamine treatment. Penicillamine therefore should be reserved for patients with a recent onset of the disease (within 2 years) in whom noticeable progression of skin disease occurs over a period of months.

Treatment with penicillamine should not be undertaken lightly because its toxicity is great. The range of toxicity observed in patients with scleroderma who are taking penicillamine is similar to that observed in those with rheumatoid arthritis treated with this drug and includes rash, dysgeusia, stomatitis, blood dyscrasias, and proteinuria due to membranous nephritis. Patients with scleroderma seem to have a higher incidence than do patients with rheumatoid arthritis of developing pemphigus and myasthenia gravis secondary to penicillamine treatment. In about one patient in five the drug must be permanently discontinued within several months because of a serious side effect.

If treatment with penicillamine is begun, the initial dosage should be 250 mg per day for the average sized adult. The leukocyte count, hemoglobin level, platelet count, and urinalysis should be monitored weekly. If the drug is tolerated, the dosage should be increased gradually, no faster than 250 mg per day per month, until maximal dosages of 750 to 1500 mg per day are reached. Even with a maximal dosage it may take 6 months or more before any clinical effects are seen. There are no established guidelines for deciding when the drug dosage should be gradually tapered and then discontinued, but in patients who respond to the drug, therapy probably should be continued at the maximal dosage for at least 1 year before attempts are made to slowly reduce the daily dosage.

In general, corticosteroids and cytotoxic drugs do not have a role in the treatment of scleroderma. There are, however, several noteworthy exceptions. Corticosteroids in modest dosages (10 to 30 mg per day of prednisone) may provide symptomatic relief in the early edematous phase of skin involvement with scleroderma, before induration sets in; the dosage should be tapered rapidly to 10 mg daily or less. Likewise corticosteroids in high dosages or cytotoxic drugs may be of use in patients with early, rapidly progressive pulmonary interstitial fibrosis, as described earlier. Symptomatic myositis, with elevated muscle enzyme levels, requires corticosteroid therapy. However, many patients with scleroderma have persistent mild elevations (twice normal) of muscle enzyme levels, and corticosteroid therapy in these patients generally is not helpful. Pleuritis or pericarditis, which can accompany scleroderma, may respond to treatment with corticosteroids in modest doses.

In conclusion, systemic sclerosis presents a broad spectrum of disease activity. The underlying abnormalities causing the disease are poorly understood, and therefore therapies to treat the disease globally have so far been disappointing. With judicious use of medications to address abnormalities of specific organ systems, survival as well as the quality of life can be significantly improved. Finally the physician must spend the time to explain to the patient that although the disease cannot be cured, its worst manifestations can be controlled. Reassurance by the physician and emotional support remain an important part of the therapeutic armamentarium in this trying disease.

SUGGESTED READING

Clements PJ, et al. The relationship of arrhythmias and conduction disturbances to other manifestations of cardiopulmonary disease in progressive systemic sclerosis (PSS). Am J Med 1981; 71:38–46.

Korn JH, Leroy EC. Scleroderma. In: Cohen AS, ed. The principles and practice of medicine. Vol. 4. Rheumatology and immunology. New York: Grune & Stratton, 1979: 249–261.

Medsger TA Jr, et al. Survival with systemic sclerosis (scleroderma). A life table analysis of clinical and demographic factors in 309 patients. Ann Intern Med 1971; 75:369–376.

Smith CD, McKendry RJR. Controlled trial of nifedipende in the treatment of Raynaud's phenomenon. Lancet 1982; 2:1299–1301.

Steen VD, Medsger TA, Rodnan GP. D-penicillimine therapy in

progressive systemic sclerosis (scleroderma), a retrospective analysis. Ann Intern Med 1982; 97:652–659.

Whitman HH, et al. Variable response to oral angiotensin-converting-enzyme blockade in hypertensive scleroderma patients. Arthritis Rheum 1982; 25:241–248.

DERMATOMYOSITIS AND POLYMYOSITIS

THOMAS R. CUPPS, M.D.

Polymyositis and dermatomyositis compose a heterogeneous group of clinical syndromes that have in common the diffuse nonsuppurative inflammatory damage of skeletal muscle. The term polymyositis is used when only skeletal muscle is involved; dermatomyositis is used when skin in addition to skeletal muscle is affected. Both may occur as isolated disease processes, or they may be associated with a number of collagen vascular diseases, including rheumatoid arthritis, systemic lupus erythematosus, scleroderma, systemic necrotizing vasculitis, and overlap syndromes. Inflammatory muscle disease in the pediatric age group is most commonly associated with a vasculitic component, with frequent involvement of the gastrointestinal tract. Involvement of organ systems other than skeletal muscles in the polymyositis-dermatomyositis complex is also recognized. Pulmonary involvement with a pattern of interstitial fibrosis or cardiac involvement with conduction or rhythm disturbances is present in a subset of these patients. The polymyositis-dermatomyositis complex in patients over the age of 40 years is associated with an increased incidence of malignant disease, the highest incidence being seen in patients who develop the disease after the age of 60 years.

The diagnosis of polymyositis-dermatomyositis is based on the finding of bilateral proximal muscle weakness with supportive laboratory findings, including elevated muscle enzyme levels (such as creatine kinase or aldolase); normal endocrine function; an electromyogram showing increased insertional activity, numerous fibrillation potentials and sharp waves at rest, and bizarre high frequency repetitive discharges; and characteristic muscle biopsy findings of a mononuclear cell infiltrate between the muscle fibers and around small vessels, necrosis, phagocytosis, and regeneration. The presence of cutaneous involvement of the eyelids, cheeks, the bridge of the nose, the front and back of the chest, and

the extensor surfaces of the extremities with the characteristic erythematous to violaceous eruption completes the clinical spectrum of dermatomyositis.

The etiology of the polymyositis-dermatomyositis complex is unknown. Although viral agents have been suggested, there is little firmly established evidence of a causal role for any infectious agent. In the absence of an established infectious cause an immunologically mediated disease process has been postulated. Evidence to support a primary immunologically mediated mechanism is indirect. The presence of a predominantly mononuclear cell infiltrate in involved muscle supports the notion of immunologically mediated muscle damage. Cell mediated immune responses to myocytes have been reported in patients with inflammatory muscle disease. The association of the polymyositis-dermatomyositis complex with other apparently immunologically mediated disease processes also supports an immunologically mediated etiology.

THERAPY

General Considerations

Immunosuppressive drugs, including glucocorticosteroids and cytotoxic drugs, are the principle drugs used in the treatment of the polymyositis-dermatomyositis complex. These drugs are administered with the therapeutic goal of suppressing the inflammatory response in the skeletal muscles, restoring muscle strength and function, and preventing irreversible fibrotic changes. The use of immunosuppressive drugs in this disease is based on the assumption that the inflammatory muscle disease is immunologically mediated and on the improvement of certain patients during treatment with these drugs. There have been no long term double blinded prospective trials of these drugs to document therapeutic efficacy in the polymyositis-dermatomyositis complex. Despite this limitation, the use of immunosuppressive drugs remains the standard therapy for inflammatory muscle disease.

After the diagnosis of inflammatory muscle disease has been established, the possibility of an associated disease process should be considered as therapeutic decisions are being made. In the pediatric population the possibility of an associated vasculitic process, particularly of the bowel, should be considered. It is important to recognize that glucocorticosteroids may mask signs and symptoms of vasculitis induced bowel ischemia if present. In patients above the age of 40 years the possibility of associated malignant disease should be pursued as clinically indicated. The potential association with pulmonary and cardiac involvement should also be evaluated. The presence of an associated disease process may alter therapeutic decisions in individual patients.

Corticosteroid Therapy

Induction

Glucocorticosteroids in pharmacologic doses are the initial form of therapy in the majority of patients with the polymyositis-dermatomyositis complex. After the diagnosis has been established and an appropriate evaluation for associated disease processes considered, treatment should be expeditiously started. Prednisone therapy, started at 1 to 1.5 mg per kg as a single morning dose, is usually effective in patients with mild to moderately severe inflammatory muscle disease. Some subsets of patients may require more aggressive corticosteroid therapy.

Patients with cardiac or pulmonary involvement, severe muscle weakness, or functional impairment of the muscles of deglutition or respiration should be given split dose prednisone therapy. Prednisone, 20 mg orally four times a day, is one example of an aggressive therapeutic approach for the subset of patients with more severe involvement. In many patients started on therapy with split doses of prednisone, the dosage level can be rapidly tapered to a single daily dose during the initial weeks of therapy. It should be emphasized that the clinical response to corticosteroid therapy in this disease tends to be gradual and may not be apparent during the initial induction phase.

Management

The majority of patients with the polymyositis-dermatomyositis complex require prolonged treatment with pharmacologic doses of corticosteroids. To minimize the potential morbidity associated with long term corticosteroid therapy, the minimal effective dosage should be established for each patient. The monitoring of disease activity becomes crucial in decisions to modulate the corticosteroid dosage. Both clinical and laboratory parameters should be determined on a regular basis to define disease activity. Serial determinations of muscle strength should be recorded using the Medical Research Council scale (0, no movement of muscle groups; 1,

flicker of movement; 2, movement with gravity eliminated; 3, movement against gravity but not against resistance; 4, movement against resistance; and 5, normal). In patients with impaired respiratory muscle function, serial determinations of the forced vital capacity also may be a useful parameter to follow.

The clinical response to corticosteroid therapy is characteristically slow and gradual. The majority of patients begin to show evidence of improved muscle strength 2 to 12 weeks after starting therapy. Delayed responses 4 to 6 months after starting therapy have been reported. In patients with dermatomyositis, the heliotrope pattern of the skin rash and the eruptions on the extensor surfaces may vary regardless of the muscle weakness; consequently the cutaneous involvement should not be used as a guide in therapeutic decisions.

Serial laboratory determinations provide useful information in evaluating disease activity. Although the creatine kinase determination is the single most sensitive and most specific muscle enzyme test in the diagnosis of the polymyositis-dermatomyositis complex, the test should be used advisedly in patients treated with corticosteroids. The use of pharmacologic doses of corticosteroids "nonspecifically" decreases the creatine kinase level. This corticosteroid associated reduction of the creatine kinase level has been noted in individuals with noninflammatory muscle disease as well as in those without muscle disease. A decrease in the level after starting corticosteroid therapy may reflect this nonspecific response rather than a true decrease in the skeletal muscle inflammation. Of note, another muscle associated enzyme, aldolase, does not appear to be affected "nonspecifically" by corticosteroid therapy. Serial aldolase levels, if initially elevated, may be a more reliable guide to underlying disease activity. Although elevated in some patients presenting with the polymyositis-dermatomyositis complex, the erythrocyte sedimentation rate is not a reliable indicator of disease activity in the majority of patients.

In cases of generally slow clinical responses to the corticosteroids, every effort should be made to establish the minimal effective dosage of this drug. Following the initial clinical improvement one should consider a gradual tapering of the corticosteroid dosage. The tapering should be carried out gradually because of the striking tendency to exacerbate the underlying inflammatory muscle disease during rapid tapering of corticosteroid dosages. An alternate day corticosteroid regimen produces less drug associated morbidity than the daily regimens and is preferable if this therapeutic approach is effective in treating the underlying disease.

Although the precise tapering schedule should be established on a patient by patient basis, the following approach is one example of a gradual tapering to an alternate day program. Starting from a single daily morning dose of 60 mg of prednisone, decrease the alternate day dosage of prednisone by 10 mg, resulting in a schedule of 60 mg as the single morning dose alternating with 50 mg as the single morning dose. After

2 weeks again drop the alternate day dose, resulting in a schedule of 60 mg alternating with 40 mg. Clinical and laboratory assessment of the disease activity should be carried out on a regular basis and the pace of the tapering adjusted accordingly. If the patient remains clinically stable, continue the tapering. A 10 mg dose of prednisone is dropped from the low day dosage regimen every 2 weeks until a dosage regimen of 60 mg alternating with 20 mg is established. At this point the tapering schedule is slowed to a reduction of 5 mg of prednisone from the low dose day every 2 weeks until a dosage of 60 mg alternating with 10 mg is obtained. Finally the alternate day low dosage is reduced by 2.5 mg every 3 to 4 weeks until a schedule of 60 mg alternating with an "off" day is established. The alternate day high dose may then be gradually tapered as tolerated. Not all patients tolerate tapering to an alternate day regimen. If the inflammatory muscle disease cannot be adequately controlled on an alternate day regimen, the prednisone dosage should be increased back to a level that was effective in controlling the disease and tapering to a low dosage daily regimen initiated once the disease process is adequately controlled.

The taper to a low dosage daily regimen should be done gradually also. The following is one example of such a prednisone taper. Starting from a single dose of 60 mg of prednisone, taper the dosage 10 mg every 2 weeks until the patient is taking 40 mg a day. At this point the tapering is slowed to lowering the dosage of prednisone by 5 mg every 2 weeks until a dosage of 20 mg a day is established. From 20 mg a day the prednisone dosage is tapered by 2.5 mg every 2 weeks until a maintenance dosage of 10 mg is reached. It is important to emphasize that these suggested corticosteroid tapering schedules are examples and will undoubtedly require some modification when used in individual patients.

Although the optimal duration of treatment varies with each patient, extended treatment periods are characteristically required. The majority of patients require treatment for 2 to 3 years. A subset of patients may respond to shorter periods of therapy. In patients who obtain complete clinical remission rapidly, an attempt to taper and discontinue the corticosteroids after 1 year of therapy should be considered. Although some patients require more prolonged therapy, approximately 75 percent can stop therapy within 5 years after starting treatment. A subset of patients require more prolonged corticosteroid therapy to suppress disease activity and may remain corticosteroid dependent for an extended period.

The management of patients with polymyositis-dermatomyositis who develop recurrent or progressive proximal muscle weakness after an established response to corticosteroid therapy requires special consideration. The use of daily pharmacologic doses of corticosteroids is associated with type 2 muscle fiber atrophy. In some patients progressive atrophy results in a clinically significant corticosteroid myopathy characterized by proximal weakness similar in pattern to the weakness seen in active myositis. The presence of prominent atrophy,

proportionately greater weakness in the lower extremities, prolonged use of daily or split dose regimens, and normal serum muscle enzyme levels suggest the possibility of corticosteroid induced myopathy. Reduction of the corticosteroid dosage results in a gradual increase in muscle strength if the weakness is due to drug induced myopathy. By contrast, if the weakness is secondary to the underlying myositis, reduction of the corticosteroid dosage will result in increasing muscle weakness and rising enzyme levels.

In some patients the drug and inflammatory myopathies may contribute to clinical weakness; consequently a follow-up muscle biopsy may provide useful information by identifying the dominant pathologic process. In addition to drug induced myopathy, patients with the polymyositis-dermatomyositis complex associated with malignant disease may respond initially to corticosteroids and then develop progressive muscle weakness despite continued treatment with previously effective dosages of corticosteroids. In older patients with refractory myositis or progressive disease after an initial therapeutic response, the possibility of an underlying neoplastic process should be reconsidered.

Morbidity

Prolonged daily corticosteroid therapy can produce significant associated morbidity. The potential side effects of prolonged corticosteroid therapy are summarized in the chapter *Temporal Arteritis*. Although the nature and extent of adverse side effects vary from individual to individual, higher dosages, increased frequency of administration, and prolonged therapy increase the likelihood of corticosteroid induced morbidity. To minimize the morbidity associated with this drug, the minimal effective dosage should be established for each individual. Limiting the patient's exposure to corticosteroids decreases the likelihood of development of dose related side effects. Clinical concerns for the management of patients treated with corticosteroids are summarized in Table 1.

Cytotoxic Therapy

Cytotoxic drugs have been widely used in conjunction with corticosteroid therapy in polymyositis-dermatomyositis. There appears to be little difference in the therapeutic effects of the two most commonly used drugs, methotrexate and azathioprine. A cytotoxic drug is generally added to the prednisone regimen when the latter produces an inadequate response after 2 to 4 months. Anecdotal experience suggests that patients with disease that is more severe or of longer duration obtain greater benefit if combined therapy with prednisone and a cytotoxic drug such as azathioprine is started simultaneously. The cytotoxic immunosuppressive drugs may

TABLE 1 Management Considerations in Patients Treated with Corticosteroids

Problem	Clinical Considerations
Increased risk of infection	Intermediate PPD skin test with anergy panel prior to therapy; clinical follow-up of opportunistic infection
Glucose intolerance	Urinalysis for glucose; serum glucose level
Cushingoid features, truncal obesity	Dietary counseling to avoid weight gain; follow weights closely
Osteopenia	Prophylactic therapy: calcium 500 mg p.o., t.i.d., or q.i.d.; vitamin D 25,000 to 50,000 units twice weekly
Gastric distress	Antacids, H$_2$ blockers, sulcralfate
Hypothalamic-pituitary-adrenal axis suppression	Educate patient about the potential for Addisonian crisis and need for parenteral corticosteroid therapy if he is unable to take oral medication >24 h

produce an "additive" as well as a "corticosteroid sparing" therapeutic effect.

Methotrexate

Methotrexate is a folic acid analogue that inhibits thymidine and hence DNA synthesis by suppressing dihydrofolate reductase function. Therapy has been reported to result in clinical improvement in more than half the corticosteroid unresponsive patients. The drug can be administered with prednisone or by itself. Intravenous administration may cause fewer side effects. Drug administration is started on a once a week schedule with an initial dosage of 10 to 12 mg (approximately 0.2 mg per kg). The dosage is increased by the same weekly increment to a maximum of 40 to 50 mg (0.7 to 0.8 mg per kg). A clinical response may be seen as early as 6 weeks, but the maximal response may not be realized for 3 to 5 months. As the patient responds clinically, the frequency of administration can be decreased to every 2 weeks and then every 3 weeks until a maintenance schedule of once a month administration is realized. As the patient responds to the methotrexate, the prednisone dosage also can be tapered in the majority of cases. The total duration of therapy may extend from months to 2 years. Intramuscular administration should be avoided because of the potential for local muscle injury and noninflammatory elevations of muscle enzyme levels.

A program of intermittent oral administration of methotrexate has also been tried in patients with inflammatory muscle disease. Drug administration is started at 2.5 mg orally every 12 hours for a total of three doses over 1½ days once a week. If this level is tolerated, the individual dose can be increased to 5 mg. The total weekly dosage should not exceed 20 mg of methotrexate.

Information about the relative safety and efficacy of intravenous versus oral administration of methotrexate in patients with polymyositis-dermatomyositis is currently not available. Side effects such as stomatitis, diarrhea, and intestinal ulceration may necessitate dosage reduction, particularly in the setting of decreased renal function. More severe side effects of methotrexate therapy include necrotizing alveolitis and hepatic fibrosis leading to cirrhosis. Liver cirrhosis is a significant long term complication of methotrexate therapy and the risk is related to the cumulative dosage of the drug. Liver function studies are not particularly sensitive indicators of hepatic fibrosis, and some authors recommend liver biopsies after a total dosage of 1.5 g of the drug has been administered. Optimal management of this potential drug related problem has not been clearly defined. Because ethanol consumption, diabetes mellitus, and obesity appear to be risk factors for the development of methotrexate associated fibrosis, the presence of these parameters is a relative contraindication to use of this drug. Patients with one of these risk factors who are treated with methotrexate should be followed with liver biopsies. Liver function studies should be carried out and a hemogram should be obtained every 2 to 4 weeks.

Azathioprine

Azathioprine is a purine analogue that inhibits purine biosynthesis. Therapy may be effective in one third of the patients with polymyositis-dermatomyositis that are refractory to corticosteroid therapy. Azathioprine generally is used in conjunction with prednisone to produce the so-called "corticosteroid sparing effect." The drug is administered orally at a dosage of 1.5 to 2.5 mg per kg. The clinical response to azathioprine does not appear to be as rapid as that with methotrexate, the maximal effect requiring 6 to 12 months. Attempts to taper the prednisone dosage can be initiated after about 3 months of azathioprine therapy. Prolonged use of low dose azathioprine therapy is feasible for several years if clinically indicated. The most common potential side effects include myelosuppression and drug induced hepatitis. Rare drug associated complications include pulmonary fibrosis, acute febrile reactions, and a slightly increased risk of malignant disease. Serial hemograms should be obtained and liver function studies done every 2 weeks during the initiation of therapy and every 4 weeks after the first 6 months of therapy.

Cyclophosphamide

Cyclophosphamide (a DNA alkylating drug) may be useful in treating refractory cases of inflammatory disease. Because of the potential for greater drug associated toxicity, the use of cyclophosphamide is reserved for patients who prove to be refractory to methotrexate, azathioprine, and prednisone. Cyclophosphamide therapy is started as a single morning dose of 2 mg per kg. Subsequently the dose is modified to maintain the total white cell count above 3,500 cells per cubic mm. The clinical response to cyclophosphamide is more rapid than that to azathioprine. Tapering to an alternate day prednisone regimen should be initiated 2 to 3 weeks after starting cyclophosphamide therapy. It should be emphasized that the combination of daily prednisone and cyclophosphamide is a very immunosuppressive regimen with a substantially increased risk of opportunistic infections. By contrast, a properly managed regimen of alternate day prednisone and cyclophosphamide therapy is generally well tolerated by the majority of patients. The side effects of cyclophosphamide include bone marrow suppression, hemorrhagic cystitis, bladder fibrosis, neoplastic transformation (acute myelocytic leukemia, bladder carcinoma), risk of infection, ovarian failure, sterility, and alopecia. The clinical management of patients treated with cyclophosphamide is discussed in more detail in the chapter on *Temporal Arteritis* in this book. Chlorambucil has been used in severe refractory cases and in patients who have developed unacceptable side effects with cyclophosphamide.

Alternative Therapies

A number of therapeutic approaches have been tried in patients with polymyositis-dermatomyositis who are refractory to the more standard forms of treatment. Anecdotal experience suggests that these approaches may work in selected individual cases, although none is uniformly successful in all refractory patients. High dose "pulse methylprednisolone" can be tried in unresponsive patients. Methylprednisolone (30 mg per kg) should be infused over 30 to 45 minutes. Different infusion protocols have been suggested. One approach is to carry out three infusions on 3 consecutive days. A second approach is infuse on alternating days for a total of six infusions. The infusion protocols generally are used in addition to other immunosuppressive therapy. The clinical management of patients treated with pulse methylprednisolone protocols is discussed in more detail in the chapter on *Temporal Arteritis* in this book.

Plasmapheresis has been used in refractory cases with limited success at some centers. Levamisole (a single 100 mg dose once a week) has been added to standard immunosuppressive regimens (prednisone with a cytotoxic drug) in refractory cases. The combination of corticosteroids, chlorambucil, and methotrexate has been used successfully in patients with refractory inflammatory muscle disease.

The successful use of cyclosporin A in the treatment of refractory polymyositis-dermatomyositis has also been reported. Drug therapy was started initially at a dosage of 7.5 to 10 mg per kg per day but was reduced to a level of 5 mg per kg per day because of associated renal toxicity. Rapid clinical and laboratory improvements after 1 to 2 weeks of therapy have been noted. Of particular importance is the high frequency of renal toxicity in patients treated with this particular protocol. Because marked individual variability in the metabolism of cyclosporin A has been reported, drug blood level determinations are required for safe administration. Close monitoring of the blood pressure and renal function parameters (blood urea nitrogen and creatinine levels) is advised.

Physical Medicine

Physiotherapy is an important aspect of the treatment of patients with the polymyositis-dermatomyositis complex. During the period of acute inflammation, excessive muscle strain should be avoided. It is, however, important to maintain flexibility with passive range of motion exercises. As the inflammatory process is controlled, the patient can progress to an active range of motion program. The increase in physical activity should be gradual as the disease is put into remission. Extreme muscle exertion should be avoided.

SUGGESTED READING

Ansell BM. Management of polymyositis and dermatomyositis. Clin Rheum Dis 1984; 10:205–213.
Bendtzen K, Tvede N, Andersen V, Bendixen G. Cyclosporin for polymyositis. Lancet 1984; 1:792–793.
Bradley GW. Inflammatory diseases of muscle. In: Kelley WN, Harris ED Jr, Ruddy S, Sledge CB, eds. Textbook of rheumatology. 2nd ed. Philadelphia: WB Saunders 1985.
Henriksson KG, Sandstedt P. Polymyositis—treatment and prognosis. A study of 107 patients. Acta Neurol Scand 1982; 65:280–300.

MIXED CONNECTIVE TISSUE DISEASE

ROBERT T. SCHOEN, M.D., F.A.C.P.
JOHN A. HARDIN, M.D.

Mixed connective tissue disease, described by Sharp in 1972, is a syndrome that includes clinical features suggestive of scleroderma, systemic lupus erythematosus, and polymyositis that occur in patients with a specific serologic marker—antibodies to extractable nuclear antigens. Since this initial report, arthritis similar to that seen in rheumatoid arthritis has been added to the spectrum of this disease.

BASIC IMMUNOLOGIC FEATURES

As a better understanding of the immunology of autoantibodies to nuclear components has evolved, additional serologic findings have been reported in mixed connective tissue disease. Early studies indicated that extractable nuclear antigens contain both a ribonuclease (RNase) sensitive antigen, referred to as nuclear ribonucleoprotein (RNP), and a second antigen that is resistant to RNase, the Sm antigen. High titers of anti-RNP characterize mixed connective tissue disease, whereas anti-Sm antibodies are almost always associated with systemic lupus erythematosus. Recent investigations have shown that the RNP and Sm antigens are the U1, U2, U4, U5, and U6 small nuclear ribonucleoprotein (snRNP) particles that mediate the excision of introns (noncoding segments) from newly synthesized premessenger RNA. Immunoprecipitation studies have demonstrated that sera of the so-called RNP specificity bind the U1 snRNP, whereas anti-Sm antibodies bind the U1, U2, and U4-6 snRNPs (Table 1).

Recently it has been observed that the most characteristic autoantibody for mixed connective tissue disease is the specificity that binds the 68K polypeptide of the U1 particles. Typically antibodies to the U series of

snRNPs produce the speckled pattern of nuclear staining when sera are studied in the indirect immunofluorescence assay. The observation of a speckled nuclear staining pattern in very high titers (greater than 1:10,000) is almost pathognomonic for antibodies to the U1 snRNP and should lead the clinician to consider a diagnosis of mixed connective tissue disease.

CLINICAL FEATURES

Since the description of mixed connective tissue disease by Sharp and his associates in 1972, there has been controversy whether the disease justifies recognition as a distinct disease with characteristic clinical features. In the original group of patients, arthritis, sometimes in association with sausage-like swelling of the hands and Raynaud's phenomenon, was the most frequent clinical manifestation and was present in most patients. Esophageal dysmotility, myositis, and lymphadenopathy were also common. Approximately one third of the patients had fever, hepatomegaly, serositis, or splenomegaly. Renal disease was not noted in the initial report. Anemia and leukopenia were common, and hypergammaglobulinemia was present frequently. The syndrome therefore was described as having features of scleroderma, systemic lupus erythematosus, and polymyositis, but the patients were said not to have renal disease. From a therapeutic point of view, good outcomes were reported with low dosages of corticosteroids given in short duration. Since this initial study, additional series of patients, including a large multicenter study, have helped to establish mixed connective tissue disease as a specific syndrome.

Several generalizations can now be added to the original clinical picture. A large percentage of patients mainly have arthralgias, but a deforming arthritis similar to rheumatoid arthritis can occur. Pulmonary disease, including not only pleuritis and pericarditis but also interstitial lung disease and primary pulmonary hypertension, has been recognized. Although most reports have continued to emphasize that renal disease is less common in mixed connective tissue disease than in systemic lupus erythematosus or scleroderma, it has been found with increasing frequency.

In a 5 year follow-up of 22 of the original 25 patients reported by Sharp in 1972, it was found that in many of the patients there had evolved a clinical picture most consistent with scleroderma or the patients had become asymptomatic.

TREATMENT OF SPECIFIC MANIFESTATIONS

Constitutional Symptoms

Many patients present with vague nonspecific constitutional symptoms. Malaise and decreased exercise

TABLE 1 Components of RNP Particles Recognized by Anti-U1 RNP and Anti-Sm Antibodies

Antibody	RNA	Polypeptides*
Anti-U1 RNP, anti-Sm	U1	<u>68K</u>, <u>A</u>, B'/B, <u>C</u>, D, E-G
Anti-U2 RNP, anti-Sm	U2	<u>A'</u>, B'/B, <u>B''</u>, D, E-G
Anti-Sm	U4	<u>B'/B</u>, <u>D</u>, others
Anti-Sm	U5	<u>B'/B</u>, <u>D</u>, others
Anti-Sm	U6	<u>B'/B</u>, <u>D</u>, others

*The major autoantigenic polypeptides on each particle are underlined.

tolerance are common. Some patients have a low grade fever, and mixed connective tissue disease can present as a fever of unknown origin. There may be weight loss, headaches, hepatosplenomegaly, and arthralgias.

The treatment of these systemic symptoms depends on their severity. Many patients are helped by a sympathetic understanding of their disease and other supportive measures, including rest. At this stage of the illness it may be helpful for the physician to define some modifications in life style that allow the patient to cope with his illness. Low grade fever may be treated with aspirin or nonsteroidal anti-inflammatory drugs. The complication of hepatic toxicity often observed in patients with active systemic lupus erythematosus treated with aspirin also may occur in patients with mixed connective tissue disease. Profound fatigue, weight loss, and high fever may necessitate the judicious use of corticosteroids. For these indications, prednisone can be given in a low dosage of 5 to 20 mg daily and, by titrating the dosage against the patient's symptoms, may be tapered and discontinued relatively quickly. Not all patients tolerate alternate day corticosteroid therapy, but if it can be used successfully, the possibility of side effects is lessened.

Skin Involvement

Most patients have some skin involvement in mixed connective tissue disease. The spectrum of involvement is broad and includes changes seen in systemic lupus erythematosus, scleroderma, and dermatomyositis. Many patients have Raynaud's phenomenon in association with arthralgias and swelling of the hands. There may be skin thickening, sclerodactyly, and telangiectasias that are similar to the changes seen in scleroderma and the CREST syndrome. Also found are skin lesions commonly associated with systemic lupus erythematosus, such as erythematous malar rashes and discoid plaques. Alopecia, vitiligo, photosensitivity, and urticaria are also seen, as are nasal septal perforation, mouth ulcers, and the sicca complex. Less common are skin changes typical of dermatomyositis, such as heliotrope eyelids and periungual telangiectasias. Cutaneous nodules and erythema nodosum have been described.

Raynaud's phenomenon, which is common, often responds to such simple measures as avoiding cold exposure. For more severe symptoms, nifedipine, 20 to 60 mg daily in divided doses, often alleviates symptoms and may contribute to the healing of digital ischemic necrosis or ulceration. Nifedipine is usually well tolerated, although side effects such as dizziness and reflex tachycardia can be further minimized by beginning with a low dosage and increasing the intake as necessary. Some patients with digital ulcers have also been found to respond to captopril and more recently to enalapril given in low dosages. Raynaud's phenomenon, swelling of the hands, and sclerodactyly often are accompanied by discomfort that is decreased by nonsteroidal anti-inflammatory drugs.

For patients with skin manifestations that are more like those commonly seen in systemic lupus erythematosus such as malar rashes and discoid plaques, topical corticosteroid therapy can be helpful. A small group of patients with more diffuse skin lesions can be helped with oral corticosteroid therapy, usually given in low dosages. When lesions suggestive of systemic lupus erythematosus are encountered, treatment with hydroxychloroquine (Plaquenil) should be considered (see following section).

Joint Involvement

Almost all patients with mixed connective tissue disease have symptoms related to joints. These symptoms compose a spectrum ranging from vague migratory arthralgias with morning stiffness to erosive deforming arthritis. Fifty percent of the patients with mixed connective tissue disease have been reported to have rheumatoid factors, and in this group especially features consistent with rheumatoid arthritis may appear. Rheumatoid changes in the hands, such as the swan neck deformity and ulnar deviation, have been described as has arthritis mutilans.

In patients with milder joint involvement, aspirin and nonsteroidal anti-inflammatory drugs are appropriate. Some patients with more severe symptoms can be treated with hydroxychloroquine (Plaquenil), 200 to 400 mg daily. This drug may cause photosensitivity, and the patient should be made aware that he needs to limit sun exposure. A rare complication of therapy with hydroxychloroquine is retinal maculopathy. Since patients who develop hydroxychloroquine retinal toxicity typically develop funduscopic or visual field changes before they develop visual symptoms, it is recommended that patients being treated for long periods with hydroxychloroquine undergo periodic ophthalmologic examination while taking this medicine.

We have not regularly treated patients with mixed connective tissue disease with the remittive drugs such as gold and penicillamine used in the treatment of rheumatoid arthritis, even though these patients sometimes present with features suggesting rheumatoid arthritis. When one is confronted with disabling arthritis, the judicious use of corticosteroids seems appropriate for certain patients. If difficulty is encountered in tapering corticosteroid dosages and cushingoid features emerge, it may be appropriate to consider the use of azathioprine (Imuran), methotrexate, or cyclophosphamide as steroid sparing therapy; little information exists about the role of these drugs in mixed connective tissue disease.

Muscle Involvement

As already discussed, myalgia is a common constitutional symptom in mixed connective tissue disease, often associated with a generalized flare of disease. Another frequent feature of the disease is an inflammatory myositis clinically and pathologically identical to polymyositis. Patients may have proximal muscle weakness and elevations of the serum creatine phosphokinase and aldolase levels. Electromyograms demonstrate myopathic changes, and muscle biopsy shows fiber degeneration and perivascular and interstitial infiltrates identical to those seen in polymyositis.

When polymyositis occurs in mixed connective tissue disease, corticosteroids are the appropriate therapy. Required dosages are typically in the range of 40 to 60 mg of prednisone daily and should be given in divided doses. The dosage is titrated downward according to the clinical response, including both subjective improvement and objective testing (such as the number of times a patient can rise from a chair in the sitting position in 1 minute), and also by following serial determinations of serum muscle enzyme levels. Often it is necessary to treat patients with moderate to severe manifestations of polymyositis for a prolonged period, and over time the potential for iatrogenic corticosteroid myopathy increases as do other serious complications of corticosteroid administration.

Gastrointestinal Involvement

Esophageal dysmotility similar to that seen in scleroderma has been described in many patients with mixed connective tissue disease. It is frequently found on cine-esophagrams and does not always cause symptoms. Most commonly, if symptoms are present, patients complain of reflux esophagitis, with swallowing difficulty occurring less often. Involvement of the small bowel with dilation, malabsorption secondary to a bacterial overgrowth syndrome, and colonic hypomotility is less common.

Patients with symptomatic esophageal dysmotility are frequently benefited by metoclopramide (Reglan), 10 mg three times daily, to improve lower esophageal sphincter tone and peristaltic motility in the esophagus. Also helpful in the management of reflux esophagitis are the H_2 antagonists ranitidine (Zantac), 150 mg twice daily, and cimetidine (Tagamet), 300 mg three times daily.

Pulmonary Involvement

It is well recognized that the lung is frequently involved in mixed connective tissue disease. The most common pulmonary manifestation of the disease is pleurisy, which is sometimes accompanied by the development of pleural effusions. Also common is the finding of abnormalities on pulmonary function testing not always associated with clinical symptoms, which include decreased vital capacity and decreased carbon monoxide diffusion capacity. Chest x-ray views may show interstitial parenchymal disease, reticulonodular infiltrates, pleural effusions, and pleural thickening. Cardiomegaly, when present, may be secondary to pulmonary hypertension. Pulmonary hypertension may be present as the result of interstitial fibrosis or as a pulmonary vascular disorder with intimal proliferation and medial muscular hypertrophy in the pulmonary arterioles. This complication may be rapidly progressive and is difficult to treat; several fatal cases have been reported.

In some patients pleurisy is a self-limited problem that requires no specific treatment. With mild symptoms nonsteroidal anti-inflammatory drugs are often helpful in hastening the resolution of pleurisy and small pleural effusions. Corticosteroid therapy given as prednisone—20 to 60 mg daily—may be necessary in patients with more severe involvement. The ability to taper the prednisone dosage in this clinical setting varies considerably. In some patients pleuritic manifestations resolve promptly, and the prednisone dosage can be tapered over several weeks. For other patients this therapy may be a longer term commitment.

As with other forms of interstitial lung disease, the use of corticosteroids is advocated in patients with mixed connective tissue disease to shorten the period of involvement and to limit the development of interstitial fibrosis. Therapy is likely to be more successful in individuals with active inflammation, a feature that may be detected as measured for example by observing increased uptake of gallium in radionuclide scans.

The treatment of pulmonary hypertension resulting from primary increased vascular resistance is uncertain. Success has been reported with corticosteroids and cytotoxic drugs such as cyclophosphamide, and there may be a role for peripheral vasodilators such as hydralazine, nifedipine, or captopril. Often these patients are gravely ill and require care in an intensive care unit setting.

Cardiac Involvement

Cardiac involvement is less common than pulmonary involvement. The most common manifestation is acute pericarditis, sometimes associated with pericardial effusion. Myocarditis also occurs and when studied pathologically has been associated with perivascular and myocardial mononuclear cell infiltrates. Coronary artery hyperplasia and mitral valve prolapse were seen frequently in a recent series in which cardiovascular manifestations in mixed connective tissue disease were studied. Less common are conduction disturbances, including complete heart block and valvular heart disease. In children particularly, aortic insufficiency has been noted. Left and right sided heart failure may develop in response to systemic or pulmonary hypertension.

The treatment of pericarditis and pericardial effusion is similar to the treatment of pleurisy and pleural effusion. Some patients may be managed with nonsteroidal anti-inflammatory drugs. However, most patients with significant features of pericarditis and certainly those with large pericardial effusions require corticosteroid therapy. In most cases prednisone—20 to 60 mg daily in divided doses—is appropriate.

Myocarditis has been more common at autopsy than expected from clinical findings. In symptomatic patients with myocarditis, corticosteroids are usually indicated. The treatment of cardiac dysrhythmias, mitral valve prolapse, and valvular disease in mixed connective tissue disease is similar to the treatment of these disorders when they occur in other settings. In mixed connective tissue disease, as in scleroderma, digoxin should be used with caution since the conduction system may be more sensitive to its adverse effects. The treatment of patients with systemic hypertension and to a lesser extent pulmonary hypertension in mixed connective tissue disease often incorporates the use of angiotensin converting enzyme inhibitors such as captopril and enalapril. Occasionally other peripheral vasodilators such as nifedipine also may be useful.

Kidney Involvement

Most reports have emphasized that renal disease is less common and less severe in mixed connective tissue disease than in systemic lupus erythematosus. A number of patients have been described, however, with membranous glomerulonephritis. These patients often have responded to corticosteroids and in some cases azathioprine. They generally have not been treated with cyclophosphamide, which has been advocated in patients with more aggressive glomerular lesions. As already described, renal vascular hypertension occurs in mixed connective tissue disease as well as in scleroderma and is treated with aggressive antihypertensive therapy, often with captopril or enalopril.

Neurologic Involvement

Neurologic involvement is less commonly seen in mixed connective tissue disease than in systemic lupus erythematosus. As in scleroderma, trigeminal neuralgia has been reported. Also seen are a vascular headache syndrome similar to migraine headaches and occasionally aseptic meningitis. It has been suggested that aseptic meningitis occurs with unexpected frequency in patients with mixed connective tissue disease who are given ibuprofen and that this drug should be avoided, although we have not had this experience. Seizures, psychosis, peripheral neuropathy, and cerebrovascular accidents are uncommon in mixed connective tissue disease.

The treatment of these problems is similar to the treatment of these disorders in other settings. Patients with aseptic meningitis have responded well to corticosteroid therapy.

CONCLUSION

With few exceptions the treatment of the manifestations of mixed connective tissue disease as described in this article is similar to the treatment of these problems as they arise in other collagen vascular diseases. For many of the more severe manifestations of mixed connective tissue disease, such as deforming arthritis, interstitial pulmonary disease, pulmonary hypertension, myocarditis, and renal involvement, the therapeutic efficacy of corticosteroids and cytotoxic drugs is anecdotal and not supported by controlled clinical trials. However, in the settings described, many authorities agree that these drugs have a useful role. On the other hand, complications attributed to steroid therapy in the original 25 patients with mixed connective tissue disease reported by Sharp at 5 years of follow-up included aseptic necrosis of bone, osteoporosis, diabetes mellitus, and infection. Of these patients, eight died. In two cases death was unrelated to mixed connective tissue disease. Two deaths were attributed to progressive renal disease. In two patients complications of corticosteroid therapy, including infection and severe diabetes mellitus, contributed significantly to death. Finally, two patients died as a result of suicide. This complication is worth emphasizing in a disease for which medical treatment is often imperfect and supportive therapy important.

SUGGESTED READING

Bennett RM, O'Connell DJ. Mixed connective tissue disease: a clinical pathologic study of twenty cases. Semin Arthritis Rheum 1980; 10:25–51.

Nimelstein SH, Brody S, McShane D, Holman HR. Mixed connective tissue disease: a subsequent evaluation of the original 25 patients. Medicine 1980; 59:239–248.

Sharp GC, Irvin WS, May CM, Holman HR, McDuffie FC, Hess EV, Schmid FR. Association of antibody to ribonucleoprotein and Sm antigens with mixed connective tissue disease, systemic lupus erythematosus and other rheumatic diseases. N Engl J Med 1976; 295:1149–1154.

Sharp GC, Irvin WS, Tan EM, Gould RG, Holman HR. Mixed connective tissue disease—an apparently distinct rheumatic disease syndrome associated with a specific antibody to an extractable nuclear antigen (ENA). Am J Med 1972; 52:148–159.

Singsen BH, Bernstein BH, Kornreich HK, King KK, Hanson V, Tan EM. MCTD in childhood. J Pediatr 1977; 90:893–900.

Sullivan WD, Hurst DJ, Harmon CE, Esther JH, Agia GA, Maltby JD, Lillard SB, Held CN, Wolf JF, Sunderrajan EV, Maricq HR, Sharp GC. A prospective evaluation emphasizing pulmonary involvement in patients with mixed connective tissue disease. Medicine 1984; 92–107.

SYSTEMIC VASCULITIS

ANTHONY S. FAUCI, M.D.
RANDI Y. LEAVITT, M.D., Ph.D.

Vasculitis is a clincopathologic process characterized by an inflammatory response within the blood vessel. Associated with this inflammatory process is a compromise of the vessel lumen with resulting ischemic changes in the tissues that are supplied by the blood vessels in question. It is predominantly this ischemia that constitutes the vasculitic syndrome. Since any size, location, and type of blood vessel may be involved in the vasculitic process, and since virtually any organ system can be involved, the vasculitic syndromes comprise a heterogeneous category of diseases, some of which have unique and distinguishing characteristics and others of which manifest overlapping clinical and pathologic features. Before one can apply a therapeutic protocol to a patient with a vasculitic syndrome, it is essential to appreciate the need to categorize as well as possible the syndrome with which one is dealing, particularly with regard to the real and potential extent of organ system involvement.

CATEGORIZATION OF THE VASCULITIC SYNDROMES

On one hand, the remarkable heterogeneity as well as the obvious overlap among the vasculitic syndromes must be appreciated by the treating physician, but on the other hand, it should not deter one from implementing the most appropriate therapeutic regimen for the particular syndrome the patient displays, as well as for the particular features within a given syndrome that the patient is manifesting. In approaching the classification of the vasculitic syndromes from the standpoint of therapy, it is helpful to realize that the vasculitis may be the primary disease process without an existing underlying disease to which it might be secondary; may be a secondary component of another underlying disease; may not be life threatening and, for example, may be limited to the skin without major organ system involvement; or may involve vital organ systems, leading to either irreversible organ system dysfunction or death. The latter type is referred to as severe systemic vasculitis, the treatment of which is the subject of this article.

An updated classification scheme for the vasculitic syndromes is shown in Table 1. Apart from the category referred to as "hypersensitivity vasculitis," which is generally associated either with a recognized antigenic stimulus, such as an infection, or with ingestion of a

TABLE 1 Classification of the Vasculitic Syndromes

Systemic necrotizing vasculitis: involves multiple organ systems with potential for irreversible organ system dysfunction
  Systemic vasculitis of the polyarteritis nodosa group
    Classic polyarteritis nodosa
    Allergic angiitis and granulomatosis (Churg-Strauss disease)
    Polyangiitis overlap syndrome
  Wegener's granulomatosis
  Giant cell arteritides
    Cranial or temporal arteritis
    Takayasu's arteritis
  Hypersensitivity vasculitis with predominantly extracutaneous involvement
    Related to known antigenic stimulus, such as drug or infection
    Secondary to another underlying disease
      Associated with connective tissue disease, such as systemic lupus erythematosus, rheumatoid arthritis, or Sjögren's syndrome
      Associated with neoplasm or infection
      Associated with other underlying diseases
    Unknown origin
  Miscellaneous systemic vasculitic syndromes
    Behçet's disease
    Mucocutaneous lymph node syndrome (Kawasaki's disease)
Predominantly cutaneous vasculitis
  Hypersensitivity vasculitis with predominantly cutaneous involvement
    Related to known antigenic stimulus, such as drug or infection
    Secondary to another underlying disease (see above)
    Unknown origin

drug (particularly antibiotics such as penicillin and sulfa drugs), virtually all the other vasculitic syndromes are primary, i.e., unassociated with other underlying disease. In the latter groups, the major distinction to be made regarding therapy is whether the disease is potentially life threatening and deserves an aggressive therapeutic approach or whether it will be confined to the skin and will not extensively and seriously involve other organ systems. This brings one to the most fundamental aspect of the treatment of the vasculitic syndromes. The physician must use information based on experience reported in the literature (to be summarized), together with clinical judgment related to the individual patient, in implementing a therapeutic regimen commensurate with the real and potential seriousness of the syndrome.

THERAPEUTIC APPROACH TO THE VASCULITIC SYNDROMES

The following discussion is directed toward the vasculitic syndromes that are truly systemic, i.e., those that involve multiple organ systems with the potential for serious organ system dysfunction. The approach to vasculitic syndromes that are confined to the skin or that manifest only minimal or insignificant renal involvement will not be discussed.

When possible, the treating physician should proceed in an orderly fashion from the most conservative therapeutic approach to a more aggressive approach, which, by definition, is generally associated with more serious toxic side effects. However, under certain circumstances when dealing with vasculitic syndromes, such as Wegener's granulomatosis and severe polyarteritis nodosa, whose usually fulminant courses are well recognized, the physician should immediately institute the aggressive therapeutic approaches (as will be discussed) that are of proved efficacy in these syndromes, as opposed to first attempting more conservative approaches. The obvious reason for this is that irreversible organ system dysfunction may occur during the period, however short, that conservative therapy is attempted. In addition, it is important to manage aggressively the hypertension that is frequently associated with the systemic vasculitides; this is often facilitated by the successful treatment of the underlying vasculitis. In Takayasu's arteritis, surgical bypass of a stenosed renal artery is sometimes required to treat the renovascular hypertension.

The following is a stepwise approach to the vasculitic syndromes.

Vasculitis Potentially Associated with a Recognized Antigen Stimulus

A substantial proportion of vasculitic syndromes associated with recognized antigenic stimuli, such as an infection or drug ingestion, manifest predominantly cutaneous features. Under certain circumstances, however, systemic and multiple organ system involvement is seen. The initial approach to this type of systemic vasculitis is the same as that for the cutaneous manifestations: withdrawal of the drug or specific treatment for the underlying infection. Unlike the cutaneous syndromes, however, which generally require only symptomatic treatment, in these cases it might be necessary to administer a brief course of corticosteroids, particularly if organ system dysfunction, such as renal function impairment, is seen. The corticosteroid administered should be prednisone, 1 mg per kilogram of body weight per day in three divided doses for 3 to 5 days, followed by consolidation to a single morning dose for an additional 2 to 3 days, followed by daily tapering by 10 mg decrements down to a total daily dosage of 30 mg per day, at which point the daily tapering should be by 5 mg decrements over a 3 week period until the dose is completely discontinued at approximately 1 month. If the patient cannot tolerate this relatively rapid tapering schedule, one can convert to an alternate day regimen, to be described, with tapering of the dosage according to the individual response. If the vasculitic process proves not to be self-limiting and organ system dysfunction persists without improvement over this period, the corticosteroid should be administered in the regimen described in Table 2 under Prednisone Component. A small percentage of patients with vasculitis associated with a recognized stimulus develop a vasculitic syndrome indistinguishable from the severe systemic ne-

TABLE 2   Combined Cyclophosphamide-Prednisone Therapy for Severe Systemic Vasculitis*

Cyclophosphamide component: cyclophosphamide, 2 mg/kg per day orally; adjust dosage such that the leukocyte count remains above 3000–3500 per cubic mm (neutrophil count of 1000–1500 per cubic mm). Continue therapy with frequent downward adjustments of dosage so that severe neutropenia does not occur. Continue therapy for 1 year following induction of complete remission, at which point dose is tapered by 25 mg decrements every 2 months until discontinued.

Prednisone component: prednisone, 1 mg/kg per day in three to four divided doses for 7 to 10 days; consolidate to single morning dose by 2 to 3 weeks; continue single morning daily dose until 1 month of total corticosteroid treatment is reached. Convert to alternate day prednisone over the second month; maintain alternate day regimen over third month, followed by gradual tapering of alternate day dose over the next 3 to 6 months.

* Precise details of this regimen are given in the text. The cyclophosphamide and prednisone are begun simultaneously. For regimens that call for corticosteroids alone, the "prednisone component" of this protocol should be employed alone in the regimen indicated.

crotizing vasculitis group within which polyarteritis nodosa falls (see Table 1). Under these circumstances, the patient should be treated with the aggressive regimen described for that category (see Table 2).

Vasculitis Associated with Another Underlying Disease

Vasculitic syndromes may be a secondary manifestation of a recognized underlying disease, such as a connective tissue disease (rheumatoid arthritis, systemic lupus erythematosus, Sjögren's syndrome), an underlying neoplasm (particularly a lymphoproliferative disease), or an infection as already mentioned. Under these circumstances, the underlying disease should be specifically treated if possible, and if this is successful, the vasculitic syndrome usually resolves. If the vasculitis is confined predominantly to the skin, potential inciting antigens such as drugs are removed and therapy is primarily symptomatic. Since there is no consistently effective therapy for isolated cutaneous vasculitis, toxic regimens should be avoided. Occasionally short courses of corticosteroids are of benefit in this disorder. If the vasculitis involves multiple organ systems and does not resolve as the underlying disease is being treated, the approach should be similar to that already described, in which mild disease is treated with a brief course of corticosteroids and persistent or fulminant disease is treated more aggressively.

Primary Systemic or Multisystem Vasculitic Syndromes

An effective chemotherapeutic protocol for the severe systemic necrotizing vasculitides is a long term low dose therapy with a cytotoxic drug administered in combination with corticosteroids. The latter drug is given initially on a daily basis, with conversion to an alternate day regimen such that the patient is maintained on daily doses of the cytotoxic drug and alternate day corticosteroids. Clearly the cytotoxic drug of choice in these syndromes is cyclophosphamide, which is an alkylating agent, and the corticosteroid used most frequently is prednisone. The precise details for the initiation and modification of the cyclophosphamide-prednisone therapeutic protocol are outlined in Table 2. Certain systemic vasculitic syndromes can be successfully treated with just the prednisone component of the protocol. However, if rapid remission is not induced with prednisone alone and if organ system dysfunction progresses with this regimen, cyclophosphamide should be added. Furthermore, and most importantly, certain syndromes, such as Wegener's granulomatosis and fulminant systemic necrotizing vasculitis of the polyarteritis nodosa group (see Table 1), should be treated with the cyclophosphamide-prednisone combination from the beginning, since long term studies have now unequivocally demonstrated the superiority of the combination regimen over prednisone alone, particularly in the treatment of Wegener's granulomatosis.

Cyclophosphamide-Prednisone Combination

Cyclophosphamide should be administered in a dosage of 2 mg per kg of body weight per day orally. If the disease is rapidly fulminant, one can give 4 mg per kg per day for the first 2 to 3 days and then convert to the 2 mg per kg per day dosage. In individuals who cannot tolerate oral medications and in patients in whom there is a question of intestinal involvement with the vasculitic process, the drug should be administered intravenously; the intravenous dose is equivalent to the oral dose. The underlying strategy of cyclophosphamide therapy in patients with non-neoplastic diseases, such as systemic vasculitis, is to suppress the disease activity without lowering the peripheral leukocyte count below a level that would cause a significant host defense defect with regard to neutropenia. It is common experience that if the leukocyte count is maintained about 3000 to 3500 cells per cubic mm, which usually results in a neutrophil count of 1000 to 1500 cells per cubic mm, patients rarely, if ever, develop opportunistic infections provided they do not have a host defense defect for another reason, such as the administration of daily corticosteroid therapy. As is to be discussed, this is one of the major reasons for the use of alternate day prednisone in combination with cyclophosphamide. For reasons that are still unclear, the disease activity of the vasculitic syndromes is almost invariably suppressed prior to the point when the leukocyte count drops below the level of 3000 to 3500 per cubic mm. Given this observation, together with the fact that cytotoxic drug induced neutropenia is associated with a significant incidence of infectious disease complications, particularly with gram

negative opportunistic infections, it is extremely important that the physician carefully monitor the leukocyte count and adjust the dosage frequently, if necessary, to maintain the count in the "safe" level. In this regard, it should be remembered that there is generally a lag of several days from a given dose to the time when the full effect on the leukocyte count is seen. In adjusting the dosage, the physician should be aware of the slope of the decline in leukocyte count as well as the absolute count so as to better guide the precise timing of the adjustment in dosage.

Daily cyclophosphamide should be continued with the frequent adjustments of dosage as already indicated for 6 months to 1 year from the time that it is believed that the patient has achieved a complete remission. When this point has been reached, the cyclophosphamide should be tapered by 25 mg decrements every 1 to 2 months until the drug has been discontinued. If flares of disease activity occur, the drug should be increased to 25 mg per day above the dosage that had been maintaining the remission. This dosage should be maintained for an additional 3 to 6 months, depending on the extent and severity of the relapse, and attempts at tapering should again be instituted as already indicated. Although there is a good deal of variability among patients with various systemic vasculitic diseases as well as among patients with a given vasculitic syndrome, it has been our experience that patients with Wegener's granulomatosis clearly require the full year of therapy following the induction of complete remission to avoid relapse. Despite the fact that the cyclophosphamide-prednisone therapeutic protocol has induced remissions in more than 90 percent of the patients with Wegener's granulomatosis, there is a substantial incidence of mild relapse if the drug is withdrawn too soon following induction of remission.

Prednisone therapy should be instituted together with the cyclophosphamide protocol, which is described herein, in the treatment of severe systemic vasculitis. The combination has proved to be quite effective, and mechanistically it is essential for prednisone to be included in the induction-of-remission protocol, since its anti-inflammatory and immunosuppressive effects are realized almost immediately, whereas cyclophosphamide in the dosage given takes 10 days to 3 weeks before producing significant immunosuppression. Therefore, the corticosteroid serves as an essential component of the early induction and can be withdrawn as the cyclophosphamide maintains the remission (as will be discussed).

Prednisone is given in a dosage of 1 mg per kg per day in divided doses for 7 to 10 days, with consolidation to a single morning dose by 2 to 3 weeks. This daily dosage is continued for an additional week, for the total daily corticosteroid regimen of 3 to 4 weeks. Over the second month of therapy, the prednisone is gradually converted to an alternate day regimen by decreasing the dose on the ultimate "off" day by 10 mg every one to two alternate day cycles. For example, on alternate days the patient is given 60 mg, 50 mg, 60 mg, 40 mg, 60 mg, and 30 mg. When 30 mg is reached on the "low" day, the tapering is changed to 5 mg decrements, that is, 60 mg, 30 mg, 60 mg, 25 mg, 60 mg, 20 mg, and so on. This is continued until the low dose is 10 mg, at which point the low day dose is tapered by 2.5 mg until the patient is receiving 60 mg alternatively with 0 mg, i.e., an alternate day regimen. The entire conversion to an alternate day regimen usually takes approximately 1 month, for a total corticosteroid treatment time of 2 months. Over the next (third) month the patient is maintained on 60 mg of prednisone on alternate days.

Hence, during the first 2 months of induction with cyclophosphamide, the patient receives 1 month of daily corticosteroid therapy to provide induction and 1 month of "modified daily" corticosteroid therapy over the period of time that the cyclophosphamide has achieved substantial immunosuppression. At the end of 2 months, the patient is receiving a true alternate day prednisone regimen with its significantly decreased incidence of opportunistic infections as well as other corticosteroid side effects (as will be discussed), which makes the synergistic host defense defect of corticosteroid and cyclophosphamide much less of a problem. Following this initial 3 month period of daily corticosteroid administration converted to alternate day therapy, the prednisone dosage is gradually tapered over 3 to 6 months until the drug is discontinued and the patient is receiving cyclophosphamide alone.

It is important to emphasize that during periods of corticosteroid tapering, the leukocyte count may decrease, necessitating appropriate reductions in cyclophosphamide dosage. As already mentioned, the cyclophosphamide should be continued for 6 months to preferably 1 year following the induction of complete remission. Since complete remission induction often takes several months, the total duration of therapy is usually about 2 years for patients with diseases such as Wegener's granulomatosis and somewhat less for others with the severe systemic necrotizing vasculitides.

The plan just delineated should be followed fairly strictly with regard to the induction phase. Once induction has been achieved, however, the precise timing of the tapering schedule should remain flexible and adjustments made according to the individual patient's response. For example, certain patients, although in complete remission, require much slower tapering of the alternate day prednisone, to the extent that it is difficult to get them off the final 10 to 20 mg every other day. Under these circumstances, one should merely be patient and continually attempt to taper the dose to the lowest possible level. Ultimately, virtually all patients who have achieved remission will be able to have their immunosuppressive regimen discontinued, or at least tapered to an extremely low dose regimen that maintains remission without causing serious side effects.

The capacity of the myeloid elements of the bone marrow to tolerate cyclophosphamide during induction and maintenance of remissions varies greatly from patient to patient and appears to be less in older patients.

We have noticed in a few patients that neutropenia occurs sooner than expected; the patients may not yet have achieved remission, but the cyclophosphamide dose must be lowered owing to neutropenia. In these patients we increase the dose of alternate day prednisone or reinstitute alternate day prednisone if it had already been discontinued. This usually results in a significant marrow sparing effect such that a higher dose of cyclophosphamide then can be given without serious neutropenia.

Other Cytotoxic Drugs

Other cytotoxic drugs, such as azathioprine (purine analogue) and chlorambucil (alkylating agent), have been used in the vasculitic syndromes. Most studies, however, indicate that they are inferior to cyclophosphamide in the treatment of the vasculitic syndromes, particularly Wegener's granulomatosis. Nonetheless, one must remember that the real and potential toxic side effects and complications of cyclophosphamide therapy are substantial (as will be discussed), and this must be taken into account when one embarks upon such a therapeutic protocol. We have used alternative cytotoxic drugs, particularly azathioprine, in situations in which cyclophosphamide could not be used, as in patients who developed severe cystitis and who still needed longer treatment with a cytotoxic drug or patients who could not accept the almost invariable gonadal dysfunction associated with chronic cyclophosphamide therapy. The dosage of azathioprine is 2 mg per kg per day, with the same adjustments being made for leukopenia as indicated for cyclophosphamide. We have found that although azathioprine is clearly not as effective as cyclophosphamide in the induction of remission in the vasculitic syndromes, it can be quite useful in the maintenance of remission in someone whose disease has been put into remission by cyclophosphamide but who cannot tolerate the drug for an additional period of required therapy.

Chlorambucil has been used in the therapy of Wegener's granulomatosis but is somewhat less effective than cyclophosphamide, especially in patients with renal disease.

A few reports have indicated that methotrexate can be effective in the vasculitic syndromes, but the experience is not extensive.

Bolus Corticosteroid and Bolus Cyclophosphamide

Bolus corticosteroid administration in the form of 1 g of methylprednisolone intravenously for 1 to 3 consecutive days has been attempted in certain inflammatory and immune mediated diseases, including the vasculitic syndromes. Since controlled studies have not been performed, it is difficult to establish the efficacy of this regimen. Initial reports indicate that such an approach may be beneficial in patients with systemic lupus erythematosus with acutely deteriorating renal function and in patients with rapidly progressive glomerulonephritis. We have occasionally used a 1 g intravenous bolus of methylprednisolone during the first few days of the induction phase of therapy in patients with fulminant vasculitis while implementing the cyclophosphamide-prednisone protocol already described; the efficacy of this approach is not established. Nonetheless, since the side effects of 1 to 3 days of bolus corticosteroid administration are minimal, it is not unreasonable to employ this regimen during the first few days of treatment of life-threatening fulminant vasculitis.

Bolus cyclophosphamide in a dosage of 0.5 to 0.75 g per square meter of body surface has been employed with and without plasmapheresis in certain inflammatory diseases. It is currently being subjected to clinical trials in cases of systemic lupus erythematosus. It has not been used in controlled trials for the vasculitic syndromes, and our experience has been that bolus intravenous cyclophosphamide therapy is ineffective in inducing remissions in the vasculitic syndromes, which seem to require significant periods of prolonged low dose therapy. It is not known, however, whether the intravenous bolus approach would be effective on an intermittent basis to maintain a remission that has been induced by the standard regimens.

Plasmapheresis and Lymphoplasmapheresis

At the present time it is unclear whether plasmapheresis or lymphoplasmapheresis will have a useful role in the treatment of the systemic vasculitic syndromes. In general, this approach has not been effective in inducing and maintaining remissions in the severe vasculitic syndromes in the few uncontrolled reports that are available. However, we have noted several patients with severe systemic vasculitis associated with Sjögren's syndrome who have responded dramatically to plasmapheresis with or without concomitant bolus cyclophosphamide. We have employed daily 3 liter plasma exchanges for 1 to 2 weeks followed by alternate day exchanges for variable periods of time (up to a few weeks). This approach is currently being further evaluated in the vasculitis of Sjögren's syndrome and the severe vasculitis that can be seen with rheumatoid arthritis. However, plasmapheresis can be used in addition to corticosteroids and cyclophosphamide in patients with fulminant vasculitis.

Cyclosporin A

Cyclosporin A, a cyclic endecapeptide, is an effective immunosuppressive drug used in patients undergoing renal transplantation. It primarily affects T lymphocyte function and has been documented to inhibit the production of interleukin 2 in T cells. Cyclosporin A has been reported to be effective in certain patients with vasculitis, but the data are preliminary and no follow-up data are available.

Miscellaneous Therapy

A number of miscellaneous therapeutic approaches have been tried in patients with vasculitic syndromes, including dapsone, antihistamines, and indomethacin, and these are usually applicable to patients with isolated or predominant cutaneous disease.

In patients who have experienced end stage renal failure and in whom the disease activity has been subsequently suppressed, renal transplantation has proved to be an eminently feasible and successful modality of treatment for vasculitic syndromes, particularly Wegener's granulomatosis. Recurrence of disease in the graft, although it may occasionally occur, does not represent a contraindication to transplantation.

It should be mentioned that nonspecific symptoms of inflammation, such as joint manifestations, generally respond to nonsteroidal anti-inflammatory drugs, such as aspirin, 600 mg every 6 hours, or ibuprofen, 300 mg every 6 hours. However, these drugs should never be substituted for the immunosuppressive regimens described, since nonsteroidal anti-inflammatory drugs are not effective in treating the vasculitic components of the severe systemic vasculitic syndromes. The only clear exception to this appears to be the treatment of the mucocutaneous lymph node syndrome (Kawasaki's disease), in which corticosteroid therapy has been reported to result in an increased incidence of coronary artery aneurysm; aspirin therapy alone remains the treatment of choice at present.

It has been reported that several patients with Wegener's granulomatosis have responded to therapy with trimethoprim-sulfa. These reports are intriguing but anecdotal, and more data certainly need to be accumulated regarding the efficacy of trimethoprim-sulfa in the treatment of this disease before any conclusions can be drawn.

TOXIC SIDE EFFECTS AND COMPLICATIONS OF THERAPY

As discussed, the two mainstays of therapy for the severe systemic necrotizing vasculitides are corticosteroids and cytotoxic drugs, particularly cyclophosphamide. Although these drugs are effective in inducing and maintaining remissions in most of the systemic vasculitides, both are associated with significant toxic side effects (Table 3). It is essential for the physician to be aware of these side effects and to follow a regimen that will, when possible, minimize their occurrence.

TABLE 3   Complications of Corticosteroid and Long Term Cyclophosphamide Therapy

Corticosteroid Therapy:

Central nervous system
- Pseudotumor cerebri
- Psychiatric disorders

Musculoskeletal
- Osteoporosis with spontaneous fractures
- Aseptic necrosis of bone
- Myopathy

Ocular
- Glaucoma
- Cataracts

Gastrointestinal
- Peptic ulceration
- Intestinal perforation
- Pancreatitis

Cardiovascular and fluid balance
- Hypertension
- Sodium and fluid retention
- Hypokalemic alkalosis

Hypersensitivity reactions
- Urticaria
- Anaphylaxis

Endocrinologic
- Suppression of hypothalamic-pituitary-adrenal axis
- Growth failure
- Secondary amenorrhea

Metabolic
- Hyperglycemia and unmasking of genetic predisposition to diabetes mellitus
- Nonketotic hyperosmolar states
- Hyperlipidemia
- Alterations of fat distribution (typical cushingoid appearance)
- Fatty infiltration of liver
- Drug interactions (decreased anticoagulant effect of ethyl biscoumacetate)

Fibroblast inhibition
- Inhibition of wound healing
- Subcutaneous tissue atrophy (striae, purpura, ecchymosis)
- Suppression of host defenses
  - Immunosuppression, anergy
  - Effects on phagocyte kinetics and function
  - Increased incidence of infections

Chronic Cyclophosphamide Therapy:
- Marrow suppression—particularly neutropenia with resulting secondary infection
- Hemorrhagic cystitis
- Gonadal dysfunction
- Alopecia
- Oncogenesis

There is no question that most, if not all, of the side effects of daily corticosteroid therapy can be significantly minimized and in some cases avoided (as with infectious disease complications) if an alternate day regimen is employed as soon as feasible following induction of remission with daily corticosteroid therapy as already indicated. Certain of the toxic side effects of cyclophosphamide can also be avoided to some extent, although some are completely unavoidable. The toxic side effect that can best be controlled by physician awareness is severe leukopenia, which is avoided by careful monitoring of the leukocyte count and consequent adjustment of dosage as already detailed.

Avoidance of significant leukopenia together with the use of alternate day as opposed to daily corticosteroid therapy has resulted in virtually no increase in the incidence of opportunistic bacterial or fungal infections in patients with vasculitis treated with this regimen. However, we have noted an increased incidence of cutaneous herpes zoster infections in patients treated with cyclophosphamide, which was not related to leukopenia. The zoster never viscerally disseminated and did not require significant modification of the cyclophosphamide regimen. Careful attention to adequate hydration has been thought to lessen the incidence of hemorrhagic cystitis due to cyclophosphamide; however, the incidence of this complication is still disturbingly high. Both pulmonary and bladder fibrosis have been reported. Oncogenesis does not seem to occur as frequently as in patients who develop a second tumor following treatment of the original tumor with high dose cyclophosphamide, and this complication in patients who are treated with the long term low dose cyclophosphamide regimen outlined is surely rare. However, cases of leukemia, lymphoma, and bladder carcinoma following cyclophosphamide therapy for vasculitis have been reported, and this possibility should be recognized.

Gonadal dysfunction and sterility are serious and frequent problems in younger individuals treated with cyclophosphamide. Over the past few years, semen has been stored in sperm banks for male patients prior to the institution of cyclophosphamide therapy, and we have been administering birth control pills to women of childbearing age who wish to procreate after discontinuation of therapy. The latter approach is based on recent reports that suppression of cyclic ovarian function during therapy may protect the ovaries from the sterilizing effects of the drug. However, there are not sufficient data at present to determine the efficacy of this approach.

SUGGESTED READING

Cohen DJ, Loertscher R, Rubin MF, Tilney NL, Carpenter CB, Strom TB. Cyclosporin: a new immunosuppressive agent for organ transplantation. Ann Intern Med 1984; 101:667–682.
Fauci AS. Cytotoxic and other immunoregulatory agents. In: Kelly

WN, Harris ED Jr, Ruddy S, Sledge CB, eds. Textbook of rheumatology. Philadelphia: WB Saunders, 1985: 833–857.
Fauci AS, Dale DC, Balow JE. Glucocorticosteroid therapy: mechanisms of action and clinical considerations. Ann Intern Med 1976; 84:304–315.
Fauci AS, Haynes BF, Katz P. The spectrum of vasculitis: clinical,

pathologic, immunologic, and therapeutic considerations. Ann Intern Med 1978; 89:660–676.
Fauci AS, Haynes BF, Katz P, Wolff SM. Wegener's granulomatosis: prospective clinical and therapeutic experience with 85 patients for 21 years. Ann Intern Med 1983; 98:76–85.

CUTANEOUS VASCULITIS

NICHOLAS A. SOTER, M.D.

Clinical disorders designated as necrotizing vasculitis combine segmental inflammation with fibrinoid necrosis of the blood vessels. The vascular damage may involve inflammatory or immunologic mechanisms. Clinical syndromes are based on criteria that include the gross appearance and histologic alterations of the vascular lesions, the caliber of the affected blood vessels, the frequency of involvement of specific organs, and the presence of hematologic, serologic, and immunologic abnormalities. Necrotizing vasculitis is frequently visually recognized in the skin, involves predominantly venules, and is known as cutaneous necrotizing venulitis. This cutaneous form of vasculitis also has been called leukocytoclastic vasculitis because of the histologic features of an infiltrate of neutrophils with fragmentation of nuclei known as leukocytoclasis or karyorrhexis.

CLINICAL FEATURES

The signature skin lesions of cutaneous necrotizing venulitis are erythematous papules that do not blanch when the skin is pressed and are known as palpable purpura. The vascular lesions are polymorphous, however, and also may consist of papules, urticaria-angioedema, pustules, vesicles, ulcers, necrosis, and livedo reticularis. Subcutaneous edema may occur in association with the dermal lesions. The eruption most often appears on the lower extremities or over dependent areas, such as the back and gluteal regions. Although the vascular lesions may occur anywhere on the integument, they are uncommon on the face, palm, soles, and mucous membranes.

The cutaneous lesions occur in episodes that may recur over weeks to years. Palpable purpura persists for 1 to 4 weeks and usually resolves leaving hyperpigmentation or atrophic scars. Lesional symptoms include

pruritus or burning and less commonly pain. An episode of cutaneous vascular lesions may be attended by fever, malaise, arthralgias, or myalgias. Coexistent systemic involvement of the small blood vessels most commonly occurs in joints, the gastrointestinal tract, muscles, peripheral nerves, and the kidneys and has been designated as hypersensitivity angiitis.

Cutaneous necrotizing venulitis may occur in association with an underlying chronic disease, may be precipitated by infections or drugs, or may develop for unknown reasons (Table 1). This form of vasculitis has been associated with a variety of collagen-vascular diseases, notably rheumatoid arthritis, Sjögren's syndrome, and systemic lupus erythematosus. Other disorders associated with cutaneous necrotizing venulitis include hypergammaglobulinemic purpura, certain lymphoproliferative disorders, cryoglobulinemia, inflammatory bowel disease, and cystic fibrosis.

Cutaneous necrotizing venulitis also can be precipitated by certain infections and drugs. Recognized infectious agents include hepatitis B virus, group A

TABLE 1   Cutaneous Necrotizing Venulitis

Coexistent chronic disorders
  Rheumatoid arthritis
  Sjögren's syndrome
  Systemic lupus erythematosus
  Hypergammaglobulinemic purpura
  Lymphoproliferative disorders
  Cryoglobulinemia
  Ulcerative colitis
  Cystic fibrosis
Recent precipitating events
  Certain bacterial and viral infections
  Drug induced reactions
Idiopathic disorders
  Henoch-Schönlein syndrome
  Chronic urticaria and/or angioedema and variants
  Erythema elevatum diutinum
  Nodular vasculitis
  Livedoid vasculitis
  Inherited C2 deficiency
  Idiopathic

hemolytic streptococci, and *Staphylococcus aureus*. Various forms of cutaneous vasculitis have been reported with a variety of viruses, *Mycobacterium tuberculosis*, and *Mycobacterium leprae*. In perhaps 50 percent of the patients the cause of cutaneous necrotizing venulitis remains unknown. The Henoch-Schönlein syndrome is the most widely recognized idiopathic disorder.

DISTINCTIVE FORMS OF CUTANEOUS VASCULITIS

Episodes of recurrent (chronic) urticaria or angioedema are an uncommon but important clinical manifestation of necrotizing venulitis. This edematous form occurs in patients with serum sickness, certain collagen-vascular disorders, physical urticaria, infections, and as an idiopathic condition. In the idiopathic group the variety of skin lesions and systemic manifestations has led to a plethora of diagnostic appellations, such as urticarial vasculitis, atypical erythema multiforme, systemic lupus erythematosus-like syndrome, hypocomplementemic vasculitis, and hypocomplementemic urticaria-vasculitis syndrome.

The skin lesions appear as erythematous, occasionally indurated, circumscribed areas of edema (wheals). Other skin manifestations include angioedema, macular erythema, foci of purpura in the wheals, livedo reticularis, nodules, and bullae. The individual urticarial lesions often last fewer than 24 hours but may last up to 3 to 5 days; this long lasting nature of the wheals is an important clinical feature. The lesions are pruritic or possess a burning quality. The episodes of urticaria range in duration from months to years and vary in frequency. General features include fever, malaise, enlargement of the lymph nodes, liver, and spleen, myalgia, and notably arthralgias. The upper airway may be affected, with the danger of death from laryngeal edema. Chronic obstructive pulmonary manifestations may develop that are more severe in individuals who smoke cigarettes. Conjunctivitis, episcleritis, and uveitis are noted in some individuals. Central nervous system involvement occurs as headaches and pseudotumor cerebri (benign intracranial hypertension).

Erythema elevatum diutinum presents as indolent erythematous plaques predominantly disposed over joints and the gluteal area that may be accompanied by arthralgias. Systemic manifestations are absent.

Nodular vasculitis occurs as painful red nodules over the lower extremities, especially the calves, without systemic manifestations. This disorder is more common in females; recurrent episodes with ulceration are common. Erythema induratum, which was associated with tuberculosis in the past, probably represents a form of nodular vasculitis.

Livedoid vasculitis occurs in women as recurrent painful ulcers of the lower extremities in association with livedo reticularis of a persistent nature. Many patients experience arteriosclerosis or stasis of the lower extremities. Healing results in sclerotic pale areas surrounded by telangiectases called atrophie blanche. Livedoid vasculitis is especially prominent in patients with systemic lupus erythematosus and central nervous system involvement. Atrophie blanche, however, probably represents the end stage of a variety of forms of vascular damage in the skin.

Inherited deficiency of the second complement protein (C2) has been noted in some patients with cutaneous necrotizing venulitis.

LABORATORY FINDINGS

An elevated erythrocyte sedimentation rate is the most frequent abnormal laboratory finding in patients with cutaneous necrotizing venulitis. The platelet count usually is normal. Other abnormalities reflect either a coexistent underlying disorder or the involvement of additional organ systems. The serum complement system is usually normal. Acquired hypocomplementemia may develop in patients with concomitant collagen-vascular diseases or cryoglobulinemia. In these instances the complement abnormalities reflect the features of the associated disease or the immunoglobulin content of the cryoglobulin. Hypocomplementemia also occurs in some patients with idiopathic cutaneous necrotizing venulitis. Patients should be evaluated for the extent of internal organ involvement, the presence of coexistent disorders associated with cutaneous vasculitis, and any precipitating causes.

THERAPEUTIC APPROACH

When the eruption is associated with a defined precipitating event, withdrawal of the medication or treatment of the infection results in resolution of the cutaneous lesions. If a coexistent chronic disorder is present, treatment of the underlying disease may be associated with improvement of the skin lesions.

H_1 antihistamines may be used to alleviate cutaneous lesional pruritus and burning sensations in patients with various forms of cutaneous necrotizing venulitis, but there are no controlled studies to indicate that any of these drugs influences the natural history of the disease. The addition of an H_2 antihistamine also has not been the subject of controlled studies in this disorder. The administration of colchicine, dapsone, corticosteroid preparations, nonsteroidal anti-inflammatory drugs, and various immunosuppressive drugs has been reported to be of benefit in small numbers of patients, but controlled clinical trials still are not available. The topical application of medicaments is not of value; however, cutaneous ulcers are generally managed by local measures.

In urticarial vasculitis, H_1 antihistamines alone or in combination with H_2 antihistamines may be administered to alleviate the pruritus. Both skin and joint manifestations may respond to indomethacin or other nonsteroidal anti-inflammatory drugs. The oral administration of corticosteroids may relieve the urticaria, uveitis, episcleritis, abdominal pain, arthritis, and renal disease. Colchicine, hydroxychloroquine, dapsone, and cyclophosphamide have been used in uncontrolled patient reports.

In patients with erythema elevatum diutinum, the administration of dapsone is effective and is the drug of choice. The treatment of nodular vasculitis consists of therapeutic trials of indomethacin and dipyridamole, a saturated solution of potassium iodide (SSKI), colchicine, intralesional corticosteroid therapy, dapsone, and prednisone. The treatment of livedoid vasculitis consists of therapeutic trials of anticoagulants, corticosteroids, nicotinic acid, low molecular weight dextran, colchicine, aspirin, dipyridamole, phenphormin, and ethylestranol.

SUGGESTED READING

Cupps TR, et al. Chronic recurrent small-vessel cutaneous vasculitis: clinical experience in 13 patients. JAMA 1982; 247:1994–1998.
Fauci AS, et al. The spectrum of vasculitis: clinical, pathologic, immunologic, and therapeutic considerations. Ann Intern Med 1978; 89:660–676.
Monroe EW. Urticarial vasculitis: an updated review. J Am Acad Dermatol 1981; 5:88–95.
Wolff K, Winkelmann RK, eds. Vasculitis. London: Lloyd-Luke, 1980.

TEMPORAL ARTERITIS

THOMAS R. CUPPS, M.D.

Temporal arteritis is a systemic panarteritis predominantly affecting elderly individuals. Although any medium or large sized muscular artery may be involved, the majority of clinical signs and symptoms result from vasculitis in the distribution of the cranial arteries. The terms cranial arteritis and giant cell arteritis are also used to describe this syndrome. Because this disease may present with a relatively nonspecific pattern, a high index of suspicion for the diagnosis of temporal arteritis should be maintained in evaluating elderly individuals with poorly characterized complaints.

The more common initial manifestations of temporal arteritis include, in descending order of frequency, headache, polymyalgia rheumatica (aching and morning stiffness of the proximal extremities, neck, and torso), fever, visual symptoms, and malaise. Less common presentations include myalgia, tenderness over the cranial arteries, jaw or tongue claudication, weight loss, and sore throat. The common laboratory findings include an abnormal erythrocyte sedimentation rate, marked elevations being characteristic. Elevations of other acute phase reactants (a_2 globulin, C reactive protein, and fibrinogen) have been reported. Other findings seen in some patients include a mild normochromic normocytic anemia with a chronic disease pattern and a mildly elevated alkaline phosphatase level.

The diagnosis is generally established by finding the characteristic pattern of panarteritis in a temporal artery biopsy specimen. The inflammatory infiltrate consists of mononuclear cells, polymorphonuclear leukocytes, and eosinophils. The major site of involvement is the media, with smooth muscle necrosis and interruption of the internal elastic membrane. Giant cells are present to varying degrees and may be relatively rare. Because of the segmental nature of the arterial inflammation, systematic evaluation of the biopsy specimen with multiple step sections increases the diagnostic yield.

THERAPY

General Considerations

Corticosteroids are the mainstay of therapy in patients with temporal arteritis. Although this group of drugs is not curative, appropriate use of corticosteroids generally suppresses the signs and symptoms of inflammation and prevents associated vascular complications. In most patients temporal arteritis is a self-limited disease with an average duration of 1 to 2 years. Although fluctuations of disease activity are commonly seen during the course of temporal arteritis, eventually the inflammatory process subsides. A subset of patients, however, may develop a more chronic process with well documented exacerbations years after the initial presentation of the disease. The therapeutic goal in the treatment of temporal arteritis is to suppress the signs and symptoms of inflammation and prevent vascular complications, particularly ischemia of the eye.

Because of the potential for adverse side effects of long term corticosteroid therapy in the elderly population affected by temporal arteritis, a systematic effort to minimize the morbidity associated with the use of this therapeutic agent is required. The potential for corticosteroid associated morbidity is related to the frequency, total dosage, and duration of therapy with this drug. Although general guidelines for the use of corticosteroids in temporal arteritis are reviewed in this article, the minimal effective corticosteroid dosage varies from patient to patient and must be established on an individual basis. The minimal effective dosage also may vary throughout the course of the disease. As disease activity decreases, the corticosteroid dosage should be adjusted accordingly, and when the condition resolves, the drug should be discontinued.

Corticosteroid Therapy Efficacy

Most patients with temporal arteritis respond dramatically to corticosteroid therapy. Within days, systemic symptoms of fever, malaise, and musculoskeletal pain begin to resolve. Focal complications of vascular disease, such as claudication, headache, or scalp tenderness, also respond. The efficacy of corticosteroid therapy in preventing blindness is well established. It should be emphasized that ischemic loss of vision, once it occurs, is frequently irreversible. Ischemia of one eye in temporal arteritis increases the risk of similar involvement in the other eye. In most cases clinical signs or symptoms of impending ocular involvement precede ischemic loss of vision by a variable period of time. In a clinical setting consistent with the diagnosis of temporal arteritis, the presence of ocular symptoms is an indication that appropriate therapy should be initiated immediately. With the exception of the ischemic loss of vision, the prognosis in temporal arteritis treated with corticosteroids is excellent. Most patients achieve complete remission and eventually can be tapered off the drug.

Induction

Once the diagnosis of temporal arteritis is made, corticosteroid therapy should be expeditiously initiated. Generally treatment is started with a dosage of 40 to 60 mg (1 mg per kg) of prednisone per day. In the absence of eye symptoms, ischemia, or severe constitutional symptoms, the prednisone therapy can be started as a single morning dose. In the presence of severe constitutional symptoms or continuing ischemia, more aggressive corticosteroid therapy is warranted. Splitting the prednisone regimen to 20 mg doses given three or four times per day increases the overall corticosteroid effect. In the setting of new onset (within 24 to 36 hours) or progressive loss of visual acuity despite use of the standard therapeutic regimen, ultrahigh dosages of corticosteroids (500 to 1,000 mg of methylprednisolone)

have been used by some investigators. An aggressive induction regimen of 1,000 mg of intravenous pulse methylprednisolone therapy every 12 hours for 5 days (followed by standard high dose oral prednisone therapy) has been used to successfully treat ocular ischemia and impaired vision that developed during treatment with the more standard pharmacologic doses of corticosteroids. Although experience with ultrahigh doses of corticosteroids in temporal arteritis remains limited, a trial of high dose pulse intravenous methylprednisolone therapy should be considered in patients with new onset or progressive ocular ischemia.

In patients started on split doses of corticosteroids, the consolidation to a single daily dose should be initiated 10 to 14 days after the start of therapy. In most of these patients the consolidation to a single daily morning dose is complete in 2 additional weeks. An example of such a consolidation would be as follows: taper from 20 mg of prednisone four times a day to 40 mg of prednisone twice a day for 3 days, 60 mg in the morning and 20 mg in the evening for 3 days, 70 mg in the morning and 10 mg in the evening for 3 days, 80 mg in the morning for 3 days followed by tapering to 60 mg as a single dose in the morning. It should be emphasized that alternate day corticosteroid therapy is not effective in inducing remissions in patients with temporal arteritis. The initial induction therapy for temporal arteritis (in the absence of ocular ischemia or altered vision) consists of 40 to 60 mg of prednisone a day for approximately 1 month.

Management

The majority of patients with temporal arteritis are in remission after the completion of the 1 month induction phase and a gradual tapering of the corticosteroids can be initiated. The corticosteroid dosage should be tapered gradually over months. The goal is to taper to the minimal dosage of the drug that maintains the remission. One of several approaches may be considered. Although alternate day prednisone is not effective during the induction phase of treatment, alternate day corticosteroid therapy effectively maintains the disease in remission following the initial induction phase. If the patient rapidly enters remission and does not have significant eye involvement, an attempt to taper the corticosteroid dosage to an alternate day regimen should be considered. The alternate day corticosteroid regimen incurs less drug associated morbidity than the daily regimens and is preferable if this therapeutic approach is effective in treating the disease.

The following approach is one example of a gradual tapering to an alternate day regimen. Starting at a dosage of 60 mg per day, drop 10 mg from the daily dosage given on alternate days, resulting in a schedule of 60 mg as a single morning dose alternating with 50 mg as a single morning dose. After 2 weeks, again drop the alternate day dose, resulting in a schedule of 60 mg alternating with 40 mg. Then 10 mg of prednisone is dropped from the low day dose every 2 weeks until a dosage of 60 mg alternating with 20 mg is established. At this point the tapering schedule is slowed to a reduction of 5 mg of prednisone from the low dose day every 2 weeks until a dosage of 60 mg alternating with 10 mg is obtained. Finally the alternate day low dose is reduced by 2.5 mg every 2 weeks until a schedule of 60 mg alternating with an "off" day is established. The alternate day high dose then may be gradually tapered. Not all patients tolerate tapering to an alternate day regimen. If the patient develops evidence of reactivation of the disease during this tapering, the dosage of prednisone should be increased back to a level that was effective in controlling the disease and tapering to a low dose daily regimen is initiated once the patient is back in remission.

Tapering to a low dose daily regimen should be done gradually also. The following is one example of such a prednisone taper. Starting from a single morning dose of 60 mg of prednisone, taper the dosage by 10 mg every 2 weeks until the patient is taking 40 mg a day. At this point the tapering schedule is slowed to lowering the dosage of prednisone by 5 mg every 2 weeks until a dosage of 20 mg a day is established. From 20 mg a day the prednisone dosage is tapered by 2.5 mg every 2 weeks until a maintenance dosage of 10 mg (or less) is obtained. It is important to emphasize that these suggested corticosteroid tapering schedules are examples and will undoubtedly require some modification when used in individual patients.

As the corticosteroid dosage is tapered, the clinician will need to follow the disease activity. Serial laboratory studies reflecting inflammation, such as the erythrocyte sedimentation rate or the C reactive protein determination, are very useful adjuncts in assessing disease activity. A follow-up sedimentation rate determination should be carried out after successful induction of remission to provide a baseline determination for comparison. One should remember that the sedimentation rate, although very sensitive, is also a nonspecific indicator of inflammation. Some variation in the follow-up determinations is to be expected, and processes other than temporal arteritis may affect the test results. It is important to emphasize the patient's clinical status in making the final assessment of the disease activity when regulating the corticosteroid dosage.

The optimal duration of therapy varies from case to case. As mentioned earlier, corticosteroids suppress the signs and symptoms of inflammation as the disease runs a self-limited course. Although selected patients may require only 6 months of corticosteroid therapy to put the temporal arteritis into sustained remission, in many patients the disease is reactivated with such a short course of therapy. The majority of patients are successfully treated with a 12 month course of corticosteroids. After completing a 1 year course of prednisone therapy, an attempt to taper the patient off corticosteroids should be initiated. The patient should be monitored closely as the maintenance dosage is gradually tapered and discontinued over several months. If evidence of recurrent disease activity develops, prednisone therapy should be restarted at a level known to control the signs and symptoms. Treatment for an additional year followed by a second attempt to taper and discontinue the prednisone should be considered. A small subset of patients may require even more prolonged therapy.

Morbidity

Prolonged daily corticosteroid therapy can have significant associated morbidity. The potential side effects of prolonged corticosteroid therapy are summarized in Table 1. Although the nature and extent of adverse side effects vary from individual to individual, higher dosages, increased frequency of administration, and prolonged therapy increase the likelihood of developing corticosteroid induced morbidity. To minimize the morbidity of this drug, the minimal effective dosage should be established for each individual. Limiting the patient's exposure to the corticosteroids decreases the likelihood of developing dose related side effects.

Prior to initiating corticosteroid therapy, the patient should have a baseline intermediate purified protein derivative (PPD) skin test together with a control anergy panel to evaluate for evidence of exposure to tuberculosis. The skin test can be carried out coincidentally with the initiation of corticosteroid therapy without markedly decreasing the diagnostic yield. A delay in the application of the skin test decreases the potential diagnostic return of this study because corticosteroid induced anergy develops. Because most patients with temporal arteritis are over the age of 60 years at the onset of the disease, most have some degree of osteoporosis when corticosteroid therapy is started. For this reason prophylactic therapy with calcium carbonate, 500 mg, on a three or four times daily schedule with vitamin D, 25,000 to 50,000 units twice weekly, is suggested. Because hypercalcemia or hypercalciuria may develop with this regimen, monitoring of the serum and urine calcium levels is advisable.

If high dose methylprednisolone infusion protocols

TABLE 1   Complications of Glucocorticosteroid Therapy

Altered mood	Hypokalemic alkalosis
Pseudotumor cerebri	Suppression of the hypothalamic-pituitary-adrenal axis
Osteoporosis	
Aseptic necrosis	Growth retardation
Proximal myopathy	Hyperglycemia
Cataracts	Weight gain
Glaucoma	Cushingoid habitus
Peptic ulceration	Striae
Hypertension	Purpura and ecchymosis
Fluid retention	Immunosuppression
	Opportunistic infection

are used, additional parameters should be evaluated. A number of sudden deaths have been reported in systemically ill patients in the postinfusion period. These deaths appear to be related to cardiac arrhythmias. A higher incidence of sudden death has been reported with rapid infusion of corticosteroids, particularly in patients with electrolyte abnormalities. During the infusion the patient may be at higher risk for developing bacteremia if an established localized infection is present. I have seen patients become bacteremic during the peri-infusion period as a result of low grade bladder infections. Finally patients with borderline or frank hypertension may develop hypertensive crises during the high dose methylprednisolone infusion protocol.

To avoid these potential complications, several precautions are suggested. Although there is some urgency in initiating corticosteroid therapy when visual symptoms are present in patients with temporal arteritis, the following parameters can be measured. While preparations are being made for the infusion, the blood pressure should be measured, baseline electrocardiography done, an electrolyte panel including a calcium and magnesium determination sent for analysis, and the urine examined for evidence of infection. If hypertension is present, appropriate therapy should be initiated. Any electrolyte abnormalities should be corrected. If there is evidence of infection, appropriate parenteral antibiotic coverage should be started. The corticosteroid should be infused slowly over a 30 to 60 minute period. The use of peripheral rather than deep central lines has also been suggested. If there is going to be any appreciable delay in safely starting the infusion, oral corticosteroid therapy should be started. When any existing problems have been addressed, the patient can then be switched to high dose infusion protocol if needed.

In the setting of continuing eye related symptoms, corticosteroid therapy may be started on the basis of a presumptive clinical diagnosis of temporal arteritis prior to carrying out a biopsy. However, the diagnostic yield in temporal artery biopsy may decrease following treatment with corticosteroids. In one series of 132 patients with a clinical diagnosis of temporal arteritis, the following biopsy results were obtained. Prior to corticosteroid therapy, patients with "clinically genuine temporal arteritis" had positive biopsy findings 82 percent of the time. During the first week of corticosteroid therapy the positive temporal artery incidence dropped to 60 percent. After 1 week of corticosteroid therapy the yield of positive results decreased dramatically to 10 percent. Thus, when corticosteroids are started on clinical grounds, a temporal artery biopsy should be performed as soon as possible after the medication has been started.

Alternative Therapies

In a very small subset of patients the dosage of corticosteroids with an acceptable morbidity does not totally suppress the signs and symptoms of temporal arteritis. This small percentage of patients represents a significant management problem, because no other group of drugs has manifested documented efficacy in the treatment of temporal arteritis. Although experience is limited, several drugs have been added to the corticosteroids to produce the so-called "steroid sparing effect." Anecdotal experience suggests that cytotoxic drugs, such as azathioprine or cyclophosphamide, when added to continuing corticosteroid therapy are effective in putting the refractory cases of temporal arteritis into clinical remission. Moreover, lower dosages of corticosteroids are generally effective when combined with cytotoxic drugs.

Azathioprine can be used at 1 to 2 mg per kg given as a single daily dose. Although this drug is generally well tolerated, hepatitis, bone marrow suppression, and an increased risk of neoplastic transformation have been reported. The patient should be appropriately monitored for these potential toxic effects. Alternatively, cyclophosphamide can be added at 1 to 2 mg per kg given as a single morning dose. Toxic effects associated with the use of cyclophosphamide include bone marrow suppression, hemorrhagic cystitis, bladder fibrosis, neoplastic transformation (acute myelocytic leukemia, bladder carcinoma), risk of infection, ovarian failure, sterility, and alopecia. Patients with temporal arteritis treated with cyclophosphamide should be monitored closely for drug related toxic effects.

During the induction phase with cyclophosphamide, the complete blood count should be monitored regularly for evidence of marrow suppression. Normally a reduction of the total leukocyte count to the 4,000 cells per cubic mm range is associated with a clinical response to cyclophosphamide. One should avoid letting the total granulocyte count drop below the 1,000 to 1,500 cells per cubic mm level because of the increased risk of infection.

The elderly population with temporal arteritis may be particularly sensitive to the marrow suppressive effects of this drug and may require a reduced dosage. The patient should be encouraged to drink enough fluid to maintain a urine output of approximately 3 liters per day. Drinking several glasses of water prior to retiring prevents the concentration of toxic metabolites in the overnight urine. Because incomplete emptying of the bladder may predispose a patient to cyclophosphamide induced bladder toxicity, a clinical history of obstructive urinary tract symptoms should be evaluated. If the patient is taking prednisone on a daily schedule when the cyclophosphamide is started, 2 weeks into the cyclophosphamide induction tapering to an alternate corticosteroid regimen should be initiated.

It should be emphasized that the prolonged daily use of prednisone and cyclophosphamide is associated with a substantial increase in the risk of opportunistic infections. By contrast, the use of cyclophosphamide and alternate day prednisone has been associated only with an increased risk of developing herpes zoster. The tapering to alternate day prednisone should be complete within 3 months after starting the cyclophosphamide therapy. During the tapering to an alternate day regimen there is a tendency for the leukocyte count to drop; consequently the dosage of cyclophosphamide must be decreased appropriately. Appropriate use and close monitoring for drug associated toxicity decrease the morbidity associated with the use of cyclophosphamide. The relative efficacy of azathioprine or cyclophosphamide when used as a corticosteroid sparing drug in temporal arteritis has not been systematically evaluated and should be considered only when it is absolutely clear that the corticosteroid regimen has failed.

Anecdotal experience with several other drugs used as "steroid sparing" therapy in temporal arteritis has also been reported. Dapsone at a dosage of 100 mg per day has been used with some success in reducing the corticosteroid dosage required to control the signs and symptoms of temporal arteritis. Cyclosporin A at a dosage of 3 mg per kg per day was used successfully in the treatment of a patient who was unresponsive to prednisone, cyclophosphamide, and dapsone. Patients treated with cyclosporin A require close monitoring, including drug level determinations and serial renal function studies. Treatment for the relatively rare case of corticosteroid resistant temporal arteritis should be evaluated on a case by case basis.

SUGGESTED READING

Allen NB, Studenski SA. Polymyalgia rheumatica and temporal arteritis. Med Clin North Am 1986; 70:369–384.
Allison MC, Gallagher PJ. Temporal artery biopsy and corticosteroid treatment. Ann Rheum Dis 1984; 43:416–417.
Cupps TR, Fauci AS. Giant cell arteritides. Major Probl Int Med 1981; 21:99–107.
Hunder GG, Hazelman BL. Giant cell arteritis and polymyalgia rheumatica. In: Kelley WN, Harris ED Jr, Ruddy LS, Sledge CB, eds. Textbook of rheumatology. 2nd ed. Philadelphia: WB Saunders, 1985.
Rosenfeld SI, Kosmorsky GS, Klingele TE, Burde RM. Treatment of temporal arteritis with ocular involvement. Am J Med 1986; 80:143–145.

TAKAYASU'S ARTERITIS

RANDI Y. LEAVITT, M.D., Ph.D.
ANTHONY S. FAUCI, M.D.

Takayasu's arteritis is a form of arteritis that typically involves the aorta and its branches and the pulmonary arteries. The disease can occur in three phases, which in any given patient presents as distinct stages, as stages that overlap each other, or in a form that remains subclinical.

The "prepulseless" or systemic phase is characterized by constitutional symptoms such as fever, malaise, weight loss, arthralgias, arthritis, myalgias, nightsweats, and skin rash. This stage of the disease is not usually associated with signs and symptoms of specific vessel inflammation, and laboratory findings are usually nonspecific and are indicative of a chronic inflammatory disease including an elevated erythrocyte sedimentation rate, anemia, leukocytosis, and thrombocytosis.

The vessel inflammatory phase is associated with pain over an inflamed vessel and ultimately results in stenosis or aneurysm formation. Nonspecific laboratory abnormalities are seen, similar to those described in the systemic phase of the disease.

The "burnt out" or chronic occlusive phase of the illness is marked by signs and symptoms of obliteration of major arteries such as bruits, absence of pulses, claudication, and hypertension. Laboratory findings in the "burnt out" stage of Takayasu's arteritis are usually completely normal. During the inflammatory stages of the disease (systemic and vessel inflammatory stages), the sedimentation rate is generally elevated and is a good indicator of disease activity and the response to therapy. In many patients the systemic findings precede the recognition of vascular insufficiency by a prolonged period of time. A significant number of patients first present during the occlusive phase of the illness. Angiography is important in establishing a diagnosis of Takayasu's arteritis and in following disease progression.

Takayasu's arteritis can involve any region of the aorta, its major branches, and the pulmonary arteries (Table 1). Cerebrovascular manifestations are seen secondary to involvement of the carotid and vertebral arteries. Loss of palpable pulses can result from aortic coarctation, subclavian, carotid, or iliac disease; aortic, subclavian, and iliac disease can result in limb claudication. Aortic insufficiency, aortic aneurysms, and renal vascular hypertension can be seen and may require both medical and surgical therapy. Pulmonary artery involvement is seen in approximately half the patients and can result in pulmonary hypertension but is rarely symptomatic. Coronary artery disease secondary to occlusion of the coronary ostia is rare but can result in angina and myocardial infarction. The abdominal aorta (including the iliac and mesenteric arteries) can be affected, resulting in abdominal pain.

Since pathologic documentation of Takayasu's arteritis is rare, arteriography is essential in establishing the initial diagnosis and in following patients. Total

TABLE 1 Frequency of Arterial Involvement in Takayasu's Arteritis and Resultant Sequelae*

Arterial Involvement	Clinical Manifestations†
Frequent (>40%)	
Subclavian	Arm claudication, Raynaud's phenomenon
Carotid	Altered vision, retinal changes, syncope, stroke
Renal	Renal vascular hypertension, renal failure
Descending aorta	—
Intermediate frequency (10–40%)	
Ascending aorta	Aortic root dilation, aortic insufficiency
Abdominal aorta	Abdominal pain, nausea and vomiting
Vertebral	Altered vision, dizziness, stroke
Iliac	Leg claudication
Innominate	—
Pulmonary	Atypical chest pain radiating to back
Mesenteric	Abdominal pain, nausea and vomiting
Infrequent (<10%)	
Coronary	Angina, myocardial infarction
Femoral	Leg claudication
Brachial	Hand and wrist claudication, Raynaud's phenomenon

* From Volkman DJ, Fauci AS. Takayasu's arteritis. In: Lichtenstein LM, Fauci AS, eds. Current therapy in allergy and immunology. Philadelphia: BC Decker, 1983: 143–147.
† Sequelae listed are those especially associated with narrowing of the indicated artery. Complications such as pain over the affected artery, bruits, pulselessness, and aneurysmic rupture can occur with any affected artery.

aortography is necessary to adequately evaluate these patients because the disease affects the aorta and its branches both above and below the diaphragm. Typically the angiograms revealed stenotic lesions, which may result in vascular occlusion and aneurysm formation. The presence of both types of lesions involving different areas of the aorta and its branches is diagnostic of Takayasu's arteritis. Although the angiogram sometimes can resemble those in atherosclerotic disease, Takayasu's arteritis usually affects young women who do not have any predisposition toward atherosclerotic disease. In this regard, establishment of the diagnosis of Takayasu's arteritis often requires clinical correlation. In our experience conventional arteriograms have been superior to digital subtraction studies in following patients because they provide better visualization of multiple vessels in a single study. In addition, we have found the conventional studies more reproducible in following serial examinations. In the absence of clinical symptoms we do not routinely perform cardiac or pulmonary angiography.

The major goals in treating a patient with Takayasu's arteritis are to accurately establish the extent and activity of the disease using both clinical observation and arteriography, stop progression of the vascular disease by suppressing the inflammatory process, and aggressively treat the sequelae of previous vascular inflammation.

Once a diagnosis is established, the physician must establish whether the patient has a continuing inflammatory process or "burnt out" disease; symptoms secondary to systemic disease and those secondary to specific vessel occlusion must be distinguished. In this regard the approach to therapy is use of a combination of anti-inflammatory drugs with surgical bypass of affected vessels.

GENERAL THERAPEUTIC APPROACH TO TAKAYASU'S ARTERITIS

Our approach to the therapy in patients with Takayasu's arteritis is shown in Figure 1.

Takayasu's Arteritis Associated with Active Inflammation

As mentioned previously, some patients with Takayasu's arteritis present with unequivocal active inflammatory disease, and these patients should be treated initially with corticosteroids daily and then given an alternate day regimen (to be described). A subset of patients present without symptoms but with elevated erythrocyte sedimentation rates and abnormal angiograms. We consider these patients to have active inflammatory disease and treat them with corticosteroids.

At the outset it is important to completely document the extent of disease by physical and laboratory examination and angiography. The patient should be followed in conjunction with a vascular surgeon since ischemic complications are a major cause of morbidity in Takayasu's arteritis. Although the optimal time to perform surgery is when the patient has inactive disease and is no longer taking corticosteroid therapy, surgery to prevent imminent ischemia of a vital organ should not be delayed because of continuing ischemia or immunosuppressive therapy. However, elective procedures should not be done until the patient is taking the lowest possible corticosteroid dosage. A therapeutic response to corticosteroid therapy is marked by a normalization of the sedimentation rate, improvement in systemic systems, and stabilization of vascular disease documented by angiography.

In this regard there is one instance in which the angiogram can show progressive vascular disease and not imply active arteritis. This is the setting of progressive vessel stenosis in a previously diseased area as a result of scarring. Under these circumstances, if the patient has no signs of active disease (e.g., elevated sedimentation rate, systemic symptoms, or new areas of vascular involvement), we do not change our therapeutic protocol but continue to follow the patient carefully. Failure to respond to corticosteroid therapy is defined as disease progression during daily corticosteroid therapy

**Patient evaluation for extent of disease including history,
physical, laboratory evaluation (including ESR)
and total aortography**

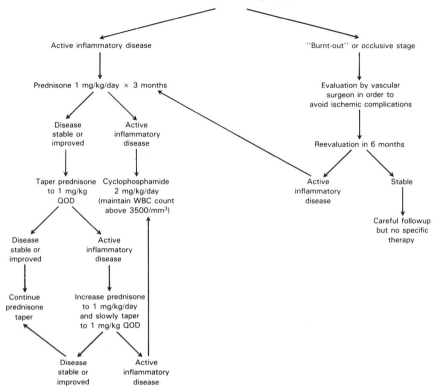

Figure 1 Approach to therapy in patients with Takayasu's arteritis.

or the inability to maintain a remission once the corticosteroid dosage has been tapered to an alternate day regimen; these patients require cyclophosphamide therapy (to be described). If the disease flairs either during the prednisone taper or while alternate day prednisone therapy is being used, the dosage can be increased back to 1 mg per kg per day (see later discussion) and tapered more slowly. If the disease flairs again during the corticosteroid taper, cyclophosphamide therapy is indicated.

In the absence of clear-cut angiographic disease progression, it sometimes can be difficult to decide whether a patient is responding to therapy. If a patient has an increasing sedimentation rate while the corticosteroid dosage is being tapered without systemic complaints and a stable angiogram, we slowly taper the corticosteroid dosage and follow the patient closely with angiograms at 6 month intervals. In our experience patients do not have systemic symptoms secondary to active arteritis without an elevated erythrocyte sedimentation rate. In addition, systemic symptoms can develop secondary to corticosteroid withdrawal, and these can mimic a flare of Takayasu's arteritis. In this situation the physician must make a clinical judgment and follow the individual patient carefully.

Takayasu's Arteritis in the "Burnt Out" Stage

Some patients with Takayasu's arteritis present in the "burnt out" stage with signs of vessel occlusion but no active inflammation. Many have a history of systemic complaints preceding the diagnosis. In the absence of active arteritis (no systemic symptoms and a normal sedimentation rate), no specific anti-inflammatory therapy is indicated. These patients should be followed closely to confirm that the disease is inactive. In addition, they should be treated aggressively both medically and surgically for problems related to the existing vascular disease (see following discussion).

SPECIFIC THERAPEUTIC APPROACH TO TAKAYASU'S ARTERITIS

Although many drugs such as anticoagulants, salicylates, vasodilators, antimalarial drugs, and antituberculous drugs, have been advocated in the treatment of Takayasu's arteritis, there is no consistent role for them in this disease. Therapy combining anti-inflammatory and immunosuppressive drugs (corticosteroids and cytotoxic drugs) with an aggressive medical and surgical approach to the vascular complications of the disease has been effective in controlling the disease.

Anti-inflammatory Therapy

Corticosteroids have potent anti-inflammatory and immunosuppressive effects and are used in treating many of the vasculitic syndromes (see article on systemic vasculitis). Prednisone is the corticosteroid of choice in treating Takayasu's arteritis, since it has a relatively short half-life and causes less suppression of the hypothalamic-pituitary-adrenal axis than other longer acting preparations; it therefore can be used in an alternate day regimen, which minimizes corticosteroid induced side effects.

Prednisone is given initially at a dosage of 1 mg per kg per day but usually not exceeding 80 mg per day. In order to provide a maximal anti-inflammatory effect it is first given in divided doses for 1 week and then consolidated and given as a single daily morning dose. Daily prednisone therapy is continued for 3 months with the patient under close observation. After 3 months the patient undergoes a complete re-evaluation, including angiography and an assessment to determine whether the disease is progressing, stable, or improving. Patients suffering from progressive disease while receiving corticosteroids should be given cyclophosphamide therapy (see next section).

In patients with stable or improving disease, after 3 months of corticosteroid therapy the prednisone dose should be tapered gradually to an alternate day regimen over approximately 1 month by maintaining the "on" day dosage at 1 mg per kg and tapering the "off" day dosage in 10 mg decrements until a dosage of 30 mg is reached, then by 5 mg decrements until it reaches 15 mg, and finally decrements of 2.5 mg are used until a dosage of 1 mg per kg on alternate days is reached. This dosage is maintained for 1 month, and if the remission is maintained, the dosage is tapered as previously described at 4 week intervals; the total duration of therapy should be 1 year following the induction of remission. If after initially responding to daily corticosteroid therapy the disease flairs during tapering to an alternate day regimen, the dosage should be increased to 1 mg per kg daily and then tapered more slowly. Under these circumstances, if the disease can be controlled only with daily corticosteroid therapy, cyclophosphamide therapy should be instituted.

Prolonged daily corticosteroid therapy is associated with many potential complications (discussed in detail in the article on systemic vasculitis). Commonly encountered corticosteroid induced side effects include psychiatric disorders, osteoporosis, aseptic necrosis of bone, myopathy, cataracts, hypertension, suppression of the hypothalamic-pituitary-adrenal axis, hyperglycemia, and an increased incidence of infection. Alternate day therapy minimizes virtually all the undesirable side effects of corticosteroids while maintaining an anti-inflammatory effect.

Cytotoxic Therapy

As mentioned previously, cytotoxic therapy is recommended in patients who have inflammatory disease that progresses with daily corticosteroid therapy or in whom the disease cannot be suppressed with tapering doses of alternate day prednisone and who therefore require daily corticosteroid therapy.

Extrapolating from therapeutic experience in systemic vasculitis, cyclophosphamide is the cytotoxic drug of choice. Cyclophosphamide is an alkylating drug that is activated in the liver and excreted by the kidneys. In this setting, it is given orally as a single dose of 2 mg per kg per day, but the same dose can be given intravenously. The drug does not induce maximal immunosuppression until approximately 2 to 3 weeks after initiating therapy, and therefore daily corticosteroid doses are continued during the first month of cyclophosphamide therapy. The corticosteroid dosage is then tapered to an alternate day regimen and finally tapered and discontinued as previously described. Once the disease is controlled with cyclophosphamide therapy, the corticosteroid dosage can be tapered over 3 to 6 months as tolerated. As in other vasculitic syndromes, cyclophosphamide therapy is continued for 1 year following the induction of remission and then tapered in 25 mg decrements per month.

Since cyclophosphamide causes leukopenia, one must balance its effect on the underlying disease with the resulting neutropenia. We aim to maintain the total white blood cell count above 3500 cells per cubic mm, resulting in a neutrophil count of greater the 1000 cells per cubic mm; neutrophil counts in this range are not associated with an increased risk of opportunistic infection. Since the maximal leukopenic effect of a given dose of cyclophosphamide lags 8 to 12 days, one must anticipate the drop and make dosage adjustments when the white blood cell count is beginning to decrease; neutropenia results if no adjustment is made before the white blood cell count reaches 3500 cells per cubic mm.

Patients maintained on cyclophosphamide have an increased incidence of herpes zoster infection. In addition to bone marrow suppression, side effects of cyclophosphamide therapy include hemorrhagic cystitis, bladder fibrosis and malignant disease, gonadal dysfunction resulting in sterility, leukemia, lymphoma, pulmonary fibrosis, and hypogammaglobulinemia.

Azathioprine, a purine analogue, is an alternative in patients who cannot tolerate cyclophosphamide. It is given at a dosage of 2 mg per kg per day.

Other Medical Therapies

Patients with Takayasu's arteritis can develop renal vascular hypertension secondary to renal artery disease. These patients are treated with conventional antihypertensive drugs or surgery (see next section). We do not routinely use captopril in Takayasu's arteritis with renal vascular hypertension because of its association with nephrotoxicity. However, captopril can be used cautiously in patients who fail to respond to more conventional therapy.

Other medical problems that arise in patients with Takayasu's arteritis such as congestive heart failure are treated with conventional drugs.

Surgical Therapy

Vascular surgery plays a major role in avoiding the ischemic complications associated with Takayasu's arteritis. We believe that an early aggressive approach to surgery in these patients has significantly improved survival. Conditions that often require surgical intervention in Takayasu's arteritis include renal vascular hypertension, cerebral hypoperfusion, limb claudication, aortic valve disease, and repair of aneurysms. In general, surgery is directed at bypassing the obstructed arteries using synthetic grafts. Although there is a higher inci-

dence of vessel or graft occlusion in patients with active arteritis, most procedures are effective and should not be delayed if deemed necessary. The graft should be placed in an area of uninvolved vessel, and the patient should continue taking corticosteroid and/or cytotoxic therapy. Elective procedures should be delayed until the patient is in remission and no longer taking corticosteroid therapy.

Although the experience with transluminal angioplasty is limited in Takayasu's arteritis, we believe that this procedure may play a role in the management of selected patients. However, at this point there are no long term follow-up data relating to patients undergoing this procedure.

SUGGESTED READING

Hall S, Barr W, Lie JT, Stanson AW, Kazmier FJ, Hunder GG. Takayasu's arteritis: a study of 32 North American patients. Medicine (Baltimore) 1985; 64:89–99.

Parrillo JE. Takayasu's arteritis. In: Lichtenstein LM, Fauci AS, eds. Current therapy in allergy, immunology and rheumatology. Philadelphia: BC Decker 1985:206–211.

Shelhamer JH, Volkman DJ, Parrillo JE, Lawley TJ, Johnston MR, Fauci AS. Takayasu's arteritis and its therapy. Ann Intern Med 1985; 103:121–126.

Volkman DJ, Fauci AS. Takayasu's arteritis. In: Lichtenstein LM, Fauci AS, eds. Current therapy in allergy and immunology. Philadelphia: BC Decker, 1983:143–147.

BEHÇET'S SYNDROME

J. DESMOND O'DUFFY, M.D.

The diagnosis of Behçet's disease is confirmed when chronically recurrent oral aphthous ulcerations coexist with at least two of the following clinical manifestations: genital ulcerations, uveitis, synovitis, cutaneous vasculitis, meningitis or meningoencephalitis, and phlebitis or large vessel arteritis (Table 1). The differential diagnosis includes Crohn's disease of the colon, less commonly herpes simplex and Reiter's syndrome, and rarely variants of pemphigus and the hypereosinophilic syndrome. Uveitis is confirmed by slit lamp biomicroscopy and funduscopy, whereas meningitis and meningoencephalitis are confirmed by neurologic examination and the finding of cerebrospinal fluid pleo-

cytosis. The disease typically affects young adults, with women predominating in a ratio of 2:1 in North America. The disease is most common in the Orient and Middle East where males predominate.

The best management is multidisciplinary. Such a team might include a rheumatologist, ophthalmologist, dermatologist, neurologist, vascular radiologist, or surgeon depending on the phase of the disease. The treatment is tailored to the severity of the disease. Serious phases of the disease such as uveitis, meningoencephalitis, or arteritis may require immunosuppressive therapy with alkylating drugs, whereas mucous membrane ulcerations, cutaneous vasculitis, and synovitis are usually treated with corticosteroids.

Histologic study of aphthous ulcerations shows a chronic inflammatory reaction with lymphocytes and monocytes infiltrating the basal and prickle cell layers of the epidermis. Since vasculitis is a prominent feature of the posterior uveal and central nervous system phases of the disease, it was logical that immunosuppressive drugs including corticosteroids and cytotoxic drugs would be used. Although there is no cure, most patients ex-

TABLE 1 Frequency of Clinical Features of Behçet's Disease

	Percentage
Recurrent aphthous stomatitis	100
Genital aphthous ulcers	75
Cutaneous vasculitis	50–60
Uveitis	50–60
Synovitis	40
Meningoencephalitis	20–30
Phlebitis	10
Large vessel arteritis	<10

perience a phase of partial remission after years of fluctuating disease, particularly if treatment has been vigorous.

THERAPEUTIC APPROACH

Skin and Mucous Membrane Involvement

The most common problem in Behçet's disease is chronically recurrent, painful oral aphthous ulcerations in the buccal mucous membrane and on the tongue, soft palate, and pharynx. Patients often report that certain foods such as nuts precipitate flares; these should be avoided. Sucralfate topically or in a chalky suspension, is in vogue as treatment. One formulation is 1 g of Carafate suspended in 15 ml of sorbitol and water.

Corticosteroids

These anti-inflammatory immunosuppressive 21-carbon steroid molecules include prednisone, which has a keto group at the 11 position. Prednisone is activated in the liver to prednisolone, the active compound. Topical preparations, for example, 0.1 percent triamcinolone as Kenalog in Orabase, may be applied to the emerging oral ulcerations. However, most patients find topical corticosteroid therapy disappointing. Likewise, most patients will not adhere to regimens of topical 2 percent viscous Xylocaine therapy except in severe flares. Oral solutions of tetracycline, diphenhydramine, and dexamethasone are preferred. Such preparations are variously concocted by pharmacies of hospitals where large numbers of patients with cancer receiving chemotherapy are subject to severe stomatitis. Oral doses of corticosteroids suppress the inflammatory response of the delayed-type hypersensitivity reaction that is mimicked in Behçet's disease. Oral prednisone therapy suppresses aphthous ulcerations in the mouth and genitalia if given in adequate doses. A few patients with discrete episodes use a brief tapering daily schedule of prednisone, such as 40-30-20-10-0 mg for attacks. Unfortunately many patients become steroid dependent in that cessation of prednisone leads to prompt flare-ups of painful ulcerations.

Levamisole

Levamisole, an antihelminthic drug, has been used for Behçet's disease since it has been reported to normalize impaired immune responses. This drug has not been released for use because it can cause severe granulocytopenia. Mucosal ulcerations may heal, but levamisole will not prevent blindness or recurrences of meningoencephalitis.

Dapsone

Dapsone is a sulfone that is bacteriostatic to *M. leprae*. In some patients it has a beneficial effect on the mucocutaneous lesions. It was used in seven men with Behçet's disease in one uncontrolled study in the Middle East. It is not known whether dapsone has any benefit in cases of major organ involvement. The initial dosage is 50 mg daily and may be gradually increased to 200 mg daily. At dosages of 100 mg or less there is usually no hemolysis unless glucose-6-phosphate dehydrogenase deficiency coexists. Monitoring of the hemoglobin level in the early months of treatment is suggested.

Thalidomide

The ill-fated sedative of the 1960s that was associated with phocomelia may yield benefit in treating the mucosal and cutaneous lesions of Behçet's disease. It is not effective in suppressing uveitis. The mechanism of action is unknown, but thalidomide may inhibit neutrophil chemotaxis or block the action of activated T lymphocytes. Thalidomide suppresses the erythema nodosum leprosum reaction that is seen in leprous patients given sulfones. Skin and mucous membrane lesions of Behçet's disease usually respond to dosages of 100 to 200 mg daily. Unfortunately the drug is not presently available because the World Health Organization strictly controls the supply and provides it only to leprosariums. Moreover, thalidomide causes a peripheral neuropathy in about 20 percent of long-term users.

Colchicine

Colchicine is an anti-inflammatory alkaloid that is commonly used in gout because it binds to microtubular proteins, interferes with the function of mitotic spindles, and reduces the motility of granulocytes. It has been used chiefly by Japanese physicians who noticed that polymorphonuclear chemotactic function in Behçet's disease was increased over that in normal subjects. They reported modest clinical improvement in uncontrolled studies and a reduction in the number of attacks of uveitis. Nevertheless most patients with Behçet's disease do not respond well to colchicine irrespective of the clinical manifestations.

Joint Involvement

Oligoarthritis, typically of short duration and non-deforming, may occur in Behçet's disease. Arthrocentesis and intra-articular corticosteroid therapy may be helpful in cases involving the knees, and nonsteroidal anti-inflammatory drugs such as indomethacin, up to 75 mg twice daily, are useful. Synovitis responds to prednisone in dosages of up to 20 mg daily.

Cutaneous Vasculitis

The various skin lesions in Behçet's disease include pustules, nodules, and papules, which typically resemble those of erythema nodosum. Biopsies often reveal perivascular inflammation of veins or arteries. Necrotizing vasculitis can also occur. For mild cutaneous vasculitis indomethacin, up to 150 mg daily can be tried. If this is ineffective, prednisone, 20 mg daily, is usually beneficial. The dermal vasculitis usually responds to moderate doses of prednisone, and these are rapidly reduced as the lesions come under control. Patients who have severe cutaneous involvement are exceptional in Behçet's disease. Such involvement should lead the clinician to suspect an alternative diagnosis, such as Crohn's disease.

Uveitis

Blindness from uveitis is the main threat of Behçet's disease. Until 20 years ago Middle Eastern patients often became blind within 4 years after the onset of the uveitis. Hypopyon, pus in the anterior chamber of the eye, is a severe form of anterior uveitis and is prevented by topical corticosteroid therapy. In anterior uveitis, cells in the anterior chamber are seen on slit lamp biomicroscopy, whereas cells are seen in the vitreous chamber in posterior uveitis. Anterior uveitis may be treated successfully by the topical application of corticosteroid drops, such as 1 percent Pred-Forte (prednisolone acetate ophthalmic suspension), one or two drops in the affected eye twice daily.

The management of a patient with posterior uveitis is often conducted jointly by an ophthalmologist and an internist. Uveitis in Behçet's disease is more likely to occur in males than in females and typically occurs 6 years after the first manifestation. It is usually bilateral and retinal infarctions, vitreous hemorrhages and cataracts are common. The ophthalmologist employs fundus photographs after the intravenous administration of fluorescein to reveal evidence of vascular permeability. Corticosteroid drops do not provide benefit in posterior uveitis because the molecules do not reach the vitreous and retina.

Posterior uveitis with associated retinal disease is only ameliorated (i.e. not adequately suppressed) by oral or subtenon corticosteroid therapy. Therefore, if the patient has either unilateral or bilateral posterior uveitis, both of which threaten blindness, chlorambucil, 0.1 mg per kilogram per day, should be used. Chlorambucil in an initial dosage of 0.1 to 0.2 mg per kilogram per day is effective, usually within 3 months. Patients who have lost one eye from uveitis usually maintain the vision in the other affected eye while this regimen is continued. Treatment typically lasts for 1 to 2 years. The dosage is slowly reduced to 2 mg daily and then treatment is stopped. Bonnet believes that chlorambucil is more effective when given alone than when given in conjunction with corticosteroids, and I agree with her.

Central Nervous System Involvement

Meningitis is manifested as headache, fever, and stiff neck and responds to treatment with prednisone, 30 to 60 mg daily. After one or more episodes of meningitis, meningoencephalitis with parenchymal lesions in the brain typically supervene. In either event the cerebrospinal fluid count exceeds 5 cells per cubic millimeter (mostly lymphocytes), and there is a mild increase in protein. Focal neurologic deficits with hemiparesis, cerebellar ataxia, or cranial nerve involvement can occur. Computed tomographic scanning or magnetic resonance imaging may demonstrate areas of infarction in the cerebrum, cerebellum, or brainstem. Most of these central nervous system lesions are due to vasculitic infarcts.

In an acute episode of meningoencephalitis, prednisone, 60 mg daily, may be used; the dosage is tapered as the erythrocyte sedimentation rate and neurologic deficits are controlled. I favor using concomitant chlorambucil, 0.1 mg per kilogram per day, and begin tapering prednisone therapy after 2 months. Patients embarking on immunosuppressive regimens between episodes of meningoencephalitis typically have a normal cerebrospinal fluid. They may be given chlorambucil, 0.1 mg per kilogram per day, to prevent recurrences. Typically such patients are treated for 1 or 2 years, again in a tapering regimen as with uveitis, already described. In patients taking prednisone simultaneously with chlorambucil, the corticosteroid dosage should be tapered first, with subsequent reduction and tapering of chlorambucil therapy. However, because up to 2 months is required for chlorambucil to take effect, it is wise to hold concomitant prednisone dosing steady for that period.

Phlebitis and Arteritis

In phlebitis and arteritis, thromboses of large veins and arteries with arterial aneurysms or infarctions may occur. Although a hypercoagulable state has been proposed in Behçet's disease, the elevated clotting factor levels merely represent acute phase reactants of inflammation. Profound recurrences of lower extremity phlebitis may not respond to anticoagulation with heparin or warfarin. Pulmonary embolism is rare. Treatment with either prolonged prednisone suppression or, in our limited experience, chlorambucil can prevent recurrences.

Intracranial venous sinus occlusion is responsible for the syndrome of benign intracranial hypertension that afflicts a few patients with Behçet's disease. These patients present with chronic headache and may be found to have papilledema when they are examined for visual defects. Cerebrospinal fluid examination shows few cells, but the pressure is usually greater than 300 mm as recorded during lumbar puncture. Here the diagnostic test is digital subtraction angiography. Prednisone, 30 to 60 mg daily, if given early can result in lysis of the clot. In some patients occlusion is irreversible, and relief of headache and visual symptoms only occur when shunting of the cerebrospinal fluid through a lumboperitoneal shunt is done by the neurosurgeon.

Large vessel arteritis is the most treacherous phase of the disease because usually there is no warning until rupture or infarction occurs. Aneurysms resulting from vasculitis can arise in any artery, and occlusions of inflamed arteries can lead to infarctions. Thus, patients may die suddenly of myocardial infarction or hemoptysis from rupture of a pulmonary artery into the tracheobronchial tree. Recurrent episodes of hemoptysis can predict the latter disaster. Major artery involvement suggests prompt treatment with prednisone, 60 mg daily, along with chlorambucil, 0.1 mg per kilogram per day. In a few patients emergency vascular surgery such as aneurysmectomy and thrombectomy have been life saving. If extremity arteries have to be replaced in surgery, synthetic grafts are preferred over venous grafts, since the latter may thrombose.

Other Manifestations

Gastrointestinal involvement in Behçet's disease may produce discrete aphthous ulcers at any site from the mouth to the anus. Crohn's disease of the colon is excluded by barium enema or colonoscopy with biopsy. Discrete aphthous ulcers may bleed, typically in the terminal ileum or right side of the colon. Blood trans-

fusions may be needed. Occasionally ileal ulcers perforate, and then surgical resection of the diseased bowel is indicated. In Japanese studies ileotransverse colostomy has been done to treat such perforations. The pathologic findings are different from those of the granulomatous enteritis of Crohn's disease. Other serious but rare events include aortic valve insufficiency as well as glomerulonephritis and pericarditis. The latter inflammatory episodes are probably best treated with prednisone, but a decision whether to use chlorambucil must still be made.

Preferred Approach

The patient is thoroughly interviewed and examined. Routine blood studies are done to rule out obvious mimics. Crohn's disease must be excluded if diarrhea is present. Mucosal ulcers are treated symptomatically by the topical application of steroids such as triamcinolone dental paste (in Orabase) or dexamethasone oral solutions. Synovitis and cutaneous vasculitis are treated with prednisone in dosages of 10 to 20 mg daily tapered by 5 to 10 percent every 3 to 7 days if tolerated (Table 2).

Patients with posterior uveitis or meningoencephalitis are treated with chlorambucil. In patients embarking on chlorambucil therapy a careful explanation of the toxicity of the drug and instructions about its use are required. Arrangements are made for toxicity monitoring. Because chlorambucil is likely to cause azoospermia in men and premature menopause in women when used beyond 6 to 12 months, reproductive counseling is indicated. Young males taking chlorambucil or cyclophosphamide are given an opportunity to store sperm in a sperm bank. Antiovulatory drugs have been proposed to protect women from ovarian toxicity, but there is as yet no proof that they do so.

Immunosuppressive Therapy: Chlorambucil Versus Corticosteroids

Prednisolone acetate suspension (Pred-Forte), given hourly as drops into the conjunctival space, is effective for anterior uveitis. Because topical steroid therapy increases the intraocular pressure, this needs to be checked during ophthalmology visits. Rebound inflammation may occur as the Pred-Forte dosage is reduced; therefore reduction should be gradual.

The ophthalmologist may well have treated the posterior uveitis with prednisone, 40 to 60 mg daily in single or divided doses or in alternate day double dosage. Periocular injections of dexamethasone sodium phosphate, 4 mg per milliliter, also may have been tried. After many months of use, the familiar corticosteroid complications of hypertension, diabetes mellitus, osteoporosis, avascular necrosis of bone and cataracts occur. It is best to hold initial dosages below 40 mg daily in

TABLE 2 Treatment Options

Drug	Indications	Initial Dosage	Toxic Effects
Prednisone	Aphthous disease (severe) Synovitis Cutaneous vasculitis	20–40 mg/day	Osteopenia Cushing's syn- drome
Chlorambucil	Posterior uveitis Meningoencephalitis	0.1 mg/kg/day	Leukopenia Thrombocytopenia Amenorrhea Azoospermia
Cyclosporine	Resistant uveitis	5 mg/kg/day	Interstitial nephritis Hirsutism Infections
Empiric drugs Dapsone	Aphthous disease	100 mg/day	Hemolytic anemia

treating mucous membrane, cutaneous, and joint inflammation. For acute meningoencephalitis or major arteritis, prednisone, 60 mg daily, is justified but seldom prevents recurrences. Therefore, chlorambucil therapy should be initiated to make possible prednisone dosage tapering. Women receiving high dose prednisone therapy should take 1000 mg of elemental calcium daily along with 400 units of vitamin D. The prednisone dosage is reduced as the disease is controlled; alternate day therapy may be tried toward the end of withdrawal. In posterior uveitis, however, systemic prednisone therapy may be avoided because chlorambucil alone, 0.1 mg per kilogram per day, is effective. Chlorambucil is given in a single dose in the morning.

The multidisciplinary approach in a patient with Behçet's disease with uveitis and meningoencephalitis could be exemplified by a cooperative triumvirate of rheumatologist, ophthalmologist, and neurologist. In this way visual acuity scores and uveitis activity are documented and the cerebrospinal fluid cell count and assessment of the neurologic status are provided during long-term immunosuppression.

Chlorambucil

Chlorambucil is a bifunctional alkylating drug that is related to nitrogen mustard. As with cyclophosphamide, it undergoes an electrophilic chemical reaction through the formation of carbonium ion intermediates that form covalent linkages with compounds of the DNA molecule. Lymphocytes are particularly susceptible to alkylating drugs, and lymphopenia and impaired lymphocyte function result. All but one of the reports dealing with chlorambucil in Behçet's disease suggested that it was effective in a dosage of 0.1 mg per kilogram per day. At least three patients treated with chlorambucil for Behçet's disease have developed acute myeloblastic leukemia. All these patients had been started on a chlorambucil dosage of 0.2 mg per kilogram per day.

About half of all fertile women beginning chlorambucil therapy with 0.1 mg per kilogram per day become amenorrheic within 1 year. However, uveitis or meningoencephalitis is controlled within 3 to 6 months. At that point a reduction in the dosage of 25 to 33 percent is begun. A decision to use prednisone along with chlorambucil is controversial but is justified in patients with active meningoencephalitis or active large vessel arteritis.

Toxicity monitoring is imperative while patients are taking chlorambucil. Complete blood counts are advised every 2 weeks for 3 months and then every month indefinitely. It is best to withhold chlorambucil when the leukocyte count is below 3000 per cubic millimeter and the platelet count is below 100,000 per cubic millimeter. When the counts return to normal, the drug is cautiously reinstituted at a lower dosage. Twenty-five percent of the patients cannot continue chlorambucil therapy because of toxicity, typically thrombocytopenia or leukopenia. Pneumococcal vaccine should be given before treatment is begun, and an annual influenza vaccination is advised. Fertile women about to take chlorambucil should first be given birth control therapy in order to avoid conceiving a defective fetus. Although most patients can taper and withdraw from chlorambucil after 1 to 2 years, a few require prolonged therapy, such as 2 mg daily or every other day for 3 or more years. Prolonged leukopenia should be avoided if possible. The alkylating compounds predispose to leukemia and carcinomas. Of particular concern is acute myelogenous leukemia, which may evolve from a dysmyelopoietic bone marrow after chlorambucil therapy.

Cyclosporine

Cyclosporine is a cyclic undecapeptide, originally discovered as a soil fungus metabolite that inhibits the clonal expansion of T helper inducer subsets while sparing T suppressor function. Cyclosporine is not cytotoxic to bone marrow cells, however, and is used to prevent rejection of grafted organs such as kidney transplants. There is usually rapid and dramatic improvement in posterior uveitis and oral ulcerations when cyclosporine, 5 mg per kilogram per day, is given. The dosage is tapered so that trough levels of cyclosporine are kept below 300 ng per millileter. Nephrotoxicity is the most serious side effect. Renal function is followed with serum creatinine determinations and the dosage must be reduced if the level rises above 1.6 mg per deciliter. Other side effects are hirsutism, paresthesias, gum hypertrophy, and a coarsening of facial features. The annual cost of cyclosporine, $5,000 to $10,000, also must be considered. Whether oncogenesis is also provoked is not yet known.

Other Remedies

Some therapies in the past that did not prove to be beneficial include Azulfidine, transfusion of blood or plasma, vitamin E, hydroxychloroquine, colchicine, transfer factor, and fibrinolytic therapy with phenformin and estradiol. Methotrexate, 25 mg per square meter every 4 days for 6 weeks, reduced uveitis activity, and cyclophosphamide when given intravenously at a dosage of 1 g per square meter of body surface weekly for 6 weeks also reduced uveitis. The efficacy of azathioprine is not proven.

PROS AND CONS OF TREATMENT

Because the prognosis for saving vision is poor in untreated patients with bilateral posterior uveitis, chlorambucil is recommended for them. North American patients fare better in all the aspects of the disease than Eastern Mediterranean and Japanese patients. It is not clear why the disease runs a more severe course in the latter countries. The only clue that matches both incidence and severity is the association of HLA-B$_5$ or BW$_{51}$, prevalent in those regions. There is no increased association of HLA-B$_5$ or any other HLA-A, B, C, or D antigen with Behçet's disease in North American patients or in English patients. Because there is risk to life and sight in Behçet's disease, there is a clear choice for alkylating treatment when bilateral posterior uveitis, meningoencephalitis, or large vessel arteritis exists. Moreover, many patients treated with chlorambucil for 2 years or so and then weaned from it may find that suppression of the uveitis or meningoencephalitis persists indefinitely.

SUGGESTED READING

Mishima S, Masuda K, Izawa Y, Mochizuki M. Behçet's disease in Japan: ophthalmologic aspects. Trans Am Ophthalmol Soc 1979; 77:225–279.
Nussenblatt RB, Palestine AG, Chan C, Mochizuki M, Yancey K. Effectiveness of cyclosporin therapy for Behçet's disease. Arthritis Rheum 1985; 28:671–679.
O'Duffy JD, Bowles CA, O'Fallon WM. The immunosuppressive treatment of Behçet's disease with emphasis on chlorambucil. In: Lehner T, Barnes CG, eds. Recent advances in Behçet's disease. Congress and Symposium Series No. 103. London, England: Royal Society of Medicine Service, 1986:130–133.
O'Duffy JD, Robertson DM, Goldstein NP. Chlorambucil in the treatment of uveitis and meningoencephalitis of Behçet's disease. Am J Med 1984; 76:75–84.
Sharquie K. Suppression of Behçet's with dapsone. Br J Dermatol 1984; 110:493–494.

COGAN'S SYNDROME

BARTON F. HAYNES, M.D.

Typical Cogan's syndrome is a rare clinical entity of unknown origin that is characterized by nonsyphilitic interstitial keratitis and vestibuloauditory dysfunction. Cogan's syndrome occurs primarily in young adults, although patients can be affected at any age. The vestibuloauditory symptoms consist of the sudden onset of hearing loss, nystagmus, tinnitus, and vertigo, which when untreated usually progress rapidly to complete deafness and persistent labyrinth dysfunction.

The primary ocular manifestation of typical Cogan's syndrome is chronic bilateral interstitial keratitis, which may vary in intensity from day to day and from eye to eye. The keratitis is manifested by patchy infiltrates of the deep corneal stroma followed by a variable degree of corneal vascularization; in the acute stage it often is associated with pain, photophobia, hyperemia, and mild uveitis. Ten percent of the patients with Cogan's syndrome present with scleritis or episcleritis associated with vestibuloauditory dysfunction instead of interstitial keratitis. This presentation of the disease has been termed "atypical Cogan's syndrome."

The primary systemic complication of typical Cogan's syndrome (interstitial keratitis and vestibuloauditory dysfunction) has been life-threatening aortic valvular disease with acute aortitis or a large vessel Takayasu-like arteritis in 10 percent of the patients. Systemic medium or small vessel vasculitis, once thought to be a complication of typical Cogan's syndrome, is rarely seen. In contrast, atypical Cogan's syndrome (scleritis, episcleritis, or types of inflammatory eye disease other than interstitial keratitis associated with vestibuloauditory dysfunction) is associated with systemic vasculitis and other systemic symptoms in up to 25 percent of the cases.

PREFERRED THERAPEUTIC APPROACH TO TYPICAL COGAN'S SYNDROME

Interstitial Keratitis

The topical application of 1 percent atropine solution or ointment is often necessary in the management of acute uveitis and keratitis; it may be applied three or four times daily. Topical steroid therapy may be indicated to control ocular inflammation. A solution of 1 percent prednisolone may be applied every 2 hours during acute states of the disease and then rapidly tapered after symptoms resolve. Between flares of interstitial keratitis, no topical ophthalmic therapy is usually necessary. Systemic corticosteroid therapy is indicated only rarely to control the symptoms of acute interstitial keratitis. Occasionally patients with typical Cogan's syndrome have persistent or severe interstitial keratitis requiring systemic corticosteroid therapy.

Vestibuloauditory Dysfunction

Corticosteroids are indicated in the early treatment of acute deafness associated with Cogan's syndrome. Some patients with Cogan's syndrome, when treated early after the onset of vestibuloauditory dysfunction, respond to corticosteroid therapy with improved hearing. Therefore, a short course of daily oral corticosteroid therapy (1 to 2 mg per kg of prednisone for 2 weeks) is warranted for patients with Cogan's syndrome with a recent onset of severe hearing impairment. If hearing is improved by this treatment, corticosteroids should be continued in an alternate day regimen followed by tapering of the dosage. If hearing does not improve after 2 weeks of daily prednisone therapy, the corticosteroid dosage should be tapered rapidly and discontinued. Immunosuppressive therapy of acute hearing loss in Cogan's syndrome has been tried in rare cases with variable results. In some cases high dose steroid therapy has improved hearing when cyclophosphamide has not.

Patients with typical Cogan's syndrome who have been treated at the onset of hearing loss with systemic corticosteroid therapy frequently are left with a permanent high frequency hearing loss and fluctuating hearing loss in the mid and low frequencies. Fluctuating hearing loss occurring in Cogan's syndrome months to years after the initial acute stage of the disease is usually due to the presence of cochlear hydrops rather than to active inflammation. Thus, although corticosteroid administration can preserve hearing acuity when administered at the onset of hearing loss, during the later quiescent stage of Cogan's syndrome, corticosteroids may not be of use and indeed may exacerbate hearing fluctuations because of salt retaining side effects. Late episodes of fluctuating hearing loss frequently can be controlled by the periodic administration of thiazide diuretics or in some cases simply by institution of a low sodium diet.

Frequently women with otherwise quiescent Cogan's syndrome experience exacerbations of vestibuloauditory dysfunction during menstruation; these symptoms nearly always respond to the administration of small doses of thiazide diuretics for 2 or 3 days.

Patients with Cogan's syndrome with sudden hearing loss should be given a trial of corticosteroid therapy in the following regimen: At the onset of vestibuloauditory dysfunction, oral doses of prednisone, 20 mg every 6 hours, should be administered for 4 to 5 days, followed by oral doses of 60 to 80 mg once daily for 1 week. If at the end of this time no improvement in hearing is noted, the steroid dosage should be rapidly tapered and stopped. If hearing improves with corticosteroid therapy, the dosage should be rapidly tapered (over 2 to 3 weeks) to an alternate day regimen. The alternate day dosage then should be tapered gradually over a 2 to 6 month period; fluctuations in hearing that occur during this time are usually due to cochlear hydrops and do not require increased dosages of corticosteroids. Hydrochlorothiazide in oral doses of 25 to 50 mg once daily is usually sufficient to alleviate hearing fluctuations due to cochlear hydrops.

The mechanism of action of corticosteroids in acute hearing loss of Cogan's syndrome is unknown. During the acute interstitial keratitis of Cogan's syndrome, the cornea is infiltrated with lymphocytes, monocytes, and plasma cells. Presumably corticosteroids improve hearing in acute Cogan's syndrome by limiting a similar type of inflammatory infiltrate in the cochlea.

Aortitis and Large Vessel Vasculitis

If aortitis with aortic insufficiency or a Takayasu-like large vessel vasculitis is present, treatment should be instituted with prednisone, 2 mg per kg, and cyclophosphamide, 2 mg per kg. We continue such therapy until manifestations of aortitis or large vessel vasculitis are stable or quiescent and then treat for 1 additional year. In cases of hemodynamically significant aortic insufficiency, aortic valve replacement should be considered. In Takayasu arteritis-like syndromes, vascular bypass surgery may be indicated to prevent ischemic tissue damage. If cyclophosphamide cannot be tolerated because of side effects or the large vessel vasculitis syndromes do not completely respond to cyclophosphamide, consideration should be given to discontinuing cyclophosphamide and instituting cyclosporin A therapy, 5 mg per kg orally daily. In the setting of Cogan's syndrome and large vessel vasculitis, with either cyclophosphamide or cyclosporin A, prednisone initially daily, and subsequently in alternate day doses, should continue to be administered.

Atypical Cogan's Syndrome and Systemic Necrotizing Vasculitis

In patients with atypical Cogan's syndrome with documented systemic necrotizing vasculitis, both prednisone and cyclophosphamide, 1 to 2 mg per kg per day, may be necessary. Data are now available that show that remissions as well as long term cures of systemic necrotizing vasculitis can be effected by the judicious use of short courses of prednisone and prolonged courses of low oral dosages (1 to 2 mg per kg per day) of cyclophosphamide.

DRUG SIDE EFFECTS

Systemic Corticosteroid Therapy

The side effects of systemic corticosteroid administration are numerous and serious, including osteoporosis, immunosuppression and susceptibility to infection, weight gain, cataracts, myopathy, and psychosis. Strict criteria therefore should be used for systemic steroid administration in Cogan's syndrome. Steroids should be used in a therapeutic trial to alleviate hearing loss as early as possible in the course of the disease. Months to years later in the course of Cogan's syndrome, corticosteroids may exacerbate hearing fluctuation if cochlear hydrops is present. Thus, steroids should be administered only late in Cogan's syndrome if the hearing loss is sudden or severe, or if manifestations of the original inflammatory process return, such as an elevated erythrocyte sedimentation rate, anemia, or leukocytosis. If hearing loss is complete or hearing fluctuations do not respond to steroids, there is no evidence that steroids should continue to be administered.

Two diuretics that are commonly used to treat cochlear hydrops in Cogan's syndrome are chlorthalidone and hydrochlorothiazide. The common side effects of both drugs are potassium depletion and volume depletion, as well as a variety of manifestations of drug allergy.

Cyclophosphamide

Cyclophosphamide is indicated for the rare patients with systemic necrotizing vasculitis and atypical Co-

gan's syndrome or typical Cogan's syndrome associated with large vessel vasculitis. An alkylating drug, cyclophosphamide is associated with severe bone marrow suppression and infection, hemorrhagic cystitis, gonadal dysfunction, gastrointestinal disturbances, and myeloid malignant disease. Therefore this drug should be used only for immune mediated hearing loss and eye disease associated with biopsy proven systemic necrotizing vasculitis or with the large vessel vasculitis syndrome associated with typical Cogan's syndrome. When used, dosages of 1 to 2 mg per kg of body weight are required; the dosage should be titered to keep the white blood cell count greater than 3000 per cubic mm and the polymorphonuclear leukocyte count greater than 1 to 2000 per cubic mm.

Cyclosporin A

Cyclosporin A is a potent immunosuppressive drug that profoundly inhibits normal T cell activation and function. The primary toxic effects of cyclosporin A include opportunistic infections and renal toxicity. The renal toxicity involves primarily drug induced interstitial nephritis and subsequent irreversible renal fibrosis. Therefore, careful monitoring of serum cyclosporin A levels should be undertaken, keeping the trough serum levels below 200 ng per ml. The serum creatinine level should be followed monthly and the dosage of cyclosporin A reduced or stopped according to the magnitude of creatinine rise. Some investigators advocate renal biopsy to monitor renal damage during long term cyclosporin A therapy. Other potential side effects of cyclosporin A are an increased risk of lymphoid malignant disease, hypertension, tremor, paresthesias, seizures, hypomagnesemia, anorexia, and nausea.

PROS AND CONS OF THERAPY

Since typical Cogan's syndrome has an excellent prognosis, corticosteroid therapy in most cases poses the greatest threat to long term patient survival. Thus, it is imperative to continue to attempt to taper corticosteroid dosages in Cogan's syndrome, preferably with the use of intermittent rather than continuous long term administration. Most patients require steroids only for the first 2 to 6 months after the onset of the disease, with chronic hearing fluctuations due to cochlear hydrops rather than to active cochlear inflammation. Intermittent topical ocular administration of corticosteroids nearly always controls interstitial keratitis. Because of the risk of herpetic keratitis, intermittent rather than long term continuous ocular steroid administration is preferred.

SUGGESTED READING

Cogan DG, Dickersin GR. Nonsyphilitic interstitial keratitis with vestibuloauditory symptoms. A case with fatal aortitis. Arch Ophthalmol 1964; 71:172–175.

Haynes BF, et al. Cogan syndrome: studies in thirteen patients, long-term follow-up, and a review of the literature. Medicine 1980; 59:426–441.

Haynes BF, et al. Successful treatment of sudden hearing loss in Cogan's syndrome with corticosteroids. Arthritis Rheum 1981; 24:501–503.

Norton EWD, Cogan DG. Syndrome of nonsyphilic interstitial keratitis and vestibuloauditory symptoms. A long-term follow-up. Arch Ophthalmol 1959; 61:695–697.

DERMATITIS HERPETIFORMIS

RUSSELL P. HALL, M.D.

Dermatitis herpetiformis is an extremely pruritic papulovesicular disease that most often begins in the second to fourth decade. It is a chronic disease, and although brief clinical remissions do occur, the patient and physician should be aware that lifetime therapy is required in almost all cases. Patients with dermatitis herpetiformis most often present with a severe itching or burning sensation, although in the rare patient only mild itching is described. Patients typically present with papules and vesicles, which occur in groups on extensor surfaces (elbows, knees, buttocks, scapula) and the scalp.

Biopsy of an early papule of dermatitis herpetiformis reveals collections of neutrophils at the dermal-papillary tips (papillary microabscesses) leading to subepidermal blister formation. This histologic picture, however, is not diagnostic for dermatitis herpetiformis, having been noted to occur in some patients with bullous pemphigoid and in patients with the bullous eruption of systemic lupus erythematosus. Biopsy of frankly vesicular lesions of dermatitis herpetiformis or of crusted papules most often does not show the characteristic papillary microabscesses. Direct immunofluorescence of normal appearing perilesional skin reveals either granular deposits of IgA (85 percent of the patients) or a linear band of IgA at the dermal-epidermal junction (15 percent of the patients). Deposits of the third component of the complement system can be seen in patients with dermatitis herpetiformis, but other immunoreactants (IgG, IgM, IgE) are rarely found. Although the clinical presentation and histologic appearance of lesions are for the most part identical in patients with linear or granular IgA deposits, the pattern of the IgA deposits is an important factor in choosing from the therapeutic options available.

Patients with dermatitis herpetiformis and granular IgA deposits have an associated asymptomatic gluten sensitive enteropathy and a high prevalence of the histocompatibility antigens HLA B8 and DR3, and their skin disease often responds to a gluten free diet (to be discussed). Patients with linear IgA deposits, however, do not have an associated gluten sensitive enteropathy; in these cases there is a normal prevalence of HLA antigens B8 and DR3, and there is no evidence to suggest that they respond to a gluten free diet. This finding has resulted in patients with linear IgA deposits being designated as having "linear IgA dermatosis," the term dermatitis herpetiformis being reserved for those with granular IgA deposits.

Because of the severe pruritus that is often present, patients with dermatitis herpetiformis may present with multiple excoriations and crusted lesions and not the typical papules and vesicles. Thus, the correct diagnosis often rests on direct immunofluorescence examination of the skin. Most false negative immunofluorescence tests are a result of obtaining lesional skin for the direct immunofluorescence examination. If normal appearing perilesional skin does not reveal IgA deposits in a patient thought to have dermatitis herpetiformis, direct immunofluorescence examination should be repeated using fresh tissue (without "transport media"), with multiple sections being evaluated for IgA deposits. The clinical response to dapsone therapy is not a useful criterion for the diagnosis of either dermatitis herpetiformis or linear IgA dermatosis.

DRUG THERAPY

The cornerstone of the treatment of both dermatitis herpetiformis and linear IgA dermatosis is the sulfone, dapsone (diaminiodiphenylsulfone). Although sulfapyridine can also be used, it is generally much less effective. Diasone (sulfoxone) is a water soluble derivative of dapsone, and although it is effective in the treatment of dermatitis herpetiformis, it is no longer available in this country. Most patients note a rapid response to dapsone with a marked decrease in the pruritus and cessation of the appearance of new lesions within 12 to 48 hours. Some physicians report that patients with linear IgA dermatosis often require the addition of systemic corticosteroid therapy to control the eruptions, but I have not found that to be necessary.

Although dapsone is an effective drug for the treatment of dermatitis herpetiformis, the presence of potentially serious adverse hematologic effects necessitates careful pretreatment evaluation and close follow-up in all patients taking dapsone. Dapsone causes a dose related hemolysis, which can be severe in patients with glucose-6-phosphate dehydrogenase deficiency. Glucose-6-phosphate dehydrogenase deficiency is most frequently found in blacks, Asians, and those of southern Mediterranean descent. In all these individuals a glucose-6-phosphate dehydrogenase level should be obtained before institution of dapsone therapy. Despite normal glucose-6-phosphate dehydrogenase levels, all patients experience some hemolysis when they take dapsone, which results in a decreased hemoglobin level. Although the amount of hemolysis is minimal at a dosage of 25 to 50 mg of dapsone per day, patients who take 100 to 200 mg of dapsone per day can show up to a 2 g reduction in the hemoglobin level. When the patient is not iron, folate, or vitamin B$_{12}$ deficient, a compensatory reticulocytosis occurs and the hemoglobin level often rises nearly to pretreatment levels. Since the degree of hemolysis is dose related and predictable, it is important to determine that patients with cardiac or pulmonary disease will not be compromised by the expected fall in the hemoglobin level that occurs with dapsone therapy.

Methemoglobinemia also occurs during dapsone therapy in a dose related fashion. This may result in a slate blue discoloration that in general is well tolerated at the levels normally encountered during therapy with 100 to 200 mg of dapsone per day (12 percent methemoglobin or less). However, patients must be made aware of this side effect and carry a card detailing their medication in order to avoid confusion during any possible medical emergency. Symptoms of methemoglobinemia can occur and include weakness, tachycardia, nausea, headache, and abdominal pain, but usually methemoglobin levels of 20 percent or more are required for such symptoms to occur. It is also important to be aware that patients with severe pulmonary or cardiac disease can be symptomatic at relatively low levels of methemoglobin.

The other side effects of dapsone are either idiosyncratic or allergic in nature and are listed in Table 1. For the most part these side effects decrease on discontinuation of the drug. The severe nature of many of these side effects, however, makes it extremely important to follow patients closely and to carefully question and examine patients regarding potential side effects during follow-up visits. Agranulocytosis has been reported in patients taking dapsone but appears to be a rare complication. The agranulocytosis associated with dapsone has always occurred within the first 3 to 4 months of therapy. When this agranulocytosis is recognized promptly, it appears to be reversible following withdrawal of the dapsone. Dapsone has been classified as a "weak carcinogen" in rats; however, similar evidence of carcinogenicity does not exist in humans.

TABLE 1 Adverse Reactions to Dapsone

Pharmacologic reactions
  Hemolysis
  Methemoglobinemia

Idiosyncratic or allergic reactions
  Headache
  Gastric irritation
  Anorexia
  Hepatitis, infectious mononucleosis-like
  Cholestatic jaundice
  Morbilliform eruption
  Erythema nodosum
  Erythema multiforme
  Toxic epidermal necrolysis
  Psychosis
  Leukopenia
  Agranulocytosis
  Hypoalbuminemia
  Peripheral neuropathy (most commonly motor)

The significant pharmacologic and idiosyncratic side effects that can occur during dapsone therapy dictate that before the institution of therapy a complete pretreatment evaluation should be done. This should include a history and physical examination, a complete blood count with a differential, liver and renal function tests, a urinalysis, and when indicated a glucose-6-phosphate dehydrogenase level. After this pretreatment evaluation, I begin therapy with 50 to 100 mg of dapsone per day. The long half-life of dapsone allows most patients to take a single daily dose. Dapsone is well absorbed, and the presence of gluten sensitive enteropathy does not appear to significantly decrease its absorption. Complete blood counts with a differential should be obtained weekly for the first 4 to 6 weeks, then bimonthly for an additional 2 to 3 months, and finally at 8 to 12 week intervals when the patient is taking dapsone. By following the hematologic status closely in the early stages of therapy, it is possible to detect early signs of agranulocytosis before serious morbidity develops and to monitor the expected hemolysis and anemia that occur with dapsone therapy.

Since dapsone is metabolized by the liver and excreted by the kidneys and occasionally can cause hepatitis, it is important to monitor hepatic and renal function at 4 to 6 month intervals. Patients should also be examined at all follow-up visits for distal motor weakness or sensory deficits, because dapsone can cause peripheral neuropathy.

Most patients respond quickly to dapsone, with a marked decrease in both itching and new lesion formation within 24 to 48 hours. After 1 to 2 weeks the dosage should be adjusted to the minimum needed to control symptoms by changing the daily dosage by 25 to 50 mg per day every 1 to 2 weeks. Most patients with dermatitis herpetiformis are controlled by 100 to 150 mg of dapsone per day.

Both the patient and the physician should be aware that some lesions continue to occur during dapsone therapy and that this normal variation in disease activity should not prompt an automatic increase in the dapsone dosage. Patients should be told to expect that they may develop two to four lesions every 1 to 2 weeks and that increasing the dosage of dapsone to eliminate these lesions may result in more significant side effects. When patients experience long periods without any active skin disease, I recommend that the dosage of dapsone be decreased slowly in order to re-establish the minimal amount needed to control symptoms. It should be emphasized to all patients that dapsone is an effective drug that is well tolerated by most patients, but that it has potentially severe side effects that are dose related. In this way the hazards of self-medication are emphasized as is the need for close follow-up.

Sulfapyridine is also an effective drug in the management of dermatitis herpetiformis. Although the side effects of sulfapyridine are less severe than those of dapsone, the drug is also less effective. Therapy can be begun with 500 mg twice daily, and the dosage can be increased to 3 to 4 g per day. Sulfapyridine cannot be taken by patients who are allergic to sulfa drugs, and it must be taken with adequate fluid and close monitoring of renal function because renal calculi can occur. Although in general patients who are thought to be allergic to sulfapyridine can take dapsone and vice versa, rare cases of cross reactivity have been reported. A history of allergy to sulfa drugs is not thought to represent an absolute contraindication to dapsone therapy, but these patients should be observed much more closely for potential adverse effects.

Dermatitis herpetiformis often affects women of childbearing age, and the question of the use of dapsone during pregnancy frequently occurs. There are few data documenting the safety of dapsone during pregnancy. I discuss this issue with the patient at the time of the initial diagnosis and suggest that she adhere to a gluten free diet (to be discussed) during pregnancy. Ideally the diet should be instituted 6 to 12 months before pregnancy so that the dapsone can be totally withdrawn prior to conception and the pregnancy. If this is not possible, I recommend low dose sulfapyridine therapy (500 to 1,000 mg per day) or low dose dapsone therapy (25 to 75 mg per day). The patient's other physicians, including the pediatrician, should be advised of the use of dapsone, and the patient should be told that dapsone is secreted in breast milk and can cause hemolytic anemia in the newborn.

opathy. This association led to trials of a gluten free diet for control of the skin disease. Strict adherence to a gluten free diet can allow a decrease in the dapsone dosage by 50 percent or more after use of the diet for 9 to 16 months in 60 to 80 percent of the patients with dermatitis herpetiformis. Thirty-five to 60 percent of the patients can stop the dapsone therapy by adhering to a gluten free diet. It should be emphasized that there is no evidence to support the use of a gluten free diet in patients with linear IgA dermatosis.

The successful use of a gluten free diet in patients with dermatitis herpetiformis requires the strict avoidance of all foods containing wheat, oats, rye, and barley. Wheat additives are often found in some ice cream, sauces, and other foods, making it imperative that the patient read all labels and consult a dietician regarding the complexities of this diet. Patients also should be made aware of the fact that it may take up to 2 years to notice benefit from the diet and that as many as 25 to 30 percent of the patients may not respond to the diet. Despite these drawbacks the gluten free diet is a means of controlling dermatitis herpetiformis without medication in the well motivated patient. Patients who are interested in trying the gluten free diet should be made aware of the resources available from the National Celiac-Sprue Society (5 Jeffrey Road, Wayland, MA 01778), which can help in the planning and executing of such a diet.

In summary, the mainstay of treatment of dermatitis herpetiformis with both granular IgA deposits and linear IgA dermatosis remains dapsone. In the well motivated patient with dermatitis herpetiformis and granular IgA deposits, a gluten free diet may allow the patient to substantially decrease the dosage of dapsone needed to control the disease. At the time of the initial diagnosis I discuss with the patient the therapeutic options available, and if no contraindications are found in the initial evaluation, I begin therapy with 100 mg of dapsone per day. It the patient is willing to follow a gluten free diet, I suggest that he also begin the diet at this time with the goal of decreasing the dapsone dosage over the following 6 to 18 months. It is important to realize that dermatitis herpetiformis is a chronic disease marked by unexplained periods of increased severity and that in many patients it is impossible to totally control the occurrence of blisters without intolerable drug side effects. Neither the physician nor the patient should regard the occasional occurrence of lesions (two to three per week) as an indication to increase the dosage of dapsone. A constant effort must be made to reduce the medication to the minimal dosage needed to control the symptoms of dermatitis herpetiformis and therefore minimize many of the adverse effects of dapsone.

DIETARY MANAGEMENT

Patients with dermatitis herpetiformis and granular IgA deposits have an associated gluten sensitive enter-

SUGGESTED READING

Fry L, Leonard JN, Swain F, Tucker WFG, Haffenden G, Ring N, McMinn RMH. Long-term follow-up of dermatitis herpetiformis with and without dietary gluten withdrawal. Br J Dermatol 1982; 107:631–640.

Hall RP. Dietary management of dermatitis herpetiformis. Arch Dermatol 1987; 123:1378a–1380a.

Katz SI, moderator, Hall RP III, Lawley TJ, Strober W, discussants.

Dermatitis herpetiformis: the skin and gut. Treatment: drugs and diet. Ann Intern Med 1980; 93:857–874.

Lang PG Jr. Sulfones and sulfonamides in dermatology today. J Am Acad Dermatol 1979; 1:479–492.

HERPES GESTATIONIS

KIM B. YANCEY, M.D.

Herpes gestationis is a rare nonviral subepidermal blistering disease of pregnancy and the puerperium. Its designation is a misnomer, since it has no association with a viral infection; instead this term refers to the herpetiform or grouped distribution of lesions in patients with this disorder.

Herpes gestationis may begin during any trimester of pregnancy or may present shortly after delivery. Lesions are usually distributed over the abdomen (frequently within the umbilicus) and the extremities. Although widespread involvement may affect the palms, soles, chest, and back, mucous membrane lesions are rare. The morphology of the lesions can be varied and may include erythematous urticarial papules and plaques, vesiculopapules, or frank bullae. Lesions are almost always very pruritic. Severe exacerbations frequently occur after delivery (i.e., within 24 to 48 hours), and the patient should be carefully evaluated at this time even if the disease was previously controlled by treatment or was inactive.

Herpes gestationis tends to recur in subsequent pregnancies, often beginning earlier during these gestations. In addition, it may flare briefly with the resumption of menses after delivery and may recur if the patient is exposed to oral contraceptive therapy. Occasionally infants born of affected mothers also demonstrate cutaneous lesions; however, these lesions are usually transient and last no longer than the first few weeks of life. Although somewhat controversial, several groups of investigators currently believe that herpes gestationis is associated with an increased risk of fetal morbidity and mortality.

Herpes gestationis is thought to be immunologically mediated. Direct immunofluorescence microscopy of normal perilesional skin from patients with herpes gestationis reveals the immunologic hallmark of this disorder—linear deposits of C3 (the third component of complement) in the epidermal basement membrane zone. Biopsy specimens from 40 to 50 percent of these patients also demonstrate linear deposits of IgG at the same location, and it is hypothesized that an avid complement

fixing IgG autoantibody is responsible for C3 deposits in both patients and their offspring. The cause of autoantibody formation in this disease is unknown, but its relationship to pregnancy suggests that it may be hormonally modulated.

To make the diagnosis of this disorder, it is advisable to obtain skin for demonstration of immunoreactants in situ (specifically, linear deposits of C3 in the epidermal basement membrane zone). This diagnostic approach is favored over attempting to demonstrate a circulating IgG autoantibody directed against the epidermal basement membrane, since this factor is found with routine indirect immunofluorescence microscopy techniques in a minority of these patients.

It is essential that the patient's obstetrician be informed about this skin disease, its potential complications, and its treatment regimen. In herpes gestationis the goal of therapy is to prevent the development of new lesions, relieve the intense pruritus associated with this disorder, and care for any erosions at sites of blister formation. Specific therapeutic measures depend on the character, extent, and severity of the eruption. Most patients with herpes gestationis require treatment with moderate daily doses of systemic corticosteroids. Twenty to 40 mg of prednisone daily usually provides substantial clinical and symptomatic relief within several days; divided doses (i.e., given every 12 hours) may hasten initial improvement in more symptomatic or extensive cases. When the eruption and symptoms have been controlled, the prednisone dosage should be tapered by approximately 5 mg every 1 to 2 weeks until only an occasional lesion develops or symptoms recur. If a postpartum exacerbation of herpes gestationis occurs, prednisone therapy should be restarted at a dosage of 20 to 40 mg daily; postpartum patients who are unable to tolerate oral medication can be treated with an equivalent daily amount of hydrocortisone given intravenously. Rarely postpartum exacerbations of herpes gestationis are severe and may require treatment with high doses of systemic corticosteroids (i.e., greater than or equal to 100 mg of prednisone daily) or immunosuppressive drugs. All patients receiving treatment after delivery should be counseled about appropriate nursing practices.

Exacerbations associated with the resumption of menses are usually mild and normally can be managed by a small daily dose of prednisone (e.g., 20 mg) or vigorous topical use of a corticosteroid cream alone. In mild cases of herpes gestationis, the vigorous topical use of potent corticosteroids such as fluocinonide, 0.05 percent (Lidex), or triamcinolone acetonide, 0.5 percent

(Aristocort), four to six times each day may control the eruption and obviate the need for systemic treatment. As with systemic therapy, topical treatment with corticosteroids in patients with herpes gestationis should be tapered gradually to the least effective dose. Weeping moist skin lesions can be dried with open wet dressings of saline or tap water used for 10 minutes three to four times each day. Erosions should be carefully inspected for sites of secondary infection.

Although patients with herpes gestationis receiving systemic corticosteroid therapy usually demonstrate prompt clinical improvement, it is not known whether this therapy affects fetal prognosis. Current evidence suggests that there is no significant difference in the incidence of uncomplicated live births between patients treated with systemic corticosteroid therapy and those treated with topical corticosteroid preparations. At present there are few human data to substantiate the notion that the treatment of pregnant patients with systemic corticosteroid therapy places the fetus at increased risk. However, as emphasized earlier, the minimal effective dose of these drugs is the preferred regimen, and modest disease activity (i.e., a few vesicles or plaques) is clearly acceptable in these patients. The decision to treat a pregnant patient with systemic corticosteroid therapy should be made in conjunction with the patient's obstetrician and should be based on the extent, severity, and symptomatology of skin disease. If systemic corticosteroid therapy is used, the prospective pediatrician should be aware of this treatment, since reversible adrenal insufficiency may occur in these infants following delivery.

SUGGESTED READING

Holmes RC, Black MM. The fetal prognosis in pemphigold gestationis (herpes gestationis). Br J Dermatol 1984; 110:67–72.

Katz SI, Provost TT. Herpes gestationis. In: Fitzpatrick TB, et al., eds. Dermatology in general medicine. 3rd ed. New York: McGraw-Hill, 1987: 586–589.

Lawley TJ, Stingl G, Katz SI. Fetal and maternal risk factors in herpes gestationis. Arch Dermatol 1979; 114:552–555.

Shornick JK, Bangert JL, Freeman RG, Gilliam JN. Herpes gestationis: clinical and histologic features of twenty-eight cases. J Am Acad Dermatol 1983; 8:214–224.

Sharnick JK. Herpes gestationis. J Am Acad Dermatol 1987; 17:539–556.

ATOPIC DERMATITIS

KEVIN D. COOPER, M.D.
ALAIN TAÏEB, M.D.

Treating a patient with atopic dermatitis is largely a matter of teaching skills. Educating the patient—or the parents if the patient is a child—is a time consuming task, especially at the beginning, but generally turns out to be the most rewarding approach when a satisfactory degree of self-management can be achieved.

Atopic dermatitis is the most common chronic skin disorder in infancy and childhood. Later onset cases may occur in early adulthood, are generally more recalcitrant, and bear an overall worse prognosis. Diagnostic criteria have been established for the diagnosis of atopic dermatitis. The major criteria include a positive family history of atopy, a chronic or chronically relapsing course, eczematous lesions of symmetrical distribution (involving mostly extensor surfaces in infants and flexural lichenification later), and low thresholds for pruritogenic stimuli, such as external irritants, sweating, and emotions. Before 3 months of age, pruritus is not noticeable and the rash may present as a recalcitrant bipolar seborrheic dermatitis.

Clinical and in vitro studies in atopic dermatitis point to a polygenic inherited defect involving abnormalities of the immune system, transduction of biochemical and hormonal signals into cells, and vascular reactivity. In combination with environmental influences these abnormalities result in a vicious cycle of self-perpetuating pathologic changes in the skin and immune system.

Certain of these abnormalities, listed in Table 1, offer potential sites of action for systemic drug therapy. However, there remains a large gap in the understanding of the relationship between the data gathered from in vitro studies and the clinical manifestations. Therefore, treatment remains largely supportive and palliative. The management of atopic dermatitis includes assessment of severity and factors of prognosis (summarized in Table 2), skin care and therapy adapted to age, type, site, and stage of lesions (acute versus chronic), and prevention of complications, with special emphasis on herpetic and staphylococcal superinfections, as well as prevention of exposure to irritants and allergens.

Two general principles ought to guide the physician. First, simplicity of therapeutic measures allows better adherence to prescriptions. The patient given too many topical medications may become confused as to their appropriate time and site of application, and accumulation of prescriptions may lead to long term storage, which in turn may compromise the efficacy of the drugs.

Second, clear and complete explanations about

TABLE 1 Pathophysiologic Data and Possible Targets for Therapy

Abnormal humoral immunity

Hyper IgE, frequent if atopic dermatitis is associated with asthma: Avoid exposure to airborne, contact, and food allergens? Specific desensitization beneficial only in rare cases.

Increased intestinal permeability and transient IgA deficiency in infancy: Elimination of potent food allergens in the first year of life? Treat any diarrhea vigorously.

Abnormal cell mediated immunity

Decreased T suppressor-cytotoxic cells and cutaneous delayed type hypersensitivity: Immunomodulators? Antibiotics and antiviral therapy as needed for complications.

Impaired neutrophil and monocyte chemotaxis: Antibiotic therapy for infectious complications.

Pharmacologic and metabolic anomalies

Altered cyclic nucleotide (cAMP) metabolism in leukocytes: Phosphodiesterase inhibitors (topical caffeine use).

"Easy releasability" of mast cells: Avoidance of triggering agents and events, mast cell stabilization: Cromolyn? Steroids, antihistamines.

bathing, skin care, prescription use, and topical medicament use are needed. Prescriptions should be explained thoroughly, and a handout may be useful to reinforce the most important points (available from the American Academy of Dermatology, Evanston, IL). For example, even techniques for bathing infants require instructions in order to avoid adverse consequences. In severe cases demonstration of appropriate handling of topical treatment by specialized personnel on an outpa-

TABLE 2 Initial Assessment: Factors Influencing Prognosis and Management

Genetic background

Bilateral atopic heredity

Atopic dermatitis symptomatic of primary immunodeficiency (Wiscott-Aldrich syndrome, hyper IgE syndrome)

Associated ichthyosis vulgaris

Clinical features

Age at onset >2 yr

Inverted pattern of lesions

Hand eczema

Severity of rash (surface involved, acuteness of lesions, duration of attacks)

Delay and degree of response to correctly administered treatment

Severe herpetic infection

Environmental factors

Poor psychologic environment

Exposure to irritants and allergens (inhalant or cutaneous)

Biologic features

Generally clinical evaluation and history suffice; high and very high (>10,000) IgE levels generally associated with severe disease

tient basis is the best choice for children, but hospitalization is sometimes required for a more complete assessment of the disease and the therapeutic response.

DERMATOLOGIC MANAGEMENT

Since atopic dermatitis has a spontaneous course of relapsing acute exacerbations followed by more or less durable periods of improvement, a two step approach is detailed here (acute disease and maintenance management). Whatever the case, treatment is aimed at relieving pruritus, cutaneous inflammation, and superinfection. The rational use of topical corticosteroid therapy dominates all stages of therapy, but antibiotic therapy, skin hydration, the use of antihistamines, recognition of complicating conditions, and counseling are all important in the management of atopic dermatitis. Some of the myriad of corticosteroid preparations available are presented in Table 3, and an outline regarding their use can be found in Table 4. Familiarity with a single formulation from each category is generally sufficient. In the authors' experience combinations of corticosteroids with antimicrobial drugs for topical application are not particularly useful. Bases containing sensitizing compounds are also best avoided.

Acute Dermatitis

Acute flares of atopic dermatitis can occur as weeping crusted eruptions or in other cases may occur as erythema with or without scales, which can be so extensive as to constitute a generalized exfoliative erythroderma. The initial assessment should always survey previous treatments with special attention directed toward the possible deleterious effects of topical therapy. Application of nonprescription drugs can aggravate a case of moderate severity because of idiosyncratic intolerance, use of irritants or inappropriate drugs, or in rare instances allergic contact dermatitis. Examples of contact allergens include balsam of Peru, lanolin, neomycin, and preservatives contained in creams. In patients with rapid aggravation associated with wet vesiculopustular or crusted lesions, herpes simplex superinfection must be suspected (eczema herpeticum). Especially in cases of dramatic skin changes associated with fever and malaise in an infant, the most severe form of eczema herpeticum, Kaposi's varicelliform eruption, should be considered. Bacterial and viral culture results may take several days, but Giemsa or Wright stained smears of scrapings of the base of vesiculopustular lesions (Tzanck's smear) may provide rapid confirmation of the diagnosis by revealing the presence of multinucleated keratinocytes.

The rapid institution of combined antiherpetic-antistaphylococcal therapy is indicated. Parenteral admin-

TABLE 3 Classification of Corticosteroids for Topical Use

Potency	Concentration*	Base†	Quantity Supplied‡
Very potent			
Clobetasol propionate (Temovate)	0.05	C, O	15, 30
Betamethasone dipropionate (Diprolene)	0.05	O	15, 45
Potent			
Triamcinolone acetonide (Kenalog, Aristocort)	0.5	C O	15, 20, 240 15, 20
Halcinonide (Halog)	0.1 0.1	C, O L	15, 30, 60, 240 20, 60 ml
Fluocinonide (Lidex)	0.05 0.05 0.05	C, CE, O L Gel	15, 45, 110, 430 20, 60 ml 15, 30, 60, 120
Betamethasone 17-valerate (Valisone)	0.1 0.1 0.1	C O L	15, 45, 110, 430 15, 45 20, 60 ml
Desoximetasone (Topicort)	0.25 0.25	CE O	15, 60; 4 oz 15, 60
Diflorasone diacetate (Florone, Maxiflor)	0.05	C, O	15, 30, 60
Amcinonide (Cyclocort)	0.1	C, O	15, 30, 60
Moderately potent			
Triamcinolone acetonide (Aristocort, Kenalog)	0.1 0.1 0.1	C O L	15, 60, 80, 240; 1, 5 lb 15, 60, 80, 240; 1, 5 lb 15, 60
Fluocinolone acetonide (Fluonid, Synalar)	0.025 0.025	C, O L	15, 30, 60, 120, 425 20, 60 ml
Flurandrenolide (Cordran)	0.05	C, O L	15, 30, 60, 225 15, 60 ml
Hydrocortisone butyrate (Locoid)§	0.1	C, O	15, 45
Mildly potent			
Triamcinolone acetonide (Aristocort, Kenalog)	0.025	C	15, 60, 80, 240; 1, 5 lb
Desonide (Tridesilon)§	0.05	C O	15, 60; 5 lb 15, 60
Hydrocortisone valerate (Wescort)§	0.2	C O	15, 45, 60, 120 15, 45, 60
Alclometasone dipropionate (Aclovate)§	0.05	C, O	15, 45
Weak			
Hydrocortisone (Hytone)§	1.0	C O	1, 4 oz 1 oz

*Concentration in % w/w. For clarity, only triamcinolone acetonide has been indicated in three different concentrations. The other molecules appear only in their highest available concentration.
†C, Cream. O, ointment. CE, cream-emollient.
‡Quantity supplied expressed in grams if no other mention.
§Non-fluorinated molecules.

istration of acyclovir (15 mg per kg per day) and methicillin (25 mg per kg every 6 hours) can be changed to oral therapy after 5 days. Milder forms of eczema herpeticum are not unusual in older patients; they are recognizable as punctate erosions that may be associated with more typical vesicles distributed over involved cutaneous areas. Simple acute bullous staphylococcal impetigo sometimes masquerades as eczema herpeticum.

Once these complications have been ruled out, treatment of acute flares of disease can proceed as follows:

TABLE 4   Topical Use of Corticosteroid in Atopic Dermatitis

TABLE 4   Topical Use of Corticosteroid in Atopic Dermatitis

Contraindications

Current cutaneous infection

Potent fluorinated corticosteroid on face

Diaper area: risk of systemic toxicity by plastic diaper occlusion: local side effects potentiated by maceration (infection, granuloma gluteale infantum)

General rules of use

Acute oozing lesions: creams, nonalcoholic lotions of moderate potency

Chronic lichenified lesions and skin of extremities: cream or ointment of potent or very potent CS; occlusion helpful in some instances

Scalp: gels and lotions

Consider comfort of patient: ointments indicated in cases of dry skin or associated ichthyosis but difficult to treat on an outpatient basis

Prefer use of commercially available preparations rather than custom compounding

Adapt quantity to involved surface

Two applications per day are sufficient (tachyphylaxis); with potent and very potent derivatives, one application per day may suffice

Monitoring of prescription

Note quantity used at each follow-up visit

Do not allow numerous automatic renewals

Check for local side effects (atrophy, infection, depigmentation) and systemic side effects (hypercorticism), especially in infants or if large quantities and occlusion are required

Acute Weeping Crusted Eczematous Dermatitis

This manifestation is most frequent in children and is almost always associated with heavy colonization and superinfection with *Staphylococcus aureus*. Initial management should be directed toward reduction of cutaneous *Staphylococcus aureus,* since this is an inciting source of inflammation as well as a source of further recontamination through scratching.

1. An antibacterial liquid soap (chlorhexidine) can be applied by gently rubbing crusted areas with soap gauze.

2. Rinse completely in the tub, since retention of this type of soap results in dry itchy skin, gently removing remaining crusts after a few minutes of soaking.

3. The skin is partially dried by patting with a smooth towel. Then an antibiotic cream such as silver sulfadiazine or gentamicin is immediately applied to affected sites and covered with gauze (tubular gauze dressings are very convenient in infants).

4. This treatment is justified twice daily in severe cases for the first day or couple of days. After sufficient disinfection (24 to 36 hours), topical corticosteroid therapy can be introduced, using a cream at the beginning, twice a day, from the moderately potent category (Table 3).

5. Quantities should be monitored precisely. A recent survey of severe cases in infants admitted as inpatients showed that 30 to 50 g of a moderately potent corticosteroid cream can clear the rash within a 4 to 6 day period in most instances. The quantities used can be reduced by application to moist, lightly pat-dried skin, allowing better spreading.

6. Accessory measures include oral doses of antistaphylococcal antibiotics, mainly erythromycin and dicloxacillin. In addition, antihistamines are useful to minimize pruritus and excoriation.

Maintenance Therapy

Once clearing of an acute flare occurs, proper skin care is essential for long term maintenance in chronic dermatitis. During the transition period topical steroid therapy is gradually tapered over a period of several weeks. In moderate disease generally two to three applications per week of a moderately potent steroid suffices. In children a 30 g tube is often enough for 6 to 8 weeks, whereas adults may require up to two 60 g tubes for a similar period. To reduce costs, adult patients with extensive disease can be given prescriptions for generic triamcinolone, 0.025 or 0.1 percent cream in 1 pound sizes.

The patient's bathing habits should be strictly regulated: Bathing should be restricted to an every other day or every third day frequency. The patient should be instructed that the baths are not to be scalding, that the shower is preferable to the bath, and that the duration of the shower or bath should not be excessive. The patient should be instructed that soaps are to be used only in the axilla and groin, using a mild soap such as Dove or Basis, and that the soap is to be rinsed off completely. Foam or bubble baths should be avoided.

Immediately upon exiting from the bath or shower the patient should apply emollients, such as a heavy cream based emollient (Eucerin cream). Some patients with heavily lichenified, thickened skin can tolerate heavier preparations, such as Aquaphor, but the occlusive properties of ointment-like preparations are uncomfortable for most patients with atopic dermatitis. Some cannot tolerate even a cream based emollient such as Eucerin and can only tolerate lotions such as Shepherd's lotion, Lubriderm, or Keri lotion. Bath oils also can be directly applied to the skin. Emollients applied to inflamed skin can be irritating.

Patients should be instructed to repeat application of the emollient as many times during the day as is necessary to keep the skin moist. For extreme xerosis, as in atopic dermatitis associated with ichthyosis vulgaris, a lactic acid containing emollient is helpful (Lacticare, Lac-Hydrin). Recommendations for emollients may have to be altered in response to changing climatic conditions. The extreme dryness and low humidity of winter often require heavy creams and more frequent applications than in summer months. Steroid preparations for topical use should not be substituted for emollients. Children who are unable to be tapered off topical steroid therapy with proper skin care should be re-evaluated.

As regards clothing, wool or acrylic sweaters should not be in direct contact with skin. Most patients do not tolerate handling raw foods or wet work with the hands, and patients who must be involved in such situations are advised to use cotton liners under protective rubber or plastic gloves. Atopic dermatitis is a common cause of occupational hand eczema. In some patients sweating associated with excessive physical exercise is poorly tolerated, but counseling in this respect should emphasize that the goal is to allow the patient a life as normal as possible.

SYSTEMIC THERAPY

Systemic Antihistamine Therapy

The systemic administration of antihistamines can benefit the patient by reducing pruritus and excoriations, particularly at night. For adults, hydroxyzine, 25 to 200 mg at bedtime, or diphenhydramine in similar doses is often a useful starting point. Pediatric doses of 5 mg per kg per day in syrup or elixir are used. However, the use of antihistamines in children should be limited to flares. Poor responses to these can be followed by the use of antihistamines from each of the major antihistamine categories. Another useful class of drugs is the tricyclic antidepressants, which exert potent anti-H_1 and H_2 activity. These can be used in adults in 25 to 75 mg oral doses at bedtime (e.g., doxepin hydrochloride or amitriptyline hydrochloride).

Antibiotics

As already stated, the use of antibiotics is helpful in acute exacerbations. In some cases with associated nummular lesions, the long term administration of erythromycin or dicloxacillin may reduce the frequency of flares.

Phototherapy

Patients with large surface area involvement and recalcitrant disease (adolescents and adults mostly, but also occasionally children) may benefit from a course of biweekly or thrice weekly exposure to banks of ultra-violet light emitting bulbs. UVB, UVB with UVA, and UVA in combination with oral doses of methoxypsoralen (PUVA) have been used successfully. Results are not long lasting.

Ketoconazole

Ketoconazole has been advocated in patients with prominent face and neck involvement and an immediate hypersensitivity to *Pityrosporon ovale*.

Corticosteroids

In extremely severe, disabling cases unresponsive to topical management in which compliance with all aspects of the regimen has been verified, systemic prednisone therapy can be used. A 2 week course of prednisone, 40 to 60 mg a day, will result in improvement. However, tapering of the prednisone dosage often results in a rebound flare, and repeated uses of 2 week bursts of prednisone to manage acute flares of the disease often results in the inability to taper the patient off prednisone and patients become committed to long term oral steroid therapy. For this reason it is best to avoid the systemic use of steroids for atopic dermatitis except in the most severe cases, when infection is under control.

ALLERGY MANAGEMENT

The role of allergen avoidance in atopic dermatitis is at best controversial. Food allergy resulting in histamine release and skin lesions has been documented in a small percentage of patients with atopic dermatitis.

The food allergens most commonly implicated are cow's milk, eggs, fish, and nuts. Although conventional breast feeding does not seem to be superior to formula in clinical trials, in cases of a clear atopic hereditary predisposition a preventive diet avoiding those items may be recommended for both the feeding mother and her child. An artificial formula devoid of cow's milk proteins (soybean hydrolysate or a similar product) is an alternative. The introduction of potential allergens should be delayed for up to 6 months for cow's milk and 12 months for eggs and fish. In severe cases with a suspicion of food allergy, a more complete work-up may be indicated, including exclusion diets and food challenges. However, since the likelihood of successful therapy using dietary manipulation is low, this approach should be used rarely in order to avoid malnutrition in the child.

Maintaining a low level of airborne allergens in the environment is not easy, but preventing asthma or allergic rhinitis is perhaps worthwhile in the ''at risk'' baby. This can be achieved by using frequent vacuum cleaning with water vacuum or wall vacuum vented to the outside to avoid aerosolization of small dust mite allergens, removing dust with a wet sponge, and avoiding carpets and other known shelters for house dust mites. Pet animals are not recommended. When present, they should be kept outside the home. An allergic cough or asthma may begin before the end of the second year and deserves a search for causative allergens. Allergen desensitization is generally not effective in clearing the skin of patients with active atopic dermatitis. Therefore, specific densensitization is rarely worth attempting, since only rare patients show some improvement.

PSYCHOLOGIC SUPPORT

Psychologic support is crucial for the patient and family. Flares are often associated with life stresses, and patients are often grateful to be asked about such recent stress events. Presentation of an overly optimistic prognosis to patients and families of atopic patients may result in frustration. Patients and the families of patients with severe disease must make adjustments for dealing with a chronic disease. Patients or their parents should be given continued positive reinforcement and encouragement to maintain their efforts toward skin care, since this may affect the overall course of the disease, and since their efforts may provide an acceptable life for themselves or their child. Psychologic counseling is indicated for families contending with frustration, depression, guilt, and manipulative behavior.

SUGGESTED READING

Hanifin JM, Cooper KD, Roth HL. Atopy and atopic dermatitis. J Am Acad Dermatol 1986; 15:703–706.
Rajka G, Braathen LR, eds. Proceedings of first international symposium on atopic dermatitis. Acta Dermatol Venereol (Suppl) (Stockh) 1980; 92:1–136.
Sampson HA, Jolie PL. Increased plasma histamine concentrations after food challenges in children with atopic dermatitis. N Engl J Med 1984; 311:372–376.
Taieb A, Body S, Astar I, du Pasquier P, Maleville J. Clinical epidemiology of symptomatic primary herpetic infection in children: a study of 50 cases. Acta Paediatr Scand 1987; 76:128–132.
Waersted A, Hjorth N. Pityrosporum orbiculare—a pathogenic factor in atopic dermatitis of the face, scalp and neck? Acta Dermatol Venereol (Suppl) (Stockh) 1985; 114:146–148.

CONTACT DERMATITIS

FRANCES J. STORRS, M.D.

Contact dermatitis is one of the most common job related skin diseases. Both at home and in the work place it is caused by irritants approximately 80 percent of the time and by allergens 20 percent of the time. Once an individual has developed chronic irritant or allergic contact dermatitis, full recovery is not likely. Consequently early aggressive treatment of acute disease and palliative or ameliorating therapy for chronic disease are all the more important. Such an approach returns workers to their jobs and people to their lives more rapidly and assists in minimizing the multimillion dollar costs of job related skin disease.

Irritant dermatitis is usually associated with life situations characterized by water abuse of the skin. It is not mediated immunologically. Housewives, dentists and dental hygienists, food handlers, machinists, and hospital workers frequently develop irritant hand dermatitis. Atopic patients with a childhood history of hand dermatitis are especially likely to develop hand dermatitis in wet work jobs.

Allergic contact dermatitis is a delayed hypersensitivity reaction of the type IV sort, which requires the interaction of complete antigen, Langerhans' cells, lymphocytes, and cytokines for its induction and expression.

The simplest treatment of acute irritant dermatitis is removal of the person from the wet work environment, coupled with some topical maneuvers. It may be prevented if predisposed atopic patients are encouraged to secure dry employment. Acute allergic contact dermatitis requires systemic corticosteroid therapy as well as identification and removal of the offending allergen. Learning about sources for allergen replacement is essential in treating and preventing allergic contact dermatitis.

The management of chronic irritant and allergic contact dermatitis is more difficult and may require the diagnostic and therapeutic skills of a dermatologist.

THE ROLE OF WATER

Water applied to and slowly evaporated from the skin initially helps "dry up" the vesicles associated with acute allergic contact dermatitis. Overuse of water on predisposed skin results in a fractured stratum corneum (xerosis or eczema craquelé), erythema, and associated inflammation of the underlying skin (irritant dermatitis). "Dishpan" hands are a result of such frequent wetting and drying. By the same token, chapped lips (licking) or dry body skin (too many baths in an overheated, low humidity environment) might be understood as "dishpan" face or "dishpan" body.

Such a simple understanding of water's effect on the skin allows a physician to instruct his patient more rationally about its role in therapy.

Wet Dressings and Soaks

Vesiculating allergic contact dermatitis or oozing irritant dermatitis benefits from intense but brief wet dressings. These may be applied as immersion soaks or as thin wet fabric dressings. Dryness is effected by wetting and slow evaporation. A dermatitic extremity might be placed in an aluminum sulfate, povidone-iodine, chlorhexidine, or silver nitrate solution for 20 to 30 minutes (Table 1). It is removed and air dried only to be reimmersed until dryness is achieved, which seldom takes more than 2 days. Overtreatment results in a secondary irritant dermatitis.

Fabric dressings utilize textiles such as loosely woven gauze (Kerlix) or thin fabrics no thicker than a sheet. The fabric is soaked with plain water or with aluminum sulfate, povidone-iodine, or silver nitrate solution applied wet, but not dripping, as a single or two or three layered covering on the affected body part (see Table 1). Ideally the dressing is removed, rewetted, and reapplied before it has fully dried on the patient (every 20 to 30 minutes). This maneuver dries, debrides, and vasoconstricts by cooling. Solution may be added to the in-place dressing for efficiency, but if this is done too frequently, it increases the solute's concentration to an irritating level. Covering a wet dressing with plastic, as

TABLE 1 Solutions for Wet Dressings or Soaks

Aluminum sulfate and calcium acetate (Burows)

One tablet or packet (Domeboro) in 1 pint of water makes a 1:40 dilution (compresses); 1:20 dilution is better for soaks

Silver nitrate, 10% solution*

1/2 oz. in 1½ quarts of water makes a 1:1000 dilution; good for soaks and compresses; stains most surfaces

Povidone-iodine solution*

Betadine solution may be used full strength as a soak; dilute 1:5 for in-place wet dressings; watch for irritation

Chlorhexidine gluconate*

Hibiclens is a 4% solution of chlorhexidine gluconate in a sudsing base; use as a 1:8 dilution for soaks only

* Useful for secondarily infected contact dermatitis.

is often done in hospitals to retard drying and protect bed clothing, can accentuate the concentration problem and provoke maceration as an additional side effect. Diaper dermatitis is an example of such a wet dressing "gone wrong." Like immersion therapy, wet dressings also result in secondary irritant dermatitis if used too long. Few skins benefit from more than 2 days of therapy.

Water in Cream Bases

A cream that is white contains water. If a cream or lotion "rubs into the skin" and leaves "no greasy film," it does that because it is mostly water and the water has evaporated. It is not hard to understand that the frequent use of a very watery cream or lotion in either irritant or allergic contact dermatitis can act like a chronically applied wet dressing and perpetuate or worsen any dermatitis even if that cream contains a potent corticosteroid. Additionally the presence of water in the cream requires humectants such as propylene glycol, preservatives, surfactants, and fragrances, all of which can cause irritation or sensitization.

Thus, in treating a more chronic irritant dermatitis, and especially in a chronic and undiagnosed case of probable allergic contact dermatitis, the use of ointment formulations based on plain petrolatum or Plastibase (Squibb; a mineral oil polymer) avoids the drying effects of water and the irritants and potential sensitizers used in cream formulations. Not all ointments are based simply on petrolatum or Plastibase and thus labels must be read. Aristocort (Lederle), Locoid (Owen), Westcort (Westwood), and Kenalog and Halog (Squibb) are petrolatum or Plastibase based, corticosteroid containing ointments.

To "trap" water in the stratum corneum, ointments should be applied when the skin is wet (after washing or in a humid bathroom). Some jobs (e.g., secretarial) make the use of ointments impractical. In such situations compromises are developed that utilize cream formulations during working hours and ointments on breaks and at night.

Often chronic irritant dermatitis can be treated successfully by stopping the use of watery creams and lotions and using only ointments (petrolatum) or creams that contain less water and leave a greasy film on the skin (do not "rub in").

Water Avoidance

Switching to a dry job is the best way to treat irritant dermatitis resulting from wet work. Water abuse worsens and perpetuates both irritant and allergic contact dermatitis. Occasionally a person with irritant dermatitis in a wet work job can avoid water enough to continue working. A significant decrease in hand washing frequency helps. Substituting a mild cleansing liquid such as Cetaphil (Owen) for hand washing is also useful; the Cetaphil is wiped off without adding water. Some waterless cleansers used in dirty industries are based on strong solvents and contain a good deal of water and may actually worsen irritant dermatitis.

Rubber gloves help minimize irritant dermatitis if separate cotton gloves are worn inside the water repellent gloves. Inexpensive, thin cotton gloves can be purchased in notion departments and from photography supply stores. Rubber gloves may cause secondary allergy, in which case vinyl gloves* may save the day. As soon as gloves are removed, the dermatitic hands must be treated with an ointment to trap the water.

The use of protective clothing, including gloves, is essential in protecting workers from chemical and physical irritants. Numerous types of barrier creams are available. They offer little protection from water, irritants, or allergies.

SYSTEMIC CORTICOSTEROID THERAPY

Acute allergic contact dermatitis that is extensive and severe is effectively treated by the prompt use of systemic corticosteroid therapy. Severe irritant dermatitis also can be treated with corticosteroids, but it is seldom necessary.

Corticosteroids work within 12 to 24 hours to "turn around" allergic contact dermatitis if the dose is high enough. Untreated allergic contact dermatitis such as poison oak or poison ivy dermatitis lasts 2 to 3 weeks. Thus, too short a duration and too low a dose are the commonest reasons for treatment failures.

Oral therapy with prednisone is the corticosteroid of choice because of its long record of use, extensive study, and low cost. It is short acting and thus can be given twice a day for the first few days of therapy. Single morning doses are also effective, however, and are unlikely to significantly blunt the pituitary-adrenal axis. There is little or no evidence to support the tapering of systemic doses of steroids when they are given to healthy persons for 2 weeks or less. The "dose packs" of longer acting, very expensive, elaborately packaged, tapering oral doses of steroids are an unnecessary indulgence. The dose drops too low too fast and the disease flares.

An average adult with acute allergic contact dermatitis responds promptly to 60 to 80 mg of prednisone given each morning for 1 week and then 30 or 40 mg each morning for an additional week. The only reason to lower the dose the second week is that with doses above 60 mg many people experience mood changes (elation or depression), agitation, sleeplessness, and increased appetite. Once the dermatitis is controlled, the prednisone dose can be lowered to a more comfortable level. These dose levels are not rigid and may be adjusted up or down depending on the patient's response. Because corticosteroids work rapidly, prescribing the 5 mg tablet allows the physician more flexibility. If prednisone must be given in high doses for more than 3 weeks to control dermatitis, the diagnosis should be suspect and a dermatologic consultation should be obtained.

Short courses of prednisone are all but side effect-free. Nevertheless people with diabetes, hypertension, peptic ulcer disease, infections, and recent myocardial infarcts should be treated very cautiously or not at all. In this regard it is noteworthy that on occasion 60 to 100 mg of prednisone given for only one to three doses may benefit acute allergic contact dermatitis so much that it can then be managed topically. This manipulation can be of value in promptly treating people with recurrent allergic contact dermatitis resulting from a known allergen that cannot be avoided.

Some physicians treat acute allergic contact dermatitis with intramuscular corticosteroid therapy. It is impossible to accurately control or adjust the steroid dose or to manage side effects when the intramuscular route is used.

TOPICAL CORTICOSTEROID THERAPY

Acute weeping irritant or allergic contact dermatitis does not respond to topical steroid therapy used alone. One therapeutic maneuver uses a topically applied corticosteroid cream under a wet dressing. The wet dressing holds the steroid against the skin, which is more easily penetrated because it is wet; this can be very useful in children.

Steroid creams that "rub in" are used for more acute dermatitis and for chronic dermatitis in people whose work makes greasy hands untenable, such as individuals working with paper. Creams without propylene glycol irritate less. Creams that mix antibiotics and steroids are generally avoided in irritant and allergic contact dermatitis because there is little convincing evidence of their increased efficacy. They cost more, and they are likely to be associated with the development of allergic sensitization.

Chronic irritant dermatitis, allergic contact dermatitis, and contact dermatitis that is suspect for an as yet unidentified associated allergen are best treated topically with a steroid ointment based on plain petrolatum or a plain mineral oil polymer. Steroid creams and ointments need be used no more than twice a day unless they are frequently washed off.

There are endless numbers of topical corticosteroid preparations available, with "new" ones appearing monthly. Although the very strong ones (betamethasone dipropionate and clobetasol propionate) are worth re-

---

*Allerderm Laboratories, 28 Glen Drive, Mill Valley, CA 94941; 415-381-0106.

membering because of their enhanced potential for producing benefit as well as side effects, and their greatly inflated cost, it is probably most helpful to remember an example of a single low potency (1 percent hydrocortisone) and a single medium potency (0.1 percent triamcinolone) steroid for day to day generic prescribing. Usually generic prescribing provides economy and efficacy for the patient. In some instances, however, steroid creams and ointments must be prescribed by brand name in order to insure a specific vehicle.

Plain hydrocortisone can be used with relative impunity on the face and in skin flexures for long periods of time. In recent years hydrocortisone esters (butyrate and valerate) have been developed. These substances are clearly stronger than plain hydrocortisone and no cheaper than medium strength corticosteroids. Their potential for causing side effects is not yet fully known.

On occasion topically applied corticosteroids formulated in lotions, gels, or sprays may be of value in treating irritant or allergic contact dermatitis in flexural or hairy areas. When a stronger corticosteroid is necessary, the menu to choose from is lengthy. Such strong steroids may be useful in treating allergic contact dermatitis that is likely to be of short duration. The slightly increased efficacy is probably not worth the expense or the increased risks inherent in treating chronic and extensive contact dermatitis.

Side Effects

Almost any small molecule applied to abnormal skin will partially penetrate it. Clobetasone propionate creams have been shown to significantly blunt (not suppress) the pituitary-adrenal axis when used on an entire extremity even without occlusion. In general, fluorinated steroids applied to large body areas under occlusion for long periods of time can also blunt the pituitary-adrenal axis. Recovery from this blunting occurs within days and its clinical effect is doubtful. Single case reports of more significant blunting are controversial. The use of high dose topical steroid therapy for long periods in infants and small children may cause somewhat more percutaneous penetration because of the relative increase in surface area.

The development of atrophy resulting from strong topical steroid therapy is not disputed. In body flexures this can occur within 3 to 4 weeks and last for years. On the face it tends to be associated with telangiectasias. On the hands it is often accompanied by purpura, especially when occlusive gloves have been used. The diaper area in babies may develop erosions, granulomas, and secondary candidosis in addition to the induced atrophy. For all practical purposes, plain hydrocortisone cream does not cause atrophy.

Cataracts, glaucoma, depigmentation, and even sensitization have also been associated with topical steroid therapy. Even plain hydrocortisone can do this, and

thus the skin around the eyes should always be treated cautiously.

The "topical steroid addiction" syndrome is associated on the face with the development of telangiectasias and an acneiform eruption that actually worsens when steroid therapy is stopped. Plain hydrocortisone is unlikely to cause acneiform facial reactions.

The problems that can be associated with the additives of steroid creams have been discussed.

OTHER SYSTEMIC THERAPY

Antihistamines

Many physicians treat acute allergic contact dermatitis and even irritant dermatitis with antihistamines. Antihistamine plays essentially no role in the pathogenesis of allergic contact or irritant dermatitis, and thus antihistamine therapy is irrational. If the antihistamine is very sedating, it may decrease the itching associated with any contact dermatitis. Hydroxyzine (25 to 50 mg) and Doxepin (10 to 50 mg) are useful in that they both sedate and provide some relief from anxiety. Both drugs may oversedate the elderly.

Miscellaneous Drugs

Antibiotics are used when appropriate.

Imuran has been used to treat very severe and chronic airborne plant dermatitis in Europe but is seldom used in the United States.

The dietary management of chronic nickel and chromate dermatitis is highly controversial.

OTHER TOPICAL THERAPY

Creams containing menthol (0.25 to 2 percent) and phenol (0.5 to 2 percent) help relieve the chronic itching of irritant dermatitis. If the cream base has too much water in it, the benefits of the antipruritic drug are lost and drying results.

Topical antihistamine therapy and anesthetics work briefly and can be sensitizing. Dermatologists seldom use them.

Crude coal tar (3 to 5 percent) in creams and ointments and in combination with steroids can help in treating chronic irritant dermatitis that is not responding.

Topical antibiotic therapy is seldom recommended.

Lotions containing powder, like zinc oxide (Calamine lotion), are not recommended because they are drying and messy. On the other hand, zinc oxide in a petrolatum and detergent base (plain Lassar's paste) can be just the thing to treat an intractable irritant or allergic contact dermatitis. The paste absorbs serum from wet lesions but is not too drying for dry lesions. It puts the skin "at rest" and eliminates the external environment.

Lassar's paste is applied thickly, like "frosting on a cake," over the top of a steroid ointment or by itself. A gelatin zinc oxide gauze dressing (Dome-paste bandage) holds the paste in place and a dry dressing is placed over it all. Such a dressing (the Unna's boot) can be left in place for up to 1 week and reapplied. In 2 to 4 weeks normal skin appears. Infected skin lesions cannot be treated with Unna dressings.

PHYSICAL AGENTS

Ultraviolet light alone and ultraviolet light with added psoralens systemically have been used to treat chronic irritant and allergic contact dermatitis. Grenz ray (superficial x-ray) therapy is also of value. These physical modalities can be managed by a dermatologist.

SUGGESTED READING

Adams RM. Occupational skin diseases. New York: Grune & Stratton, 1983.
Arndt KA. Manual of dermatologic therapeutics. Boston: Little, Brown, 1983.
Burrows D. The effect of systemic and implanted metals on metal dermatitis. Dermatol Clin North Am 1984; 2:603–617.
Fisher AA. Contact dermatitis. 3rd ed. Philadelphia: Lea & Febiger, 1986.
The leading work-related diseases and injuries. Morbid Mortal Weekly Rep 1986; 35:561–563.
Rystedt I. Hand eczema and long-term prognosis in atopic dermatitis. Edsbruk: Holms Gards Tryckeri, 1985.
Storrs FJ. Use and abuse of systemic corticosteroid therapy. J Am Acad Dermatol 1979; 1:95–105.

PEMPHIGUS

LYNNE H. MORRISON, M.D.
GRANT J. ANHALT, M.D.

The term pemphigus refers to a group of intraepidermal bullous diseases that share common features. They all present with mucocutaneous blisters and erosions resulting from loss of normal epidermal intercellular adhesion, which is mediated by an autoantibody of the IgG class directed against a cell surface antigen. Routine histologic study thus shows acantholysis, that is, separation of adjacent keratinocytes from each other, and immunofluorescence studies of skin biopsy specimens show IgG and often C3 deposited in the intercellular spaces. The majority of these patients also demonstrate circulating autoantibodies.

Pemphigus vulgaris is the most common form of pemphigus on the North American continent and the most severe form of the disease. Its variant, pemphigus vegetans, is characterized by large fungating lesions arising predominantly in flexural areas. Pemphigus foliaceus is a more benign form of the disease, the epidermal split occurring more superficially. Pemphigus erythematosus is a variant of pemphigus foliaceus in which some features of lupus erythematosus are present. Brazilian pemphigus foliaceus (fogo selvagem) is an endemic form of pemphigus occurring primarily in central Brazil.

PEMPHIGUS VULGARIS

Pemphigus vulgaris usually begins in middle adult life, presenting with painful erosions characteristically starting in the oral mucosa before progressing to glabrous skin. The blisters are flaccid, are typically distributed over the scalp, face, and trunk, and demonstrate a positive Nikolsky sign (extension of a blister or denuding of perilesional skin by lateral pressure). The acantholytic separation in pemphigus vulgaris occurs deep in the epidermis, immediately above the basal cell layer, which accounts for the weeping erosions seen clinically.

In the presteroid era pemphigus vulgaris carried a substantial mortality, half the patients dying in the first year of the disease from infection, cachexia, and fluid and electrolyte imbalance. Mortality is now much less common and is largely related to complications of therapy. Pemphigus vulgaris is a serious disorder, requiring aggressive systemic therapy, which is most effective if started early in the course of the disease. A desirable response to therapy can be judged by cessation of formation of new bullae, loss of the Nikolsky sign, and finally by healing of the existing lesions. The circulating pemphigus antibody titer generally correlates with disease activity, but overall is less important in monitoring the therapeutic response than the patient's clinical status. Under certain circumstances the titers may be useful in management. For example, if a patient who has been under good control develops a minor flare of the disease, a rising antibody titer may indicate that a medication change is required, whereas a stable antibody titer favors continuation of the same treatment schedule.

Corticosteroids are the mainstay of therapy in pemphigus vulgaris, prednisone being the medication most frequently used. Cytotoxic drugs may need to be added in some patients in order to reduce the side effects of corticosteroids. Before starting steroid therapy, it is necessary to determine whether the patient has a history of diabetes, hypertension, gastric or duodenal ulcers, or exposure to tuberculosis. A routine cell count with a differential, chest x-ray examination, fasting glucose level, and urinalysis are also obtained, and PPD is given. If diabetes or hypertension is present, careful monitoring during steroid therapy is necessary, and if evidence of tuberculosis is found, the management should be coordinated with an infectious diseases specialist. We prefer having our patients use antacids routinely while taking high doses of steroids in order to reduce the risk of inducing ulcers. If cytotoxic therapy is anticipated, a chemistry screen prior to beginning therapy is indicated, since these drugs are generally metabolized via the hepatic or renal route.

It has been advocated that therapy of pemphigus vulgaris be initiated with dosages of prednisone in the range of 180 to 360 mg daily, continued for 6 to 10 weeks to induce remission, and then tapered. We believe, however, that this regimen puts the patient at too high a risk of life threatening infection.

Most patients respond well to initial dosages of prednisone in the range of 1 to 2 mg per kg per day in divided doses. Evidence of disease control is usually evident within the first 2 weeks after starting therapy, at which time the prednisone therapy can be consolidated to a single morning dose. The dosage then can be tapered, rather rapidly at first (5 to 10 mg per week) but then more slowly as the dosage approaches 40 mg per day. Once this is achieved, an alternate day regimen should be started, by tapering the dosage given every other day to zero. When the patient is stable on doses of 40 mg and 0 mg on alternate days, the high dose day then can be tapered to zero. At this point in therapy the disease is most apt to flare, and management of such relapses needs to be individualized. Although some patients develop clinical remission following steroid therapy, others may need to be maintained on low dosages of prednisone for years. Alternate day therapy in this situation helps reduce the well known side effects of long term steroid treatment.

If a patient is not responding uniformly to oral prednisone therapy, the lack of response may be related to variation in bioavailability of the drug. Using deltasone rather than generic prednisone may help eliminate this problem.

If high maintenance doses are required or if the patient is not tolerating prednisone, addition of a cytotoxic drug should be considered. Cytotoxic drugs that are beneficial in the treatment of pemphigus include cyclophosphamide (Cytoxan), azathioprine (Imuran), and methotrexate. It is safest to initiate therapy with these drugs when tapering of the prednisone dosage has begun, since their addition during the initial therapy with high dosages of prednisone can result in a profound and hazardous immunosuppression. When the disease is controlled by prednisone and the immunosuppressive drug, an attempt should be made to decrease the prednisone dosage by 5 to 10 mg weekly. It is often necessary to continue low dose, alternate day maintenance therapy in the range of 10 mg of prednisone every other day. Finally, the dosage of the immunosuppressive drug should be tapered over a several month period.

Cyclosphosphamide is an effective immunosuppressive drug, having a greater capacity to reduce immunoglobulin synthesis than does azathioprine or methotrexate and reasonably predictable side effects. For these reasons it is generally our choice when a cytotoxic drug is indicated. Cytoxan is used in dosages of 1 to 2 mg per kg daily. Significant adverse side effects include bone marrow suppression, hemorrhagic cystitis and bladder fibrosis, sterility, and an increased long term risk of the development of malignant disease. These effects mandate routine monitoring of the cell counts with a differential and routine and microscopic urine examination. Some degree of bone marrow suppression is commonly seen with Cytoxan and is dose dependent. In general, elderly patients are more sensitive to the drug than younger patients. It is important to be aware of the fact that although steroids blunt the leukopenic effects of Cytoxan, the circulating neutrophils will not function normally because of the steroid effect, and a significant host defense defect may be present in the face of an apparently normal leukocyte count. The risk of developing hemorrhagic cystitis can be minimized by having the patient maintain an oral fluid intake of at least 2 liters daily. The possibility of developing latent malignant disease is the most concerning side effect. Although the exact chance of this occurring is uncertain, this drug is, in general, best reserved for older patients.

Azathioprine is another immunosuppressive drug that is useful in controlling pemphigus vulgaris. Like cyclophosphamide, it is given in dosages of 1 to 2 mg per kg per day and may be useful in patients with bladder problems or those who do not tolerate or respond to Cytoxan. It shares with Cytoxan the adverse effect of bone marrow suppression and increased risk of causing malignant change and should be used with the precautions already mentioned regarding these side effects. Unlike cyclophosphamide, it has been associated with hepatotoxicity and therefore should be avoided in patients with liver disease. A complete blood count with a differential and chemistry profile should be carried out before beginning therapy with this drug, and test results should be followed routinely during its use.

Methotrexate, although previously a more popular adjunctive drug because of its familiarity, is currently used less often. It is not believed to be as effective as either cyclophosphamide or azathioprine. Methotrexate is used on a weekly basis; generally either 25 to 30 mg is given in a single intramuscular dose or 12.5 to 15.0 mg is given orally, divided into three doses given 12 hours apart over a 36 hour period. Because of hepatotoxicity, routine chemistry screens are necessary. If long term treatment is anticipated, liver biopsies, both pretreatment and yearly during treatment, should be considered.

Gold has also been useful both as a steroid sparing drug and as sole therapy for pemphigus vulgaris. Both gold sodium thiomalate (Myochrysine) and gold thioglucose (Solganal) have been used successfully, but the latter is preferred by some dermatologists because of a lower incidence of nitroid reactions. The treatment regimen is similar to that used for rheumatoid arthritis; a 10 mg test dose is given, followed by a 25 mg dose given 1 week later. If this is tolerated well, 50 mg is given weekly; a therapeutic effect usually is not seen until after a cumulative dosage of 500 mg has been given. When adequate control has been achieved, maintenance therapy is instituted, which varies from 25 to 50 mg of gold every 2 to 8 weeks. Approximately one-third of the patients taking gold therapy develop some type of adverse effect. Generally the side effects are not serious, but they can be significant, such as nephritis, leukopenia, and thrombocytopenia. These reactions can be identified early if the complete blood count with a differential and urinalysis are monitored routinely. It is important to obtain these laboratory data before each gold injection. Additional adverse effects include nitroid reactions (flushing and weakness occurring soon after injection) and a persistent pruritic dermatitis.

Plasmapheresis also has been of short term benefit in controlling pemphigus vulgaris. This process decreases the titer of circulating pathogenic autoantibodies, which is thought to be the basis for its therapeutic effect. This modality, however, is very expensive and time consuming and produces only temporary improvement. Removal of the circulating IgG can actually stimulate autoantibody production and cause a rebound flare when the exchanges are discontinued. For these reasons the use of plasmapheresis should not be considered a routine therapeutic option. It is useful mainly for quickly decreasing antibody titers while waiting for systemic therapy to take effect.

Topical care of the eroded and crusted skin lesions should include application of Domeboro compresses three to four times daily to help debride gently and decrease discomfort. This should be followed by application of an antibacterial ointment or cream such as silver sulfadiazine cream (Silvadene) to minimize colonization of the erosions and also provide some pain relief. During the acute phase of the disease, frequent cultures of the skin lesions and appropriate antibiotic therapy when indicated are important to reduce the risk of systemic infection and facilitate local healing.

Patients with extensive oral lesions usually require a soft diet and Benadryl solution prior to meals. Topical application of a steroid in a gel base, such as fluocinonide gel, may be of some benefit.

PEMPHIGUS FOLIACEUS

Pemphigus foliaceus differs from pemphigus vulgaris histologically by showing a more superficial epidermal split, which occurs just below the stratum corneum. The clinical picture reflects this, showing more superficial scaling and crusted lesions, which are reminiscent of widespread impetigo. The face, scalp, and trunk are involved most frequently, with mucous membranes being rarely affected. This variant represents a more benign form of pemphigus and has a better prognosis.

The therapeutic approach is similar to that with pemphigus vulgaris, but generally is less aggressive because of the more benign nature of this pemphigus variant. The disease in most patients can be controlled with a combination of low dose oral steroid therapy with potent topical steroid therapy. The use of an immunosuppressive drug is rarely required, but when it is, the options for pemphigus foliaceus are the same as outlined for pemphigus vulgaris.

DRUG INDUCED PEMPHIGUS

Both D-penicillamine and captopril have been reported to cause lesions resembling pemphigus foliaceus and less commonly pemphigus vulgaris. There are two subsets of patients with drug induced pemphigus: those with and those without demonstrable autoantibodies. In either group, examination of a lesional skin biopsy specimen by light microscopy shows acantholysis similar to that seen in the idiopathic disease. In patients lacking autoantibodies, direct immunofluorescence examination of perilesional skin shows only complement components deposited in the epidermal intercellular spaces. Indirect immunofluorescence examination of the serum for circulating autoantibodies yields negative findings. In these cases it is possible that the acantholysis is due to a toxic effect of the drug on the epidermal cells. It has been possible to recreate this acantholysis in organ culture studies, incubating human skin with either penicillamine or captopril in the absence of human antibodies. In these patients the treatment is primarily to stop the drug; the disease should resolve after approximately 2 months. Systemic steroid therapy is not necessary in these cases, but potent topically applied steroids such as fluocinonide, 0.05 percent, may be helpful.

In patients who develop circulating autoantibodies, the immunoglobulins can be detected both in perilesional skin and in the patient's serum. The significance of this association is unclear at present. These patients must be treated as if they had idiopathic pemphigus foliaceus.

SUGGESTED READING

Aberer W, et al. Azathioprine in the treatment of pemphigus vulgaris: a long term follow-up. J Am Acad Dermatol 1987; 16:527–533.
Ahmed AR. Pemphigus: current concepts. Ann Int Med 1980; 92:396–405.

Jordon RE. Pemphigus. In: Fitzpatrick TB, Eisen AZ, Wolff K, Freedberg IM, Austen KF, eds. Dermatology in general medicine. 3rd ed. New York: McGraw-Hill, 1987: 571.
Lever WF, Schaumburg-Lever G. Immunosuppressants and prednisone in pemphigus vulgaris. Arch Dermatol 1977; 113:1236–1241.
Penneys NS, et al. Management of pemphigus with gold compounds, a long term follow-up report. Arch Dermatol 1976; 112:185–187.

BULLOUS PEMPHIGOID

ROBERT E. JORDON, M.D.

Bullous pemphigoid is a chronic, self-limited, inflammatory blistering skin disease that afflicts primarily patients who are in the sixth, seventh, and eighth decades of life. First recognized as a distinct clinical entity by Lever in 1953, this disease process was called bullous pemphigoid because of the close clinical similarity to pemphigus vulgaris, but with the absence of histologic evidence of acantholysis. Until recently bullous pemphigoid has long been confused with other blistering diseases affecting the skin.

The major clinical feature of bullous pemphigoid is the presence of large tense blisters, which may arise on normal appearing skin or on erythematous bases. Lesions are commonly present on the inner aspect of the thighs, the flexure surfaces of the forearms, the axillae, the groin, and the lower abdomen. The mucous membranes are less commonly involved and are rarely the site of initial manifestation of the disease process. When present, oral lesions usually appear as intact blisters. The anus, vagina, and esophagus also may be involved.

Histopathologically bullous pemphigoid is characterized by subepidermal bulla formation with an infiltrate usually consisting of eosinophils and lymphocytes. The subepidermal appearance of microvacuoles may be the earliest pathologic event. By electron microscopy, blister formation is seen to occur in the area of the cutaneous basement membrane zone between the basal cell membrane and the basal lamina, an area referred to as the lamina lucida region of the basement membrane zone.

Like many other blistering diseases of the skin, bullous pemphigoid is an autoimmune disease. Patients with this disease have serum autoantibodies that react with a component of the lamina lucida region of the basement membrane zone of skin. These antibodies are present in approximately 75 percent of active cases, are of the IgG type, and are capable of fixing various components of the complement system. Unlike the situation in pemphigus, however, measuring levels of these antibodies is not particularly useful in monitoring therapeutic success. In addition to circulating antibodies, IgG and complement components are almost universally present, bound to the basement membrane zone of skin lesions. Because of these immunopathologic investigations, these circulating IgG autoantibodies and complement have been implicated in the pathogenesis of this interesting blistering skin disease.

THERAPY

The mainstay of therapy for bullous pemphigoid, as with other blistering diseases of the skin such as pemphigus, remains systemic corticosteroid therapy. In contrast to pemphigus, however, lower doses of corticosteroids are usually sufficient to suppress the disease process. Patients with widespread bullous lesions may be ill and require hospitalization, especially if the patient is elderly and debilitated and has other medical problems. Starting dosages of 50 to 100 mg of prednisone daily in such patients usually suppress new blister formation. This dosage should be maintained until cessation of formation of new blisters. Once control has been achieved, I usually wait about 2 weeks before tapering the initial prednisone dosage. During this acute period, when the dosages of prednisone are relatively high, a constant vigil for the development of infection, including opportunistic organisms such as gram negative bacteria, fungi, and tubercle bacilli, should be maintained. Secondary infection is a leading cause of death in bullous pemphigoid, particularly if the patient is debilitated and lesions are widespread.

Once effective control has been achieved, I gradually reduce the prednisone dosage over 6 to 8 weeks to about 30 mg daily. At this level of prednisone several different approaches may be entertained. The first approach I usually take is to reduce the amount of prednisone taken on alternate days; i.e., switch to alternate day steroid therapy. In most instances this approach is sufficient to control the disease in this maintenance period. If this approach is not successful, one can add an immunosuppressive drug such as azathioprine, cyclophosphamide, or methotrexate. Of the three, I favor azathioprine in dosages of about 100 to 150 mg per day, but cyclophosphamide, 100 to 200 mg per day, or methotrexate, 25 to 30 mg per week, also may be utilized. Immunosuppressive drugs, however, are not useful in the acute phase of the disease because they do not exert an effect for about 3 to 4 weeks. After 3 to 4 weeks of their use, however, the prednisone dosage usually can be reduced much further and faster. In some instances corticosteroids may be discontinued, and the disease may be controlled by immunosuppressive drugs alone. Periodic laboratory evaluation, including a complete blood count, liver and kidney chemistry profile, and urinalysis should be performed to monitor for side effects of the medications.

Sulfapyridine or sulfones also may be of value in the therapy of bullous pemphigoid, particularly in patients whose skin biopsy specimens demonstrate a predominance of neutrophils. The notion that such patients represent bullous pemphigoid rather than another bullous skin disease, however, has recently been challenged. Gold therapy also has been attempted in patients with bullous pemphigoid, with results less effective than in patients with pemphigus. Plasmapheresis and cyclosporin also have been utilized in these patients with some success.

Topical measures, used with and without systemic therapy, may also be of benefit in these patients. In very mild cases such measures may replace systemic therapy altogether. Topical therapy with fluorinated corticosteroids, with and without wet dressings, applied two to three times daily are of value. Cleansing baths and cool compresses are also beneficial. A powdered bed (cornstarch) may be utilized for hospitalized patients with widespread denuded lesions. This measure prevents denuded surfaces from sticking to the bedding. A powdered bed is especially useful in the acute or early healing phase of the disease.

SUGGESTED READING

Goldberg NS, Robinson JK, Roenigk HH, Marder R, Rothe M. Plasmapheresis therapy for bullous pemphigoid. Arch Dermatol 1985; 121:1484–1485.

Jordon RE, Beutner EH, Witebsky E, Blumental G, Hale WL, Lever WF. Basement zone antibodies in bullous pemphigoid. JAMA 1967; 200:751–756.

Jordon RE, Kawana S, Fritz KA. Immunopathologic mechanisms in pemphigus and bullous pemphigoid. J Invest Dermatol 1985; 85:72s–78s.

Lever WF. Pemphigus and pemphigoid. J Am Acad Dermatol 1979; 1:2–31.

Person JR, Rogers RS. Bullous pemphigoid responding to sulfapyridine and sulfones. Arch Dermatol 1977; 113:610–615.

Thivolet J, Barthelemy H, Rigot-Muller G, Bendelac A. Effects of cyclosporin on bullous pemphigoid and pemphigus. Lancet 1985; 1:334–335.

ERYTHEMA MULTIFORME

KIRK D. WUEPPER, M.D.

Erythema multiforme is a cutaneous reaction, usually self-limited, that follows the time course of an immunologic reaction. It is expressed as erythematous macules, papules, annular or iris (target shaped) lesions, or bullae. The inciting causes of erythema multiforme may be ingestion or contact with chemicals or drugs, the occurrence or recurrence of infectious agents, or the treatment of tumors with ionizing radiation.

The extent of lesions and tissue damage varies from banal to generalized and life threatening. The former (erythema multiforme minor) may represent only a few erosions on mucous membranes of the mouth, eyes, and genitalia or symmetrically distributed papules and annular lesions on the dorsum of the hands and knees. More severe reactions (erythema multiforme major) may represent generalized erosions and sloughing of mucosal epithelium with or without generalized skin involvement. The latter reactions may require management usually reserved for the extensively burned individual.

EVALUATION

I try first to ascertain whether I am dealing with minor or major erythema multiforme. A detailed history and physical examination allow one to determine the extent and degree of injury already present and to decide whether the disease is progressing, stabilized, or showing some degree of resolution. Fiery red lesions are often new or rapidly evolving where milder hues toward a salmon pink suggest a tendency toward resolution. Lesions appear predominantly during a 2 to 4 day interval and heal over the course of 10 to 14 days. It is useful to review the many inciting causes of erythema multiforme. These have been recently updated to include references to many newly introduced chemotherapeutic drugs capable of causing erythema multiforme.

THERAPEUTIC ALTERNATIVES

An identifiable cause should be removed immediately or management instituted promptly. This may require antibiotics for bacterial or Mycoplasma infections or withdrawal of drugs introduced 9 to 14 days previously. For the minor forms of erythema multiforme, still considered to be evolving and worsening, I prefer to initiate therapy with prednisone or prednisolone, 40 to 60 mg, immediately and then repeat daily as a single morning dose. The 20 mg tablet is convenient for this purpose. The dosage is reduced by 20 mg at 5 to 7 day intervals and then discontinued.

During the active phase of lesion development, care should be taken to avoid traumatizing the skin or mucous membranes since the Koebner phenomenon occurs in erythema multiforme. If the lesions seem to have stabilized or have begun healing at the initial evaluation, I am less likely to use anti-inflammatory corticosteroids and may provide symptomatic care only as well as education and reassurance of the patient.

Because the public has become widely educated about Herpesvirus hominus infection, I frequently describe how recurrent herpes can trigger erythema multiforme in some individuals. This sometimes provokes the patient to remember a trivial herpes simplex virus infection that was not reported, or it provides a concrete example that the patient can relate to. If a drug or another agent has been responsible for the current bout of erythema multiforme, the patient is admonished to remember the name(s) of the agent and to alert other physicians whom he sees about the nature of his sensitivity to it.

Erythema multiforme major must be approached aggressively in an attempt to minimize tissue damage. Severe erosions in the eyes, mouth, or genitalia may lead to excessive pain, superinfection, or blindness. The most severe cases should be managed with a team of experts and may require temporary grafting to cover denuded skin, expert ophthalmic care, cleansing of the mouth with antibiotic solutions (tetracycline suspension, clotrimazole troches), and catheterization to prevent urinary retention or stenosis. With evolving and progressing disease I use moderately high doses of corticosteroids, 60 to 120 mg of prednisone or prednisolone daily, with consideration given to the patient's age and weight and the severity of the disease.

PREVENTION

When a chemical or substance is identified as the cause of erythema multiforme, avoidance of that substance may be possible, thus preventing the repeated occurrence of erythema multiforme. Examples are 9-bromofluorine (a compound synthesized in college laboratory chemistry classes) or the emulsifier added to butter in the Netherlands that caused a widespread outbreak of erythema multiforme.

By far the most common cause of erythema multiforme that can be identified is recurrent Herpesvirus hominus infection. If the factors that induce a recurrence are known, it may be possible to avoid them, e.g., excessive sun exposure in photoreactivated herpes. In addition, photoprotection may be offered by application of sunscreen containing skin lotion or lip balm. Agents with a protective factor (SPF) of 15 or greater should be recommended.

If protection or prevention fails, herpes generally is heralded by sensations of tingling or hyperesthesia at the site where recurrences usually occur for 6 to 24 hours before the herpetic lesions actually begin to appear. Erythema multiforme lesions follow the recurrent herpes lesions by 2 to 5 days and then persist for 7 to 10 days.

There has been recent success in the treatment of recurrent herpes with acyclovir (Zovirax), 200 mg orally four or five times daily for 1 week, beginning at the earliest recognition of the recurrence; this often aborts the herpetic lesions and prevents recurrent erythema multiforme.

Before acyclovir became available, another strategy to minimize erythema multiforme following recurrent herpes was to give 40 to 60 mg of prednisone (20 mg tablets) orally as a single morning dose for 7 to 10 days at the onset of prodromal sensations or any sign of early lesions. Most individuals seem to grasp the cause-effect relationship between herpes and erythema multiforme and warrant the physician's trust in prescribing medication before the onset of overt disease.

CONTINUOUS ERYTHEMA MULTIFORME

Occasional patients subject to recurrent herpes simplex infections associated with menses, dental abscess, or unknown factors may experience erythema multiforme 10 to 12 times yearly. In such individuals lesions barely heal before the next bout of erythema multiforme. We have observed two such individuals who had been treated with corticosteroids for symptomatic improvement. Later, withdrawal of steroids provoked extensive erythema multiforme. One of these individuals then exhibited persistent viral vesicles on the skin and persistent and continuous erythema multiforme. Acyclovir appears to be an excellent choice for therapy in such patients.

Leigh and associates recently described three patients with recurrent and continuous erythema multiforme. Although Huff does not include such individuals by his definition of erythema multiforme, I believe that this is an entity that occasionally must be dealt with. The patients of Leigh et al responded to intramuscular pooled human gamma globulin, 750 mg once monthly, with clearing within 2 to 8 weeks after the initiation of therapy. An alternative treatment for continuous erythema multiforme may be the use of Imuran, 100 mg as a daily oral dose.

SUGGESTED READING

Huff JC, Weston WL, Tonnesen. MG. Erythema multiforme: a critical review of characteristics, diagnostic criteria, and causes. J Am Acad Dermatol 1983; 8:763–775.

Jones RR. Azathioprine therapy in the management of persistent erythema multiforme. Br J Dermatol 1981; 105:465–467.
Kazmierowski JA, Peizner DA, Wuepper KD. Herpes simplex antigen in immune complexes of patients with erythema multiforme. JAMA 1982; 247:2547–2550.
Leigh IM, Mowbray JF, Levene GM, Sutherland S. Recurrent and continuous erythema multiforme—a clinical and immunological study. Clin Exp Dermatol 1985; 10:58–67.
Lemak MA, Duvic M, Bean SF. Oral acyclovir for the prevention of herpes-associates erythema multiforme. J Am Acad Dermatol 1986; 15:50–54.
Shelley WB. Herpes simplex virus as a cause of erythema multiforme. JAMA 1967; 201:153–156.

IMMUNOLOGICALLY MEDIATED NEPHROTIC RENAL DISEASE

SHARON ADLER, M.D.
RICHARD J. GLASSOCK, M.D.

The nephrotic syndrome may be defined as a constellation of abnormal clinical and biochemical abnormalities brought about by the persistent loss of plasma proteins in the urine due to a defect in glomerular permeability. The quantity of proteins lost in the urine usually, but not invariably, exceeds 3.5 g per day per 1.73 square meter of body surface area.

The nephrotic syndrome may be due to a wide variety of disorders, only some of which are believed to be immunologically mediated (Table 1). The evidence implicating immune mechanisms is largely indirect (e.g., deposits of immunoglobulin or complement in glomeruli), and the details of the processes that trigger an immune reaction and lead to glomerular injury and thus proteinuria are for the most part unknown. Even so, strategies of management of many forms of the nephrotic syndrome involve drugs that have potent and often lasting effects on the immune system. Such therapy has evolved in a highly empiric fashion. Since therapeutic efforts are not always successful in abolishing the nephrotic state, it is also important to consider the general management of the condition even in the face of continuing high levels of proteinuria. Such management may forestall complications that can arise secondary to the biochemical disturbances brought about by persistent heavy losses of protein or that under some circumstances may delay or retard the progression of disease to end

TABLE 1 Nephrotic Syndrome—Classification Based Upon Etiology

Idiopathic
  Minimal change disease
  Focal and segmental glomerulosclerosis
  Mesangial proliferative glomerulonephritis
  Membranous glomerulonephritis
  Membranoproliferative glomerulonephritis
  IgA nephropathy (Berger's disease)
  Crescentic glomerulonephritis (rare)

Secondary
  Autoimmune disease: systemic lupus erythematosus, rheumatoid arthritis, mixed connective tissue disease, dermatomyositis, Henoch-Schönlein purpura, Goodpasture's syndrome, vasculitis
  Infections: Poststreptococcal glomerulonephritis, infective endocarditis, "shunt" nephritis, syphilis, hepatitis B, human immunodeficiency virus, cytomegalovirus
  Drugs: Gold, mercury, penicillamine, probenecid, trimethadione, captopril, nonsteroidal anti-inflammatory drugs, "street" heroin
  Neoplasia: Hodgkin's disease, nonHodgkin's lymphoma, leukemia, carcinoma of the colon, breast, lung, thyroid, kidney, melanoma
  Metabolic: Diabetes mellitus types 1 and 2, hypothyroidism
  Multisystem: Amyloidosis, Sjögren's syndrome, sarcoidosis
  Heredofamilial: Congenital nephrotic syndrome, Fabry's disease, sickle cell disease
  Other: Toxemia of pregnancy, renal allograft rejection, malignant hypertension, renal arterial stenosis, vesicoureteric reflux

stage renal failure independent of an effect on the fundamental pathogenic mechanisms responsible for initiating the disorder.

As always, proper management rests on accurate diagnosis. In the case of immune mediated nephrotic renal disease this often requires an examination of renal tissue obtained by biopsy. However, the need for renal biopsy in the evaluation of the nephrotic syndrome is not without controversy. Some have argued that, in the main, empiric therapy with glucocorticoids without biopsy is just as effective as therapy guided by biopsy findings.

This view may be supported by the following observations:

1. For the most part, truly specific therapies for the nephrotic syndrome based upon histopathologic diagnoses have not yet been fully devised.

2. There is little morbidity or mortality associated with short courses of high dose glucocorticoid therapy, especially when they are administered on an alternate day basis.

3. Renal biopsies are costly, require hospitalization, and under rare circumstances may cause morbidity and mortality.

We advocate a trial of glucocorticoids in patients with idiopathic nephrotic syndrome who do not have medical contraindications against the use of these drugs. This approach thus categorizes patients with idiopathic nephrotic syndrome into steroid responsive, steroid resistant, or steroid dependent groups based on the success of empiric therapy. This expedient approach works well in the pediatric population, in which the underlying causes of the idiopathic nephrotic syndrome are more restricted than in adults and the predominant lesion encountered is steroid responsive.

When possible and when an individual skilled and experienced in the biopsy technique is available, our recommendation continues to include the performance of a renal biopsy in adult patients prior to the initiation of glucocorticoid or cytotoxic therapy for the treatment of the idiopathic nephrotic syndrome. A study performed at our institution demonstrated that in this clinical setting, renal biopsies frequently identify previously unsuspected systemic diseases (e.g., amyloidosis). The renal biopsy also offers additional information useful in predicting the prognosis. Finally, although it is true that specific therapies for the idiopathic nephrotic syndrome based on histopathologic findings are still forthcoming, both university based and private practice nephrologists use information obtained from renal biopsies to alter treatment plans in their patients. Thus, we believe that renal biopsies continue to be valuable in guiding management in adults with the nephrotic syndrome.

BIOCHEMICAL DISTURBANCES IN THE NEPHROTIC SYNDROME

The defect in glomerular permeability underlying the nephrotic syndrome leads to a perturbation in plasma protein and lipid metabolism consequent to urinary protein loss. Compensatory changes in plasma protein synthesis and specific protein deficiency states develop. The changes in plasma protein and lipid concentrations that characterize the nephrotic syndrome are given in Table 2. In addition, the nephrotic syndrome is accompanied

TABLE 2 Nephrotic Syndrome: Plasma Protein and Lipid Disturbances

Increased concentration
  Alpha and beta globulins:
  Fibrinogen
  IgM (some cases)
  IgA (Berger's disease)
  Very low density lipoproteins
  Low density and intermediate density lipoproteins
  Factor VIII (antihemophilic globulin)
  Factor X
  Factor VII
  Factor V
  Alpha$_2$ macroglobulin

Decreased concentration
  Albumin
  IgG
  C1q (some cases)
  C3 (some cases)
  Transferrin
  Cholecalciferol binding protein
  Zinc and copper binding proteins
  Thyroxine binding globulin
  Cortisol binding globulin
  Lipoprotein lipase
  Lecithin cholesterol acyltransferase
  Alpha-1 antitrypsin
  Factor IX
  Factor XII
  Factor XI
  Protein C (some cases)
  Antithrombin III (some cases)

Variable or unchanged concentration
  High density lipoproteins
  Factor II

by a tendency for sodium chloride and water retention to develop, which, depending on the underlying disease, may be due to a primary mechanism or be secondary to a perceived defect in the intravascular volume. Such deficiencies of effective intravascular volume could be due to a translocation of fluid into the interstitial compartment as a consequence of the reduced plasma oncotic pressure, leading to a disturbance of the Starling dynamics within the peripheral capillary circulation. Notwithstanding these considerations, the majority of adult patients with the idiopathic nephrotic syndrome have a normal or expanded plasma volume and probably have sodium chloride and water retention resulting from some primary disturbance of renal excretion.

The biochemical disturbances that accompany the nephrotic syndrome deserve careful attention, especially since even aggressive therapies aimed at correction of the fundamental abnormality may fail to ameliorate the urinary losses of protein. Thus the biochemical milieu of the nephrotic syndrome may persist and produce disabling symptoms and signs.

GENERAL MANAGEMENT OF THE NEPHROTIC SYNDROME

Management of Edema

The degree of edema in patients with the nephrotic syndrome ranges from none to anasarca, and rarely even marked pulmonary congestion may develop. Patients with minimal or no edema require no therapy. Mild to moderate edema is often well controlled by restricting the dietary sodium level to approximately 2 g per day and the dietary sodium chloride level to 4 g per day. Water restriction is usually unnecessary.

Diuretics may be indicated in patients compromised by scrotal or labial edema, lower extremity pain, superimposed cellulitis, the inability to wear shoes, or other unacceptable cosmetic effects. Patients with volume dependent hypertension, tense ascites restricting diaphragmatic movement, pleural effusions, or pulmonary vascular congestion have clear-cut indications for the use of potent diuretics in association with rigorous sodium chloride restriction. Thiazide diuretics, often in combination with potassium sparing drugs such as spironolactone, triamterene, or amiloride, may suffice to control edema. Potassium sparing drugs should be used with great caution in patients with azotemia.

With more severe volume overload, initial intravenous therapy with loop acting diuretics (e.g., furosemide, bumetanide) may be necessary if gastrointestinal edema impairs the absorption of orally administered drugs. Subsequently, loop acting diuretics given orally twice daily may be required to maintain a stable body weight. Alternatively, a loop acting diuretic in combination with metolazone (2.5 to 10 mg per day) may produce a dramatic diuresis in patients who are refractory to loop acting diuretics as monotherapy. Since these potent combinations can produce severe intravascular volume depletion, hypokalemia, and metabolic alkalosis, close follow-up during initiation of this therapy is imperative.

Finally, in some patients with severely compromised pulmonary function due to tense ascites, pleural effusions, or pulmonary vascular congestion, paracentesis, thoracentesis, or intravenous albumin administration combined with loop acting diuretics may be indicated. The major disadvantage in employing these procedures is that the benefit derived is short-lived. In addition, in the case of paracentesis and thoracentesis, repeated removal of fluid and protein potentially can lead to malnutrition. Sudden removal of large amounts of fluid may also precipitate hypotension and even acute renal failure.

In rare patients, severe volume overload due to the nephrotic syndrome may persist in the presence of advanced azotemia. In this setting, if end stage renal disease is imminent, the nephrotic syndrome may be terminated by renal ablation. This has been achieved by angiographically controlled embolization of the kidneys, balloon catheter renal infarction, and medical nephrectomy induced by aminoglycosides, mercurial diuretics, or nonsteroidal anti-inflammatory drugs. The use of the latter reduces protein excretion by approximately 50 percent in nearly one-half of the patients with severe nephrotic syndrome, although the glomerular filtration rate often frequently falls concomitantly. Converting enzyme inhibitors, careful control of the systemic arterial pressure, or protein restriction may also reduce urinary protein excretion in some patients.

Management of Proteinuria

Several approaches have emerged that reportedly diminish proteinuria. Indomethacin (50 to 100 mg orally three times daily) and meclofenamate (50 to 100 mg orally three times daily) are said to decrease proteinuria more than they decrease the glomerular filtration rate in patients with the nephrotic syndrome. The precise mechanism for this effect remains undetermined. In our experience these drugs have limited value in decreasing the clinical complications of proteinuria in nephrotic subjects.

Angiotensin converting enzyme inhibitors, including captopril, enalapril and lisinopril, reduce proteinuria in animal models of nephrotic disease and in some instances in humans. Their effects appear to be related to their capacity to reduce intraglomerular hypertension. They are of particular value in hypertensive nephrotic patients because of their dual beneficial effects on systemic and intraglomerular pressures. In this clinical setting we use angiotensin converting enzyme inhibitors as the antihypertensive drugs of choice. Their use in nonhypertensive nephrotic subjects is less clear, especially since angiotensin converting enzyme inhibition in nephrotic patients with diminished intravascular volume may be associated with significant postural hypotension. Since angiotensin converting enzyme inhibition is achieved with relatively small doses of these drugs, it is possible that they may yet prove to be useful and safe even in nonhypertensive patients with the nephrotic syndrome.

Finally, dietary protein restriction is a nonpharmacologic means of diminishing proteinuria. A decline in the magnitude of proteinuria with restriction of protein intake has been observed in experimental models of the nephrotic syndrome in rats, in diabetic man, and in cases of immunologically mediated nephrotic syndrome in man. In one study patients with abnormal proteinuria and serum albumin levels as low as 0.9 g per deciliter were given diets restricted in protein to 0.8 g per kilogram of ideal body weight per day, supplemented with multiple vitamins, calcium, and iron for 2 weeks. Proteinuria diminished significantly while serum albumin levels remained stable or increased. There was no evidence of malnutrition during this brief study.

The mechanism of diminished proteinuria in patients consuming a diet restricted in protein has not been well defined. A diminished glomerular filtration rate is probably only partially responsible for the effect. Decreased intraglomerular pressure is the most likely explanation. At present we prefer the use of angiotensin converting enzyme inhibitors over dietary protein restriction as a means of diminishing proteinuria. However, we do prescribe dietary protein restriction more readily in normotensive nephrotic patients. The effects of a combination of dietary protein restriction and angiotensin converting enzyme inhibitors on the nephrotic syndrome remains to be determined. High protein diets, on the other hand, only aggravate the magnitude of proteinuria and do not regularly increase plasma protein levels.

Nutritional Prescription

As already noted, dietary protein restriction may diminish urinary protein loss and enhance renal survival while maintaining adequate nutrition provided urinary losses of protein are not massive (e.g., more than 10 g of protein per day). The caloric intake in protein restricted diets is kept constant by increasing the ingestion of simple and complex carbohydrates. At our current state of knowledge, protein restriction (dietary protein intake of 0.6 to 0.8 g per kg of ideal body weight, 60 to 75 percent of which is of high biologic value) should be used with some caution in patients with the nephrotic syndrome. Frequent measurements of the serum albumin and transferrin levels, measurement of the body weight, and anthropometry should be performed to monitor the nutritional adequacy of the diet.

Hypocalcemia is common in nephrotic patients. It is most often associated with hypoalbuminemia and requires no therapeutic intervention if the corrected total serum calcium and measured ionized calcium levels are normal and there is no evidence of renal osteodystrophy. However, owing to urinary losses of the cholecalciferol binding protein and 25-hydroxycholecalciferol, a state of vitamin D deficiency is sometimes present. Thus, although a decrease in vitamin D is common in patients with azotemia, it may also occur in nephrotic patients without azotemia. The resultant compromise in the gastrointestinal absorption of calcium may lead to secondary hyperparathyroidism and renal osteodystrophy. The dietary calcium level should be maintained at about 1.5 g per day. Vitamin D supplements should be considered in patients with low measured vitamin D levels or decreased ionized serum calcium levels. In nephrotic patients without profound azotemia, supplemental 25-hydroxyvitamin D in dosages of 20 to 40 μg per day compensate for urinary losses. Patients with azotemia may also require 1,25-dihydroxyvitamin D. The use of these drugs is more strongly indicated in patients with concomitant renal osteodystrophy and in those with a protracted nephrotic syndrome unresponsive to therapy.

Low levels of iron, zinc, and other trace metals may be present as a result of urinary losses of metals along with serum transport proteins. Further study is required before specific recommendations for supplementation can be made. In rare circumstances a profound hypochromic microcytic anemia may be seen; this is due to urinary losses of transferrin and deficiencies in the iron transport system. Parenteral iron therapy may be of value in the treatment of this condition.

Treatment of Hyperlipidemia

Type IIA or IIB hyperlipoproteinemia is commonly observed in the nephrotic syndrome. Very low density lipoprotein levels increase as a result of enhanced hepatic synthesis and impaired conversion to low density lipoproteins. Low density lipoprotein levels also rise owing to increased production. High density lipoprotein levels are variable. Severe proteinuria and hypoalbuminemia associated with structural glomerular lesions are often accompanied by a decreased high density lipoprotein cholesterol level. The resultant increase in the low density–high density cholesterol ratio may predispose to atherosclerosis and to an increased risk of coronary artery disease. Unfortunately, therapy directed at correcting this lipid disorder in the nephrotic syndrome is of uncertain value. Some lowering of the total serum cholesterol level (10 to 30 percent) can be achieved by resins, such as cholestyramine and colestipol. However, these drugs are not well tolerated and could have undesirable effects on vitamin D absorption. Niacin is also an effective hypolipidemic drug, but its long-term benefits are unknown. Clofibrate and gemfibrozil have their primary effects on triglycerides and may cause muscle injury if given in the usual dosages because of decreased albumin binding. Probucol is also modestly effective in reducing the total serum cholesterol level, but no long-term studies of its safety and efficacy have yet been reported. Mevinolin may be the drug of choice; however, its use in the nephrotic syndrome has not been widely tested, and side effects (e.g., cataracts, liver damage) may limit its overall value. Nonetheless preliminary studies have shown significant decreases in the total cholesterol and low density lipoprotein cholesterol levels on the order of 35 to 40 percent, often accompanied by a modest increase in the high density lipoprotein cholesterol level with the use of mevinolin, gemfibrozil, or probucol. Dietary management is usually unsuccessful, but a prudent diet consisting of a reduced cholesterol intake and an increased ratio of monounsaturated to polyunsaturated fat is indicated. It is seldom possible to normalize the total serum cholesterol or low density lipoprotein cholesterol level in patients with unremitting nephrotic syndrome with either diet or pharmacologic agents.

Management of Hypercoagulability

The nephrotic syndrome is a hypercoagulable state characterized by reduced levels of inhibitors of coagulation (e.g., antithrombin III, protein C, protein S) and increased procoagulant factors (platelets, fibrinogen). Spontaneous arterial and venous thromboses are not uncommon. Management involves regular exercise, avoidance of venostasis, and prophylactic low dose heparin therapy during periods of immobilization. Long-term warfarin therapy may be indicated if an episode of proven thrombosis or embolism occurs (e.g., renal vein thrombosis). The presence of hypoalbuminemia and the concomitant use of other drugs may alter the absorption or metabolism of warfarin, requiring careful monitoring with prothrombin time measurements.

THERAPIES SPECIFIC FOR THE PRIMARY GLOMERULAR LESION

Spectrum of Minimal Change Disease, Mesangial Proliferative Glomerulonephritis, and Focal and Segmental Glomerulosclerosis

These entities are considered together because there is a growing consensus that they may represent points in a spectrum of disease severity. Systemic factors associated with their presence should be ruled out prior to instituting treatment. These include Hodgkin's disease or the use of nonsteroidal anti-inflammatory drugs in cases of minimal change disease; systemic lupus erythematosus in cases of mesangial proliferative glomerulonephritis; or intravenous drug abuse, vesicoureteral reflux, acquired immunodeficiency disease, unilateral renal agenesis, and morbid obesity in cases of focal and segmental glomerulosclerosis.

Prednisone is the mainstay of therapy for minimal change disease, 85 percent or more of adults achieving a remission in proteinuria. Ninety-five percent of the children similarly treated achieve a complete remission of proteinuria. Administration may begin on a daily basis (60 mg daily) or on an alternate day basis (120 mg every other day), less adrenal suppression and other side effects occurring with the latter method. Disease in most pediatric patients remits during the first month of high dose steroid therapy. The response to steroids usually takes longer in adults, and higher dosages (80 mg per day or 150 mg every other day) may be required. Tapering of the steroid dosage should begin about 1 week after complete remission is achieved, and complete withdrawal can be accomplished within the next 1 to 2 months, unless a relapse occurs.

Approximately 40 to 60 percent of adult patients and a similar number of pediatric age patients have at least one relapse. The older the patient at the time of diagnosis, the less the likelihood of relapse. Initial relapses may be treated with increased doses of steroids alone or with a combination of steroids and cytotoxic drugs. Chlorambucil, 0.1 to 0.2 mg per kilogram per day of ideal body weight, and cyclophosphamide, 2 mg per kilogram per day of ideal body weight, are the cytotoxic drugs most commonly recommended. These may be employed for approximately 2 months during which the induction of a new remission is attempted with steroids.

The use of cytotoxic drugs for the treatment of a relatively benign condition such as minimal change disease remains controversial. One should remember that spontaneous remissions in untreated patients occur in approximately 25 to 40 percent of the cases, although such remissions may require several months to develop. We recommend the use of cytotoxic drugs only for the treatment of incapacitating, frequently relapsing, steroid dependent, or steroid resistant nephrotic syndrome. Three or more relapses in any 1 year period would be sufficient to define the disease as frequently relapsing. Approximately 50 percent of the patients treated with cytotoxic drugs in this fashion are rendered relapse free for at least 5 years. Patients who experience relapses during steroid tapering or shortly thereafter (the steroid dependent patient) may not fare as well, with only about 20 to 30 percent of such patients treated with cytotoxic drugs remaining relapse free for at least 5 years.

Some investigators have employed cyclosporine, 3 to 7 mg per kilogram per day for 4 weeks, to induce remission in steroid dependent, frequently relapsing, or steroid resistant cases. Although this drug may induce a remission in these circumstances, a relapse almost invariably occurs upon discontinuation of the drug. Unfortunately cyclosporine may be too nephrotoxic to be used over long periods of time. Further work is needed to define the specific role of this drug in the treatment of the nephrotic syndrome.

At our center, patients with mesangial proliferative glomerulonephritis and focal and segmental glomerulosclerosis are treated by protocols similar to those just described for minimal change disease, unless there are independent contraindications against the use of glucocorticoids or cytotoxic drugs. The expectation of a beneficial response is lower in these patients than in those with minimal change disease (approximately 50 to 60 percent benefit for mesangial proliferative glomerulonephritis and 25 to 30 percent for focal and segmental glomerulosclerosis). A complete remission of proteinuria is generally not observed; a diminution in proteinuria to non-nephrotic levels is more commonly found. Finally, when prescribing potentially toxic drugs, such as cytotoxic drugs, it is imperative to carefully and completely review the possible benefits and risks with the patient and his family.

Membranoproliferative Glomerulonephritis

Membranoproliferative glomerulonephritis is an uncommon form of glomerulonephritis in adults, occurring in less than 2 percent of the patients undergoing biopsy for the nephrotic syndrome. The disorder is also known as mesangial capillary glomerulonephritis. Several subtypes exist based upon findings in electron microscopy and immunofluorescence microscopy. The clinical features of these subtypes are similar, although one subtype, dense deposit disease or type II membranoproliferative glomerulonephritis, is commonly associated with a profound reduction in the serum concentration of the C_3 component of complement and detectable levels of an autoantibody to the C_3 convertase (C_3 nephritic factor). Depression of the serum C_3 level may be seen in the other subtypes of membranoproliferative glomerulonephritis but less commonly.

The majority of adult patients with light microscopic findings suggesting idiopathic membranoproliferative glomerulonephritis have underlying systemic illnesses. These include, but are not limited to, systemic lupus erythematosus, cryoglobulinemia, postinfectious glomerulonephritis, chronic hepatitis B infection, intravenous drug abuse, sickle cell anemia, and partial lipodystrophy. Most studies evaluating therapy involve patients with the form of membranoproliferative glomerulonephritis known as type 1 or subendothelial deposit membranoproliferative glomerulonephritis.

The appropriate treatment for membranoproliferative glomerulonephritis has long been an area of controversy. Uncontrolled early studies suggested benefit from a combination of dipyridamole, warfarin, and cyclophosphamide. Prospective controlled studies, however, have failed to demonstrate benefit from this regimen. Uncontrolled studies also have claimed that long-term survival and remission of the nephrotic syndrome are associated with glucocorticoid therapy, especially when this is begun early in the course of the disease. However, these studies have been criticized because of their uncontrolled design, the exclusion of a signficant number of patients from the final analysis, and the use of cytotoxic drugs in addition to glucocorticoids in approximately one-quarter of the patients reported. Limited controlled studies employing glucocorticoids have failed to confirm a substantial benefit. Prospective controlled studies have demonstrated marginal preservation of the glomerular filtration rate but no decrease in proteinuria in patients taking aspirin, 325 mg, and dipyridamole,

75 mg three times daily. In the absence of definitive proof of benefit from glucocorticoids or cytotoxic drugs, we take a conservative approach and treat patients with this disorder with aspirin and dipyridamole. Further prospective clinical studies are needed in this group of patients, since the prognosis is poor and the benefit of aspirin-dipyridamole therapy is marginal.

IgA Nephropathy (Berger's Disease)

IgA nephropathy is a common disorder that does not often evoke the nephrotic syndrome. Most patients present with recurring bouts of macroscopic hematuria, often in association with an upper respiratory infection and sometimes accompanied by a transient reduction in renal function. Progressive renal failure develops in approximately 30 percent of the patients followed for 20 years. The remainder either retain normal renal function or have stable but abnormal renal function.

Approximately 5 to 10 percent of the patients develop the nephrotic syndrome. These fall into two groups based upon findings in light microscopy. Those with no or mild glomerular changes, resembling minimal change disease, respond to glucocorticoids in the same way that patients with minimal change disease respond, as already described. Patients with well developed mesangial proliferation, focal and segmental glomerulosclerosis, or segmental crescentic disease respond poorly if at all to glucocorticoids. At present there is no satisfactory therapy for the latter group of patients. Numerous approaches have been tried but none have produced consistent success. The protracted course of the disease and the slow evolution of renal failure make prospective controlled trials difficult.

The long-term use of glucocorticoid or glucocorticoid-cytotoxic drug combinations is probably not of great value, except in the patients with the nephrotic syndrome and minimal change disease, and may be associated with increased complications. Their use is not recommended until prospective clinical trials can define a subset of responsive patients in addition to those with minimal change disease.

Intensive plasma exchange combined with glucocorticoids and azathioprine or cyclophosphamide could be used for the rare patient with the nephrotic syndrome, rapidly progressive renal failure, and extensive glomerular crescents. Patients with acute renal failure associated with microscopic hematuria and upper respiratory infection, in whom renal biopsies demonstrate only occasional segmental crescents (usually involving less than 50 percent of glomeruli) and extensive tubulointerstitial alterations, should be treated conservatively, since nearly all achieve spontaneous complete recovery of renal function.

Long-term trials involving combinations of warfarin, dipyridamole, and cyclophosphamide, currently in progress, may provide a rationale for a more aggressive approach in subsets of patients with IgA nephropathy. Occasional patients benefit from a gluten free diet if they can be shown to have circulating antigliadin antibodies or intestinal biopsy findings consistent with celiac disease. Patients with nephrotic range proteinuria or impaired renal function may benefit from modest protein restriction or treatment with angiotensin converting enzyme inhibitors. Cyclosporine may have a short-term benefit; however, it is too toxic a drug to be widely recommended. Broad spectrum antibiotics may be used in patients with recurring infections and episodes of macroscopic hematuria, although there is no evidence that they alter the true natural history of the disease. Dilantin, dapsone, and tonsillectomy have all been used to some extent, but there is no convincing evidence of efficacy. High oral doses of eicosapentaenoic acid (fish oil) have been recommended. There is anecdotal evidence for a reduction in the frequency of bouts of hematuria, but no prospective control trials have been conducted thus far to demonstrate long-term efficacy. Such agents may also be deleterious to the course of renal failure, since they may produce renal vasodilation and aggravate glomerular capillary hypertension.

Cromolyn sodium has been advocated, but there is no evidence of long-term efficacy.

In short, except for the patient with the nephrotic syndrome and minimal change disease and perhaps the patient with rapidly progressive glomerulonephritis due to extensive crescentic disease, no therapy is of proven effectiveness in IgA nephropathy. At present such patients are probably best treated conservatively, awaiting the results of continuing prospective clinical trials.

SUGGESTED READING

Cameron S, Glassock R, eds. The nephrotic syndrome. New York: Marcel Dekker, 1988.
Glassock R, Adler S, Ward H, Cohen A. The primary and secondary glomerular diseases. Chapters 22 and 23. In: Brenner B, Rector F, eds. The kidney. Philadelphia: WB Saunders, 1986: 929.
Jacquot C, Baran D, Vendeville B, et al. Update on immunosuppressive therapy in human and experimental glomerulonephritis. Adv Nephrol 1988; 17:77–100.
Schrier RW, Gottschalk C. Diseases of the kidney. Fourth Edition. Section X, Chronic glomerulonephritis and chronic interstitial nephritis. Boston: Little, Brown, 1987: 1827.

ACUTE INTERSTITIAL NEPHRITIS

GERALD B. APPEL, M.D., F.A.C.P.
MICHAEL I. LEVINE, M.D.

The term acute interstitial nephritis describes a pattern of renal failure characterized by rapid deterioration of renal function and associated with typical clinical and renal histologic findings. Although there are many more common causes of renal dysfunction, acute interstitial nephritis remains an important cause since it is often iatrogenic, is clinically and histologically distinct, and is potentially treatable. The following discussion focuses on the therapeutic decisions concerning this pattern of renal disease.

Acute interstitial nephritis initially was described in the postmortem examinations of patients dying from systemic infectious diseases such as diphtheria and scarlet fever. In these disorders the interstitial inflammatory cell infiltrates and edema between the glomeruli and tubules were thought to be secondary to the systemic infection rather than due to direct invasion by the organisms. With the advent of effective antimicrobial drugs such causes of acute interstitial nephritis have

become far less common and of minor clinical importance. Over the last 25 years it has become clear that the majority of cases of acute interstitial nephritis are medication associated. Although the beta lactam antibiotics, and especially methicillin, were major offenders in the past, numerous other drugs, including other antibiotics, diuretics, H_2 blockers, and the nonsteroidal anti-inflammatory drugs, have been implicated in producing acute interstitial nephritis. In some patients acute inflammation of the renal interstitial space has also been associated with autoimmune or collagen diseases, such as systemic lupus erythematosus. In others acute interstitial nephritis appears to be idiopathic with no known offending medication or associated illness.

Appropriate diagnosis of acute interstitial nephritis is crucial in reaching appropriate decisions concerning treatment and management. Fortunately in many cases, and especially in those related to the administration of medications, the clinical features are helpful in establishing the diagnosis. The "hypersensitivity triad" of rash, fever, and eosinophilia is found in many cases of acute interstitial nephritis seen with penicillins and other drugs. The rash is often maculopapular or morbilliform and typical of a drug rash. A febrile illness often occurs at the onset of the allergic reaction. In the case of antibiotic related acute interstitial nephritis the original infectious febrile illness abates only to be followed by a recrudescence of fever several weeks later at the onset of the acute interstitial nephritis. Eosinophilia is present on peripheral blood smears in many patients.

All three features of the hypersensitivity triad need not be present simultaneously, and indeed they may occur in any combination or sequence. Most typically they occur after several weeks of therapy. Other systemic findings such as arthralgia, arthritis, lympadenopathy, and hepatomegaly are less common in acute interstitial nephritis. The urinary findings also can be helpful and may include sterile pyuria, mild proteinuria (less than 3 g per day), and especially eosinophilia. As with peripheral blood eosinophilia, eosinophiluria need not be present in documented cases of acute interstitial nephritis; however, the greater the magnitude of the eosinophilia-eosinophiluria in a patient with acute renal insufficiency, the greater the likelihood of acute interstitial nephritis. The renal dysfunction in acute interstitial nephritis is usually acute in onset with rapidly rising blood urea nitrogen and serum creatinine levels; nonoliguric renal failure is common.

An exception to the typical clinical and laboratory features of drug induced acute interstitial nephritis are the cases associated with the use of nonsteroidal antiinflammatory drugs. In such cases the patients are often in the older age group, have taken the drug for many weeks to many months before the onset of the disease, and often do not develop rash, fever, or eosinophilia. Moreover, the acute interstitial nephritis produced by this class of drugs is often associated with nephrotic range proteinuria and "minimal change" glomerulopathy on renal biopsy.

Idiopathic acute interstitial nephritis may present as isolated acute renal failure without other clinical features. It also may be associated with uveitis or iridocyclitis and bone marrow granulomas. Acute interstitial nephritis associated with systemic infection (e.g., streptococcal disease, subacute bacterial endocarditis) usually produces only mild acute deterioration of renal function.

The exact mechanism(s) of renal dysfunction in acute interstitial nephritis is unclear. There is, however, evidence of immunologic derangements in the pathogenesis of drug induced acute interstitial nephritis. The reaction, which is typically not dose related, occurs in only a small percentage of patients treated with the drugs; it may exacerbate on rechallenge with the same or a similar drug. The presence of rash, fever, eosinophilia, eosinophiluria, and eosinophilic interstitial inflammatory infiltrates in some cases is suggestive of hypersensitivity phenomena. At times elevated IgE levels have been reported as well as IgE containing plasma cells in the interstitial renal infiltrates. In some cases granulomatous reactions or increased numbers of cytotoxic T cells are found in the renal interstitium, suggesting a cell mediated immune response; antibasement membrane antibodies and linear staining for drug hapten, immunoglobulins, or complement along the tubular basement membranes suggest a humoral mechanism of renal damage. The precise mechanism in any case may involve one or several such immune reactions.

Although the foregoing clinical and laboratory features may suggest a diagnosis of acute interstitial nephritis, only a renal biopsy can confirm the diagnosis. At times, in severely ill patients with relative contraindications to renal biopsy, deferring this procedure may be prudent. In general, if immunosuppressive therapy is to be used to treat a presumptive lesion of acute interstitial nephritis, a confirmatory renal biopsy is advisable. Likewise, if the results of the biopsy will influence the nature and course of the planned therapy, it should be undertaken. On the contrary, in a patient with the classic hypersensitivity triad, in whom renal dysfunction reverts toward normal by just discontinuing the likely offending drug, and in whom no additional immunosuppressive therapy is contemplated, a biopsy is superfluous.

The first step in the treatment of medication induced acute interstitial nephritis is to discontinue the suspected offending drug. It is not always obvious which therapeutic agent is the "offender" in patients receiving multiple drugs. Stopping administration of all such drugs is clearly a wise decision, but if this is not possible, changing the potentially offending drugs to drugs of chemically unrelated classes would be desirable (e.g., discontinue penicillin and replace with vancomycin rather than with another beta lactam antibiotic, such as a cephalosporin; discontinue furosemide and replace with spironolactone rather than with another loop diuretic with a similar structure such as bumetanide). The majority of patients, and in our experience especially those with plasma creatinine levels less than 3 mg per dl, experience a prompt return of renal function toward normal in several days to 1 week just by discontinuing the drug. In an extensive review of beta-lactam antibiotic induced acute interstitial nephritis, only a small percentage of patients had severe renal failure or failure that was prolonged enough to require dialysis. Despite the high incidence of remission on discontinuing the offending drug, some patients continue to experience a progressive rise in the blood urea nitrogen and plasma creatinine to uremic levels.

Good supportive care is crucial in the survival of this population. Dialysis may be necessary to prevent uremic symptoms, to correct acid-base and electrolyte imbalances, and to optimize the fluid status. Because the acute renal failure is typically nonoliguric, in our experience dialysis is rarely needed before the serum creatinine level reaches 10 mg per dl or the blood urea nitrogen, 100 mg per dl. With good support the majority of patients regain enough renal function in a period of days to weeks so that dialytic intervention is no longer required.

Despite multiple isolated reports of the use of corticosteroids in patients with acute interstitial nephritis, two major therapeutic questions remain concerning their use. First, do they alter the progression of acute renal failure, leading to less severe renal failure, less requirement for dialysis, and a more rapid return of renal function to normal? Second, does the use of corticosteroids prevent the acute interstitial inflammatory process from leading to chronic interstitial scarring and fibrosis?

Although many case reports have shown that patients treated with high doses of corticosteroids may experience a dramatic reversal of the acute renal failure, an equal number of reports show no major benefit from corticosteriod therapy. Such treatment does have a theoretical basis for use and appears to be effective in other immune mediated forms of acute renal interstitial inflammatory conditions (e.g., lupus interstitial nephritis, acute cellular transplant rejection).

A study comparing the use of corticosteroids with their absence in the treatment of acute interstitial nephritis included 14 patients with methicillin induced acute interstitial nephritis. Eight of the 14 received prednisone at an average dosage of 60 mg daily for approximately 10 days. The treated and nontreated groups were generally comparable in terms of severity of disease, as reflected by average peak serum creatinine levels. In a greater percentage of treated patients (⅝ compared with ⅔) the renal function returned to the premethicillin baseline level as indicated by the serum creatinine level. Additionally, the treated group had a lower final mean serum creatinine level (1.4 mg per dl versus 1.9 mg per dl), and the time for renal function to return to baseline was shorter in the treated group. However, this study was not adequately controlled or blinded, allowing for potential bias. It does strongly suggest that certain patients can benefit from steroid therapy, resulting in a shorter course of illness and greater return of function.

Likewise, a report describes seven patients who received high doses of steroids (500 to 1000 mg of prednisolone intravenously) for 2 days as treatment for acute interstitial nephritis. Each patient experienced rapid recovery of renal function. Again there was no control group. Of particular note was the successful use of cyclophosphamide along with prednisolone, with resolution of the nephrotic syndrome in one case complicated by a history of minimal change disease.

Another retrospective review examined patients with acute interstitial nephritis who received 40 to 80 mg of prednisone for 4 to 6 weeks. The maximal creatinine values were comparable in these treated patients to those in a nontreated group with acute interstitial nephritis, and there was no difference in the duration of acute renal failure. After 8 weeks from the onset of the renal failure there was a statistically lower serum creatinine level in the treated group. This suggested that steroid therapy had its greatest impact on reducing the severity of chronic renal insufficiency. This study was retrospective and included patients with a variety of etiologies of acute interstitial nephritis.

Patients with nonsteroidal anti-inflammatory drug induced acute interstitial nephritis most often experience resolution of the acute renal failure and the nephrotic syndrome with cessation of use of the offending medication. However, in patients who had an unremitting course after 4 to 5 weeks, most respond to a course of corticosteroid therapy. Similarly, although rare cases of idiopathic acute interstitial nephritis may remit spontaneously, there are also reports of cases that respond dramatically to a course of prednisone. Unfortunately, as in cases of acute interstitial nephritis caused by antibiotics, these have not been well controlled studies.

Thus, there is sufficient evidence that in certain cases steroid therapy can hasten the recovery of renal function and reduce or prevent permanent renal damage. Further studies are required to determine which cases will resolve without therapy and which patients are at risk for the development of chronic renal dysfunction.

Our approach to the patient with presumed acute interstitial nephritis includes discontinuation of any medications known to produce this pattern of renal disease. Alternative medications should include drugs of different classes that do not cross react with the potential offending drugs. Patients in whom renal failure is still progressive, those whose diagnosis is uncertain from the clinical picture, and those who will be treated with corticosteroids or other immunosuppressive medications warrant a renal biopsy unless there are strong contraindications to this procedure (bleeding diathesis, solitary kidney). Most patients respond before they require dialysis for the correction of uremia. In patients whose renal function has not reverted toward normal at this point, and in those whose renal function has not returned to baseline at 3 to 4 weeks, we have tried several therapeutic options.

First, daily high dosage corticosteroid therapy is given (approximately 60 mg of prednisone daily) for a maximum of 1 to 2 months or a shorter treatment period if there is a clear response with a decrease of the serum creatinine to the baseline value. Second, alternate day high dosage steroid therapy (120 mg prednisone every other day) is given for a similar period. Third, pulse intravenous doses of steroids are given at very high dosages (500 mg to 1 g of methylprednisolone every other day for three doses followed by no treatment or either of the first two regimens). It should be stressed that although there is suggestive evidence of therapeutic benefit with each of these regimens, none has been rigorously proven to be efficacious in reversing the acute renal failure or preventing later renal interstitial scarring. Since the latter two regimens without daily administration of corticosteroids may produce fewer steroid induced side effects such as gastrointestinal bleeding, hypertension, and risk of infections, we have found them preferable.

The decision to terminate corticosteroid treatment should be based on one of the following:

1. A clear response to treatment, with the serum creatinine level returning to the baseline value.

2. The unusual case of lack of reversal of renal failure after 1 to 2 months of treatment, at which point it is unlikely that any further short term or long term benefit will accrue.

3. Side effects related to the use of corticosteroids, which make the risks of continued therapy outweigh the benefits.

Other immunosuppressive or cytotoxic medications (e.g., cyclophosphamide, azathioprine, cyclosporine) have not yet been tried in this condition in any sizable population or in a rigorous fashion, and their use remains totally experimental. They should be reserved for patients who fail to respond to all the foregoing measures in whom the risks of intensive immunosuppressive therapy are clearly outweighed by the risks of prolonged or potentially permanent renal failure.

SUGGESTED READING

Appel GB, Kunis CL. Acute tubulo-interstitial nephritis. In: Cotran RS, ed. Contemporary issues in nephrology. Vol. X. New York: Churchill Livingstone, 1983; 151–187.

Cotran RS, Ramzi S. Tubulointerstitial nephropathies. Hosp Pract 1982; 17:79–92.

Feinfeld DA, Olesnicky L, Pirani CL, Appel GB. Nephrotic syndrome associated with use of the non-steroidal anti-inflammatory drugs. Neprhon 1984; 37:174–180.

Galpin JE, Shinaberger JM, Stanley TM, Blumerkrantz MJ, Bayer AS, Friedman GS, Montgomerie JZ, Guze LB, Coburn JW, Glassock RJ. Acute interstitial nephritis due to methicillin. Am J Med 1978; 65:758–765.

Laberke HG. Treatment of acute interstitial nephritis. Klin Wochenschr 1980; 58:531–532.

Pirani DL, Valeri A, Appel GB. Renal toxicity of nonsteroidal anti-inflammatory drugs. Contrib Nephrol 1987; 551:159–175.

Pusey, C. Drug associated acute interstitial nephritis: clinical and pathological features and the response to high dose steroids. Q J Med (New Series) 1983; 52:194–211.

RENAL TRANSPLANT REJECTION

KURT H. STENZEL, M.D.
JHOONG S. CHEIGH, M.D.
MANIKKAM SUTHANTHIRAN, M.D.

Despite significant advances in maintenance immunosuppressive therapy for renal transplants, the treatment of graft rejection remains a frequent and sometimes formidable problem. At our center the regimens for both maintenance and rejection therapy are the same for renal grafts from cadaveric and living related donors. Recipients of related living grafts, however, receive, in addition to drug therapy, pretransplant conditioning consisting of donor specific transfusions. This technique cannot yet be used for recipients of cadaveric grafts because of the limited time that such organs can be preserved. Table 1 lists our current maintenance therapy for renal transplant recipients. Using this therapeutic approach, and the rejection therapy described in this article, we have achieved graft survival incidences of over 95 percent for recipients of related living donor grafts and over 75 percent for recipients of cadaveric grafts. Patient survival incidences for both types of transplants are over 95 percent.

REJECTION REACTIONS: CELLULAR AND HUMORAL COMPONENTS

Rejection of renal grafts can occur at any time after transplantation but is most common within the first 3 months. Acute rejection is the most well defined type of rejection and is characterized by a dense cellular infiltrate within the kidney. This is an immunologically mediated event in which the host immune system becomes sensitized to and reacts against cell surface structures expressed on the transplanted organ. The most potent of these structures are collectively known as the histocompatibility, or transplantation, antigens. As host lymphoid cells circulate through the transplanted organ, or as cells from the transplant are sloughed into the circulation, an immune reaction is initiated. Foreign structures are recognized, probably via the T cell antigen receptor and in conjunction with accessory factors such as macrophages, dendritic cells, and interleukin 1, proliferation and clonal expansion of the antigen specific T cells are initiated. The cells differentiate into a variety of effectors, including cells that are destructive to the graft (cytotoxic T lymphocytes and delayed hypersensitivity type cells) and ones that tend to reduce the potency of the immune response (suppressor cells).

TABLE 1 Maintenance Immunosuppressive Therapy for Renal Transplants

	Prednisone (PO) or Methylprednisone (IV)	Cyclosporine
10–12 hours prior to transplant	0	5 mg/kg PO
Day of transplant	100 mg IV before and after transplant	1.5 mg/kg IV 3–4 hours before and 8–9 hours after transplant
Days 1–30	15 mg PO b.i.d.	8–10 mg/kg PO in two divided doses
Days 30+	Taper*	Taper†

* The prednisone dosage is tapered by 5 mg every month to a dosage of 10 mg per day in month 6. This dosage is then continued without further reduction.
† The exact dosage of cyclosporine is adjusted to keep the plasma cyclosporine level at 100 to 200 ng per ml for the first month. Thereafter the dosage is tapered to 4–6 mg per kg per day to maintain the plasma levels at 50 to 150 ng per ml.

Antibodies to transplantation antigens often develop via B cell activiation. These antibodies may also be destructive to the graft (cytotoxic antibodies or those mediating antibody dependent, cell mediated cytotoxicity), or they may block specific immune responses (blocking or anti-idiotypic antibodies). Effector cells and antibodies reach the kidney and induce an acute graft destructive inflammatory reaction. The antigen specific cells and antibodies recruit a variety of additional inflammatory cells to the kidney that contribute significantly to the overall response. Both cellular and humoral elements contribute to the inflammatory response in acute rejection.

TYPES OF REJECTION

Hyperacute Rejection

Hyperacute rejection is mediated primarily by humoral factors. This type of rejection is now, fortunately, a rare occurrence. It is seen when the recipient previously has been immunized to antigens expressed on the transplanted kidney and circulating preformed antibody to these structures is present. Hyperacute rejection is characterized by a sudden loss of function, marked deterioration in renal blood flow, and hemorrhagic necrosis of the kidney. Although plasmapheresis, anticoagulation, and other heroic measures have been tried, there is no successful treatment for this type of rejection and the transplanted kidney must be removed.

Acute Rejection

Acute rejection is often reversible. The principles of management of acute rejection include rapid and accurate diagnosis and prompt administration of immunosuppressive drugs, at a dose and for a duration that result in reversal of the rejection episode while at the same time not resulting in excessive impairment of host defense mechanisms and consequent opportunistic infection.

The diagnosis of rejection may be difficult, especially in the first few weeks after transplantation when recipients of cadaveric grafts are sometimes in acute renal failure. Fever must be differentiated from that of infection or a drug reaction, and decreasing renal function must be differentiated from obstruction of the urinary tract, arterial or venous disease of the transplanted kidney, acute renal failure from any cause, nephrotoxicity (especially as a result of cyclosporine therapy), and recurrent or de novo renal disease.

The diagnosis of transplant rejection therefore is made after excluding other causes that might be responsible for graft failure and for the systemic manifestations

TABLE 2 Identification of Renal Graft Rejection Episodes

I. Major criteria

Increase in serum creatinine level in absence of obstruction or systemic hemodynamic alterations to account for increased creatinine, and intact (although diminished) blood flow

II. Minor criteria

a. Clinical

Fever, enlarged graft, perirenal tenderness, hypertension

b. Imaging studies

1. Renal scan: decreased flow or function

2. Sonogram: lack of obstruction

3. Doppler examination: sluggish arterial flow and diminished pulsation

c. Laboratory studies

1. Immune evaluation: increased spontaneous blastogenesis, normal or increased natural killer cell activity, and intact T cell proliferative response to T cell mitogens

2. Serum cyclosporine level: <200 ng/ml (by RIA)

III. Definitive criteria

Percutaneous renal biopsy: increased mononuclear cell infiltration (cellular rejection) or vasculitis (humoral rejection)

of acute rejection. Table 2 shows our current approach. The diagnosis of rejection is straightforward in patients with functioning renal grafts. An increase in the serum creatinine level, in the presence of an intact blood flow in the major renal vessels (by renal scan) and the absence of obstruction (by sonogram) or adverse systemic hemodynamic factors, is a sufficient trigger for the initiation of antirejection therapy. The presence or absence of other additional criteria listed in Table 2 for rejection seldom influences the decision to treat the patient, except perhaps for a plasma cyclosporine level that is greater than 200 ng per ml. Such a level might be consistent with cyclosporine toxicity, but the use of cyclosporine levels is controversial.

The commonly available cyclosporine radioimmunoassay measures intact cyclosporine as well as metabolites. Although some metabolites retain immunosuppressive properties, most do not and are apparently not nephrotoxic. High performance liquid chromatography measurements can distinguish intact drug from metabolites, but this procedure is not readily available to most transplant units. We believe that radioimmunoassays of trough cyclosporine levels are of definite value, when coupled with other diagnostic methods, in assessing the possibility of cyclosporine mediated nephrotoxicity.

The absence of minor criteria for rejection should alert the clinician to the need for a definitive diagnosis by renal biopsy. This is of special importance if a second course of antirejection therapy is contemplated. We seldom perform renal biopsies prior to initiation of the first course of antirejection therapy.

The diagnosis of rejection is often difficult in patients with nonfunctioning renal allografts. Acute renal failure of transplanted cadaveric kidneys is not unusual and can result in several weeks of oliguria. The presence of multiple minor criteria listed in Table 2 is required to make the diagnosis, and renal biopsy is often indicated prior to initiation of the first course of antirejection treatment. In the absence of a definitive renal biopsy, it is conceivable that some rejection episodes may not be recognized. Alternatively some patients may receive unnecessary antirejection therapy.

Chronic Rejection

Chronic rejection is an indolent, slowly progressive loss of renal function, characterized by an obliterative arteriopathy and consequent ischemic changes, leading to glomerular sclerosis, tubular atrophy, and interstitial fibrosis. It is resistant to antirejection therapy. The relative roles of immunologic damage and hyperperfusion injury are not clearly defined and are a subject of current investigation.

TREATMENT OF REJECTION

Steroid Pulse Therapy

Once the diagnosis of rejection is made, and renal scans show adequate blood flow to the grafted organ, all patients with acute transplant rejection episodes are treated with steroid pulse therapy. Methylprednisone, 250 mg, is given as an intravenous bolus, twice a day, for 3 consecutive days. Following this, oral doses of prednisone are given, 50 mg every 12 hours and tapered 10 mg per day to a maintenance dosage of 15 mg twice a day. This therapy results in reversal in approximately 75 percent of first rejection episodes.

Prednisone has several anti-inflamatory effects, including induction of lympholysis and inhibition of interleukin 1 production. The major hazard of pulse steroid therapy is an increased incidence of infection. This increase is directly related to the dose and frequency of steroid pulse therapy. If the rejection episode does not respond to the 3 day pulse, another antirejection drug is administered, depending on the patient's clinical status.

Specifically, it is important to determine whether the patient has a significant infection or is severely immunosuppressed, as determined by immunologic monitoring assays. We routinely monitor the following responses of peripheral blood mononuclear cells: mitogen responsiveness, natural killer cell (NK) activity, and antibody dependent cell-mediated cytotoxicity (ADCC). In addition, T cell subset distribution is assessed by flow cytometry. Peripheral blood mononuclear cell activation by mitogens that is less than 25 percent of normal, a decrease in NK and ADCC activity to 10 percent or less

of normal, and reversal of T4/T8 ratios are interpreted as indications of severe immunosuppression. The most common cause of these changes is immunosuppressive therapy, but coexisting infection, especially of viral etiology (cytomegalovirus, for instance), is also possible. The treatment of life threatening infection of course has priority over the treatment of rejection. If such infections occur, immunosuppression should be severely reduced or eliminated (save for stress dose steroid administration) and appropriate antibiotics administered.

OKT3 Monoclonal Antibody

Both antithymocyte or lymphocyte globulin and OKT3 monoclonal antibody have been used for steroid resistant rejection episodes. We now use OKT3. This is a mouse monoclonal antibody directed against the T cell differentiation antigen cluster 3 (CD3) that is expressed on virtually all mature T cells and only about 10 percent of thymocytes. CD3 consists of three peptide chains and is the invariant portion of the T cell antigen receptor complex. This complex consists of the invariant CD3 and the polymorphic portion, Ti. OKT3, when added to lymphocytes in vitro, binds to the CD3 antigen and modulates the antigen receptor complex (that is, causes it to disappear from the cell surface). OKT3 induces polyclonal T cell activation (proliferation and induction of cytolytic activity). When it is administered in vivo, there is a rapid loss of CD3 bearing cells in the peripheral blood, similar to the effect of antithymocyte globulin.

OKT3 is a potent reagent, with significant toxicity, and induces marked immunosuppression. It can result in increased pulmonary capillary permeability, especially with the first several doses. For this reason it is imperative that patients be at or close to their dry weight when the drug is administered. A chest x-ray examination should be done to make sure that there is no evidence of incipient pulmonary edema or pulmonary vascular congestion.

The first dose of OKT3 often results in chills, fever, dyspnea, wheezing, and chest pain. The patient should be informed of these effects. If the patient is receiving azathioprine, this is discontinued. The cyclosporine dosage is reduced to 200 mg per day or 3 mg per kg per 24 hours, whichever is lower. The prednisone dosage is reduced to 15 mg by mouth twice a day. In addition, the patient should receive methylprednisolone, 1 mg per kg, 30 minutes prior to OKT3 administration for the first three doses. Our current regimen is to administer OKT3, 5 mg per day, for 10 days; it is given as an intravenous bolus over 1 minute. The cyclosporine dosage is readjusted to the pre-OKT3 level 3 days prior to the last dose of OKT3.

The use of low dose cyclosporine therapy, rather than azathioprine, during OKT3 therapy may be advantageous. Recent studies in our laboratory have indicated that cyclosporine and methylprednisolone are more effective in inhibiting OKT3 mediated activation of T cells than 6-mercaptopurine (the active metabolite of azathioprine). OKT3 mediated activation may be related to the adverse effects seen with administration of OKT3. Our studies provide experimental support for therapeutic strategies that include the use of low dose cyclosporine and methylprednisolone therapy in patients receiving OKT3.

Renal biopsy is clearly indicated in those who fail to respond to a second course of anti-rejection therapy. A renal scan is also performed to ensure that blood flow is maintained to the renal allograft. Our current practice is not to treat patients with more than three courses of antirejection therapy within a 1 month period because of the morbidity associated with intense immunosuppression.

Additional Antirejection Strategies

Equine ATG is used by some centers to treat acute rejection episodes. This was introduced prior to the development of OKT3 and was shown to be effective in several studies. Most transplant centers now use OKT3.

Pulse therapy with cyclosporine has been suggested as a therapy for rejection, but nephrotoxicity limits its use and we have not evaluated this technique. Plasmapheresis has also been evaluated for the treatment of rejection. Our experience and several controlled studies

failed to support the use of this technique for rejection episodes.

The addition of monoclonal antibodies, such as OKT3, to the therapeutic choices available has significantly enhanced our ability to reverse transplant rejection episodes. Fruits of recent research efforts directed at generating cell subset specific monoclonal antibodies and immunotoxins appear to be on the horizon and might further enhance our ability to reverse acute rejection episodes.

SUGGESTED READING

Cheigh JS, Suthanthiran M, Kaplan M, Evelyn M, Riggio RR, Fotino M, Schechter N, Wolf CFW, Stubenbord WT, Stenzel KH, Rubin AL. Induction of immune alterations and successful renal transplantation with a simplified method of donor-specific blood transfusion. Transplantation 1984; 38:501–510.
Ortho Multicenter Transplant Study Group. A randomized clinical trial of OKT3 monoclonal antibody for acute rejection of cadaveric renal transplants. New Engl J Med 1985; 313:337–342.
Shield CF, Cosimi AB, Rubin RH, Talkoff-Rubin NE, Henin J, Russell PS. Use of antithymocyte globulin for reversal of acute allograft rejection. Transplantation 1979; 28:461–464.
Suthanthiran M, Evelyn M, Rubin AL, Stenzel KH. A reappraisal of the effects of monoclonal antibodies directed at T cell differentiation antigens. Transplantation 1984; 38:720–726.
Suthanthiran M, Garavoy MR. Immunologic monitoring of the renal allograft recipient. Urol Clin North Am 1983; 10:315–325.
Suthanthiran M, Riggio RR, Cheigh JS, Walle A, Fotino M, Stenzel KH. Presumed assault or accommodative reactions involved in human renal transplantation. Uremia Invest 1985; 8:245–249.

LUPUS NEPHRITIS

JOHN H. KLIPPEL, M.D.

Lupus nephritis is responsible for significant morbidity and mortality in patients with systemic lupus erythematosus. The major potential risks include complications from the nephrotic syndrome, impaired renal function or hypertension induced by kidney disease, as well as the development of end stage renal failure. Essentially all patients with lupus have pathologic evidence of kidney involvement, whereas only a fraction actually develop clinical nephritis. Treatment is generally reserved for patients with clinical nephritis who are considered to be at substantial risk for a poor renal outcome. The two principal approaches to therapy involve the use of corticosteroids and various experimental

modalities that modify immune function, such as cytotoxic chemotherapy, apheresis, and total lymphoid irradiation. These immune modifying approaches may be associated with serious adverse side effects and remain the subject of considerable controversy.

CLINICAL VERSUS PATHOLOGIC LUPUS NEPHRITIS

The presence of clinical renal involvement in a patient with systemic lupus erythematosus is typically first detected on routine laboratory screening by the finding of an abnormal urine sediment, proteinuria, or evidence of impaired renal function with an elevated blood urea nitrogen or serum creatinine level (Table 1). Occasionally patients are identified on the basis of unexplained edema or, rarely, actually present with advanced renal failure. In the evaluation of patients with suspected lupus nephritis, it is important to exclude the influence

TABLE 1   Clinical and Pathologic Features of Lupus Nephritis

Clinical features

  Active urine sediment (red cells, white cells, cellular casts)

  Proteinuria

  Impaired renal function

Pathologic features

WHO classification	Quantitative scoring system
I. Normal	Activity index (0–24)
II. Mesangial nephritis	Cellular proliferation (0–3)
	Leukocyte exudation (0–3)
III. Focal proliferative nephritis	Karyorrhexis–fibrinoid necrosis (0–6)
IV. Diffuse proliferative nephritis	Cellular crescents (0–6)
	Hyaline deposits (0–3)
V. Membranous nephritis	Interstitial inflammation (0–3)
VI. Glomerulosclerosis	Chronicity index (0–12)
	Glomerular sclerosis (0–3)
	Fibrous crescents (0–3)
	Tubular atrophy (0–3)
	Interstitial fibrosis (0–3)

of various contributing nonlupus causes of renal or lower urinary tract disease. Frequent causes of the latter include hypertension, urinary tract infection, cystitis (lupus or drug related), drug induced impairments of renal function (particularly nonsteroidal anti-inflammatory drugs), and rare conditions that may coexist with systemic lupus erythematosus, such as Sjögren's syndrome, amyloidosis, or thrombotic thrombocytopenic purpura.

Opinions concerning indications for renal biopsy to determine the type of disease in a patient with clinical lupus nephritis vary widely. Several of the more accepted indications include persistent abnormality of the urine sediment, proteinuria in excess of 1.0 g per day, and accelerated loss of renal function. The same guidelines also apply to the patient with chronic unstable clinical nephritis in whom major changes in therapy are being considered and in whom renal pathology from the preceding 6 months is unavailable.

Several different classification schemes for the description or quantitation of pathologic findings in lupus nephritis have been developed. The two most widely used systems are that of the World Health Organization (WHO) and a quantitative system scoring active and chronic pathologic features of glomerular and tubulo-interstitial areas (Table 1). These provide valuable prognostic information about the projected course of clinical lupus nephritis and help to guide therapeutic decision making. The WHO system is structured around glomerular findings with subdivisions based on mesangial and intracapillary hypercellularity and inflammation, basement membrane thickening, location of immune deposits, and glomerular sclerosis. In the quantitative renal scoring system, individual pathologic features are scored and then summed to give an activity index and a chronicity index.

There are advantages and disadvantages to each of these systems. For instance, the WHO system has been the more extensively used and thus is more familiar to most physicians and pathologists. Although certain classes within this system seem to be associated with greater risks of progressive renal disease than others, each class, particularly diffuse proliferative, would seem to be heterogeneous, with patients having good and poor prognoses contained within the same class. Selected features of the quantitative scoring system such as tubular atrophy, glomerular sclerosis, and cellular crescents seem to identify patients at increased risk for progressive renal disease; in particular, the chronicity index has been reported to be a sensitive measure of a poor renal outcome. On the other hand, this pathologic classification scheme has not been extensively validated among different nephropathologists nor does it provide for the quantitation of membranous changes.

A comprehensive evaluation of a patient with lupus nephritis for determination of prognosis and therapeutic needs typically requires integration of both clinical and pathologic variables. In general, prominent clinical features associated with minimal pathologic involvement tend to respond promptly to aggressive, short term therapeutic interventions. In contrast, severe pathologic involvement independent of clinical abnormalities most often necessitates more prolonged therapy. Because the correlation between these variables is unreliable, it becomes difficult to predict either clinical or pathologic abnormalities on the basis of knowledge of one or the other. For instance, a patient might present with a pathologic urine sediment, modest proteinuria, and a slight increase in the serum creatinine level only to be found to have relatively benign abnormalities on renal biopsy. Or conversely, a renal biopsy occasionally reveals significant serious renal disease despite minimal clinical evidence of nephritis.

INDICATIONS FOR TREATMENT

Rigid, absolute criteria for the treatment of lupus nephritis have not been established. In principle, treatment needs to be directed primarily at those patients at greatest risk for progressive acute or chronic renal disease. As discussed, this determination is most often made on the basis of both clinical and pathologic data. It would seem possible to construct a therapeutic index incorporating these various features based on the logic used by clinicians in making therapeutic decisions in lupus nephritis.

A draft of a lupus nephritis therapy index scale is displayed in Table 2. Although this scheme would seem to approximate some of the logic used in therapy, it is important to emphasize that the clinical utility of this index is completely unproved. Indications are categorized as major, intermediate, and minor and assigned scores of 5, 3, and 1, respectively. The need for ag-

TABLE 2   Indications for Therapy of Lupus Nephritis—A Lupus Nephritis Therapy Index

	Major (5 Points)	Intermediate (3 Points)	Minor (1 Point)
Clinical			
Urine sediment	Hematuria (>20 red cells/ hpf) + frequent red cell casts	Hematuria (10–20 red cells/hpf) + rare red cell casts	Hematuria (<10 red cells/hpf)
Proteinuria	>3.5 g/24 h + nephrotic syndrome	3–5 g/24 h No nephrotic syndrome	<3 g/24 h, fixed
Serum creatinine level	Elevated, rapidly rising	Elevated, slowly rising	Elevated, stable
Pathologic			
WHO classification	Diffuse proliferative	Focal proliferative Mixed membranous-pro-liferative	Mesangial Membranous Glomerulosclerosis
Activity index	>10	5–10	<5
Chronicity index	>4	2–4	<2
Other		Low, falling serum com-plement	Elevated anti-DNA Male sex
		Failure to respond to or toxicity to high dose corticosteroids	Young patient

gressive therapy would be directly proportional to an increase in the cumulative index score. The cumulative index score might be based entirely on clinical criteria, pathologic criteria, or some combination. The cut-off score at which aggressive therapy would be unequivocally indicated would seem to be in the range of 10 or greater. At this level there would appear to be a definite risk of progressive renal disease to warrant aggressive therapy.

TREATMENT

The objectives of treatment of lupus nephritis may be several—reduce the abnormality of the urine sediment, reduce proteinuria, improve, stabilize, or prevent deterioration of renal function, or minimize the dependence of the patient on corticosteroids. In many patients more than one of these goals would be appropriate. The selection from the various therapeutic alternatives and the intensity and duration of treatment are largely functions of the exact indications for therapy and the desired objectives.

Corticosteroids

High dose corticosteroid therapy has been the standard of therapy of active lupus nephritis for several decades. Despite extensive clinical experience, many important issues relating to the optimal drug dose, duration of treatment, and rigorous proof of long term efficacy remain unresolved. Both high dose oral and megadose bolus intravenous corticosteroid regimens are used for the treatment of acute nephritis (Table 3). Corticosteroid toxic effects generally limit long term usage. Thus, high dose oral programs should not exceed 4 to 6 weeks in duration at which time reduction of the dose should be attempted. Patients who fail to respond to high dose oral corticosteroid therapy after this interval or who develop unacceptable toxic effects are candidates for other forms of therapy. The use of repeated bolus intravenous corticosteroid therapy in the long term management of lupus nephritis is a potentially valuable approach. Of particular concern with bolus megadose corticosteroid therapy is a variety of toxic effects not typically seen with high dose oral regimens (see Table 3).

Immunosuppressive Drugs

Various cytotoxic and antimetabolite drugs are used in the treatment of serious manifestations of systemic lupus, including nephritis. The rationale for this approach stems from the concept that products of the immune system mediate the pathologic changes seen in lupus nephritis and that these agents suppress the heightened or exaggerated immune functions responsible for the observed disease. These drugs are not selective for

TABLE 3 High Dose Corticosteroid Regimens for Treatment of Active Lupus Nephritis

	Schedule	Toxic Effects
Oral	Prednisone (or equivalent) at a dose of 1 mg/kg in single or divided daily dose; duration should not exceed 4–6 weeks	Many—Cushingoid body features, infection, cataracts, hypertension, osteonecrosis, and others
Intravenous, bolus, megadose	1 g (or 15 mg/kg) of methylprednisolone sodium succinate IV over 30 minutes; often repeated for 3 consecutive days	Minor (common): anxiety, facial flushing, metallic taste, hypertension, hyperglycemia
		Major (rare): anaphylaxis, seizures and other neurologic complications, intractable hiccups, arrhythmias

the immune system, and the effects on other cells are responsible for a host of toxic effects associated with this approach. Immunosuppressive drugs are regarded as experimental and generally are reserved for patients with serious forms of nephritis who have failed to benefit from conservative therapies, including high dose corticosteroid therapy.

Drugs of two different classes—alkylating drugs and purine analogues—are used most commonly (Table 4). These drugs should not be considered as alternatives or substitutes for corticosteroids, but rather are typically given in combination with corticosteroids. A number of formal randomized trials to evaluate immunosuppressive drugs in lupus nephritis have now been conducted. The differences in outcomes between treatment with immunosuppressive drugs and corticosteroids and treatment with corticosteroids alone have been extremely difficult to demonstrate convincingly. Recent data from an extensive long term trial at the National Institutes of Health have suggested that immunosuppressive drugs, compared to prednisone alone, prevent the progression of irreversible sclerosing and atrophic renal disease and

reduce the probability of end stage renal failure. There has been no evidence that immunosuppressive drugs significantly alter patient survival. Intermittent intravenous doses of cyclophosphamide given over prolonged periods (every 3 months for an average of 4 years) appeared to be the most effective drug regimen in these studies.

The potential complications of immunosuppressive drug therapy arise from the direct consequences of suppression of immune function as well as adverse effects unique to individual drugs. There seems to be little doubt that in choosing between azathioprine and cyclophosphamide, the two drugs most commonly used in systemic lupus, cyclophosphamide is associated with many more complications. In particular, the risks of herpes zoster, gonadal failure, hemorrhagic cystitis, and carcinoma of the bladder are all significantly increased with the use of this drug. Of perhaps greatest concern with each of these drugs, however, is the risk of late developing neoplasia. Although it seems clear that there is a definite risk, its actual magnitude remains undefined and likely extensive cooperative efforts will be required

TABLE 4 Immunosuppressive Drug Regimens Used in Treatment of Lupus Nephritis

	Schedule	Toxic Effects
Alkylating drugs		
Cyclophosphamide	PO: 1.0–4.0 mg/kg/day IV: 0.5–1.0 g per sq m; give IV over 60 minutes followed by hydration for 24 hours to induce diuresis; repeated every 1 to 3 months	Gastrointestinal distress, myelosuppression, amenorrhea-azoospermia, increased risk of infection and neoplasia Unique to cyclophosphamide—hemorrhagic cystitis, bladder fibrosis and carcinoma, cardiac and pulmonary toxicity, and inappropriate ADH
Chlorambucil	PO: 0.1–0.2 mg/kg/day	
Mechlorethamine	IV: 0.2–0.4 mg/kg	
Purine analogues		
Azathioprine	PO: 1.0–4.0 mg/kg/day	Gastrointestinal distress, myelosuppression, hepatitis, pancreatitis, aseptic meningitis, increased risk of infection and neoplasia
Combination chemotherapy		
Cyclophosphamide + azathioprine	PO: 50 mg/day, each drug	Same as for individual drugs; ? additive toxicities

over extended periods to establish a proper perspective on this issue.

Plasmapheresis

Plasma exchange reduces the intravascular concentrations of antibodies and immune complexes and in addition has been reported to have effects on cellular immunity and reticuloendothelial system function. These alterations are usually transient and confined mostly to the time during and immediately following plasmapheresis. Typically 40 ml of plasma per kg of body weight is removed at a time and replaced with a colloid solution, most often 5 percent albumin. The procedure is often repeated several times a week for 2 to 4 weeks. To prevent a prompt rebound by a stimulated immune system from the effects produced by plasma exchange, immunosuppressive drugs are usually given in conjunction with plasmapheresis.

The role of plasmapheresis in the treatment of lupus nephritis is still unclear. Although plasma exchange continues to be regarded as a potentially useful experimental adjunct to conventional therapy, clinical investigation of this modality in lupus has diminished markedly over the past several years. Preliminary results from several recent controlled trials suggest that plasmapheresis does not have a major impact in the long term management of lupus nephritis. However, there continue to be many proponents of plasmapheresis as a successful modality in the treatment of acute severe nephritis, particularly with a clinical picture of rapidly progressive glomerulonephritis.

Other Experimental Therapies

Total lymphoid irradiation, used in the treatment of Hodgkin's disease, has been studied in a small group of patients with lupus nephritis. The procedure has long term effects on both cellular and humoral immunity that appear to be mediated primarily by the depletion of helper-inducer lymphocytes. Clinically the predominant benefits reported have been a reduction in urine protein excretion, decreases in immune abnormalities as determined by laboratory testing (serum anti-DNA antibody and complement levels), as well as possible stabilization of renal function. Complications of nodal irradiation, particularly infection and cardiovascular disease, appear to pose significant limitations on this approach to therapy.

Additional experimental approaches to therapy for which limited clinical data are currently available include the immunomodulating drug cyclosporine A, the defibrinogenating drug ancrod, dietary modifications, and additives such as eicosapentaenoic acid and hormonal therapy.

END STAGE RENAL FAILURE

End stage renal failure in a patient with lupus nephritis has been very successfully managed by hemodialysis or peritoneal dialysis or transplantation. Rarely patients treated by dialysis may recover sufficient renal function to be able to discontinue dialysis. These patients with "reversible dialysis" often evolve a course leading up to dialysis as a result of abrupt and rapid deterioration of renal function. Although some of these patients are able to live without dialysis for extended periods, many eventually again develop renal failure and require long term dialysis.

An interesting clinical observation in patients with lupus undergoing hemodialysis has been a marked decrease in nonrenal manifestations as well as serologic abnormalities (anti-DNA and complement) indicative of disease activity. Whether this develops as a consequence of the effects of uremia on inflammation or immune function or dialysis per se is not clear.

The survival of patients with lupus who are managed by dialysis has been reported to be similar to that of patients with other forms of end stage renal disease, with 5 year cumulative survivals of approximately 85 percent. However, a possible exception may be in the first year of hemodialysis, in which patients with lupus appear to be highly susceptible to serious infections. In several series this has accounted for a significant mortality in the course of early dialysis.

Finally, renal transplantation has been successful in the management of end stage lupus nephritis. Transplantation is typically reserved for patients with prolonged quiescence of clinical and laboratory evidence of lupus activity. Somewhat surprisingly, recurrence of lupus nephritis in the renal allograft appears to be very infrequent.

SUGGESTED READING

Balow JE, Austin HA III, et al. Lupus nephritis. Ann Intern Med 1987; 106:79–94.

Coplon NS, Diskin CJ, et al. The long-term clinical course of systemic lupus erythematosus in end-stage renal disease. N Engl J Med 1983; 308:186–190.

Felson DT, Anderson J. Evidence for the superiority of immunosuppressive drugs and prednisone alone in lupus nephritis: results of a pooled analysis. N Engl J Med 1984; 311:1528–1533.

Kimberly RP. Pulse methylprednisolone in SLE. Clin Rheum Dis 1982; 8:261–278.

Klippel JH. Lupus nephritis. In: Pinals RS, ed. Post-graduate advances in rheumatology. Princeton: Forum Medicus, 1986:I–IX, 1.

Strober S, Field E, et al. Treatment of intractable lupus nephritis with total lymphoid irradiation. Ann Intern Med 1985; 102:450–458.

GOODPASTURE'S SYNDROME

HARRY J. WARD, M.D.
RICHARD J. GLASSOCK, M.D.

Severe glomerulonephritis mediated by autoantibodies to glomerular basement membrane is a dramatic, albeit relatively uncommon occurrence. The prototypic anti-glomerular basement membrane disease is Goodpasture's syndrome, which by definition requires the additional presence of lung purpura. The propensity for Goodpasture's syndrome to present in an explosive fashion has tended to exaggerate the importance of this disease in the grand scheme of nephrologic practice. However, the observation that anti-glomerular basement membrane disease is usually severe and frequently life threatening has ensured its niche as one of the major immunologic renal diseases with which to contend from a therapeutic standpoint. Goodpasture's syndrome and other anti-glomerular basement membrane antibody mediated glomerulonephritides may progress to oligoanuric renal failure within days, while pulmonary hemorrhage may result in the loss of up to 4 liters of blood into the lungs within a 24 hour period. Therefore, Goodpasture's syndrome represents a true medical emergency and calls for the application of definitive diagnostic and therapeutic procedures in order to effect a favorable outcome.

The identification of the autoimmune anti-glomerular basement membrane mechanism, along with an improved understanding of the kinetics of anti-glomerular basement membrane antibody production, made possible the development of more intelligent therapeutic approaches to Goodpasture's syndrome. Rational effective therapy aimed at actually removing the phlogistic antibodies and reducing their rate of synthesis turned the tide in this disease. It is gratifying to know that our enhanced understanding of the underlying immunopathogenetic mechanisms of a specific human glomerular disease has contributed substantially to the medical management.

DIAGNOSIS

In order to establish the diagnosis of Goodpasture's syndrome, the physician has to hold a high index of suspicion in any patient displaying evidence of a pulmonary-renal syndrome. Several months usually elapse between the first clue of pulmonary symptoms or hemoptysis and establishment of the diagnosis of Goodpasture's syndrome. A higher relative risk for Goodpasture's syndrome has been linked to several factors, including male sex, a patient age less than 30 years or greater than 60 years, exposure to hydrocarbon or cigarette smoke, concurrent viral disease, possession of haplotype DR-2, and certain immunoglobulin (Gm) allotypes. Cigarette smoking and intercurrent infection appear to pose particular risks to the patient with Goodpasture's disease who is already suffering from pulmonary hemorrhage.

The outcome of therapy in cases of anti-glomerular basement membrane disease is heavily influenced by the rapidity with which a diagnosis was established and the subsequent prompt institution of effective therapy. Clinical suspicion for the diagnosis of Goodpasture's syndrome should be aroused by the presence of renal abnormalities, such as a "nephritic" urinary sediment (red cell casts, white cells, proteinuria), coupled with pulmonary abnormalities. Pulmonary hemorrhage may be severe with anemia and hemoptysis, or subtle with only radiologic evidence of atypical alveolar infiltrates, increased diffusing capacity for carbon monoxide (kCO), or detection of hemosiderin laden macrophages on sputum examination. Goodpasture's syndrome is often misdiagnosed as renal failure complicated by pulmonary edema or pneumonia. The definitive diagnosis requires confirmation of the presence of circulating anti-glomerular basement membrane antibodies in serum by radioimmunoassay or by ELISA or demonstration of linear ribbon-like deposits of IgG along the glomerular basement membrane by direct immunofluorescence. One should not rely on linear alveolar basement membrane staining in lung biopsy examination, since it can be a variable occurrence in anti-glomerular basement membrane disease. Indirect immunofluorescence of normal human kidney substrate is a fast but relatively inaccurate method for the diagnosis of anti-glomerular basement membrane disease. It should be emphasized that other disorders may provoke lung hemorrhage and nephritis, including systemic lupus erythematosus, Wegener's granulomatosis, necrotizing vasculitis, cryoglobulinemia, and Schönlein-Henoch purpura.

THERAPEUTIC RATIONALE

The observation that Goodpasture's syndrome and other forms of anti-glomerular basement membrane antibody mediated glomerular disease progress in a rapid, usually relentless course to uremia or death has necessitated that one approach these diseases as medical emergencies. Fewer than 15 percent of untreated patients remain dialysis free, and mortality from pulmonary hemorrhage is high. It is now well established that the production of anti-glomerular basement membrane antibody is transient, lasting only weeks or months in most cases. More severe disease is associated with persistently high titers of antibody. Immunosuppressive drugs by themselves probably have a minimal effect on anti-glomerular basement membrane antibody production and thus have no long term role in the management of the disease. Moreover, removal of potential antigen in the

TABLE 1   Recommended Therapy of Goodpasture's Syndrome

Specific measures	
Plasma exchange	Daily 4 liter exchanges for albumin or plasma protein substitutes for 10–14 days
Cyclophosphamide	2 mg/kg/day for 8 weeks
Azathioprine	1 mg/kg/day for 8 weeks
Methylprednisone	1 g intravenous bolus for 3–5 consecutive days (optional)
Prednisone	1 mg/kg/day; then taper by 10 mg weekly until 20 mg; thereafter taper by 5 mg weekly until discontinued
Nonspecific measures	
Ventilatory support (use of CPAP, PEEP); avoid oxygen toxicity	
Dialysis (hemo- or peritoneal)	
Strict aseptic technique for extracorporeal treatment modalities	
Avoidance of cigarette smoking	
Prophylaxis or vaccination against influenza virus	

form of the kidneys (i.e., bilateral nephrectomy) should no longer be advocated as a maneuver to diminish further anti-glomerular basement membrane antibody synthesis. According to that line of reasoning, remaining lung tissue would still serve as an antigenic stimulus, leaving us with the inescapable conclusion that this approach is ineffectual and hazardous.

The therapeutic emphasis should be on the short term goal of reducing acute high concentrations of anti-glomerular basement membrane antibody and on the suppression of kidney and lung parenchymal injury. The best way to achieve this goal is by plasma exchange therapy, combined with the administration of cytotoxic drugs and steroids. Table 1 summarizes the recommended therapeutic approach.

SPECIFIC TREATMENT

Our approach to the management of Goodpasture's syndrome is derived from a modification of the standard regimen advocated by Rees and colleagues at the Hammersmith Hospital. It consists basically of daily whole plasma volume exchanges (3 to 4 liters) using 5 percent albumin or plasma protein fraction performed for 10 to 14 consecutive days. Patients with milder disease can be converted to an every other day plasma exchange regimen after five to seven exchanges. A total course of plasma exchange usually involves about 14 exchanges, although on occasion more intensive therapy may be required. We use the centrifugal method of plasma-blood separation, although membrane separation devices capable of removing IgG are probably also effective.

Plasma exchange is combined with several immunosuppressive drugs, including cyclophosphamide (2 mg per kg per day), azathioprine (1 mg per kg per day), and prednisone (1 mg per kg per day). Alternatively prednisone may be preceded by high dose intravenous

methylprednisolone therapy, 1 g daily for three to five doses. The latter approach is advocated by some authorities but is not the preference of the authors. Azathioprine or cyclophosphamide dosages are tapered in the event that marrow toxicity occurs, as metabolites of azathioprine may accumulate within a week or so in patients with compromised renal function. All immunosuppressive drugs are discontinued after 8 weeks of demonstrated undetectable anti-glomerular basement membrane antibody titers and clinical resolution of nephritis and lung purpura. Cyclophosphamide is usually discontinued earlier in older patients. Prednisone is usually reduced by 10 mg at weekly intervals until a dosage of 20 mg daily is achieved. It is then safer to proceed at a slower tapering rate by decrements of 5 mg weekly until all prednisone is discontinued. Five repeat plasma exchanges are recommended for recurrences of disease activity.

An extra note of caution is extended to the reader using the combination of cyclophosphamide and azathioprine. Aside from marrow toxicity, one should beware of troublesome stomatitis, idiosyncratic febrile reactions, and hemorrhagic cystitis (cyclophosphamide).

Complications of Plasma Exchange

The technique of plasma exchange involves the removal of whole blood from a patient and its subsequent separation into plasma and cellular constituents by centrifugation or membrane filtration. The blood cells are reinfused with fresh replacement fluid, usually in the form of albumin or plasma substitutes. The patient's original plasma is discarded, presumably ridding the individual of phlogistic antibodies (e.g., IgG complement, fibrinogen) or other soluble mediators of disease. By exchanging 4 liters of plasma, one removes up to 45 percent of the IgG fraction and can virtually eliminate a marker substance from the plasma for a short time. Immunosuppressive drugs are thus employed to maintain the low concentrations of anti-glomerular basement membrane antibody and to prevent rebound phenomena.

Vascular access is required for repeated plasma exchanges as already detailed for the treatment of Goodpasture's syndrome. Central vein double lumen catheters are our preference for both dialysis and plasma exchange. Care must be taken to avoid catheter induced infection in these immunocompromised hosts. Bleeding may occur (e.g., from a prior renal biopsy done less than 48 hours before commencing plasma exchange) if depletion of clotting factors or platelets occurs and should be corrected in the former situation with fresh frozen plasma replacement (2 units) at the end of an exchange.

Respiratory Care

Good supportive care is indispensable in the critically ill patient with Goodpasture's syndrome. Respiratory failure and literally drowning from pulmonary hemorrhage are the greatest threats to the life of the patient. Intubation for hypoxemia and active hemorrhage frequently requires treatment of the patient in the intensive care unit. Although oxygen toxicity is a concern as an exacerbating factor for pulmonary hemorrhage, there is no question that ventilator driven positive end expiratory pressure (PEEP) breathing employed to treat these patients has saved lives. Continuous positive airway pressure (CPAP) and the judicious use of inspired oxygen concentrations contribute toward improved respiratory care and patient survival in Goodpasture's syndrome.

Dialysis Therapy

During the acute stages of Goodpasture's syndrome when oligoanuric acute renal failure is not uncommon, dialysis may be indicated. Fluid overload has been reported to precipitate pulmonary hemorrhage. The requirement for dialysis therapy is a poor prognostic indicator but is usually lifesaving when employed. Hemodialysis requires dependable vascular access (as does plasma exchange) and some degree of anticoagulation with heparin. "Tight" minidoses of heparin should be used in these patients to minimize the risk of aggravating pulmonary hemorrhage. Peritoneal dialysis may avoid such a risk but is only rarely employed in modern dialysis therapy today.

General Considerations

As mentioned earlier, cigarette smoking has been reported to cause pulmonary hemorrhage or relapses of Goodpasture's syndrome. Therefore, smoking is absolutely contraindicated for the indefinite future in these patients. Intercurrent viral or bacterial infection is especially dangerous and should be prevented by the use of good sterile technique, vaccination, and isolation procedures when appropriate. The overzealous use of glucocorticoids or cytotoxic drugs increases the infection risk.

OUTCOME OF TREATMENT

The severity and rapidity of progression of Goodpasture's syndrome preclude efforts to obtain randomized controlled observations concerning the treatment that we currently employ. However, the large series of Rees and colleagues (Hammersmith) indicates that anti-glomerular basement membrane antibody disappears indefinitely after a full course of plasma exchange. Persistence of autoantibody is more prevalent in patients undergoing shorter periods of treatment (less than 12 days). Wilson and colleagues (Scripps) also reported in another large series of patients with Goodpasture's syndrome that the combination of plasma exchange and immunosuppressive drugs was superior to the drugs administered alone. They found that pulmonary hemorrhage was less protracted as the levels of anti-glomerular basement membrane antibody fell. Mild disease progressed when left untreated. From the data in over 50 patients with Goodpasture's syndrome included in these two studies, combined with our own experience, we conclude that plasma exchange and cyclophosphamide act in true therapeutic synergy to control subsequent anti-glomerular basement membrane antibody synthesis. Steroids and azathioprine act primarily as anti-inflammatory drugs employed in short intensive courses. More prolonged use of steroids adversely affects the outcome. The overall mortality still approaches 20 percent, most of which is related to pulmonary hemorrhage. Terminal renal failure is the rule in patients in whom the serum creatinine level exceeds 6.8 mg per dl or in those who go on to develop oligoanuria prior to institution of plasma exchange–immunosuppressive therapy. Therefore, upon application of this form of therapy in patients with advanced disease, one should not anticipate a favorable response with return of renal function. On the other hand, plasma exchange–immunosuppression regimens are nearly always effective in controlling pulmonary hemorrhage.

MONITORING THE PATIENT WITH GOODPASTURE'S SYNDROME

Careful clinical examination, serial urinalysis, and monitoring of the serum creatinine level are the cornerstone in gauging the progress of patients with anti-glomerular basement membrane disease. Serial chest radiographs should be assessed with changes in kCO on a twice weekly basis. Arterial blood gas levels are checked as circumstances dictate. Anti-glomerular basement membrane antibody titers are monitored initially to confirm the effectiveness of plasma exchange. Recent reports of the occasional coexistence of Wegener's granulomatosis with anti-glomerular basement membrane disease has prompted some experts to advocate the search for antineutrophil cytoplasm antibodies. Histo-logic evidence of recurrence of anti-glomerular basement membrane disease after renal transplant is not uncom-mon, whereas clinical recurrence and graft loss are rare. We generally advocate holding patients on dialysis until anti-glomerular basement membrane antibody is no longer detectable by radioimmunoassay. Such an approach, however, does not guarantee protection against recur-rences of Goodpasture's syndrome after transplant.

HYPERSENSITIVITY PNEUMONITIS

RAYMOND G. SLAVIN, M.D.

Synonyms for hypersensitivity pneumonitis include pulmonary hypersensitivity syndrome and extrinsic allergic alveolitis. The latter term is perhaps the most appropriate because it is so descriptive. "Extrinsic" refers to an exogenous allergen as the cause of the problem. "Allergic" refers to the hypersensitivity basis for the disease. "Alveolitis" refers to the part of the lung that is most affected. Despite the different terms, they all refer to the same underlying pathogenetic entity, namely, a disease process that is caused by sensitivity to an organic dust that is inhaled. The clinical presentation of the disease depends on the circumstances and degree of exposure. In the more common acute form associated with intermittent intense exposure to the organic dust, the individual responds 4 to 6 hours after exposure with low grade fever, chills, chest pain, cough, and dyspnea. In the chronic form associated with prolonged low grade exposure, the clinical presentation is much more insidious, with progressively increasing cough, dyspnea, weakness, malaise, and weight loss.

The causative antigens responsible for hypersensitivity pneumonitis can be divided into several categories, including thermophilic actinomycetes, fungi, amebae, animal products, and small molecular weight chemicals. The majority of cases are associated with occupational exposure, such as farming, mushroom packing, or grain loading. However, offending antigens may contaminate home heating or humidification units or be associated with hobbies such as pigeon breeding.

The diagnosis of hypersensitivity pneumonitis should be suspected in any patient presenting with interstitial pneumonitis or pulmonary fibrosis. Pulmonary function testing reveals a largely restrictive dysfunction, includ-ing decreases in pulmonary compliance and in carbon monoxide diffusion capacity. A careful history eliciting the onset of symptoms following exposure with remis-sion on avoidance together with positive serum precip-itins to the appropriate antigen is presumptive evidence of hypersensitivity pneumonitis. In rare instances further confirmation may have to be made by inhalation chal-lenge with the suspected antigen.

THERAPEUTIC APPROACH

Avoidance

Clearly the most important aspect in the manage-ment of hypersensitivity pneumonitis is recognition and avoidance of the causative antigen. The physician's diagnostic index of suspicion must be high, and in every case of interstitial pneumonitis or pulmonary fibrosis a careful environmental survey of the patient's occupa-tional, home, and avocational life must be carried out, searching for the presence of offending antigens. Once the disease is diagnosed and the antigen recognized, early avoidance is the definitive therapy. Hypersensitiv-ity pneumonitis ultimately may be a fatal disease due to progressive respiratory insufficiency. It is estimated that five acute episodes will be followed by pulmonary dam-age and progressive disease. Therefore, it is vital to make the diagnosis early and institute proper environ-mental precautions to prevent the inexorable conse-quences of pulmonary fibrosis and irreparable tissue damage.

A general approach to the prevention of hypersen-sitivity pneumonitis is seen in Table 1. A number of interventions will decrease the formation of antigens in conducive environments. For example, the growth of thermophilic actinomycetes spores in compost can be suppressed by treatment with a 1 percent solution of propionic acid. Water that remains for long periods of time in older air conditioning or humidification units may become a fertile source for the growth of thermo-

TABLE 1   Prevention of Hypersensitivity Pneumonitis*

Decrease formation of antigens
  Add chemicals to prevent growth
  Change water frequently in humidification or air conditioning units
  Use storage dryers on hay and straw
  Harvest crops when moisture content is low

Decrease exposure to organic dust
  Mechanically handle dusty materials within closed spaces
  Remove dusts from ambient air
  Use personal respirators or masks

Remove worker from disease producing environment

* Modified from Terho EO. Extrinsic allergic alveolitis—management of established cases. Eur J Respir Dis 1982; 123:101.

philic organisms. Therefore, the water needs to be changed and the unit cleaned on a regular basis. Contaminated ventilation systems have to be thoroughly cleaned or replaced. Blowing cool air through stored hay helps to prevent the growth of mold. Harvesting crops when the moisture content is low also results in less exposure to organic dusts.

In occupational situations in which organic dust generation is inevitable, every effort should be made to reduce the workers' exposure. In enclosed spaces extremely dusty material should be handled mechanically. The use of particular types of silos may allow for automated feeding of cattle. Materials such as sugar cane should be stored outside and cattle fed outside as much as possible so that the associated organic dusts can be diluted by the ambient air.

In terms of removal of dusts from the air, improved ventilation may aid considerably. Electrostatic air purifiers may be of help when the concentration of dust is not too great. They would be overwhelmed in an area where moldy hay is being handled in which it is estimated that there are 1600 million spores per cubic meter of air. A person doing light work with moldy hay inhales 10 liters of air per minute, which would deposit 750,000 spores per minute in the lung.

The use of personal dust respirators or masks is limited because of inconvenience. A type 2B filter is effective in filtering small particles but causes so much resistance to the flow of air that people hard at work are unable to wear them. An air stream helmet in which an electrical pump blows air through a filter and into the breathing zone is heavy and uncomfortable to wear. Even the best device has a maximal filtering capacity of 99 percent for fine particles. The remaining 1 percent can produce new attacks in a highly sensitive individual. If the disease is not yet manifest, even a filter with 95 percent filtering capacity is adequate. Good results have been reported with a 3M disposable mask model 8710.

When the foregoing environmental control measures cannot be carried out or are inadequate, the patient should be removed from that work area. This may entail

a change in the work place or type of work or in extreme cases a change in occupation.

Drug Therapy (Table 2)

In many cases no treatment is necessary other than avoidance of the causative antigen. Corticosteroid therapy, however, can greatly accelerate clinical improvement and should be considered in very ill patients with gross radiographic or physiologic abnormalities, such as hypoxemia. Oral therapy with prednisone in an initial daily dosage of 40 to 60 mg is usually adequate and should be continued until there is significant clinical, radiographic, and pulmonary function test evidence of improvement. The prednisone dosage then may be tapered slowly until resolution of clinical and radiologic signs is complete. The total duration of therapy is generally no more than 4 to 6 weeks provided exposure to the antigen is prevented. Inhaled corticosteroids are of no value in the treatment of hypersensitivity pneumonitis nor are bronchodilators or cromolyn unless bronchospasm is also present.

The dramatic response of hypersensitivity pneumonitis to corticosteroids may be a two edged sword. The rapid relief afforded by steriods may result in a false sense of security, so much so that the patient may return to the same work environment. Re-exposure will result in progression of the lung disease. It therefore must be emphasized and re-emphasized to the patient that corticosteroids are not a substitute for antigen identification and avoidance.

In cases of severe hypoxemia in the acute stage, oxygen should be administered in amounts sufficient to keep the Po_2 level between 60 and 100 mm Hg. Other supportive measures include rest, antitussives, and antipyretics.

On occasion, despite the physician's best efforts, the patient may elect to return to the same work place or occupation. This seems to be especially true of farmers, who find it particularly difficult to leave farming

TABLE 2   Treatment of Hypersensitivity Pneumonitis

Acute form
  Remove patient from exposure; may entail hospitalization
  Oxygen
  Prednisone 40–60 mg/day with slow tapering
  Supportive measures—rest, antitussives, antipyretics

Repeated acute or subacute form
  Decrease exposure as much as possible
  Long term corticosteroid therapy emphasizing alternate day therapy

Chronic form
  Trial with corticosteroids but continue only if radiographic findings and physiologic testing indicate a response

because of age, a large financial investment, and a lack of training and skills in other occupations. In these instances long term continuous corticosteroid therapy may have to be administered. One should strive for an alternate day program utilizing the lowest dosage that still controls the patient's symptoms.

The chronic form of hypersensitivity pneumonitis develops insidiously and occurs either following repeated acute episodes or as a result of long term low grade exposure. A therapeutic trial of steroids can be given but should be continued only if radiographic findings and physiologic testing indicate a beneficial response.

Appropriate treatment of the acute episode of hy-

persensitivity pneumonitis with avoidance of further antigen exposure results in an uneventful recovery with no progression to chronic untreatable disease.

SUGGESTED READING

Fink JN. Hypersensitivity pneumonitis. J Allergy Clin Immunol 1984; 74:1–9.
Terho EO. Extrinsic allergic alveolitis—management of stable cases. Eur J Respir Dis 1982; 123:101 (Suppl.).
Schatz M, Patterson R. Hypersensitivity pneumonitis—general considerations. Clin Rev Allergy 1983; 1:451–467.

IDIOPATHIC PULMONARY FIBROSIS

HERBERT Y. REYNOLDS, M.D.

The interstitial lung diseases are a heterogeneous group of diseases that affect the supporting structure of the air exchange units, especially the perialveolar tissue and alveolar walls; initially inflammation in the alveolar walls and air spaces causes an acute phase of mural and luminal alveolitis. Following prolonged or smoldering inflammation, which subsequently involves adjacent portions of the interstitium, vasculature, and respiratory bronchioles, fibrosis produces scarring and distortion of lung tissue that lead to significant derangement of gas exchange function and ventilation.

Most patients present with symptoms of breathlessness, induced by moderate exertion, and a nonproductive cough; systemic symptoms are not common unless the lung disease is a manifestation of a multiorgan illness, as found with a connective tissue disease or vasculitis. Episodic symptoms with chills and fever point to inhalational exposure to organic dusts, which could be a clue to a specific etiologic agent. A distinctive chest radiograph with symmetrical hilar adenopathy and paratracheal nodes could signal sarcoidosis. However, in many patients who have only exertional dyspnea and cough a chest radiograph shows reticular shadows in the lower lung zones, and pulmonary function tests reveal a reduction in lung volume, restrictive ventilation, and decreased diffusion capacity. After working through the broad differential diagnosis of so-called diffuse intersti-

tial lung diseases, a diagnosis of exclusion often formulated is idiopathic pulmonary fibrosis, or cryptogenic fibrosing alveolitis, as the entity is termed in Great Britain and parts of Europe.

Although the adjectives "idiopathic" and "cryptogenic" denote that the etiology is unknown, the disease is not a nebulous wastebasket diagnosis but a well defined clinical entity. This disease was described by Hamman and Rich about 50 years ago as a fulminant fatal form of the so-called alveolar-capillary block syndrome in which proliferating fibrous tissue virtually occludes the peripheral airways. In the interim, as forms of interstitial fibrosis have been recognized more frequently, it is evident that a spectrum of disease severity exists. More commonly idiopathic pulmonary fibrosis is a chronic interstitial pneumonia in which patients have respiratory symptoms for some months to several years before the diagnosis is made and thus present themselves for medical evaluation at the midstage of disease; survival afterward is in the range of 2 to 10 years. This more slowly evolving, progressive disease in middle aged adults is characteristic of most patients studied in recent clinical series.

Based upon serologic tests, histologic descriptions of lung tissue, and analyses of cells and proteins-enzymes recovered from the distal airways and alveolar surface by bronchoalveolar lavage, a composite view of immunopathogenic mechanisms has been developed (Table 1). Greatly aiding this process has been the in vitro culturing of respiratory cells, especially alveolar macrophages, with measurement of cellular mediators secreted into the culture medium and subsequent assessment of their effects on other cells, such as fibroblasts and polymorphonuclear neutrophils.

Important for management of the patient are four ingredients that must be considered by the physician: insuring the accuracy of the diagnosis to reasonably

TABLE 1   Idiopathic Pulmonary Fibrosis: Cellular and Immunologic Changes

Blood	Bronchoalveolar Fluid	Lung Tissue
Ig (IgG$_{1,3}$)	Alveolitis (characterized by more macrophages and increased percentage of PMN [20%], eosinophils [2–4%], but lymphocytes can be increased also [20%])	Interstitial inflammation Plasma cells Fibroblasts Collagen synthesis (type III > I) fibrosis but no granuloma Bronchiolitis obliterans can develop
Immune complexes		
Cryoglobulins		
Serologic titers (low)	Alveolar macrophages—active and their secretory components are numerous: Chemotaxins to attract PMN and ? muscle cells Plasminogen activator Fibroblast growth factor Fibronectin Steroid receptors increased; mitosis increased	
T lymphocytes (sensitized to type I collagen)		
	Collagenase (PMN origin)	
	IgG increased; G$_3$, G$_1$ subclasses	
	Immune complexes	
	IgG releasing cells	
	Histamine elevated	

exclude other diseases that might require a much different therapeutic approach (e.g., lymphangitic spread of carcinoma or an occupational disease such as asbestosis), staging the cellular activity of the process, initiating anti-inflammatory immunosuppressive therapy, and monitoring the disease process either by watching the natural course in an untreated patient or assessing the efficacy of therapy.

DIAGNOSIS

Although a clinical impression, various blood and laboratory tests of lung function, chest imaging (computed tomography and gallium[67] citrate lung scans), and bronchoalveolar lavage analysis suggest a diagnosis of idiopathic pulmonary fibrosis, none of these is sufficiently specific or pathognomonic to make the diagnosis unequivocally. Lung tissue is desirable for pathologic scrutiny. Multiple transbronchial biopsy specimens obtained during fiberoptic bronchoscopy from different portions of an affected lung usually may not suffice for a definitive diagnosis by a pathologist. By contrast, a granulomatous interstitial disease such as sarcoidosis may be diagnosed from such specimens in up to 70 percent of the cases. However, an attempt at diagnosis by this method is advisable because most patients are going to be subjected to bronchoscopy by a pulmonologist, a reasonably low risk invasive procedure even with transbronchial biopsy. (Approximately 1 to 5 percent of the patients develop partial pneumothorax and about 25 percent experience a postprocedure pneumonitis that is transient and usually not microbial; therefore antibiotic therapy is not required in most instances.)

In up to 25 percent of the cases of idiopathic pulmonary fibrosis, a reasonably certain diagnosis can be made on the basis of transbronchial biopsy tissue examination; histologic examination has helped to rule out many other disease processes. Microbial cultures and cytologic examination are other indispensable parts of the bronchoscopy procedure.

A frequent dilemma is whether to accept a probable clinical diagnosis of idiopathic pulmonary fibrosis in the face of an inadequate or nondiagnostic transbronchial biopsy and initiate treatment, or to proceed with an open lung biopsy. The decision is always more difficult in an elderly and frail patient. Will a short trial of corticosteroid therapy to see how the patient responds really reverse or obscure the tissue characteristics of the disease should this therapy not prove effective and it then becomes necessary to perform a thoracotomy?

My strong recommendation is to obtain an adequate tissue diagnosis before embarking on therapy even if it requires an open biopsy and the patient is not enthusiastic about having even a minithoracotomy. This bias is the result of seeing many patients in consultation in whom the tissue diagnosis is not certain and the baseline data (e.g., pulmonary function, decreased diffusion capacity) are not complete.

A frequent scenario involves a patient whose lung symptoms have progressed despite corticosteroids and the question of using a cytotoxic drug for greater immunosuppression is raised, or corticosteroids have not been helpful yet the patient now is dependent on them and has significant side effects but weaning from the drugs is difficult. Without knowing what process was occurring in the lung or how advanced it was (as judged by the cellularity of the biopsy specimen and the distribution and type of inflammatory cells present), therapy for the patient becomes guesswork.

STAGING DISEASE ACTIVITY

Typically most patients with idiopathic pulmonary fibrosis have had some respiratory symptoms (exertional breathlessness and cough) for several years before seeking or receiving a thorough evaluation. Prior chest radiographs may have shown increased linear shadows in the lung bases that were not identified then but in retrospect, as judged by a current film, the interstitial process had begun and was evident. Thus, a patient may present in a midstage of the illness when pulmonary function tests document restrictive function, loss of diffusion capacity, and arterial desaturation of oxygen if assessed during exercise. These tests all corroborate the chest radiographic findings. Physical examination at midstage reveals lung findings, principally inspiratory coarse crackles, but overt cardiac involvement (right heart hypertension due to increased pulmonary artery resistance) may be absent. Mild digital clubbing may be found at this stage (in 50 percent of the patients), but noticeable cyanosis is unusual. Unless a multisystem disease is the cause of the interstitial lung disease, other abnormal physical findings are not common. Therefore, an objective way to assess the activity of the interstitial lung process is important in forming a prognosis and gauging therapy; this involves judging the relative degree of inflammation, which might be reversible, as opposed to fibrosis, which implies a fixed nonreversible lesion. The lung biopsy specimen is still the most accurate way of obtaining such information. Special instructions should be given to the surgeon to obtain samples that will provide the most information about the disease process, preferably from several different places in a lung, and not to take the most readily available tissue (e.g., lingula or tip of the right middle lobe), which might not be optimal.

Many pathologists no longer believe that a rigid grading of the biopsy findings as representing desquamative interstitial pneumonitis or usual interstitial pneumonitis distinguishes separate forms or stages of the disease; rather they believe that these reflect a continuum of the same disease process. However, the relative cellularity of the lung tissue and other distinguishing features in the histologic examination have been found to help with the prognosis and in anticipating the response to corticosteroid therapy.

The experience of Carrington and co-workers in categorizing lung biopsy findings in this way is important (Table 2). Of note, some of the patients with desquamative interstitial pneumonitis, if untreated, had spontaneous remission of disease, but most did not; treatment with corticosteroids (prednisone, 40 to 60 mg per day, tapering after 3 months to 20 mg per day and continuing for 1 year) caused 62 percent of the patients with desquamative interstitial pneumonitis to improve. Usual interstitial pneumonitis was much worse in all respects. The experience offered in this study argues persuasively for a careful attempt at classifying patients,

TABLE 2   Outcome in Desquamative Interstitial Pneumonia and Usual Interstitial Pneumonitis*

	Desquamative Interstitial Pneumonia (%)	Usual Interstitial Pneumonitis (%)
Overall mortality		
Dead at 5 years	4.8	45
Dead at 10 years	30	72
Course		
Untreated	(32 patients)	(48 patients)
Spontaneously improved	22	0
No change	16	15
Worse	62	85
Treated with corticosteroids	(26 patients)	(26 patients)
Improved	62	12
No change	12	19
Worse	26	69

* Adapted from Carrington CB, et al. Natural history and treated course of usual and desquamative interstitial pneumonia. N Engl J Med 1978; 298:801–809.

on the basis of open lung biopsy, into the two histologic groups for prognostic and treatment purposes. These results also confirm the original postulate of Liebow and colleagues that desquamative interstitial pneumonitis represents a distinct entity among the interstitial pneumonias. Balanced against this is the prevalent concept that it is just an early gradation within the evolution to usual interstitial pneumonitis, and that desquamative interstitial pneumonitis does not distinguish patients with another form of the disease (and possibly a different etiologic agent).

However, open lung biopsy is usually a once-only procedure and is not a way to monitor a patient's future course; transbronchial lung biopsy findings may not be representative either. Other tests that can be used indirectly to assess the inflammation and cellular activity in lung tissue are to be discussed briefly: blood studies, pulmonary function tests, lung scanning with gallium, and bronchoalveolar lavage for analysis of cells and proteins retrieved from the alveolar surface.

Blood Studies

Although idiopathic pulmonary fibrosis is limited to the lungs, except for its association with collagen-vascular diseases as included in some series, the effects of chronic inflammation may be reflected systemically. An elevated sedimentation rate is usual, and low titers in certain serologic tests—rheumatoid factor, cryoglobulins, and immune complexes—can be detected. Despite initial reports that circulating immune complexes in patients with idiopathic pulmonary fibrosis correlated with cellularity of the lung biopsy specimen, this association has not proved helpful.

Pulmonary Function Tests

Routine spirometry documents reduced lung volumes and restrictive ventilation, but these simple tests are not as informative in the overall management of the patient as the carbon monoxide diffusing capacity and the arterial oxygen tension recorded during exercise. The carbon monoxide diffusing capacity, which was found to correlate with the amount of fibrosis in the lung biopsy specimen, and assessment of hypoxemia (oxygen desaturation recorded with oximetry) during exercise seem to reflect the functional capacity of the patient. The carbon monoxide diffusing capacity may increase with successful therapy. In contrast, worsening hypoxemia may signal the need for supplemental oxygen and impending right heart failure reflecting cor pulmonale; both complications indicate advanced idiopathic pulmonary fibrosis and limitation of physical activities.

Imaging Techniques

Although the routine chest radiograph is often the first test to document the presence of diffuse interstitial disease, it may not prove to be a sensitive parameter for future monitoring. Reticulolinear shadows that reflect fibrotic areas may not disappear even with therapy. Computed tomographic scans of the lungs can give a better view of cystic changes and areas of traction bronchiectasis created by fibrosis than does conventional radiography, and this may prove to be a more accurate means of documenting the extent of parenchymal disease. Moreover, computed tomography gives a better view of the pleural and mediastinal anatomy, which is important in excluding other diagnoses.

Gallium[67] lung scans have been a popular way of assessing the degree of inflammation in the parenchyma and also in revealing the extent of lung involvement and the heterogeneity or patchy nature of the disease process. The gallium isotope is taken up by inflammatory cells such as polymorphonuclear leukocytes (or in the case of sarcoidosis by activated macrophages). Although an elevated gallium scan index does seem to reflect the recovery of polymorphonuclear leukocytes in bronchoalveolar lavage fluid that indicates alveolitis or peripheral airway irritation, routine use of gallium scanning has not proved to be very helpful in the long term monitoring of patients.

Bronchoalveolar Lavage

At the time of fiberoptic bronchoscopy, the distal airways and alveolar surface, subtended by the tip of the bronchoscope wedged into a fourth generation bronchus, are washed with sequential aliquots of saline (such as 20 to 50 ml amounts up to 100 to 300 ml total volume), which are aspirated through the bronchoscope and collected for cellular and protein analyses. Details of the procedure have been reviewed elsewhere. Lavage can be done in several different portions of a lung to record the variable degree of disease involvement or in both lungs; transbronchial biopsy specimens can be obtained afterward from one side. As noted in Table 1, many components can be measured and counted in the lavage fluid in an attempt to define the degree of alveolitis. Characteristic of patients with an active phase of idiopathic pulmonary fibrosis is an increased recovery of cells in bronchoalveolar lavage fluid, including macrophages and an increased percentage of polymorphonuclear leukocytes (10 to 30 percent or more) and eosinophils (2–4 percent). In certain patients, often those with associated collagen-vascular disease, an increased percentage of lymphocytes (20 percent or so) can be present; this generally is regarded as a good sign that the patient will have some response to immunosuppressive therapy.

The status of bronchoalveolar lavage fluid analysis in idiopathic pulmonary fibrosis is uncertain at present and deserves several additional comments. Lavage is a direct means of sampling the areas involved by disease in the terminal airways and alveoli, providing an estimate of luminal inflammation. Because it does not sample the parenchymal tissue or interstitium, the information obtained is incomplete. Except for polymorphonuclear leukocytes recovered during lavage, the analysis generally underestimates the degree of tissue inflammation and infiltration with lymphoid cells. Although cellular profiles counted in bronchoalveolar lavage fluid are not diagnostic of idiopathic pulmonary fibrosis per se, the pattern helps to eliminate other complicating diseases and suggests that idiopathic pulmonary fibrosis is a feasible diagnosis.

Fiberoptic bronchoscopy coupled with bronchoalveolar lavage is not a very risky procedure for the patient and can be repeated at intervals if desired. The cost of the procedure and an analysis of the cellular components in lavage is substantial but not prohibitive and has to be factored into the cost effective balance of the diagnostic work-up. Because analysis of bronchoalveolar lavage fluid is labor intensive and requires special handling in a clinical laboratory, it is not usually performed routinely. Thus, special arrangements are required, and the logistics of transporting the specimens must be worked out. Until the role of bronchoalveolar lavage fluid analysis is confirmed in the management of patients with diffuse interstitial lung disease, it is my judgment that it should be used in the context of clinical research protocols and that the patient should not assume the cost of the analysis.

THERAPY

A trial of anti-inflammatory immunosuppressive therapy is usually offered to a patient with idiopathic pulmonary fibrosis, even though he/she has been found to have advanced fibrotic disease in the staging procedures outlined and there is little prospect for reversibility. The prognosis of the disease dictates that some therapeutic action be taken (see Table 2), and a trial of oral corticosteroid therapy is advised first (Table 3). The concept of a trial must be emphasized so that after 6 to 8 weeks of high dose prednisone therapy daily, its continuation can be justified and tapering of the dose to a maintenance level can be begun. This means having a good baseline of clinical data—blood tests, pulmonary function tests, possibly bronchoalveolar lavage fluid analysis and gallium imaging—to compare with follow-up test results that will allow the objective assessment of improvement. The side effects of corticosteroids can be significant, and a clear indication that some improvement has occurred will justify continuation (Table 4).

If the lung disease seems progressive despite an adequate trial of corticosteroids, use of cyclophosphamide for additional immunosuppression can be considered. In about 30 percent of the patients who are "steroid failures" cyclophosphamide can have a favorable effect in improving or stabilizing the disease. Because the complications of this supposed alkylating drug can be numerous and severe (see Table 4), the patient must be well informed about the risks and must be followed closely by the physician. For example, weekly white cell counts are necessary until the maintenance dosage of cyclophosphamide proves to be stable; even then biweekly counts are still advisable. A urinalysis should be performed every 6 weeks.

As a general rule for adjusting the daily oral dosage

TABLE 3 Treatment Regimens for Idiopathic Pulmonary Fibrosis

Corticosteroids

Two to 4 weeks after open lung biopsy, oral prednisone therapy is begun at a dosage of 1 mg per kg body weight daily. This dosage is continued for 6 to 8 weeks.

If lung disease (judged by pulmonary function studies, serial bronchoalveolar lavage, chest films) shows improvement, tapering to a maintenance dosage is done.

The prednisone dosage is tapered to 5.0 mg each week until a daily maintenance dosage of 0.25 mg per kg is reached.

If the disease worsens, the dosage of prednisone is increased or alternative immune suppressive treatment is considered.

Cyclophosphamide

Therapy is started when the patient is taking a daily maintenance oral dose of prednisone (0.25 mg per kg).

Cyclophosphamide is begun at a dosage of about 1.0 mg per kg body weight daily (50 to 75 mg).

Adjust dosages of cyclophosphamide as necessary, to maintain the white blood cell count at about 3000 cells per ml; the dosage can be increased by 50 mg increments at 7 to 10 day intervals if necessary.

Encourage the patient to take the medication in the morning, to drink large volumes of fluids, and to empty the bladder frequently.

Monitor the lung disease as described in the text.

TABLE 4 Side Effects of Treatment

Corticosteroid therapy
  Salt and water retention
  Increased appetite with weight gain
  Hyperglycemia
  Cutaneous ecchymoses, striae formation, and acne
  Posterior subcapsular cataract formation
  Osteoporosis
  Peptic ulcer disease
  Adrenal suppression
  Opportunistic infection

Cyclophosphamide therapy
  Hemorrhagic cystitis
  Alopecia
  Anorexia, nausea, or vomiting
  Mucosal ulcerations
  Bone marrow suppression
  Azoospermia, amenorrhea
  Increased incidence of subsequent lymphoproliferative disease
  Opportunistic infection

of cyclophosphamide, to provide a margin of safety for the patient against granulocytopenia and possible infection, and still achieve adequate immunosuppression as judged by lymphopenia, the following plan is offered: Increments of 50 mg of cyclophosphamide orally can be given each week until the desired level of leukopenia is achieved. Usually a daily dosage of 100 to 150 mg is sufficient for most medium sized adults. The total white cell count should be reduced to half the normal baseline value (i.e., from 8000 cells per ml to 3000 to 4000 cells per ml) with a distinct drop in the total lymphocyte count. However, a minimal count of 1000 polymorphonuclear leukocytes per ml should be maintained to stave off bacterial infections. If improvement in the lung disease is documented after 3 months of this therapy, it should be continued for 12 months.

Some preliminary studies suggest alternative means for giving corticosteroids and cyclophosphamide in an attempt to reduce side effects. A large weekly dose as an intravenous bolus of steroid has been suggested, but it is uncertain that the cumulative adrenal suppressive effects are any less. Because corticosteroids frequently do not seem to be helpful in treating idiopathic pulmonary fibrosis, bypassing this therapy and beginning with cyclophosphamide has been advocated. Cyclophosphamide is a more potent immunosuppressive drug than prednisone, and the initial use of such powerful therapy can be supported. However, because it seems best to use small doses of prednisone concomitantly, a preliminary trial of corticosteroids still seems justified in most patients. As a final caution, cyclophosphamide itself has been reported to cause lung disease; when this occurs, the effects may be reversed with corticosteroid therapy.

In addition to suppressing the alveolitis and stabilizing the inflammatory process, several other measures may help improve respiratory function. It is imperative that these patients stop smoking cigarettes. Although a patient can have relatively normal oxygen saturation at rest, with exercise there is frequently a marked drop in the PaO_2 value. Therefore exercise tolerance may be significantly improved with supplemental oxygen therapy. When oxygen requirements are high (more than 2 liters flow per minute), direct administration of oxygen into the trachea may be preferred. Several modes of transtracheal catheter oxygen delivery are available. In addition to attaining a high local concentration of oxygen in the lungs, the cosmetic effect of not wearing obvious nasal prongs can be important.

As the pulmonary vascular bed is ravaged by progressive fibrosis, pulmonary hypertension and cor pulmonale can develop; right sided congestive heart failure can be difficult to control. Judicious use of diuretics is advised, for a significant decrease in the intravascular volume may be deleterious for lung perfusion. Digitalis or antiarrhythmic drugs may be required, although adequate oxygenation is probably the best treatment for the heart failure. Some patients also may develop obstruction to air flow and may be troubled by wheezing and coughing, which may respond to bronchodilators. Because infection may occur during immunosuppressive therapy, it is important to maintain a high index of suspicion and to treat infection aggressively. Prophylactic use of pneumococcus and influenza vaccines is encouraged. Finally, with refractory disease limited to the chest, the question of lung transplantation arises. Recent success with single lung transplantation for diffuse interstitial lung disease will make this therapy a reality for some patients, and already more medical institutions are beginning to offer the service.

change in pulmonary function can be monitored with diffusion capacity and exercise tests that will reveal cardiac performance, oxygen delivery, and especially important, the degree of arterial hypoxemia. Overall these kinetic lung function tests performed at submaximal levels of exercise are the most helpful parameters to follow. Use of gallium[67] citrate uptake lung scanning (48 hour interval) to assess overall parenchymal inflammation is of questionable value and should not be used routinely. Likewise periodic bronchoalveolar lavage with cellular and immunologic analysis is uncertain and does not faithfully document a response to anti-inflammatory drug therapy in all patients. For selected patients with elevated lymphocyte or polymorphonuclear leukocyte counts, bronchoalveolar lavage analysis is helpful. However, enough uncertainty exists about the value of bronchoalveolar lavage in the longitudinal assessment of patients with idiopathic pulmonary fibrosis that its role should be evaluated in prospective clinical protocols. In this way the cost effectiveness of an expensive and invasive test can be determined.

It seems clear that the recovery of cells and alveolar proteins from the affected airways and alveolar surface has contributed greatly to our understanding of the immunopathogenetic mechanisms of inflammation and fibrosis (see Table 1), yet for clinical purposes merely enumerating cells or easily measured protein and enzyme levels is not sufficient. In the future, more subtle (but technically more involved to measure) secretory cell mediators (e.g., macrophage fibroblast growth factors) and the molecular expression of certain cell membrane markers will yield more sensitive and more accurate indices of cellular activity and markers for progressive disease.

MONITORING DISEASE FOR NATURAL HISTORY OR RESPONSE TO THERAPY

Longitudinal assessment of the patient with diffuse interstitial lung disease can be a difficult task unless objective parameters are established that can be reasonably measured at periodic intervals (6 to 12 months). Subjective symptoms of dyspnea and breathlessness are hard to quantitate and new physical findings may lag behind physiologic changes. Drugs, especially corticosteroids, effect transient improvement in well-being or appetite but may not actually benefit pulmonary function. Moreover, lung shadows in the chest radiograph representing fibrosis may not revert. Precise selection of the tests for monitoring, however, is controversial, for no single test can be relied upon exclusively. A panel of abnormal test results must be followed, and perhaps the test panel must be individualized for each patient.

Baseline blood counts (for immunosuppressive drug effects), erythrocyte sedimentation rate, and serologic titers, if abnormal initially, are easy to follow. Objective

SUGGESTED READING

Carrington CB, Gaensler EA, Coutu RE, Fitzgerald MX, Gupta RG. Natural history and treated course of usual and desquamative interstitial pneumonia. N Engl J Med 1978; 298:801–809.

Crystal RG, Bitterman PR, Rennard SI, Hance AJ, Keogh BA. Interstitial lung diseases of unknown cause: disorders characterized by chronic inflammation of the lower respiratory tract. N Engl J Med 1984; 310:154–244.

Dreisin RB, Schwartz MI, Theoflopoulos AN, Stanford RE. Circulating immune complexes in the idiopathic interstitial pneumonias. N Engl J Med 1978; 298:353–357.

Fulmer JD, Roberts WC, vonGal ER, Crystal RG. Morphologic-physiologic correlates of the severity of fibrosis and cellularity in idiopathic pulmonary fibrosis. J Clin Invest 1979; 63:665–675.

Rankin JA, Naegel GP, Reynolds HY. Use of a central laboratory for analysis of bronchoalveolar lavage fluid. Am Rev Respir Dis 1986; 133:186–190.

Reynolds HY. Bronchoalveolar lavage. Am Rev Respir Dis 1987; 135:250–263.

Reynolds HY. Idiopathic interstitial pulmonary fibrosis—contribution of bronchoalveolar lavage analysis. Chest 1986; 89:139S–144. (Includes review of history about IPF.)

Reynolds HY, Fulmer JD, Kazmierowski JA, Roberts WC, Frank MM, Crystal RG. Analysis of cellular and protein content of bronchoalveolar lavage fluid from patients with idiopathic pulmonary fibrosis and chronic hypersensitivity pneumonitis. J Clin Invest 1977; 59:165–175.

Rudd RM, Haslam PA, Turner-Warwick M. Cryptogenic fibrosing alveolitis: relationships of pulmonary physiology and bronchoalveolar lavage to response to treatment and prognosis. Am Rev Respir Dis 1981; 124:1–8.

Stoller JK, Rankin JA, Reynolds HY. The impact of bronchoalveolar lavage cell analysis on clinicians' diagnostic reasoning about interstitial lung disease. Chest 1987; 92:839–843.

Strumpf IJ, Feld MK, Cornelius M, Keogh BA, Crystal RG. Safety

of fiberoptic bronchoalveolar lavage in evaluation of interstitial lung disease. Chest 1981; 80:268–271.

Turner-Warwick M. Staging and therapy of cryptogenic fibrosing alveolitis. Chest 1986; 89:148S–150.

Turner-Warwick M, Haslam PL. The value of serial bronchoalveolar lavages in assessing the clinical progress of patients with cryptogenic fibrosing alveolitis. Am Rev Respir Dis 1987; 135:26–34.

Walters LC, et al. Idiopathic pulmonary fibrosis: pretreatment bronchoalveolar lavage cellular constituents and their relationships with lung histopathology and clinical response to therapy. Am Rev Respir Dis 1987; 135:696–704.

ALLERGIC BRONCHOPULMONARY ASPERGILLOSIS*

PAUL A. GREENBERGER, M.D.

Allergic bronchopulmonary aspergillosis is a complication of asthma that is more common than initially suspected and is characterized by clinical, immunologic, radiologic, and pathologic findings that range from mild bronchospasm to end stage pulmonary fibrosis. It can result in destructive lung disease such that death occurs in patients in the third decade of life. The disease is of interest in many respects because:

1. Roentgenographic infiltrates may be asymptomatic in one third of the cases.

2. Lung damage is thought to result from an array of serologic and cellular reactions in the lung.

3. The disease results from the presence of living fungi in the bronchial tree, but it is not an invasive or contagious disease.

4. The optimal pharmacologic therapy is oral doses of corticosteroids, although these drugs are not fungicidal.

5. The total serum IgE level is a valuable aid in diagnosis and management because it serves as an acute phase reactant that helps identify new infiltrates visible roentgenographically.

The major diagnostic criteria include asthma, immediate cutaneous reactivity to Aspergillus, precipitins to *A. fumigatus* (Af), an elevated total serum IgE level (higher than 1,000 ng per ml), peripheral blood eosinophilia, a history of chest infiltrates revealed by roentgenography, and proximal bronchiectasis.

Sera from patients with roentgenographic evidence of infiltrates have elevated serum IgE-Af and IgG-Af levels compared with sera from patients with asthma and immediate cutaneous reactivity to Aspergillus who do not have allergic bronchopulmonary aspergillosis. These elevations of isotypic antibodies to *A. fumigatus* can be considered the eighth criterion for the diagnosis of allergic bronchopulmonary aspergillosis. Some patients expectorate golden brown plugs, which contain *A. fumigatus* hyphae; however, with diagnoses made at earlier stages before significant bronchiectasis has occurred, this finding is less common.

If the physician waits for all the seven or eight criteria to be present, many cases will be missed. Clearly the first six criteria listed may occur in patients with asthma. In the absence of cystic fibrosis, proximal bronchiectasis is considered pathognomonic of allergic bronchopulmonary fungosis. Nevertheless, if one attempts to identify allergic bronchopulmonary aspergillosis before detectable bronchiectasis has occurred, even this sine qua non criterion cannot be used. Patients with the classic criteria of allergic bronchopulmonary aspergillosis, including proximal bronchiectasis, are identified by the notation ABPA-CB (for central bronchiectasis), whereas those with the first six listed criteria in whom bronchiectasis is not identified are identified by the notation ABPA-S (for seropositive). This distinction is made possible by the use of immunoassays that have demonstrated at least twice the levels of serum IgE-Af and IgG-Af in ABPA-S compared with sera from patients with asthma.

Allergic bronchopulmonary aspergillosis should be excluded in all cases of asthma. We believe that this is not difficult in most cases. If the patient does not have immediate cutaneous reactivity to Aspergillus, allergic bronchopulmonary aspergillosis is excluded. If the immediate skin test is positive, total serum IgE and precipitin levels for *A. fumigatus* should be determined. If the total serum IgE level is elevated, we determine whether the patient has elevated serum IgE-Af and IgG-Af levels compared with sera from patients with asthma. The latter serologic study is not routinely available. The chest roentgenogram should be reviewed as well as prior

*Study supported by USPHS grant AI 11403 and the Ernest S. Bazley grant.

films. When a patient has clinical, serologic, and roentgenographic evidence of allergic bronchopulmonary aspergillosis, hilar tomography may be carried out to search for proximal bronchiectasis. One may determine whether ABPA-CB or ABPA-S exists.

THERAPEUTIC ALTERNATIVES

The goal of treatment is to inhibit the growth of fungi in the bronchial mucus in order to minimize or eliminate the release of antigenic material associated with an intense immunologic destructive response in the bronchi as well as in the peripheral airways as a result of progressive fibrosis. A variety of pharmacologic agents have been administered to patients with allergic bronchopulmonary aspergillosis, including antifungal drugs such as amphotericin B, nystatin, clotrimazole, flucytosine, ketoconazole, as well as cromolyn sodium and inhaled corticosteroids.

The most effective therapy is oral administration of corticosteroids. We utilize prednisone, which results in resolution of roentgenographic evidence of the chest infiltrate in 2 to 4 weeks in most cases, reduction of symptoms of asthma, a decrease in sputum production and often culture recovery of incriminated fungi, at least a 35 percent decline in the total serum IgE level in 6 weeks, and resolution of peripheral blood eosinophilia. Corticosteroids decrease the pulmonary inflammatory response and appear to prevent progression to end stage pulmonary fibrosis in patients with allergic bronchopulmonary aspergillosis. In some patients with new onset disease the underlying asthma may be made worse, such that prednisone therapy cannot be discontinued without the onset of disabling wheezing that is uncontrollable with bronchodilators and the prophylactic use of anti-inflammatory medications.

Prednisone is administered at a dosage of 0.5 mg per kg as a single morning dose for 2 weeks, at which time roentgenographic evidence of the chest infiltrates will have resolved. Then we convert to the same dosage given on alternate days for about 3 months. The dosage of prednisone does not result in invasion of the fungi into bronchial walls or suprainfection. The prednisone dosage is decreased and discontinued, depending on the severity of the underlying asthma or whether there is a recurrence of roentgenographic evidence of infiltrates.

Therapy After the Initial Diagnosis

Patient education is important in several respects. In contrast to severe asthma, the patient may have mild or moderate respiratory symptoms or no symptoms despite radiographically impressive areas of consolidation or lobar collapse. The same extent of disease in a bacterial pneumonia would produce symptoms that are much more obvious to the patient. It is necessary to emphasize that although oral corticosteroid therapy is indicated, its use is not necessarily indefinite, and that a certain percentage of patients have remissions, either temporary or permanent, from allergic bronchopulmonary aspergillosis.

The patient also should be told that when recurrent infiltrates occur in patients with the disease who have not been treated effectively with corticosteroids, progressive lung damage has resulted that can necessitate home oxygen therapy, frequent antibiotic treatment because of purulent sputum production, and irreversible pulmonary obstructive and restrictive disease. Cigarette smoking must be discouraged. Antiasthma medications should be continued as indicated.

It is also recommended that the patient avoid obvious areas of potential high fungal spore concentration, such as mulches, compost piles, flooded crawl spaces, and basements. However, because aspergilli are ubiquitous and can be recovered from outdoor air in subfreezing temperatures, the exact contribution of high spore burdens to the development of new infiltrates remains unknown.

A prolonged evaluation of patients with the corticosteroid dependent asthma stage of allergic bronchopulmonary aspergillosis did not document progression to the fibrotic stage when the patients were studied for a mean of 10.2 years. One patient had been treated for 19 years. This information from eight well characterized patients suggests that although long term prednisone therapy is required in some patients, progression to irreversible pulmonary fibrosis is not inevitable.

During the first year after the diagnosis is made, the physician should attempt to identify the stage of allergic bronchopulmonary aspergillosis because this affects management. The five stages that have been recognized include I (acute), II (remission), III (exacerbation), IV (corticosteroid dependent asthma), and V (fibrotic).

We measure the total serum IgE level monthly for the first year if possible. After the initial decline of the total serum IgE level associated with prednisone administration and resolution of the acute infiltrates, the prednisone dosage is tapered and discontinued. The total serum IgE level declines but usually remains elevated, and therapy should not attempt to reduce it to normal levels. One can attempt to establish the range of baseline concentrations of IgE so that when new symptoms occur or when at least a 100 percent increase over the baseline IgE level occurs, a chest roentgenogram may be obtained to detect new infiltrates. After the first year, depending on the stage of the disease, the frequency of IgE measurements can be adjusted appropriately.

In patients with disease in the acute, recurrent exacerbation, and corticosteroid dependent asthma stages, we obtain sera for IgE determinations every 4 to 8 weeks in the second year and thereafter. Because disease in remission may evolve into recurrent exacerbations, both the patient and the physician should be alert for this possibility. Patients with disease in the fibrotic stage have irreversible decreases in pulmonary function and chest roentgenographic changes and often require high dose alternate day or daily prednisone therapy. New infiltrates with increases in the total serum IgE level are not observed frequently. These patients require observation for cyanosis, production of unusual organisms on sputum culture, and development of terminal pulmonary hypertension and cor pulmonale as a result of fibrotic lung disease.

ADDITIONAL ISSUES REGARDING ALLERGIC BRONCHOPULMONARY ASPERGILLOSIS

Pulmonary function measurements including lung volume and diffusion capacity can be undertaken at the time of diagnosis or after resolution of the acute infiltrate. These measurements often are within normal limits or show obstructive changes consistent with asthma. The measurements may be repeated annually or biannually, although they may be insensitive in reflecting bronchiectatic changes in allergic bronchopulmonary aspergillosis. The most abnormal pulmonary function measurements are observed in patients with status asthmaticus who present with infiltrates and in the end stage in patients who have severe restrictive lung disease.

Because patients with allergic bronchopulmonary aspergillosis exhibit many atopic conditions and have immediate cutaneous reactivity to many common aeroallergens, the patient may be receiving allergen immunotherapy when the diagnosis is made or may require immunotherapy for severe allergic symptoms. Although conventional allergen immunotherapy does not result in immune complex disease, we do not incorporate fungal antigens in the injection mixtures. Patients with allergic bronchopulmonary aspergillosis may develop marked immediate or late local reactions or anaphylaxis to subcutaneous injections of A. fumigatus. The concurrent administration of cromolyn sodium or the inhalation of corticosteroids does not appear to prevent repeated exacerbations of infiltrates. These drugs, however, may be utilized as antiasthma drugs.

In allergic bronchopulmonary aspergillosis, even the oral dose of corticosteroids is often greater than that required for asthma alone (in adults 35 to 50 mg of prednisone on alternate days). The patient should be warned regarding possible adverse effects of oral corticosteroid administration. Because therapy in most pa-

tients utilizes alternate day prednisone treatment, most of the potentially serious adverse effects of prednisone can be avoided. The patient should understand the consequences of not receiving effective therapy for a destructive lung disease. The patient can be advised regarding the apparent small risk that long term alternate day prednisone will cause loss of bone mass or posterior subcapsular cataracts.

Some patients have allergic bronchopulmonary syndromes in response to fungi other than A. fumigatus or other aspergilli. Making the definitive diagnosis requires the assistance of microbiologists who analyze sputum cultures and laboratory technicians who can test sera for precipitin reactions to a series of fungal antigens.

Allergic bronchopulmonary aspergillosis complicates approximately 10 percent of the cases of cystic fibrosis and should be searched for and treated in this population. Determination of elevated IgE-Af and IgG-Af levels compared with sera from patients with asthma has proved to be the most valuable diagnostic aid. Prednisone is effective in the management of allergic bronchopulmonary aspergillosis in cystic fibrosis because it helps to resolve some of the roentgenographic evidence of chest lesions attributable to allergic bronchopulmonary aspergillosis, decreases wheezing from asthma, and results in a decline in the total serum IgE level. In the doses used for the management of allergic bronchopulmonary aspergillosis, prednisone does not result in invasive aspergillosis in this population.

SUGGESTED READING

Greenberger PA, Patterson R. Diagnosis and management of allergic bronchopulmonary aspergillosis. Ann Allergy 1986; 56:444–452.
Hendrick DJ, Ellithorpe DB, Lyon F, Hattier P, Salvaggio JE. Allergic bronchopulmonary helminthosporiosis. Am Rev Respir Dis 1982; 126:935–938.
Laufer P, Fink JN, Bruns WT, Unger GF, Kalbfleisch JH, Greenberger PA, Patterson R. Allergic bronchopulmonary aspergillosis in cystic fibrosis. J Allergy Clin Immunol 1984; 73:44–48.
Lee TM, Greenberger PA, Patterson R, Roberts M, Liotta JL. Stage V (fibrotic) allergic bronchopulmonary aspergillosis: a review of 17 cases followed from diagnosis. Arch Intern Med 1987; 147:319–323.
Patterson R, Greenberger PA, Lee TM, Liotta JL, O'Neill E, Roberts M, Sommers H. Prolonged evaluation of patients with corticosteroid dependent asthma stage of allergic bronchopulmonary aspergillosis. J Allergy Clin Immunol 1987; 80:663–668.
Patterson R, Greenberger PA, Halwig JM, Liotta JL, Roberts M. ABPA—natural history and classification of early disease by serologic and roentgenographic studies. Arch Intern Med 1986; 146:916–918.

SARCOIDOSIS

PAUL KATZ, M.D.

Sarcoidosis is a disease of unknown cause that is characterized by noncaseating granulomatous inflammation of many organ systems. Although the lung is most commonly involved, this disease can affect many extrapulmonary sites. In most cases the long term morbidity and mortality of sarcoidosis are related to lung disease. Nonetheless nonpulmonary disease may necessitate therapy to provide symptomatic relief as well as to prevent the sequelae of unchecked inflammation.

The clinician confronted with a patient with newly diagnosed sarcoidosis is faced with a number of not inconsequential therapeutic decisions. Specifically, should this patient be treated and, if so, what therapy should be employed? If the physician embarks on a therapeutic course, new questions arise: How long should therapy be continued and at what dosage, and how should a clinical response be gauged? A much larger question facing the treating physician is whether the therapy selected will ultimately alter the natural history of the disease or merely provide transient symptomatic benefits. Physicians treating patients with sarcoidosis are often uncertain of the answers to these questions, which become more difficult because the primary mode of therapy, corticosteroids, can cause significant side effects.

There is general agreement that corticosteroids are the drugs of choice in most patients who require some form of therapy. As will be discussed, in certain patients with sarcoidosis long lasting suppression of many disease manifestations can be achieved through the use of nonsteroidal drugs. My indications for nonsteroidal and steroidal therapy and the regimens to be employed will be discussed. The reader should realize beforehand, however, that this area is controversial and that approaches other than those expressed here may be utilized by clinicians interested in the therapy of sarcoidosis.

INDICATIONS FOR THERAPY

Much of the dilemma regarding sarcoidosis relates to therapy, particularly which patients to treat and which drug(s) to utilize. In many patients no therapy is required and the disease is either self-limited or so mild as to warrant observation without specific treatment. However, the identification of these patients is difficult, and the guidelines to be discussed assist in the decision making process.

Indications for No Therapy

Once the diagnosis of sarcoidosis is established, a decision has to be made regarding the necessity for therapy and, if therapy is indicated, what drugs should be used. It is well known that not every patient with sarcoidosis requires therapy. Since a significant portion of patients have a spontaneous remission of the disease or have no evidence of end organ functional impairment, one must be cognizant of the fact that the establishment of this diagnosis need not necessitate therapy. All patients with sarcoidosis, however, should undergo a simple series of investigative studies performed to determine the severity and extent of organ system involvement. These are listed in Table 1. These studies enable the clinician to establish whether a need exists for more aggressive forms of therapy.

Radiographic staging of the extent of pulmonary involvement has been a useful adjunct to therapeutic decision making. Stage I sarcoidosis is characterized by hilar adenopathy alone; stage II, hilar adenopathy with parenchymal infiltrates without fibrosis; and stage III, pulmonary fibrosis. In individuals with stage I or II sarcoidosis, a period of observation for 6 to 12 months is warranted if there is no impairment of pulmonary function, no hypercalcemia or hypercalciuria, and no evidence of cardiac, renal, ocular, or central nervous system involvement. During this interval the patient should be seen periodically to assess the stability of these parameters. Should deterioration in these laboratory study results develop or should there be evidence of extrapulmonary disease activity in the organ systems just listed, therapy is indicated, and is to be outlined. The 6 to 12 month observation time enables the physician to better appreciate the natural history of a given patient's disease, and, as already indicated, many patients do well with no therapy. A hasty decision to institute corticosteroid therapy in a patient with only minimal localized pulmonary disease may be a great disservice to this individual. In such patients the resolution of disease activity may be inappropriately at-

TABLE 1 Investigative Studies in Patients with Sarcoidosis

Chest x-ray examination with staging
Arterial blood gas measurements
Pulmonary function tests (including diffusing capacity)
Electrocardiogram
Complete blood count
Serum calcium and 24 hour urine calcium levels
Serum creatinine and blood urea nitrogen levels
Liver function tests
Ophthalmologic evaluation (including slit lamp examination)
Other studies as indicated by symptoms

tributed to corticosteroids when, in fact, a benign course with a reasonable chance of spontaneous remission may have occurred in the absence of the drug.

It is often possible to identify patients with sarcoidosis who are likely to have a self-limited course. These are generally patients under 30 years of age who have an abrupt onset of stage I disease often associated with fever, arthralgias, and erythema nodosum. Evaluation often reveals little in the way of organ dysfunction and the disease resolves without therapy within 2 years. It is this group of patients in whom therapy is not required and is generally of little benefit in hastening recovery from the illness. Unfortunately only the minority of such patients fall into this class; most require some pharmacologic intervention.

Indications for Nonsteroidal Therapy

In some cases of sarcoidosis the symptomatology is severe enough to warrant therapy but less than that requiring systemic corticosteroid therapy. Some of the symptoms and signs that may be amenable to nonsteroidal regimens are listed in Table 2. It should be remembered that some of these patients may require corticosteroid therapy if nonsteroidal drugs are insufficient for control and if a particular disease manifestation progresses. In general, nonsteroidal therapy may be useful in patients with constitutional symptoms or organ system involvement that is unlikely to progress or cause permanent damage. Therapy with these drugs should not be instituted alone in patients with progressive pulmonary disease, ocular disease, hypercalcemia or hypercalciuria, hypersplenism, or cardiac, renal, or central nervous system involvement.

Aspirin and the newer nonsteroidal anti-inflammatory drugs, particularly indomethacin, are useful in the symptomatic relief of fever, erythema nodosum, arthralgias, and pain of pulmonary or lymphatic origin. Aspirin

TABLE 2 Indications for Nonsteroidal Therapy in Sarcoidosis*

Manifestations	Therapy
Fever	Aspirin, indomethacin, nonsteroidal anti-inflammatory drugs
Erythema nodosum	Aspirin, indomethacin, nonsteroidal anti-inflammatory drugs
Arthralgias	Aspirin, indomethacin, colchicine, nonsteroidal anti-inflammatory drugs
Chest pain of pulmonary origin; painful lymph nodes	Aspirin, indomethacin, nonsteroidal anti-inflammatory drugs
Nondisfiguring skin lesions	Topical corticosteroid therapy, antimalarial drugs

* These therapies do not control disease activity in all cases and more aggressive forms of therapy (for example, corticosteroids) may be necessary.

therapy is initiated with eight tablets per day in four divided doses and increased to up to 14 tablets per day as needed and tolerated. Salicylate therapy may be limited by typical gastrointestinal side effects or tinnitus. In patients who are unable to tolerate aspirin, I prefer indomethacin for these symptoms at an initial dosage of 75 to 150 mg per day in three or four divided doses. As with the salicylates, use of this drug may be curtailed by gastrointestinal symptoms. Some of the newer nonsteroidal anti-inflammatory drugs are as efficacious as indomethacin. Colchicine has been reported by some investigators to be useful, particularly for sarcoid arthropathy. However, the almost uniform development of drug induced diarrhea makes this a less than optimal medication.

Controversy exists regarding the therapy of nondisfiguring nonfacial skin lesions. As already discussed, self-limited erythema nodosum rarely requires more than therapy aimed at symptomatic relief if the lesions are painful. However, maculopapular eruptions, nodules, plaques, and lupus pernio may require therapy for cosmetic reasons. Although these lesions generally heal spontaneously without residua, many patients are self-conscious about their appearance and are anxious for some form of treatment. Topical or intralesional corticosteroid therapy (usually triamcinolone) may be useful in hastening the disappearance of cutaneous abnormalities. It has been reported that the antimalarial drugs chloroquine and hydroxychloroquine may be useful in infiltrative sarcoid skin and mucosal lesions. However, the risk of retinopathy and the necessity for periodic ophthalmologic evaluations make these drugs somewhat less desirable. Therefore, one often must decide whether the skin lesions are severe enough to warrant systemic corticosteroid therapy and, if so, what the goal of therapy is. In general, the presence of facial involvement is an absolute indication for the use of corticosteroids, to be described.

Indications for Corticosteroid Therapy

Corticosteroids have been considered by most students of sarcoidosis to be the mainstay of therapy. However, there is no general agreement concerning the goals of this therapy, the indications for the initiation of drug therapy, or whether this form of treatment alters the eventual outcome of the disease. Certainly there are disease manifestations about which there is little controversy concerning the necessity for corticosteroid therapy. Thus, evidence of cardiac, ocular, renal, or central nervous system disease should be considered an absolute indication for aggressive corticosteroid therapy (Table 3). Additionally cutaneous lesions of the face, hypercalcemia or hypercalciuria, and hypersplenism are held by most authorities to be at least relative indications for institution of therapy with these drugs.

The major question concerning corticosteroid ther-

TABLE 3 Nonpulmonary Indications for Corticosteroid Therapy in Sarcoidosis

Cardiac involvement

Ocular involvement

Renal involvement

Central nervous system involvement

Cutaneous facial lesions

Hypercalcemia

Hypercalciuria

Hypersplenism

Relief of symptoms not controlled by nonsteroidal drugs

apy is in regard to the treatment of pulmonary disease. There is virtually uniform agreement that corticosteroids can ameliorate pulmonary symptoms if given in adequate doses for a reasonable length of time (3 to 6 months) early in the course of the disease. What is less clear, however, is whether early aggressive corticosteroid therapy improves lung function or alters the ultimate outcome of pulmonary involvement. The lack of carefully controlled, prospective studies to evaluate this question has contributed to the lack of a therapeutic consensus.

Recently new technologies have been developed that may assist in the determination of disease activity and ultimately in the decision to institute therapy. During active pulmonary inflammation an alveolitis develops that is characterized by helper T lymphocytes and macrophages. While this alveolitis is continuing, corticosteroid therapy may be particularly useful and may result in clearing of pulmonary infiltrates. Conceivably if this inflammation is untreated, fibrosis may ensue, at which time corticosteroids will be of no benefit. The degree of alveolitis can be readily assessed via fiberoptic bronchoscopy with saline lavage. Cells so retrieved can be phenotyped and the degree of inflammation ascertained. However, the precise utility of this procedure in choosing therapeutic regimens is still undefined.

Lung scanning using gallium[67] may indicate active alveolitis by incorporation of this isotope into macrophages. This noninvasive test can be used serially to assess activity. Elevations in serum angiotensin converting enzyme levels are reported in 50 to 70 percent of the patients with active sarcoidosis, particularly those with active lung involvement. The presence of elevated levels in other conditions has limited its usefulness as a diagnostic test; however, in patients with angiotensin converting enzyme levels above normal, the determination may be a marker of disease activity that can be utilized in selecting therapy.

If corticosteroids are to be considered in a given patient, it is incumbent upon the clinician to consider how these drugs will affect the pathologic process. Corticosteroids have well described effects on the circulatory kinetics and functional capabilities of immunoregulatory leukocytes. Conceivably, then, in cases of sarcoidosis with active alveolitis comprised primarily of T lymphocytes and mononuclear phagocytes, one can postulate that corticosteroids could modify the composition or function of the white cells involved in the alveolitis. This in turn could negate the formation of granulomas and ultimately the fibrotic lung disease that lead to significant morbidity and mortality. Once interstitial fibrosis and parenchymal damage have occurred, corticosteroids are generally of no benefit. It would seem reasonable, therefore, to institute corticosteroid therapy at a time of active alveolitis and prior to the development of irreversible end stage fibrotic pulmonary disease.

In general, stage III sarcoidosis is considered an absolute indication for at least a trial of corticosteroid therapy. In these patients there is evidence of pulmonary fibrosis and impaired lung function. Although these drugs are of no benefit for the already fibrosed lung, therapy is initiated in the hope that some potential for disease reversibility is still possible. Therapy at this stage might then prevent further fibrosis and lessen the likelihood of right sided heart failure. Therapy should be started with prednisone (to be outlined) after baseline chest radiography, arterial blood gas measurements, and pulmonary function tests have been carried out. It should be noted that patients often report a diminution in symptoms (for example, decreased dyspnea on exertion) even in the absence of objective evidence of clinical improvement. Therapy in these patients therefore should be continued. In patients not reporting an amelioration of pulmonary complaints, prednisone therapy should be continued for at least 6 months. At this time, if there is no subjective or objective evidence of a corticosteroid effect, serious consideration must be given to discontinuation of the drug in view of its potential life threatening side effects.

Greater difficulty in making the decision to institute corticosteroid therapy occurs with the individual with stage I or II disease. In many patients with stage I sarcoidosis there is spontaneous resolution of the disease within 1 to 2 years. In such patients with normal pulmonary function, a period of observation for 12 months is warranted. If at that time the chest x-ray findings and pulmonary function test results are unchanged, a trial of steroids seems warranted, since in up to 50 percent of these patients the disease resolves with such therapy without sequelae or recurrence. The patient with stage I disease with reduced lung function should be observed for 6 months if the degree of pulmonary dysfunction is minimal. Treatment is instituted if the abnormalities persist or worsen. If the patient is symptomatic or has evidence of significant respiratory impairment at the time of presentation, corticosteroid therapy is justified.

Patients with x-ray changes typical of stage II disease and normal to minimally reduced lung function should be observed and periodically reevaluated for 6 to 12 months. At the end of 1 year, if no radiographic or functional improvement is observed, corticosteroid treatment should be initiated. Deterioration of these parameters during the observation period of course necessitates corticosteroid therapy. Treatment also should

TABLE 4 Recommendations for Therapy of Pulmonary Involvement in Sarcoidosis*

Stage I: hilar adenopathy

With normal pulmonary function, observe every 3 months for 12 months. If no radiographic improvement is apparent, treat. With minimally reduced lung function at the time of presentation, observe for 6 months and treat if abnormalities persist or worsen. With pulmonary symptoms or significant respiratory dysfunction at presentation, treat.

Stage II: hilar adenopathy and pulmonary infiltrates

With normal to minimally reduced pulmonary function, observe and reevaluate every 3 months for 6 to 12 months. At 12 months, if no improvement, treat. If parameters deteriorate during observation period, treat. With pulmonary symptoms or significant pulmonary dysfunction at presentation, treat.

Stage III: pulmonary fibrosis

All patients should be treated after documentation of pulmonary function. If no subjective or objective improvement after 6 months, discontinue therapy. If there is subjective or objective improvement, continue therapy.

* The indications for corticosteroid therapy listed in Table 3 should take precedence over the indications listed here.

be instituted in patients with significant diminution in lung function at presentation. In patients with stage I and II disease who are receiving corticosteroids, treatment should be continued for at least 6 to 12 months using the protocol to be described. The continued use or tapering of therapy with these drugs is governed by the clinical response. The indications and recommendations for corticosteroid treatment for pulmonary involvement are listed in Table 4.

It should be re-emphasized that the aforementioned absolute indications for corticosteroid therapy take precedence over the indications for treatment based on radiographic staging (see Table 3). For example, the asymptomatic patient with stage I disease with normal pulmonary function would be treated if there were evidence of myocardial involvement.

Once the physician has decided to institute corticosteroid therapy, a therapeutic regimen must be devised. In general, prednisone is the drug of choice in view of its relatively short half-life and almost uniform absorption following oral administration. The use of longer acting preparations, such as dexamethasone, makes tapering of the dosage to an optimal alternate day basis impossible in view of the prolonged half-life.

Therapy is generally initiated with 60 to 80 mg per day of prednisone in a single daily dose. In patients with extremely active, potentially life threatening disease, this dosage may be divided into four equal portions throughout the day. This regimen, although often more efficacious in hastening the resolution of symptoms, is significantly more immunosuppressive and more likely to cause side effects than single dose therapy.

The duration of this relatively high dosage therapy should depend on the patient's response symptomatically, radiographically, and functionally. Most patients

who are going to respond to corticosteroids begin to show improvement within several weeks after the institution of therapy. Patients initially may report a new sense of well-being and a diminution in dyspnea and constitutional symptoms. This dosage is continued for 1 to 2 months following improvement, at which time an attempt at tapering is initiated. If no response is noted, this level of prednisone is maintained for 6 to 12 months. If neither subjective nor objective evidence of an amelioration of disease activity is apparent, consideration should be given to discontinuation of therapy with the drug.

If the patient has demonstrated a clinical response to corticosteroids, an attempt should be made to lower the dosage to an alternate day schedule. This is probably best achieved by continuing or raising the maintenance prednisone dosage on 1 day ("high" day) and lowering the dosage on the other day ("low" day). That is, if a patient is maintained on 40 mg of prednisone per day, the dosage is initially increased to 80 mg one day alternated with 40 mg the next. The 40 mg, or "low" dose day, dosage is then tapered by 5 to 10 mg decrements every 4 to 6 days as tolerated. Once the dosage reaches 80 mg every other day with no prednisone on the "low" dose day, one can attempt to taper the remaining prednisone as gauged by the disease activity. After an alternate day schedule is attained, the risk of serious corticosteroid side effects is minimal and the tapering of the drug dosage on this schedule can be done more gradually.

The side effects of corticosteroids are well known and are not unique to patients with sarcoidosis. As in all diseases treated with these drugs, the efficacy of therapy is often limited by the concomitant development of undesirable dose related effects. In these instances the necessity for continuing corticosteroid therapy at a given dosage must be weighed against the implications of the possible drug induced complications.

OUTCOME OF CORTICOSTEROID THERAPY

Although corticosteroids can decrease symptomatology, their effects on lung function and radiographic abnormalities are less predictable. Patients achieving symptomatic improvement may develop recurrence of their complaints following discontinuation or tapering of the drug dosage. In individuals with renal or ocular involvement, corticosteroids can prevent permanent functional impairment if therapy is instituted early. Cardiac and central nervous system involvement may be less responsive to treatment, and such therapy may not prevent fatal complications. Hypercalcemia and hypercalciuria secondary to increased vitamin D sensitivity usually respond promptly to corticosteroids.

Although the long term effects of corticosteroids on pulmonary sarcoidosis are somewhat difficult to discern, at least a trial of therapy is justifiable in patients with respiratory symptoms, pulmonary function abnormalities, or persistent chest x-ray abnormalities. Although one cannot predict whether a given patient will respond to such drugs, their judicious use may provide long term symptomatic and, it is hoped, functional improvement.

INDICATIONS FOR CYTOTOXIC DRUGS

Drugs other than those already discussed here have also been employed in the therapy of sarcoidosis. Sporadic reports of the use of chlorambucil, azathioprine, methotrexate, and cyclophosphamide have appeared in the literature, but the series were small and lacked controls and the patients often were only those with far advanced disease. It is therefore difficult to draw any conclusions regarding the efficacy of these drugs. However, the clinician may be confronted with a situation in which a trial of a cytotoxic drug is warranted. I believe that these drugs should be reserved for patients with advanced disease in whom corticosteroids have failed or for patients who have responded to corticosteroids but who have developed unacceptable side effects from these drugs. The treating physician and the patient should be well aware of the lack of controlled studies using these drugs and their potential for serious reactions before embarking on a therapeutic trial.

I prefer to use cyclophosphamide in patients fulfilling the aforementioned criteria for the use of cytotoxic drugs. This drug has proven effective in other immunologically mediated diseases characterized by granulomatous inflammation, such as Wegener's granulomatosis, lymphomatoid granulomatosis, and allergic angiitis and granulomatosis (Churg-Strauss syndrome), and at least theoretically this drug might be efficacious in sarcoidosis. Therapy is initiated and maintained using the protocol presented elsewhere in this text. That is, treatment is initiated with 2 mg per kg per day in a single dose with adjustment as needed to maintain the white blood cell count between 4,000 and 5,000 cells per cubic mm with at least 1,000 to 1,500 granulocytes per cubic mm. At these leukocyte levels the incidence of infection is negligible. A hiatus of 5 to 7 days before the white count starts to decrease is generally seen, and the dosage often must be lowered to prevent leukopenia. The successful institution of therapy with this drug may permit tapering of the corticosteroid dosage. Since corticosteroids partially protect the bone marrow from the leukopenic effects of cyclophosphamide, the dosage of the cytotoxic drug usually requires downward adjustment as the corticosteroid dosage is tapered.

Since controlled studies using this drug are not available, the decision as to what constitutes an adequate trial is somewhat arbitrary. I have used a 2 to 3 month trial period after the white count has been lowered to the foregoing levels. If no subjective or objective improvement is noted during this interval, the drug is discontinued.

The side effects of cyclophosphamide are well known and are not unique to this disease. The most common complications include leukopenia, hemorrhagic cystitis, alopecia, and infertility.

As an alternative to cyclophosphamide, I have used another alkylating drug, chlorambucil, in some patients. I believe that this drug is less potent than cyclophosphamide, but it may be better tolerated and has fewer side effects potentially. Chlorambucil is administered at a dosage of 6 mg per day in concert with prednisone prescribed as already indicated. Because of the potential bone marrow toxicity, the guidelines for following the white blood cell count described for cyclophosphamide should be followed. If no clinical response is observed after 3 to 4 months, I discontinue the drug.

SUGGESTED READING

Baughman RP, Fernandez M, Bosken CH, Mantil J, Hurtubise P. Comparison of gallium-67 scanning, bronchoalveolar lavage, and serum angiotensin-converting enzyme levels in pulmonary sarcoidosis. Predicting response to therapy. Am Rev Respir Dis 1984; 129:676–681.

Ceuppens JL, Lacquet LM, Marien G, Demedts M, van den Eeckhout A. Alveolar T-cell subsets in pulmonary sarcoidosis. Correlation with disease activity and effect of steroid treatment. Am Rev Respir Dis 1984; 129:563–568.

Hollinger WM, Straton GW Jr, Fajman WA, Gilman MJ, Pine JR, Check IJ. Prediction of therapeutic response in steroid-treated pulmonary sarcoidosis. Evaluation of clinical parameters, bronchoalveolar lavage, gallium-67 lung scanning, and serum angiotensin-converting enzyme levels. Am Rev Respir Dis 1985; 132:65–69.

Johns CJ, Schonfeld SA, Scott PP, Zachary JB, MacGregor MI. Longitudinal study of chronic sarcoidosis with low-dose maintenance corticosteroid therapy. Outcome and complications. Ann NY Acad Sci 1986; 465:702–712.

Spratling L, Tenholder MF, Underwood GH, Feaster BL, Requa RK. Daily vs alternate day prednisone therapy for stage II sarcoidosis. Chest 1985; 88:687–690.

Turner-Warwick M, McAllister W, Lawrence R, Britten A, Haslam PL. Corticosteroid treatment in pulmonary sarcoidosis: do serial lavage lymphocyte counts, serum angiotensin-converting enzyme measurements, and gallium-67 scan help management? Thorax 1986; 41:903–913.

MULTIPLE SCLEROSIS

BARRY G. W. ARNASON, M.D.
ANTHONY T. REDER, M.D.

The cause of multiple sclerosis is not known, but there is evidence that regulation of the immune system is disordered when the disease is active. Abnormalities in immune regulation include, but are not restricted to, a loss of T suppressor cell function. The pathologic hallmark of multiple sclerosis is destruction of patches of central nervous system myelin. Multiple sclerosis plaques surround venules; these demyelinated areas contain infiltrating T cells, B cells, and macrophages. The trigger causing immunocytes to infiltrate into the central nervous system and their activation and proliferation within multiple sclerosis lesions is not known. However, their very presence within the brain, taken together with the abnormalities of immune regulation already mentioned, provides a rationale for the employment of immunosuppressive therapy to treat multiple sclerosis. Immunosuppression does ameliorate symptoms, and there is evidence that it can slow disease progression, albeit modestly. It must be emphasized that no treatment in current use is curative, that immunotherapeutic regimens are not without risk, and that in a disease with a mean survival time of some 30 years after diagnosis, risk-benefit ratios must weigh heavily in choices of whom to treat and when to do so.

The multiple central nervous system lesions that characterize multiple sclerosis appear in various sites and evolve over time. The sites affected and the burden of disease are both highly variable. This variability finds its reflection in a wide clinical spectrum. The course of multiple sclerosis traditionally has been divided into three broad categories—relapsing-remitting disease, chronic progressive disease, and stable disease. Patients may shift from one category to another. Thus, a course that begins as a relapsing-remitting one may evolve as the years pass into a progressive one. Within subgroups the tempo of progression and the severity of deficits vary widely.

The traditional subgrouping of cases of multiple sclerosis may be overly simplistic. Recent data obtained by magnetic resonance imaging indicate that lesions can appear and disappear without evidence of clinical change even in "stable" multiple sclerosis. If immunosuppressive treatment were completely without risk, it would seem reasonable to treat all patients with long term immunosuppressive therapy. However, medical tradition and an acute awareness of the potential complications of prolonged immunosuppression have led most neurologists to settle for more restricted goals. In general, treatment has been directed toward the following: has-

tening recovery from an acute attack, reducing the frequency of relapses, slowing the rate of progression in those with rapidly progressive disease, and instituting symptomatic treatment that provides relief of particular complaints without influencing the course of the disease.

ACUTE ATTACK

The mainstay of treatment is adrenocorticotropic hormone (ACTH), which has been shown in controlled trials to reduce the recovery time from an acute attack of multiple sclerosis. ACTH to some extent may also reverse the worsening of deficits in progressive multiple sclerosis. The response to ACTH is not predictable a priori, and perhaps half the patients to whom it is given show minimal or no response. When ACTH is given in a hospital setting, there is some additional benefit from bedrest alone. ACTH therapy does not appear to affect the long term evolution of multiple sclerosis, but its short term benefit sometimes can allow patients to return to work or to recover to their pre-exacerbation baseline more rapidly than if no treatment is given.

The appearance of new symptoms or signs is not necessarily due to the development of a new multiple sclerosis plaque. Transient worsening lasting hours to a day or so may occur because of changes in the capacity of already demyelinated axons to conduct. This capacity is influenced by body temperature, and anything that increases body temperature can augment deficits or unmask subclinical lesions. Cystitis or other infections, warm weather, vigorous exercise, and even the circadian rise in body temperature that occurs in the afternoon can amplify symptoms. It is important not to mistake such variations for attacks of disease. Therefore relapses in multiple sclerosis are usually defined as new symptoms that persist for more than 24 hours and usually for several days.

Our practice is to treat acute exacerbations of multiple sclerosis with 3 days of intravenous therapy with ACTH (80 IU) in the hospital (some neurologists prefer a 10 day course). The patient is then managed as an outpatient, and ACTH therapy is continued intramuscularly with gradual tapering. It is believed that a phased reduction of the dosage over time may lessen the chance of a post-treatment recrudescence of disease. ACTH stimulates cortisol secretion, and this results in decreased edema within plaques. ACTH also lowers body temperature and in addition may directly or indirectly increase the conduction efficiency of demyelinated axons.

The ACTH schedule that we use is that described by Hier (Table 1).

Oral potassium supplements are advisable.

Glucocorticoids are preferable to ACTH in the management of most other autoimmune diseases, and some neurologists prefer to use them in multiple sclerosis rather than ACTH. There is no question that some patients with multiple sclerosis respond favorably to

*Adapted from Hier DB. Demyelinating diseases. In: Samuels MD, ed. Manual of neurologic therapeutics. Boston: Little, Brown, 1987:268.

TABLE 1 ACTH Treatment of Acute Attacks of Multiple Sclerosis*

Days 1–3	Aqueous ACTH 80 units in 500 ml of 5% dextrose in water IV over 8 hours each day
Days 4–10	ACTH gel 40 units IM every 12 hours
Days 11–13	ACTH gel 35 units IM every 12 hours
Days 14–16	ACTH gel 30 units IM every 12 hours
Days 20–22	ACTH gel 40 units IM daily
Days 23–25	ACTH gel 30 units IM daily
Days 26–28	ACTH gel 20 units IM daily
Days 30, 32, 34	ACTH gel 20 units IM each day

glucocorticoid treatment. The argument advanced in support of glucocorticoid treatment, in preference to ACTH, is that ACTH acts in multiple sclerosis solely via its stimulation of cortisol secretion, and since the effect of ACTH on the adrenal cortex is variable from patient to patient, it makes more sense to use the final vector of the response rather than a stimulator of the release of that vector. The issue remains contentious; our experience has been that the response to ACTH is greater than that to prednisone, at least at the doses of each that are commonly employed. ACTH has other effects in addition to stimulating glucocorticoid release. There are, for example, ACTH receptors on lymphocytes and astrocytes. No direct controlled comparison of ACTH with prednisone in multiple sclerosis has ever been done.

A frequently employed glucocorticoid regimen is the following: 60 mg of prednisone in divided doses for 5 days followed by a tapering over 3 weeks. Others advocate pulse therapy over 3 to 7 days with as much as 1 g of methylprednisolone given intravenously each day followed by a tapering over a period of months rather than weeks.

REDUCTION IN FREQUENCY OF ATTACKS

Azathioprine (Imuran) is the drug most commonly employed to reduce the frequency of attacks. Therapy is begun with daily oral dosages of 100 to 150 mg, and the dosage eventually is adjusted according to its effect on hematologic indices. In early studies attempts were made to maintain the white cell count between 3,000 and 4,000 per cubic mm. We find that the mean red cell volume can be used as an index of azathioprine's effect on the hematologic system without reducing the white cell count to potentially dangerously low levels. We attempt to maintain the mean corpuscular volume at 105

cubic micra (normal, 85 to 95 cubic micra). The complete blood count and alkaline phosphatase level should be monitored as well. The efficacy of azathioprine in reducing the frequency of exacerbations is a matter of controversy. Some controlled trials have shown benefit, but in others no clear-cut effect has been seen. We treat attacks in patients taking azathioprine with ACTH.

The frequency of exacerbations in relapsing-remitting multiple sclerosis may be reduced with alpha or beta interferon. Alpha or beta interferon may increase natural killer cell function, which according to some reports is deficient in multiple sclerosis. They also augment T suppressor cell function, which is defective when the disease is active. Alpha or beta interferon may also counteract to some extent the actions of gamma interferon, a possibly important point, since in a single trial, and one that is unlikely to be repeated, exogenously administered gamma interferon caused exacerbations of multiple sclerosis. Preliminary studies have shown that alpha or beta interferon may halve the incidence of exacerbation and reduce eventual disability. Side effects were deemed acceptable (flulike symptoms). Further clinical trials are in progress.

TREATMENT OF PROGRESSIVE DISEASE

Cyclophosphamide (Cytoxan) is coming into increased use as a treatment for progressive multiple sclerosis. In general, treatment is reserved for those whose disease is progressing rapidly. This seems prudent, given the hazards of the drug.

A commonly employed regimen is that introduced by Hauser et al in which 400 to 500 mg per day are given intravenously for 10 to 14 days. ACTH is given concomitantly (Table 2). Treatment is stopped immediately if the white blood cell count falls below 2,500 per cubic mm.

In published series using Cytoxan in multiple sclerosis, about one third of the cases have shown improvement, one third have shown an arrest of worsening, and one third have continued to progress. Unfortunately, even in patients who have appeared to benefit, reactivation of disease often occurs within 6 months to 3

TABLE 2 ACTH Treatment Given with Intravenous Cyclophosphamide Therapy

Dosage	Days
25 units IV	1–3
20	4–6
15	7–9
10	10–13
5	13–15
40 units IM	16–18
20	19–21; then discontinue

years. In some a repeat course again reverses progression or halts it. Alopecia, which is reversible, is invariable with the use of cyclophosphamide according to this protocol. Bone marrow suppression with its attendant increased risk of infection is an additional potential complication as is hemorrhagic cystitis. The occurrence of the latter may be decreased with good hydration. A final risk is the development of a lymphoma or other cancer.

Several other treatments for progressive multiple sclerosis have been tested over the years. Hyperbaric oxygen, initially reported to be beneficial, has failed to show benefit in subsequently performed controlled trials. Its use is discouraged. Plasmapheresis has been reported as helpful by one group (Khatri), but others have been unimpressed by it, and it should be viewed as experimental at this juncture. Total lymphoid irradiation has been reported to be helpful; we have had no experience with it. Lymphocytopheresis seems unpromising, and thymectomy is without benefit.

Cyclosporine is being tested currently, and a multicenter trial is under way. The potentially serious renal side effects of cyclosporine must be signalled.

CONTROL OF SYMPTOMS

Many patients find that lowering the body temperature reduces fatigue and increases strength. Cool showers and swimming, air conditioning, or iced beverages are often helpful and work by reversing conduction block in demyelinated areas. 4-Aminopyridine blocks potassium efflux and enhances nerve conduction in a somewhat similar manner. It appears to be effective in reducing temperature sensitive symptoms. High dosages may cause seizures and paresthesias. Proper dosages are under investigation with this promising drug.

Spasticity can be reduced by several drugs. Baclofen (Lioresol) is the most effective treatment for spasticity in multiple sclerosis. Drowsiness and weakness are its major side effects. Therapy should be begun at a low dosage (5 mg three times daily for 3 days) and then gradually increased, weighing the benefits obtained from reduced spasticity against the limitations produced by increasing weakness. The maximal dosage we employ is 20 mg four times daily.

Diazepam (Valium), 2 to 5 mg orally several times per day or whenever necessary, is sometimes helpful in reducing spasticity. Dantrolene (Dantrium) reduces chronic spasticity but has caused fatal and nonfatal hepatic dysfunction and has more associated risk than baclofen or diazepam. It also increases weakness, and in our experience this is the major limitation to its use. Liver function tests should be monitored during treatment; the drug should be stopped if laboratory values indicate hepatitis. Phenothiazines in addition to phenytoin or glycine have been reported to reduce spasticity in occasional patients.

Depression, which is frequent in multiple sclerosis, and pseudobulbar affect, which is less common, can be treated with relatively low doses of antidepressants. Amitriptyline (Elavil), 25 to 75 mg at bedtime, has been effective. This drug should be used with caution in patients with seizures, urinary retention, or cardiac disease.

Tremor is difficult to treat in multiple sclerosis. Occasional patients respond to beta-adrenergic blockers (e.g., propranolol, 40 to 240 mg per day). We also have had some success with clonazepam (Clonopin) in patients with intention tremor. The major side effect of this drug is sedation. Therapy should be begun at a dosage of 0.5 mg twice daily and gradually increased to a maximum of 10 to 20 mg per day.

SUGGESTED READING

Hauser SL, et al. Intensive immunosuppression in progressive multiple sclerosis: a randomized three-arm study of high-dose intravenous cyclophosphamide, plasma exchange, and ACTH. N Engl J Med 1983; 308:173–180.

Hier DB. Demyelinating diseases. In: Samuels MA, ed. Manual of neurologic therapeutics. Boston: Little, Brown, 1987:268.

Khatri BO, Koethe SM, McQuillen MP. Plasmapheresis with immunosuppressive drug therapy in progressive multiple sclerosis. Arch Neurol 1984; 41:734–738.

Reder AT, Arnason BGW. Immunology of multiple sclerosis. In: Vinken PJ, Bruyn GW, Klawans HL, Koetsier JC, eds. Handbook of clinical neurology. Amsterdam: Elsevier Science Publishers, 1985; Vol. 3(47):337.

Rose AS, et al. Cooperative study in the evaluation of therapy in multiple sclerosis: ACTH vs. placebo—final report. Neurology 1970; 20:1–59.

Troiano R, Cook SD, Dowling PC. Steroid therapy in multiple sclerosis: point of view. Arch Neurol 1987; 44:803–807.

MYASTHENIA GRAVIS

MARJORIE E. SEYBOLD, M.D.

Myasthenia gravis is an organ specific autoimmune disorder directed at the acetylcholine receptor of skeletal muscle. It may afflict patients of either sex at almost any age but occurs most commonly in young adult women and older men. Children born to mothers with myasthenia gravis may display transient weakness at birth (neonatal myasthenia gravis), which characteristically disappears within 1 to 2 months.

Clinically myasthenia gravis is characterized by skeletal muscle weakness and fatigability, which usually fluctuate and are asymmetric. In approximately 20 percent of the patients the disease is symptomatic only in the ocular muscles (ocular myasthenia gravis). In the remainder of the patients any skeletal muscle may be involved (generalized myasthenia gravis). Bulbar muscle weakness is particularly common and may produce nasal regurgitation, dysphagia, or dysarthria. Bulbar weakness, along with respiratory muscle involvement, represents the most dangerous manifestation of myasthenia gravis.

The symptoms of myasthenia gravis result from a loss of acetylcholine receptors on the postsynaptic membrane of the neuromuscular junction. More than 80 percent of the patients have detectable circulating antibody to acetylcholine receptor. The antibody is thought to interfere with acetylcholine receptor function in a variety of ways, including enhancement of its normal degradation, complement mediated destruction of the postsynaptic membrane, and direct and indirect blockade of the receptor. Absolute serum levels of acetylcholine receptor antibody do not correspond to clinical severity, although clinical improvement is often accompanied by decreasing levels of antibody in the individual patient.

The diagnosis of myasthenia gravis at times can be made on clinical grounds alone. More often supplementary tests are used. These include the observation of objective improvement with cholinesterase inhibitors such as edrophonium chloride (Tensilon; to be discussed), the presence of characteristic electromyographic abnormalities, and the finding of acetylcholine antibody in the serum.

Myasthenia gravis may occur in association with other autoimmune diseases, the most common of which is thyroid disease. Recognition and correction of thyroid imbalance or any other coexisting disorder are mandatory to achieve good control of myasthenia gravis as well as to aid in selection of the therapeutic approach.

TABLE 1 Sequence of Therapies in Myasthenia Gravis

Ocular myasthenia gravis
  1. Anticholinesterase therapy
  2. Symptomatic therapy, e.g., eye patch
  3. Prednisone or azathioprine every other day, if necessary
Generalized myasthenia gravis (< 50–60 year old patient)
  1. Anticholinesterase therapy
  2. Thymectomy
  3. Prednisone every other day, if necessary
  4. Azathioprine, if necessary
  5. Plasmapheresis, if necessary
Generalized myasthenia gravis (> 60 year old patient)
  1. Anticholinesterase therapy
  2. Prednisone every other day, if necessary
  3. Azathioprine, if necessary
  4. Plasmapheresis, if necessary
Crisis
  1. Respiratory support
  2. Stop anticholinesterase therapy for 24 to 72 hours
  3. Restart anticholinesterase therapy
  4. Prednisone, if necessary
  5. Plasmapheresis, if necessary

THERAPEUTIC ALTERNATIVES

Therapy in myasthenia gravis must be tailored to the needs of the individual patient. The clinical severity of the disease, the patient's tolerance of symptoms, and his or her age influence the therapies employed and their sequence. The commonly employed measures are cholinesterase inhibitors, thymectomy, corticosteroids, azathioprine, and plasmapheresis. These are generally used in the sequences and circumstances indicated in Table 1.

Patients with myasthenia gravis may experience a worsening of symptoms caused by many factors, including infection, metabolic or endocrine imbalance, menses, surgery, emotional upset, or the action of many different drugs. Neuromuscular blocking drugs must be used with extreme caution, if at all. Other drugs, including aminoglycoside antibiotics, antiarrhythmic and local anesthetic drugs, morphine and other central nervous system depressants, and d-penicillamine, should be used with caution in these patients.

Cholinesterase Inhibitors

Cholinesterase inhibitors are used first in virtually all patients with myasthenia gravis. These medications increase the synaptic concentration of acetylcholine by decreasing its degradation rate, thereby enhancing the likelihood that available acetylcholine receptors will become activated. The three available anticholinesterase preparations are pyridostigmine (Mestinon), neostigmine (Prostigmin), and ambenonium (Mytelase). Pyridostigmine is the most frequently used and is available in

60 mg tablets, 180 mg sustained release tablets (timespan), syrup, and injectable form. Neostigmine is available in tablets and injectable form, and ambenonium is available in tablet form only. Pyridostigmine taken orally has its onset of action within 10 to 30 minutes and a duration of 3 to 4½ hours. A similar onset and duration are reported for neostigmine and ambenonium.

Pyridostigmine therapy is usually initiated with 60 mg taken with meals three times daily if chewing and swallowing are not affected or 45 minutes before meals (with a small amount of food) if they are. The patient is asked to keep a record of symptoms at the peak of medication effectiveness (usually about 2 hours) and at the time immediately preceding the next dose. If the effects of the medication are noted to "wear off" before the next dose, the interval between medications is gradually shortened. If an individual dose results in only partial relief of symptoms, a larger amount may be tried (in 30 to 60 mg increments). When an increase in medication no longer produces a definite decrease in symptoms, the previous lower amount of medication is resumed. Patients rarely benefit from more than 120 mg of pyridostigmine every 3 hours. Some patients require larger amounts of medication at different times of day (for example, late afternoon) and thus each dose need not be the same. In patients with dysphagia or jaw fatigue, meal times should be adjusted to correspond to medication peaks.

Many patients experience gastrointestinal discomfort and diarrhea with anticholinesterase medications. These symptoms often lessen with time and are diminished by taking the medication with a small amount of food. When needed, diphenoxylate with atropine (Lomotil) may be taken once or twice a day for the control of diarrhea. Excessive amounts of anticholinesterase medication flood the neuromuscular junction with acetylcholine, resulting in blockade and increased weakness. Thus, any increase in medication that does not produce a clear improvement should not be continued.

Pyridostigmine timespan may be used by the patient who experiences weakness during the night or on awakening in the morning. It is not generally used during the day because of its somewhat uneven release. The pyridostigmine syrup is not commonly used but may be easier to administer in small children or in adults with marked dysphagia. However, careful observation should be made to insure that the salivation induced by the muscarinic effect of pyridostigmine (and enhanced by the sweet syrup vehicle of this form of the drug) does not lead to excessive secretions. The parenteral administration of anticholinesterase medication is reserved for occasions when oral intake is not possible (to be discussed) or for diagnostic testing.

Most patients benefit significantly from anticholinesterase medication, and some obtain relief of symptoms from this medication alone. Often some symptoms persist, especially diplopia. In this case the physician and patient must decide whether the symptoms are sufficiently severe or distressful to warrant other forms of therapy. Diplopia, for instance, may be adequately relieved by patching one eye. However, many patients find a patch disfiguring or occupationally threatening and request further treatment.

Thymectomy

The thymus gland is abnormal in most patients with myasthenia gravis. Ten to 15 percent of the patients have a thymoma, while most others demonstrate thymic hyperplasia. Hyperplasia is particularly common in younger patients with myasthenia gravis and is less frequent in the elderly.

The presence of a thymoma as suggested by chest x-ray examination, tomography, or computed tomography is considered an indication for its removal. These tumors are often locally invasive but rarely metastasize outside the chest. When it has been incompletely removed, radiation therapy is administered postoperatively. Following thymomectomy the patient may show clinical improvement in myasthenia gravis symptoms and postoperative care should be given as described below for thymectomy without thymoma. Long term improvement in myasthenia gravis after thymoma removal does occur but is unpredictable. Should symptoms worsen postoperatively, corticosteroids should be added to the therapeutic regimen (to be discussed).

Thymectomy in the absence of suspected thymoma is more controversial. The theoretical basis for thymectomy in myasthenia gravis is the suspicion that the thymus harbors a cell or cell bound material that acts in the propagation of myasthenia gravis. Well controlled studies are difficult to carry out, but most investigations suggest that thymectomy in the young patient with myasthenia gravis increases the chances for remission or improvement in the disease for at least the first 3 years after the surgery. Best results appear to occur if the surgery is done within a year after the onset of symptoms.

I favor the use of thymectomy in all patients with generalized myasthenia gravis above the age of puberty and below the age of 50. Children below the age of puberty would be considered candidates for thymectomy if they were not well controlled on anticholinesterase medication. Adults between 50 and 60 who are otherwise in good health but not responding well to anticholinesterase would also be considered. Thymectomy is generally not advised in patients with only ocular symptoms. Exception could be considered for a young patient with a recent onset of severe symptoms that are unresponsive to anticholinesterase medication. At some institutions patients over the age of 60 years with myasthenia gravis are advised to have thymectomy. I have found these patients to be very responsive to corticosteroid therapy and prefer to use this medication in older patients, rather than thymectomy, unless there is evidence of thymoma.

Thymectomy requires a skilled surgeon and anesthesiologist, with postoperative intensive care in a unit with experienced personnel and careful attention to medication needs. It is most often done through a trans-sternal approach, with removal of all thymic tissue and adjacent fat. The transcervical approach is more controversial because of the possibility of incomplete removal of thymic tissue. Although almost all my patients have been operated on by the trans-sternal approach, I believe that the transcervical approach should be considered if a surgeon skilled in this procedure is available and the patient, for reasons of better cosmetic appearance or faster recovery, requests this approach.

The medication needs of the patient with myasthenia gravis usually decrease immediately postoperatively. This may occur following any operative procedure but is especially true following thymectomy. I advise that anticholinesterase medication be discontinued postoperatively and be restarted as needed, either because of recurrence of symptoms or following a positive response to parenteral anticholinesterase therapy. The latter can be given in the short acting form, edrophonium (Tensilon) in increments of 2 mg, 3 mg, and 5 mg spaced at 1 to 2 minute intervals. Improvement can be expected within 20 to 40 seconds after injection, with a duration of action of 2 to 3 minutes. If improvement occurs with 2 or 3 mg, the test is discontinued. It is highly unlikely that a response will be obtained from a large edrophonium bolus (for example, 10 mg), if no response is obtained from a smaller injection. Additionally, muscarinic side effects are much more distressing with the larger injections.

Often anticholinesterase medication does not have to be resumed until the patient is able to take oral medications. If so, they are restarted on 60 mg of pyridostigmine three times daily, to be increased as necessary on a program similar to that used for the initiation of anticholinesterase therapy. When parenteral therapy is necessary postoperatively, it may be administered either intramuscularly, subcutaneously, or intravenously (0.5 mg of neostigmine methylsulfate every 4 hours by continuous infusion). If the patient was taking alternate day prednisone prior to surgery, he should receive an equivalent daily parenteral dose of corticosteroid therapy until oral medications can be resumed. Occasionally a patient is difficult to wean from the respirator postoperatively. In this circumstance a short course of plasmapheresis may be helpful (to be discussed).

Corticosteroids

Corticosteroids are widely accepted as a treatment modality for myasthenia gravis, although the mechanism of action is incompletely understood. Steroids decrease acetylcholine receptor antibody levels in some patients with myasthenia gravis, usually those showing the most definite improvement. Whether there are additional im-munosuppressive actions or direct effects on the neuromuscular junction that are significant is not known at present. Older male patients in particular seem to benefit greatly from prednisone therapy and often can be maintained for years in a relatively asymptomatic state. Patients with only ocular symptoms often benefit more from steroids than from anticholinesterase drugs. In these patients the risk-benefit ratio must be considered carefully by the physician and the patient before steroids are begun. If the benefits seem significant (for example, job preservation), steroids may be warranted in some patients with ocular myasthenia gravis.

The method of commencing steroid administration varies with the severity of the disease. For the patient with only ocular symptoms or with mild generalized myasthenia gravis, I begin with low dose (20 mg), alternate day prednisone therapy on an outpatient basis. The prednisone dosage is increased by 5 mg every 2 weeks to a level at which a good result is obtained. For some patients this may be as low as 25 or 30 mg. If a good result is not obtained by the time a level of 40 mg is reached, the prednisone dosage is increased in 10 mg increments at 2 week intervals until a level of 100 mg every other day is reached. The patient is maintained at this level until a satisfactory response is obtained or for 3 to 6 months, after which a slow tapering is attempted (5 to 10 mg per month). Early in treatment patients usually feel better during the day "on" prednisone. Generally a more balanced effect is achieved as time goes on. The maintenance level selected is whatever amount of prednisone is required to give the patient acceptable relief of symptoms. Rarely a patient may have no improvement with prednisone. When no improvement is observed in 3 months, a slightly more rapid tapering seems justified in anticipation of alternative therapy.

The method just described probably results in a slower improvement than that obtained from daily prednisone therapy or higher initial dosages. It has advantages, however, that seem to me to outweigh this disadvantage: patients may be treated as outpatients and continue to work while beginning therapy; exacerbations of symptoms (a common occurrence with prednisone when initiated in high daily doses) can be avoided; side effects such as a cushingoid appearance, mood change, and sleeplessness are rare; and some patients respond while taking a low dosage, thus avoiding the need to take higher dosages. Most patients show a definite response within 3 to 6 weeks after beginning prednisone by this method, and improvement may continue over several months.

When the patient has more severe symptoms, more rapid introduction of prednisone is necessary. Patients with rapidly evolving disease, or with difficulties with food intake or respiratory symptoms or signs, should be hospitalized for the initiation of steroid therapy. Patients with respiratory difficulty should be placed in an intensive care unit, while others often may be treated on the ward under careful observation. The initial dosage and rapidity of increase must be determined by the patient's clinical status. Elderly patients with bulbar symptoms often tolerate increments of 10 mg of prednisone every 5 days from an initial dosage of 20 mg without exacerbation. Only in the most desperate of circumstances would I start a patient on daily high dosage prednisone (60 to 100 mg) therapy, because this requires admission to the intensive care unit and has a high probability of inducing an exacerbation requiring respiratory support.

Long term maintenance on prednisone, as previously mentioned, should be at the lowest dosage that controls symptoms. For most patients this is 15 to 40 mg every other day. Few patients can be tapered from prednisone completely, and if exacerbation occurs during tapering, the dosage often must be raised substantially to obtain the same level of improvement seen previously. While taking prednisone, the patient may benefit from vitamin D (400 IU per day) and calcium gluconate or carbonate (1,000 mg per day).

The side effects of prednisone therapy include osteoporosis, aseptic necrosis of bone, increased risk of infection, ulcers, cataracts, hypertension, exacerbation of diabetes, and fluid retention. Periodic examination of the blood count, blood glucose and electrolyte levels, and yearly chest x-ray and eye examinations are recommended.

Azathioprine and Other Immunosuppressive Drugs

Azathioprine should be considered for the patient who has disabling symptoms despite careful regulation of anticholinesterase and steroid medications, or for the patient who is unable or unwilling to take steroids. Like steroids, azathioprine often results in a lowering of the acetylcholine receptor antibody level in the serum. Whether this reduction in the acetylcholine receptor antibody level is responsible for the therapeutic effectiveness is not known.

Azathioprine is given orally. The usual recommended dosage is 2.0 to 2.5 mg per kg per day (125 to 200 mg per day for most patients). I have found it effective to start with 50 mg per day and to increase to 100 mg after 2 weeks. As with prednisone, some patients improve with small amounts of azathioprine, obviating the need for higher dosages and diminishing the risks of the drug. Incremental increases to 2.5 mg per kg per day may be given over the following month if necessary and as tolerated by the patient. Improvement may be seen as early as 1 month after starting treatment, but often several months are required for maximal effect.

Side effects from azathioprine include leukopenia, thrombocytopenia, an increased hazard of infection, fever, nausea and vomiting, hepatic toxicity, and alopecia. A reduction in dosage or discontinuation of the drug usually results in a decrease in the side effects. Blood counts and liver function studies should be carefully monitored for the patient taking azathioprine, weekly for the first month and biweekly or monthly thereafter. Whether long term azathioprine treatment in myasthenia gravis will be associated with the development of neoplasia, as it has been in transplant patients, remains to be seen. As yet, no such association has been recognized.

I have found azathioprine particularly helpful for the patient who requires large amounts of prednisone to control myasthenia gravis. In these patients the addition of azathioprine often results in improvement and allows the prednisone dosage to be tapered to a lower maintenance level.

Other immunosuppressive medications, such as cyclophosphamide (Cytoxan) and cyclosporine, have been employed in patients with myasthenia gravis. Although this therapy is effective in some cases, the high toxicity of these drugs will probably limit their use to the most severely ill patients.

Plasmapheresis

Plasmapheresis is well accepted as a method to induce improvement in patients with myasthenia gravis. Usually a series of four to eight treatments is administered over a 5 to 10 day period. This treatment decreases the amount of circulating acetylcholine receptor antibody, but whether this is the cause of the improvement is not known. The effects of plasmapheresis often last only 2 to 4 weeks, and the patient may revert to the previous level of disease. This appears less likely to happen if prednisone and azathioprine are given concomitantly.

Indications for plasmapheresis in myasthenia gravis include respirator dependency, life threatening exacerbation of disease, and chronic severe myasthenia gravis despite high doses of prednisone and azathioprine. It may also be used prior to thymectomy in the patient with moderately severe disease in an attempt to obtain improved strength during the perioperative period.

The complications of plasmapheresis include infection, hypotension, thrombocytopenia, and hypocalcemia. It is also expensive. It should be employed only when other methods for the control of myasthenia gravis have not been successful; fortunately this is uncommon.

CRISIS

Rarely a patient with myasthenia gravis may experience an abrupt increase in symptoms, which appear refractory to medication. This may be caused by excessive anticholinesterase medications (cholinergic crisis) or by an actual deterioration in responsiveness to therapy (myasthenic crisis). In either case the patient should be hospitalized immediately and placed in an intensive care unit if ventilatory inadequacy is suspected or has occurred in the past. Patients in crisis may deteriorate extremely rapidly and precautionary support of ventilation is judicious. Once adequate ventilation is insured, assessment of cholinergic versus myasthenic crisis can be made. Treatment of the cholinergic crisis usually requires that all anticholinesterase medications be discontinued for 24 to 72 hours and then restarted as at the beginning of anticholinesterase therapy. If the patient is receiving steroid therapy, this is not altered. For a myasthenic crisis, anticholinesterase medications are also withheld for 24 to 72 hours and then restarted in the standard manner. In addition, a source for the induction of the crisis should be sought. This is often an infection, but may be attributable to medications, emotional upset, surgery, or other factors. When necessary, prednisone may be started or increased, or the patient may undergo plasmapheresis. With respiratory assistance already being provided, the danger from prednisone induced exacerbation is reduced and high dosages (60 to 100 mg of prednisone) may be used. My preference has been to use 100 mg every other day, although a daily dosage is employed in most centers.

NEONATAL MYASTHENIA GRAVIS

Twelve to 15 percent of the infants born to mothers with myasthenia gravis experience transient weakness. Symptoms are usually present on the first day of life and persist for an average of 18 days. Feeding difficulties are the most common evidence of the disorder. The child also should be carefully observed for respiratory difficulty and given support if necessary. Medications such as pyridostigmine syrup (4 to 10 mg) may be given orally or by nasogastric tube if necessary, preferably 45 minutes before feedings. Decreasing doses of anticholinesterase medication are needed as the disorder improves spontaneously and care should be taken to avoid overmedication.

SUGGESTED READING

Drachman DB, de Silvia S, Ramsay D, Pestronk A. Humoral pathogenesis of myasthenia gravis. Ann NY Acad Sci 1987; 505:90–105.
Engel AG. Myasthenia gravis and myasthenic syndromes. Ann Neurol 1984; 16:519–534.
Lisak RP, Barchi RL. Myasthenia gravis. Philadelphia: WB Saunders, 1982.
Oosterhuis HJGH. Myasthenia gravis. Edinburgh: Churchill Livingstone, 1984.
Seybold ME. Myasthenia gravis. A clinical and basic science review. JAMA 1983; 250:2516–2521.

AUTOIMMUNE UVEITIS

DOUGLAS A. JABS, M.D.

Uveitis is not one disease but several diseases, most of which are defined by their characteristic clinical picture, and only some of which are associated with a systemic disorder. An anatomic classification of uveitis has proven to be useful in the approach to therapy. Uveitis can be classified as anterior (iritis, iridocyclitis), intermediate (pars planitis), posterior (choroiditis, chorioretinitis, retinitis), or panuveitis. Anterior uveitis (inflammation involving the anterior segment of the eye) often can be treated with topically applied medications. Since such medications have little penetration capacity posterior to the lens, the treatment of intermediate or posterior uveitis generally requires the use of the periocular or systemic route.

Prior to the initiation of therapy for uveitis, it is important to differentiate between diseases of an autoimmune or presumed autoimmune origin and those due to an infectious or neoplastic process. Infectious diseases, such as toxoplasmosis, should be treated with antimicrobial drugs. Neoplastic processes, such as histiocytic lymphoma (reticulum cell sarcoma), often respond well to radiation therapy. Therapy for uveitis should be directed toward treating the active inflammation to prevent sequelae such as glaucoma, cataract formation, and macular edema. The type of treatment employed should always take into consideration the potential risks and benefits, particularly with the use of systemic therapy. The goal of therapy is to control the inflammation as rapidly as possible in patients with acute disease and to prevent recurrences in those with chronic disease.

CORTICOSTEROID THERAPY

The mainstay of therapy in patients with uveitis is corticosteroid treatment. The three routes available for the administration of corticosteroids in ocular disease are topical, periocular, and systemic. The use of steroid therapy for uveitis and the regimens employed are empiric; however, the theoretical considerations for its use are similar to those in other autoimmune diseases.

Topical Steroid Therapy

Topical steroid therapy is used to treat anterior uveitis. The advantages of topical therapy are in its application directly to the inflamed eye and the lack of systemic toxicity. Although sophisticated studies have suggested that topically applied steroid preparations are systemically absorbed, it is highly unlikely that any systemic side effects result from these drugs in the adult. Topically applied steroids penetrate the cornea and enter the anterior chamber, but have little effect on inflammation posterior to the lens.

A variety of topical corticosteroid preparations are available. Experimental data have suggested that a 1 percent suspension of prednisolone acetate is the most effective drug for suppression of anterior segment inflammation and that drops appear to be superior to ointments. Therefore, I generally initiate treatment with 1 percent prednisolone acetate every 1 or 2 hours applied during the patient's waking hours. I also add a dexamethasone containing ophthalmic ointment for use at night in order to provide anti-inflammatory medication while the patient is asleep.

Cycloplegic drugs are an important adjunct in the treatment of anterior segment inflammation. Cycloplegia not only makes the patient more comfortable, but also decreases the chance of formation of posterior synechiae and subsequent pupillary block glaucoma. For very mild inflammation I often use 1 percent cyclopentolate once or twice daily. For moderate to severe inflammation I use 1 percent atropine twice daily. Although systemic side effects from the topical application of corticosteroids are unlikely, side effects can result from the topical use of cycloplegics. One drop of 1 percent atropine contains approximately 0.5 mg of atropine, and frequent instillation of this medication can lead to systemic side effects in children.

When using topical steroid therapy, it is important that the disease activity be monitored regularly. If hourly topical therapy does not begin to decrease the inflammation within 1 week, additional therapy with either periocular or systemic doses of corticosteroids may be needed. Once the inflammation has been completely suppressed, the steroid dosage may be tapered. Abrupt cessation of topical steroid therapy frequently leads to a recrudescence of the uveitis, which may be explosive in nature. My schedule for tapering is to reduce the frequency of application of steroid drops from every 2 hours to every 4 hours, then to four times daily, then three times daily, then twice daily, and finally once daily. The initial steps in tapering can be taken every 3 to 4 days, but subsequent steps are planned at weekly intervals. I try discontinuing the topical corticosteroid

therapy after the patient has been using one drop daily for approximately 1 week. If the uveitis recurs at this point, I reinstitute therapy but taper more slowly. I then switch from 1 percent prednisolone once daily to 0.125 percent prednisolone four times daily and taper this over 3 to 4 weeks. Some patients have chronic inflammation and can be controlled only with long term therapy. Often a threshold below which inflammation routinely recurs can be determined and long term suppressive therapy instituted.

There are no absolute contraindications to topical steroid therapy. However, if active herpes simplex keratitis is present, antiviral therapy, such as the topical application of trifluorothymidine, must be used. The side effects of topical steroid use are cataracts, secondary glaucoma, impaired wound healing, and an increased susceptibility to infection. Cataracts and glaucoma are also complications of uveitis. In general, the side effects of topical corticosteroid therapy are proportional to the total amount of steroid used. Steroid induced glaucoma generally appears 2 to 4 weeks after the initiation of therapy. If secondary glaucoma develops, as a result of either uveitis or steroid therapy, some clinicians substitute a weaker steroid preparation (e.g., fluorometholone). I generally do not change treatment to a weaker steroid preparation, because this often leads to recurrence of the uveitis and leaves the clinician in the unsatisfactory situation of having both active uveitis and an elevated intraocular pressure to treat. Instead I continue with the steroid regimen just outlined and treat the elevated intraocular pressure with appropriate antiglaucoma medications.

Periocular Steroid Therapy

Periocular corticosteroid therapy is useful in patients with anterior segment inflammation who have failed to respond to topical therapy or in patients with uniocular intermediate uveitis complicated by cystoid macular edema. Experimental data have suggested that periocular doses of steroids are additive to topical corticosteroid therapy in the treatment of anterior segment inflammation. Furthermore, the systemic side effects of steroids can be minimized with a periocular injection. The injection may be given more anteriorly or posteriorly, depending upon the site of the inflammation. Although injections may be repeated, after multiple injections the orbital tissue becomes fibrotic and injection becomes more difficult. In addition, there may be a greater chance of complication from the use of multiple periocular injections.

Both soluble and depot steroid preparations are available. Soluble preparations, such as dexamethasone sodium phosphate, are rarely associated with secondary glaucoma but have a limited duration of action. Conversely, depot preparations, such as methylprednisolone acetate, have a long duration of action but may cause an uncontrollable elevation of intraocular pressure requiring surgical removal of the depot preparation. Therefore I generally use a soluble preparation initially. I reserve depot steroid preparations for patients with a clear-cut response to soluble injections, a recurrent problem, and an absence of steroid glaucoma.

The complications of periocular steroid use include steroid induced glaucoma, fibrosis of the orbit, atrophy of subcutaneous tissue, extraocular muscle atrophy leading to gaze limitation, perforation of the globe, retrobulbar hemorrhage, and retinal artery occlusion. Perforation of the globe is uncommon; however, if such perforation occurs, the eye is generally lost. The use of periocular steroid therapy is contraindicated in scleritis because it may cause scleral melting and perforation. It is also contraindicated in any infectious process unless the disease has been controlled with appropriate antibiotic therapy. Properly used, this mode of administration is useful and may avoid the side effects of systemic therapy.

Systemic Steroid Therapy

Systemic steroid therapy generally is used in patients with bilateral uveitis with posterior segment involvement in whom vision is threatened as a result of the inflammatory process. The use of steroids in unilateral ocular disease must be carefully considered and the risks of long term steroid therapy weighed against the potential visual loss. Occasionally a brief course of oral steroid therapy may be necessary in a patient with primarily anterior segment disease in order to bring the inflammation under control. This usually consists of high doses of steroids for 3 to 5 days, followed by rapid tapering and discontinuation of all systemic medications within 2 to 3 weeks. During this time intensive topical corticosteroid therapy is continued.

When using oral corticosteroid therapy, I generally begin with oral dosages of 1 mg per kg of prednisone daily. Although some patients may respond to a dosage greater than 100 mg daily, the potential for infectious complications appears to be markedly increased above this dosage level. Once the inflammation has been suppressed, I begin to taper the prednisone dosage, using visual acuity and inflammatory activity to assess the effect of the drug. I initially taper by 10 mg decreases until 40 mg daily is reached and then use 5 mg decreases. Below 15 mg daily, I often taper by using 2.5 mg decreases. The initial rate of tapering may be as rapid as every 3 to 5 days, but later steps (e.g., below 20 to 40 mg daily) are generally made at weekly intervals. If the disease flares while the steroid dosage is being tapered, I increase the dosage and taper more slowly. If the patient has a steroid responsive uveitis, but cannot be weaned and requires long term steroid therapy, I then try to institute an alternate day schedule. Alternate day steroid therapy is less effective than daily therapy but

appears to cause fewer side effects. In patients with chronic uveitis, long term steroid therapy may be needed. In this case one must clearly weigh the relative risks and benefits.

The systemic complications of long term oral steroid therapy are well known and include cataracts, glaucoma, a cushingoid habitus, fluid retention, weight gain, diabetes mellitus, hypertension, lipid abnormalities, osteoporosis, ischemic necrosis of bone, myopathy, impaired wound healing, neuropsychiatric dysfunction, and possibly peptic ulcer disease. Patients requiring long term steroid therapy should be informed about the potential complications and their physician's aid enlisted in the prevention and treatment of these problems.

NONSTEROIDAL MEDICAL THERAPY

For patients who fail to respond to the regimen just described, or in whom the side effects of steroid therapy prove intolerable, immunosuppressive drugs may be employed. The drugs most frequently used are azathioprine, chlorambucil, and cyclophosphamide. Nonsteroidal anti-inflammatory drugs, such as indomethacin, are effective in treating anterior scleritis but are ineffective in treating uveitis. Systemic cyclosporine therapy has been used in an investigational manner as an alternative to immunosuppressive drugs.

Azathioprine

I use azathioprine in patients who have steroid responsive disease but in whom the side effects of steroids have proved intolerable. In patients whose ocular inflammation is steroid dependent and who require unacceptably high systemic doses of corticosteroids, the systemic dose of steroids often can be tapered to much more acceptable levels with the use of azathioprine. Before such therapy is begun, the patient should be evaluated systemically; all possible side effects, including the risk of neoplasia, should be discussed with the patient. If such therapy is to be instituted and the ophthalmologist is not familiar with these drugs, he should seek the help of an internist. The dosage of azathioprine used is 1 to 2 mg per kg daily. The hematologic profile and liver function tests must be monitored regularly. If the peripheral leukocyte count falls below 3,000 per cubic mm, the drug should be stopped and reinstituted at a lower dosage. If there is evidence of hepatotoxicity, the drug should be discontinued. In my experience the value of azathioprine is as a "steroid sparing" drug for the patient with steroid responsive disease. Azathioprine appears much less effective in controlling uveitis that is not controlled by steroids alone.

Systemic Treatment with Alkylating Drugs

In contrast to azathioprine, alkylating drugs such as chlorambucil and cyclophosphamide may be useful in patients who have failed to respond to systemic steroid therapy. I generally employ these drugs in conjunction with systemic corticosteroid therapy and attempt to taper the steroid dosage once the inflammation has been controlled. As with azathioprine, the patient must be evaluated systemically, and all possible side effects, including the increased risk of neoplasia, must be discussed with the patient. Again the assistance of an internist is important.

Chlorambucil therapy is generally begun at a dosage of 2 mg daily and increased every 2 weeks until a therapeutic effect is noted or side effects occur. The usual therapeutic dosage is 0.1 mg per kg per day (6 to 10 mg daily). The dosage of cyclophosphamide is 1 to 2 mg per kg daily. Again the peripheral leukocyte count must be monitored frequently and drug therapy interrupted if the count falls below 3,000 per cubic mm. With cyclophosphamide treatment, the urinalysis also must be monitored for the development of hemorrhagic cystitis. If there is a good response, I generally try to treat the patient for at least 1 year and then withdraw the drug. Sometimes a long term remission may be induced. If the disease recurs, therapy is restarted.

Systemic Cyclosporine Therapy

Cyclosporine has been used on an investigational basis in patients who have failed to respond to systemic steroid therapy or cytotoxic drugs. Cyclosporine does not suppress the entire immune system or cause leukopenia; instead it affects T cell function. The dosage employed has usually been 10 mg per kg daily. The dose limiting side effect of cyclosporine therapy has been nephrotoxicity, and the creatinine clearance must be monitored regularly. Hepatic toxicity is less common, but the dosage must be adjusted for this problem as well. Other side effects include hypertension, gingivitis, hypertrichosis, paresthesias, tremor, gastrointestinal upset, and mild anemia. Although the initial results of cyclosporine therapy were encouraging, the frequent occurrence of nephrotoxicity has limited enthusiasm for use of this drug by itself. Renal biopsy specimens have demonstrated interstitial nephritis in almost all patients treated with cyclosporine, even in those in whom clinical evidence of nephrotoxicity was not apparent. Studies utilizing lower doses of cyclosporine in conjunction with systemic corticosteroid therapy are now being performed.

SURGICAL APPROACHES

There are no surgical techniques to control uveitis, but many of the complications require surgical treatment. Cataracts, glaucoma, and vitreoretinal problems sometimes require surgical therapy. In addition, retinal neovascularization as a consequence of uveitis and retinal nonperfusion may require laser treatment. Ideally the inflammation should be well controlled prior to surgery. In addition, systemic corticosteroid therapy should be used prior to intraocular surgery in order to minimize the chance of a postoperative flare-up. I generally use 1 mg per kg of prednisone daily, starting 2 to 3 days prior to surgery, and continue it through the immediate perioperative period. Subsequently the steroid dosage may be tapered rapidly.

SUGGESTED READING

Leibowitz HM, Kupferman A. Anti-inflammatory medications. Ophthalmol Clin 1980; 20:117–134.

O'Connor GR. Corticosteroids and immunosuppressives reviewed. In: Srinivasan BD, ed. Ocular therapeutics. New York: Masson, 1980: 69.

Palestine AG, et al. Renal histopathologic alterations in patients treated with cyclosporine for uveitis. N Engl J Med 1986; 314:1293–1298.

Polansky JR, Weinreb RN. Steroids as anti-inflammatory agents. In: Sears ML, ed. Pharmacology of the eye. New York: Springer-Verlag, 1984: 459.

Schlagel TF Jr. Nonspecific treatment of uveitis. In: Duane TD, Jaeger EA, eds. Clinical ophthalmology. Vol. 4. Philadelphia: Harper & Row, 1986; Ch. 43, 1.

Smith RE, Nozik RM. Uveitis: a clinical approach to diagnosis and management. Baltimore: Williams & Wilkins, 1983: 48.

AUTOALLERGIC DISEASES OF THE EXTERNAL EYE

ALAN G. PALESTINE, M.D.

The external eye is composed of the eyelids, conjunctiva, cornea, episcleral tissue, and sclera. Within this anatomic group of tissues are a wide diversity of structures capable of developing a variety of immune responses and disease. Diseases related to the skin, mucous membranes, and connective tissues may appear as external eye diseases. Some of these may be unique and isolated to the eye, whereas others are part of a systemic immune phenomenon. The primary functions of the external eye structures are to maintain corneal clarity and to provide structural support and protection for the intraocular structures. Hence, inflammatory disease of the external eye not only may be uncomfortable for the patient but may also cause visual impairment or blindness if not promptly treated. The external eye is easily examined in the office using a bright light source, although slit lamp examination is preferred because of the magnification and directed light source, which aid in the localization of lesions within the cornea and conjunctiva. This article focuses on the therapy of inflammatory external eye diseases categorized by the location of the primary inflammation.

EYELID DERMATITIS

The skin of the eyelid is soft, pliable, and thin. It is susceptible to contact dermatitis and may be more sensitive than the thicker skin elsewhere in the body. The eyelid skin is capable of developing significant swelling and redness with minor degrees of inflammation, and this frequently causes the patient to seek medical attention for inflammation that would be of less concern elsewhere on the skin.

Eyelid contact dermatitis is characterized by itching, redness, and swelling of one or both lids. It is probably a delayed hypersensitivity (type IV) immune reaction, with an onset 24 to 48 hours after exposure to the allergen. It is important to differentiate this condition from periorbital cellulitis due to bacterial infection. The presence of pain and a localized abscess is suggestive of cellulitis. The location and history are helpful in determining the cause of the allergy. For example, dermatitis of the lower lid with streaks may be due to an allergy to eyedrops. Preservatives such as thimerosal and medications such as atropine are capable of producing contact allergy of the lids and conjunctiva. Nail polish is a common contact allergen, and women who are sensitive and touch the skin around the eye before the polish is fully dry develop significant dermatitis there but rarely at other skin locations. The therapy of eyelid dermatitis consists of the topical application of a steroid cream, such as 1 percent hydrocortisone, three to four times daily, cool compresses, and identification of the cause of the allergic reaction. Potent fluorinated steroid creams should not be used to treat disorders of the eyelid.

ALLERGIC CONJUNCTIVITIS DUE TO DRUGS

Allergic conjunctivitis, like eyelid dermatitis, may also result from eyedrops or other materials such as eye cosmetics that come in contact with the conjunctiva. These may be type IV hypersensitivity reactions or possibly IgE mediated immediate hypersensitivity (type I) reactions. Therapy consists of identification of the cause and topical steroid therapy if the allergic reaction is severe. Usually a low potency steroid, such as 0.125 percent prednisolone phosphate or 1 percent medrysone, applied several times a day for 3 or 4 days is sufficient. Medrysone probably penetrates the eye less than other preparations and may cause ocular side effects less frequently.

GIANT PAPILLARY CONJUNCTIVITIS

This is a specific type of conjunctivitis characterized by large papules beneath the upper lid in addition to diffuse conjunctival injection and is associated with contact lens wear. The exact cause is still uncertain, but it appears to be due to a type I hypersensitivity to the protein deposits that can develop on the contact lens, especially soft contact lenses. Therapy consists of removal and cleaning of the contact lens or replacement with a new contact lens. Four percent disodium chromoglycate is available for topical ocular use and often leads to marked improvement when applied three to six times per day.

There is another contact lens related conjunctivitis due to type IV contact sensitivity to preservatives such as thimerosal in the contact lens cleaning solution. Patients are usually patch test positive. This form does not cause a giant papillary response visually, but the two may coexist. The condition responds to changing to cleaning solutions that are preservative free.

VERNAL KERATOCONJUNCTIVITIS

Vernal keratoconjunctivitis is characterized by a giant papillary reaction similar to that which occurs in contact lens related conjunctivitis. It is probably a type I hypersensitivity reaction with elevated tear IgE and histamine levels. However, vernal keratoconjunctivitis is a seasonal disorder occurring in the spring and fall, most commonly in the southern United States. It occurs in children and young adults and is accompanied by severe itching, tearing, and burning. There is often a thick mucoid discharge. In addition to conjunctivitis, patients can develop inflammation of the cornea. This usually occurs at the corneal limbus, but may occur centrally and impair the vision. The attacks usually last for many weeks or several months and recur for many years.

The initial therapy consists of the topical application of steroid drops, such as 1 percent prednisolone phosphate every 1 or 2 hours. After improvement occurs, use of the drops should be tapered, since prolonged topical use of steroid drops may cause glaucoma or cataract. It is often not possible to completely taper therapy with the steroid drops, and the patient must be monitored for the ocular side effects of steroids. The minimal amount and concentration of steroid that are effective should be used.

Disodium cromoglycate is also useful in this disorder. Such therapy can be started prior to the seasonal attack and used for long periods because it has few ocular side effects. Even if it is not effective as a sole therapy, cromoglycate is useful in reducing the amount of topical steroid therapy needed. Acetylcysteine drops are a useful adjunct as a mucolytic agent. Rarely a short tapering course of systemic prednisone therapy beginning at 1 mg per kg for a few weeks may be needed initially to control this conjunctivitis.

HAY FEVER ALLERGIC CONJUNCTIVITIS

During the hay fever season, patients with hay fever manifest itching, burning, and redness of the conjunctiva. The primary goal of therapy is to reduce the redness and discomfort. This often can be accomplished by the topical application of vasoconstrictors such as 0.5 to 1 percent naphazoline combined with topical antihistamine therapy, such as 5 percent antazoline given three to four times a day. Patients should avoid other eye irritants, which will enhance their discomfort. Topical therapy with 4 percent disodium cromoglycate can be started prior to the allergy season in an attempt to avert this type of conjunctivitis. As in other allergic conjunctival disorders, the topical use of steroids, such as 0.125 percent prednisolone phosphate or medrysone, is usually effective, but their use must be balanced against the possible ocular complications of long term topical steroid use. The lowest dose frequency and concentration should be used, and the patient must be followed carefully. If the patient does develop glaucoma secondary to steroid therapy, prompt discontinuation of the medication often leads to a normalization of the intraocular pressure. The posterior subcapsular cataracts that may

occur do not resolve if the steroid treatment is stopped and may progress and require surgical removal.

KERATOCONJUNCTIVITIS SICCA (SJÖGREN'S SYNDROME)

Dry eye syndrome is a very common disease in the ophthalmologist's practice. Only in some of these patients is lack of tear secretion accompanied by dry mouth and the systemic immune manifestations that can be grouped as Sjögren's syndrome. However, the treatment of dry eye, whether due to an isolated ocular disease or associated with Sjögren's syndrome, is essentially the same. Tear substitutes consisting of saline combined with a wetting and viscosity agent, such as methylcellulose or polyvinyl alcohol, can be used as often as four times an hour to provide comfort and ocular lubrication. The real danger in the dry eye is the development of epithelial erosions or corneal ulcers. The dry eye surface heals poorly and is susceptible to infection. If tear substitutes are inadequate, ointments such as Lacrilube or time release tear replacements such as Lacriserts may help.

The unresponsive patient may be treated with occlusion of the lacrimal puncta to maximize the small amount of tears produced. This occlusion is done under local anesthesia utilizing cautery to close and scar the puncta in the nasal aspect of the eyelids. If corneal decompensation occurs, lateral tarsorrhaphy can decrease the ocular surface available for evaporation and aid in protecting the cornea. Goggles that prevent evaporation may also help maintain adequate tears, but they frequently become fogged and may not help in maintaining useful vision.

Currently investigation is under way concerning the topical use of vitamin A ointment. This ointment reverses the epithelial cell metaplasia and increases conjunctival goblet cell mucus production, which enhances the capacity of the tears to wet the surface of the eye, thereby decreasing many of the symptoms of dry eye.

PERIPHERAL CORNEAL INFILTRATES AND MELTING

Patients may develop disease in the peripheral cornea, near the limbus, as a result of several disorders. The most common is the inferior peripheral corneal infiltrate associated with chronic staphylococcal blepharitis. These lesions probably occur following staphylococcal antigen-antibody deposition and secondary cellular infiltration. In severe cases the cornea may ulcerate. Treatment is directed at control of the blepharitis using lid hygiene and, if needed, topical antibiotic therapy, such as sulfacetamide. Lid hygiene is performed using 1 drop of baby shampoo in 1 tablespoon of warm water applied to a cotton applicator and used to clean the eyelids near the eyelashes once or twice a day. The peripheral corneal infiltrates may respond to these measures or may require topical steroid therapy, such as 0.125 percent prednisolone phosphate, four to six times daily. Once the infiltrates resolve, steroids and antibiotic therapy can be stopped, but the lid hygiene may need to be continued to prevent recurrences.

More serious peripheral corneal melting can occur in systemic diseases such as Wegener's granulomatosis, rheumatoid arthritis, or the isolated ocular condition known as Mooren's ulcer. These melting conditions can lead to perforation of the cornea and loss of the eye. Immunosuppressive therapy, such as 100 to 150 mg per day of cyclophosphamide, in combination with prednisone is indicated. If perforation occurs, it can be managed by corneal grafting, but the condition may recur within the grafted tissue.

Another form of corneal infiltrate is termed phlyctenular keratoconjunctivitis. These nodules appear at the limbus and extend into the cornea and conjunctiva. The nodules last approximately 2 weeks and may ulcerate. The disease is thought to be a hypersensitivity reaction to tuberculin, or more commonly in the United States to staphylococcal antigen similar to the marginal infiltrates already described. Phlyctenules differ from staphylococcal peripheral infiltrates in that with phlyctenules there is usually not a clear space between the cornea and conjunctiva and they tend to extend more centrally with more vascularization. Lid hygiene and topical therapy with corticosteroids, such as medrysone or prednisolone, in combination with topical therapy with sulfacetamide or gentamicin four times daily usually control the condition. If the condition becomes chronic and recurrent and is associated with permanent corneal scarring, oral tetracycline therapy is effective in controlling the disease.

Herpes simplex infection of the cornea is a common cause of corneal disease with many manifestations and must be ruled out prior to initiating therapy because corticosteroids cause this form of corneal disease to worsen.

OCULAR PEMPHIGOID

Of the bullous skin diseases, only cicatricial pemphigoid commonly affects the eye. This disease is a serious progressive disease of the conjunctiva with eventual secondary corneal scarring. This disease is probably due to type II antigen-antibody reactions, but T cells may also participate in the inflammatory response. There is no clinical bullous formation in ocular pemphigoid. Rather there is progressive scarring of the conjunctiva with loss of the mucus producing goblet cells and loss of the fornices. The cornea opacifies as the eye becomes increasingly dry. Symblepharon, an adhesion between the bulbar and palpebral conjunctiva, is the hallmark of this disease. In addition to the secondary dry eye that occurs, the lashes may turn inward (trichiasis), resulting in corneal abrasion.

The nonimmune complications of pemphigoid should be treated aggressively. The treatment of dry eyes has been outlined already. If a soft contact lens can be tolerated, it can protect the eye from trichiasis. Aberrant lashes must be removed and an effort made to prevent corneal ulceration or opacification. The ocular immune disease has responded better to therapy with cyclophosphamide than to corticosteroids, although these may also be helpful. A dosage of 100 to 150 mg per day adjusted to keep the absolute neutrophil count above 2,000 may be effective. However, patients with pemphigoid are elderly, and the risk of this therapy must be weighed individually for each patient. Once corneal scarring or other structural damage has occurred, immunotherapy does not repair the damage. Corneal grafting results are poor in these patients because of the dry eye condition and the continuing disease. A complicated and risky procedure, keratoprosthesis, has been used to replace the cornea with a metal or plastic prosthesis with a lens system. Vision often can be restored, but the eyes frequently succumb to glaucoma, infection, or retinal detachment.

ERYTHEMA MULTIFORME

The conjunctiva is frequently and severely affected in erythema multiforme. There may be only mild conjunctivitis, or the disease may progress to severe conjunctival scarring. As in pemphigoid, the scarring leads to loss of goblet cells, dry eye, trichiasis, and corneal opacification. Unlike pemphigoid, the scarring is generally not progressive after the acute inflammation has resolved. The acute lid and conjunctival disease can be treated with wet soaks for comfort and debridement. Systemic corticosteroid therapy (1.0 to 1.5 mg per kg per day) has been suggested, but it is unclear whether these drugs modify the eventual outcome of the disease; they should be used if there are no other contraindications. Lysis of the symblepharon with a glass rod in the acute stage of the disease may prevent conjunctival obliteration but does not prevent goblet cell loss. After the acute disease is quiescent, the patient will have continuing problems with dry eyes, trichiasis, and blepharitis, which should be managed as outlined in other sections of this article.

CORNEAL GRAFT REJECTION

The cornea is avascular, and 90 percent of primary grafts are not permanently rejected. However, 25 percent of the patients with grafts have an immunologic rejection episode requiring treatment. Furthermore, in regrafts or in primary grafts in which the cornea is vascularized from previous disease, the incidence of rejection is much higher. Graft rejection must be differentiated from mechanical problems such as glaucoma or corneal endothelial damage during surgery. Treatment of a graft rejection should begin immediately with the hourly use of 1 percent prednisolone drops supplemented by a subconjunctival injection of triamcinolone or a short course of oral prednisone therapy (1 mg per kg per day). Other antirejection regimens employed in other organ transplants, such as cyclosporine, have not been evaluated in corneal transplantation. In part this is because the systemic toxicity outweighs the benefit in most patients. Donor tissue matching is also rarely done, but appears to be useful in grafts in which there is a high likelihood of failure because of previous graft failure.

SCLERITIS AND EPISCLERITIS

Episcleritis refers to inflammation of the connective tissue between the conjunctiva and the sclera, whereas scleritis refers to inflammation of the deeper, denser scleral tissue. Both tissues may develop inflammation in isolated ocular disease or in conjunction with a systemic immune disorder such as Wegener's granulomatosis or rheumatoid arthritis. In both tissues the inflammation may be nodular or diffuse. Episcleritis presents as a red, somewhat painful eye in which the inflammation is located deep to the conjunctiva and only over the globe of the eye. It does not present a threat to vision. The inflammation usually responds to the application of 1 percent prednisolone four to six times per day or to systemic therapy with nonsteroidal drugs such as indomethacin.

Scleritis is usually much more painful than episcleritis and results in a reddish purple color. It may extend over into the cornea or deeper into the choroid of the eye. The topical use of 2.5 percent phenylephrine constricts the conjunctival vessels and makes it easier to examine the sclera. The disorder may be associated with intraocular inflammation. In advanced scleritis, especially a painless variety known as scleromalacia,

there is a risk that the marked scleral thinning will result in ocular perforation. Because of the potential for visual loss as well as because of the pain, oral therapy with corticosteroids (1.0 to 1.5 mg per kg per day) or cyclophosphamide (100 to 150 mg per day) is indicated. The disease is chronic, and long term therapy may be needed. Alternate day steroid therapy may be useful in some but not all patients. The presence of scleritis should prompt a search for other systemic immune mediated disease, and a flare-up of the scleral inflammation may be associated with increased systemic disease activity. We have utilized cyclosporine successfully in several patients with scleritis that was not responsive to other immunosuppressive therapy. If scleral perforation occurs or is imminent, scleral patch grafting using donor sclera can be utilized to reinforce the wall of the eye.

Diseases of the external eye are not infrequently first seen by the nonophthalmologist, who may be in the best clinical position to correlate the ocular diagnosis with systemic findings and to coordinate therapy by considering the overall medical status of the patient.

SUGGESTED READING

Allansmith MR, Ross RN. Ocular allergy and mast cell stabilizers. Surv Ophthalmol 1986; 30:229–244.
Foster CS, Forstot SL, Wilson LA. Mortality rate in rheumatoid arthritis patients developing necrotizing scleritis or peripheral ulcerative keratitis. Effects of systemic immunosuppression. Ophthalmology 1984; 91:1253–1263.
Foster CS, Wilson LA, Elkins MB. Immunosuppressive therapy for ocular cicatricial pemphigoid. Ophthalmology 1982; 89:340–352.
Kelley CG, Guss RB, Franklin RM. Immunologic diseases of the external eye. In: Easty DL, Smolin G, eds. External eye disease. London: Butterworth, 1985: 215.
Mondino BJ, Brown SI. Ocular cicatricial pemphigoid. Ophthalmology 1981; 88:95–100.
Sanfilippo F, MacQueen JM, Vaughn WK, Foulks GN. Reduced graft rejection with good HLA-A and B matching in high-risk corneal transplantation. N Engl J Med 1986; 315:29–35.

ULCERATIVE COLITIS AND CROHN'S DISEASE

FERGUS SHANAHAN, M.D., F.R.C.P.(C), M.R.C.P.(UK), M.R.C.P.I.
STEPHAN TARGAN, M.D.

The term idiopathic inflammatory bowel disease is used to encompass two chronic intestinal inflammatory diseases of unknown etiology—ulcerative colitis and

Crohn's disease. Excluded are the acute specific inflammatory disorders of known infectious, toxic, or ischemic etiology, which occasionally may mimic ulcerative colitis and Crohn's disease.

There is no specific treatment for either form of idiopathic inflammatory bowel disease. The emphasis therefore is on supportive measures and the judicious use of potentially toxic anti-inflammatory and immunosuppressive drugs. Our purpose here is to provide some guidelines for the management of these disorders, beginning with an account of the therapeutic measures and drugs available and then providing an overview of their use in the clinical settings that are frequently encountered. Although ulcerative colitis and Crohn's disease are considered together because of their overlapping features, important differences between them are emphasized. The approach to patients with ulcerative colitis and Crohn's disease should not be algorithmic but rather should be individualized. We believe that as with other chronic inflammatory diseases in which specific therapy is unavailable, the single most important aspect of patient management is the availability of a physician who is interested in the disease, sympathetic, and committed to the long term care of those who suffer from it.

THERAPEUTIC MODALITIES

Patient Education and Support

As with all chronic illnesses, patient education is an important component of a successful long term management program. This should include specific instruction regarding the nature of the disease, its clinical spectrum, and reasonable expectations from its therapy. We encourage all patients to learn about their disease and its management and advise them to enroll with The National Foundation for Ileitis and Colitis (National Headquarters, 444 Park Avenue South, New York, NY 10016). The Foundation publishes some excellent brochures and books about Crohn's disease and ulcerative colitis. When colectomy is being considered, the advantages and disadvantages of the types of operations available should be discussed as early as possible, and an enterostomal therapist should discuss stoma management with the patient well in advance of the operation. The United Ostomy Association (2001 West Beverly Boulevard, Los Angeles, CA 90057) is an excellent source of information and support for patients.

Although stress and other psychosomatic factors do not cause inflammatory bowel disease, stress may exacerbate the disease and perhaps trigger relapse, particularly in patients with proctitis. The patient and his family should be aware of this. Anxiolytic and antidepressant drugs occasionally may be indicated, but we prescribe them only for specific psychiatric problems and only in consultation with a psychiatrist with a knowledge and interest in patients with chronic organic disease. Many patients have difficulty in accepting their disease. Such individuals frequently benefit considerably from continuing regular counseling by a psychiatrist or psychologist and by participating in patient support group activities.

Diet and Nutrition

Patients with inflammatory bowel disease constantly ask about dietary instructions. However, we encourage as normal a diet as possible, with minimal restrictions. Emphasis is placed on maintaining adequate caloric intake and avoidance of excessive weight loss or malnutrition. The possibility of food allergy, although often raised, is rarely if ever a cause of relapse. For patients with known lactose intolerance, a reduction in lactose intake or the use of lactose digested dairy products is recommended. A reduction in dietary residue is indicated in patients with strictures.

The indications for specific dietary supplements include iron for patients with chronic blood loss, calcium for patients with ileal disease or lactose intolerance, folic acid for patients taking long term sulfasalazine therapy, and parenteral doses of vitamin B_{12} for patients with extensive ileal disease or previous ileal resection. Additional vitamin and trace elements may have to be supplemented in patients with extensive small bowel Crohn's disease. However, in the absence of a documented specific deficiency, or risk of such, we do not routinely prescribe multivitamins and discourage indiscriminate use of "megavitamin therapy." Since the irritable bowel syndrome frequently coexists with inflammatory bowel disease, supplementation with dietary fiber or synthetic roughage such as methylcellulose or psyllium may be helpful in the management of diarrhea in certain patients.

Drug Therapy

A limited number of drugs that are capable of reducing the inflammatory process in ulcerative colitis and Crohn's disease are available. The major limitation with each of these drugs is either the frequency or the severity of side effects.

Sulfasalazine and 5-Aminosalicylic Acid

Sulfasalazine has proven efficacy in the management of mild attacks of ulcerative colitis and Crohn's colitis and in reduction of the frequency of relapses of ulcerative colitis. We also use it in Crohn's disease of the small intestine, although its role here is not clear. Sulfasalazine consists of one molecule of sulfapyridine linked by an azo bond to one molecule of 5-aminosalicylate (5-ASA). 5-ASA is the therapeutically active moiety of the drug. Sulfapyridine, which is clinically inactive, is thought to be responsible for most of the side effects of sulfasalazine. Although sulfasalazine is absorbed intact through the intestinal mucosa, most of it is broken down by bacteria in the colon to its component molecules. The released sulfapyridine is then absorbed and is metabolized in part by acetylation in the liver before excretion in the urine. The rate of acetylation is the major determinant of sulfapyridine levels and thus the frequency of side effects. In contrast, 5-ASA is not well absorbed from the colon, and therefore most of it remains at its site of action.

The major limitation to the use of sulfasalazine in inflammatory bowel disease is the frequency of side

TABLE 1   Spectrum of Adverse Effects of Sulfasalazine*

Hematologic	Hemolysis, sulfohemoglobinemia, methemoglobinemia, cytopenia(s), aplasia(s)
Hepatic	Acute hepatitis, cholestasis, granulomatous hepatitis
Gastrointestinal	Dyspepsia often mimicking peptic ulceration Pancreatitis Bloody diarrhea and exacerbation of ulcerative colitis†
Pulmonary	Fibrosing alveolitis, tracheolaryngitis, eosinophilic pneumonia
Cardiac	Tachycardia
Dermatologic	Rash, toxic epidermal necrolysis, "cyanosis," Stevens-Johnson syndrome, hair loss
Miscellaneous	Reversible male infertility (hypospermia), "lupus-like" syndrome

* This is intended as a representative but not comprehensive list of all side effects that may occur with sulfasalazine.

† In contrast to the majority of side effects that are related to sulfapyridine, the exacerbation of colitis appears to be attributable to the salicylate moiety.

effects associated with its use (Table 1). However, in the majority of patients the side effects tend to be mild and transient. They usually can be minimized or avoided if the drug is introduced in a low dosage that is gradually increased. We usually begin with a dosage of 250 to 500 mg four times daily and gradually increase to 1 g four times daily. At the higher dosages discoloration of the urine may be noted, and patients should be warned of this in advance. Dyspeptic symptoms are particularly frequent and may be reduced by giving the drug with an antacid or by prescribing an enteric coated preparation of sulfasalazine. Sulfasalazine induced malabsorption of folic acid has been described, but in our experience it is rarely a problem and may be avoided by supplementation with folic acid, 1 mg per day, in patients taking the drug for long periods.

For individuals who are intolerant of the drug, two approaches may be adopted: "desensitization" and use of the active salicylate moiety. The term sulfasalazine desensitization is used loosely because most of the side effects for which it is prescribed do not involve allergic or immunologic sensitization. Several "desensitization" programs have been described, and all involve the cautious introduction of the drug in milligram dosages (e.g., 100 to 200 mg per day) with gradual increments every 1 to 2 weeks until the standard dosage of 2 to 4 g per day is reached. It is important to note that any form of desensitization is absolutely contraindicated in patients who have sustained serious life threatening side effects or organ damage, such as hemolysis or hepatic, cardiac, or pulmonary toxicity.

A variety of salicylate preparations including 5-ASA and 4-ASA (which is more stable and more soluble than 5-ASA) are currently being evaluated and will be useful for patients who are intolerant to sulfasalazine. Indeed as new formulations of salicylate become available, it is likely that these drugs will be increasingly used as alternatives to sulfasalazine for many patients. 5-ASA enemas have been particularly effective in patients with predominantly left sided colitis, although up to 10 percent of the patients experience salicylate induced diarrhea. Because of its nearly complete absorption in the upper gastrointestinal tract, unmodified 5-ASA is not given orally but rather by enema. Effective oral preparations of 5-ASA require either a "carrier" molecule, to deliver it intact to the colon where bacterial degradation can release it, or a delayed release formulation. One solution to this has been to couple two molecules of 5-ASA in linkage through an azo bond (azodisalicylate). 5-ASA also has been linked through the azo bond to a variety of inert nonsulfa carrier molecules. Slow release preparations of 5-ASA, which do not involve azo bond formation but in which the drug is coated with an acrylic based resin (Asacol) or with a semipermeable membrane of ethylcellulose (Pentasa), also have been developed recently. These and similar preparations probably will be available for clinical use in the United States in the near future.

Oral and Topical Corticosteroid Therapy

Systemic corticosteroid therapy is effective in the management of acute exacerbations of both ulcerative pancolitis and Crohn's disease. Unlike sulfasalazine, however, these drugs are of no use in the prevention of relapses. Corticosteroid therapy is usually commenced at oral dosages ranging from 40 to 60 mg of prednisolone per day, given as a single oral dose, for 2 to 4 weeks and then tapered according to the clinical activity. The precise regimen is individualized and varies considerably from patient to patient. However, it should be noted that the most frequent cause of steroid failure is a tapering program that is either premature or too rapid. For hospitalized patients the intravenous administration of adrenocorticotropic hormone (ACTH) may be considered as an alternative to corticosteroids. There is evidence that for patients with severe ulcerative colitis who have not previously received oral corticosteroid therapy, intravenous therapy with ACTH (120 units per 24 hours) may be more effective than systemic steroid therapy and less likely to cause side effects.

Topical corticosteroid therapy should be used in preference to systemic doses in patients with predominantly left sided colitis or proctitis. We also use it for troublesome symptoms such as urgency and rectal pain in patients with pancolitis, and in this situation it may help minimize the systemic dose of steroid required. Topical steroid therapy may be given as a retention enema (Cortenema, hydrocortisone aqueous suspension 10 percent) or as a foam (Cortifoam, hydrocortisone acetate foam 10 percent). With both these preparations it is essential that the patient be instructed and clearly understand the correct method of their application. Enemas are effective and generally well tolerated by patients who are properly instructed. They should be used once (or twice) daily, usually before bedtime and retained overnight. The hydrocortisone foam appears to be equally effective. It is also given once to twice daily and has the advantage of being less expensive and more easily retained in the bowel.

As with systemic steroid therapy, topical steroid preparations are not indicated for maintenance therapy; prolonged use leads to adrenocortical suppression and even cushingoid features. New topical steroid preparations such as tixocortol pivalate or beclomethasone dipropionate, which have minimal systemic effects because of either poor systemic absorption or rapid metabolism, are currently being developed and tested. The major advantage of such drugs will be that potentially they may be given in higher dosages without risk of suppression of the hypothalamic-pituitary-adrenal axis.

Immunosuppressants: Azathioprine and 6-Mercaptopurine

The immunosuppressive purine analogues, azathioprine and its active metabolite, 6-mercaptopurine, have been shown in recent studies to be clinically effective in some patients with Crohn's disease. These drugs appear to be particularly useful in ameliorating or healing fistulas. We use 6-mercaptopurine in chronically active Crohn's disease uncontrolled by corticosteroids and in patients requiring persistently high doses of steroids over long periods for the control of disease activity. In our experience only a minority of patients with Crohn's disease (about 10 percent) require treatment with these drugs at some stage during the course of the disease. Such patients should be referred to a specialist gastroenterologist experienced in using these potentially toxic drugs. Clinical experience with these drugs in treating ulcerative colitis is minimal, but we use 6-mercaptopurine in the occasional patient requiring continuous high doses of steroids in whom surgery is contraindicated or vetoed by the patient.

It should be recognized that these immunosuppressant drugs do not produce clinically beneficial effects rapidly, and the mean response time in patients with Crohn's disease is approximately 3 months. This implies that immunosuppressants are not likely to be useful in critically ill patients and that steroid therapy should not be stopped until sufficient time has elapsed for the immunosuppressant effect to become established.

6-Mercaptopurine is used in a dosage of 1 to 1.5 mg per kg daily. Patients must be carefully instructed about the details and importance of follow-up and vigilance for possible side effects. The major early risk of toxicity is bone marrow suppression, and patients must be followed with weekly blood counts for the first 2 months of therapy and monthly thereafter. Infection is a constant threat, and patients must be told to stop taking the drug at the first sign of infection and report to their doctor. Therapy with the drug may be temporarily stopped and restarted in a few days when intercurrent infection is treated or ruled out. The risk of neoplasia is not clear but may not be a significant problem at these low dosages. Infertility and teratogenicity are also important considerations, and therapy with the drug should be stopped when patients are contemplating having children. The most frequent short term complication of 6-mercaptopurine and azathioprine is pancreatitis, which occurs in 3 to 4 percent of patients. This usually occurs within the first month of therapy. It appears to be an allergy-hypersensitivity phenomenon and is a contraindication to reintroduction of the drug. A dangerous drug interaction may occur when 6-mercaptopurine is given to a patient who is already taking the xanthine oxidase blocker allopurinol. 6-Mercaptopurine is metabolized by xanthine oxidase, and the concomitant use of drugs that block this enzyme leads to dangerously high levels.

Antibiotics

The use of antibiotics is reserved for patients with severe fulminant colitis and for those with complications such as intra-abdominal or perineal sepsis. Although long term use of antibiotics such as ampicillin has been advocated by some physicians for patients with Crohn's disease, we have not found this to be helpful. Antibiotic therapy may exacerbate diarrhea by simply altering bowel flora or by predisposing to *C. difficile* toxin induced diarrhea. In addition, alteration in bowel flora might impede the metabolism of sulfasalazine. Metronidazole has been found in recent studies to be beneficial in Crohn's disease and particularly in patients with perineal and perirectal fistulas and abscesses. Dosages up to 750 mg orally three times daily may be required. In our experience few patients can tolerate the drug at this dosage, and it must be tapered to 250 mg three to four times daily after 7 to 10 days. Adverse effects include nausea, taste distortion, peripheral neuropathy, and disulfiram-like effects with alcohol. Metronidazole is potentially teratogenic and should not be used in pregnant women.

Antispasmodic and Antidiarrheal Drugs

We do not use antispasmodic-anticholinergic drugs because of their minimal efficacy and frequent side effects. Antidiarrheal drugs such as diphenoxylate (Lomotil) or loperamide (Imodium) may be of temporary benefit in selected patients. However, they are prescribed only sparingly on a short term basis. These drugs should never be given to patients with acute symptoms or severe colitis. Major hazards associated with their use include the precipitation of toxic megacolon in patients with acute severe colitis and their tendency to be habit forming.

TABLE 2   Spectrum of Clinical Severity of Ulcerative Colitis

Feature	Mild	Moderate	Severe
Daily frequency of bowel movements	Up to five	More than five	Hourly (liquid)
Rectal bleeding	Intermittent	Usually	Continuous and severe
Weight loss	Minimal	Less than 10 lb	Usually more than 10–20 lb
"Toxic" appearance	No	No	Yes
Fever	No	May have	Yes
Tachycardia	No	Frequently	Yes
Abdominal tenderness	No	Frequently	Yes
Bowel sounds	Normal	Normal or increased	Reduced or silent
Anemia	Usually no	Hematocrit >30	Hematocrit ≤25–30
Leukocytosis	No	Yes	Yes
Left shift	No	Yes	Yes
Albumin	Normal	Normal or slightly reduced	Reduced
Bacteremia	No	Usually no	Frequently

TREATMENT OF ACUTE ULCERATIVE COLITIS

The treatment of acute ulcerative colitis depends on the clinical severity of the condition. Table 2 outlines the spectrum of clinical signs and symptoms that help determine the degree of disease activity.

Mild and Moderate Ulcerative Colitis

Most patients with mild ulcerative colitis can be successfully treated with oral doses of sulfasalazine given alone or with a topically applied steroid. The latter are particularly useful for patients with left sided colitis and proctitis and for those with pancolitis in whom symptoms of proctitis such as urgency, frequency, rectal pain, and bleeding are particularly troublesome.

Patients with moderately severe ulcerative colitis require close outpatient follow-up to assess the progress of disease activity and to provide support and encouragement. The goals of treatment are to prevent progression to severe or fulminant disease and to achieve a reduction in inflammatory activity or full remission. It is important that intervention begin early and that one obtain remission as promptly as possible. Full dosages of sulfasalazine (1 to 1.5 g four times daily) are indicated. In addition, systemic corticosteroid treatment generally is required. Once the clinical assessment indicates that the colitis is moderately severe, there is nothing to be gained from postponing steroid medication. Steroid therapy should be commenced at a relatively high dosage (prednisolone, 40 to 60 mg per day) to bring the inflammation under control, and the dosage then should be tapered as the clinical course permits. For a given patient

the rate at which the steroid dosage is tapered is not fixed. Thus, we taper from 60 to 20 mg per day over a relatively short period (e.g., 5 to 10 mg every 1 to 2 weeks), but when a dosage of 20 mg per day is reached, the period over which it is tapered may be extended. This helps minimize side effects and reduces the risk of early relapse. Although the majority of patients have pancolitis, the most troublesome symptoms (tenesmus, urgency, bleeding) may be due to left sided disease or proctitis. For such patients the addition of topical steroid therapy may produce prompt improvement and allow tapering of the systemic steroid dosage more rapidly.

Severe Fulminant Ulcerative Colitis

Patients with acute severe ulcerative colitis should be admitted to the hospital for treatment and close observation. The emphasis should be on clinical assessment. Because of the risk of sudden deterioration with toxic megacolon, these patients may need to be assessed on an hourly basis. Abdominal roentgenography performed once to twice daily is a useful guide to the presence of toxic dilation. There is no place for colonoscopy or barium enema in the assessment of patients at this stage of the disease; these procedures are not necessary and may precipitate toxic megacolon. Surgical consultation should be obtained at the outset, for these patients are best managed by a physician-surgeon team approach.

The essential points in management include intravenous fluid therapy to correct dehydration and electrolyte abnormalities, broad spectrum antibiotic coverage, and intravenous corticosteroid therapy (for example, methylprednisolone) in a dosage equivalent to 80 mg of prednisone daily. Intravenous ACTH therapy may be considered as an alternative to corticosteroids in patients who have not been treated with corticosteroids and therefore do not have adrenal suppression. Finally, all opiate medications and anticholinergic or antispasmodic drugs are contraindicated and should be discontinued because they may precipitate toxic megacolon.

Sulfasalazine is not likely to have a significant therapeutic effect at this stage of the disease. Parenteral alimentation may be required if the prehospital clinical course has been prolonged and associated with significant malnutrition. We consider total parenteral nutrition with bowel rest as an adjunct to therapy but not as a primary form of management.

Surgical intervention should not be delayed if after 48 hours there is failure of medical therapy or clinical deterioration occurs despite aggressive medical therapy. Indeed, for these acutely ill patients surgery is often the conservative approach and safer than prolonged medical therapy. The procedure of choice in this situation is a standard ileostomy.

Toxic Megacolon

Acute dilation of the colon or toxic megacolon is a medical emergency and may occur as a complication of any form of severe ulcerative colitis. Occasionally it may be the presenting feature. Factors implicated in precipitating toxic megacolon include anticholinergics, opiates, hypokalemia, and barium enema or colonoscopic procedures. Dilation may involve the entire colon but is usually maximal in the transverse colon. In affected areas the bowel is thinned, and the inflammatory process extends into the muscle layer perhaps because of bacterial overgrowth. This inflammatory process leads to paralysis of motor function. Perforation and septic shock are major threats, with mortality incidences up to 30 percent reported. Abdominal tenderness, guarding, tympany, and reduced or lack of bowel sounds are the cardinal clinical features. Colonic dilation is best demonstrated by a plain abdominal radiograph with dilation beginning in the transverse colon. A continuous column of colonic air usually precedes this. There is a loss of haustral markings, and the luminal border is irregular, with nodular defects indicating islands of necrotic mucosa alternating with areas of ulceration. Gas shadows within the wall of the colon are a particularly ominous sign. It is important to note that the time sequence leading to toxic dilation and perforation may be rapid, occurring over a period of hours.

Immediate treatment includes the elimination of all precipitating drugs, resuscitation with intravenous fluid and electrolyte replacement, and broad spectrum antibiotic coverage. Colonic decompression should be attempted using a soft rectal tube and a long nasoenteral tube. The colonic gas can be effectively redistributed by intermittently repositioning the patient from the supine to the prone position for 10 to 15 minutes every 1 to 2 hours. Unless prompt resolution occurs with this regimen, ileostomy and subtotal colectomy or proctocolectomy should be performed.

LONG TERM MANAGEMENT OF ULCERATIVE COLITIS

The long term goal of treatment is to maintain the patient in remission and minimize the frequency of exacerbations of colitis. The effectiveness of medical therapy is judged in terms of quality of life and the ability to work and function socially. Assessment of disease activity at regular follow-up visits is done primarily on a clinical basis. Emphasis should be placed on the nature and severity of symptoms and not endoscopic or biopsy findings. Patients should not be subjected to repeated radiologic or endoscopic procedures just "to see what is going on."

The only drug that has been shown to reduce the frequency of relapses is sulfasalazine. There is no general agreement concerning how long or at what dose patients should continue taking the drug after remission of symptoms has occurred. Again this must be decided on an individual basis, depending on the severity and frequency of relapses. For patients planning to have children, the issue of sulfasalazine induced reversible oligospermia must be considered. In general, we use sulfasalazine in a full dosage (1 g four times daily) for at least 3 months after remission of symptoms has occurred and then taper to 500 mg four times daily, which is maintained indefinitely.

Dysplasia and Cancer Surveillance

Patients with ulcerative colitis are at increased risk of developing colonic carcinoma. The risk is greatest in patients with pancolitis and a disease duration of 10 years or more. The diagnosis of established colonic cancer in patients with ulcerative colitis may be difficult or delayed because the lesion is often clinically silent or because symptoms are obscured by the underlying disease. Colitis associated cancer lesions may be multifocal, small, flat, and difficult to detect endoscopically or radiologically. Annual colonoscopic surveillance for precursor dysplastic lesions therefore is recommended after 7 to 10 years for patients with pancolitis and after 15 to 20 years for patients with left sided colitis.

The term dysplasia is used to describe epithelial cell changes that are unequivocally neoplastic and therefore may precede invasive carcinoma. The diagnosis and classification of colonic dysplasia in ulcerative colitis have recently been comprehensively reviewed by an international panel of pathologists. Interpretation of biopsy findings may be difficult in the presence of active inflammation. Therefore, multiple biopsy specimens must be taken from the entire colon and should be examined by an interested and experienced pathologist. Patients with biopsy findings that are indefinite should be followed closely with early repeat biopsy. Low grade dysplasia requires confirmation by repeat biopsy. If dysplasia is unequivocally confirmed, colectomy should be considered. If surgery is considered to be a relative contraindication for medical or psychologic reasons, follow-up biopsies should be performed every 3 months. If high grade dysplasia is found, colectomy must be strongly advised.

The Role of Surgery in Ulcerative Colitis

Surgery for ulcerative colitis, unlike the situation in Crohn's disease, eliminates the disease and the risk of recurrence. Emergency indications for surgery include massive hemorrhage, perforation, and established toxic megacolon. We believe that patients with fulminant colitis that progresses or fails to improve despite 48 hours of aggressive medical management is also an indication for emergency colectomy. Elective indications for colectomy include the development of colonic dysplasia and failure of medical therapy to control symptoms. Three types of colectomy are available:
1. First is the standard (Brooke) ileostomy.
2. Second is the continent ileostomy or Kock pouch, which consists of an ileal reservoir rendered continent with a nipple valve. No external appliance is required, but the pouch must be emptied by regular catheterization several times daily. Complications include inflammation of the pouch ("pouchitis") and obstruction or malfunction of the nipple valve.
3. Finally there is the endorectal ileal pouch–anal anastomosis. In this procedure the colon is removed, leaving the rectum, from which the mucosal lining is stripped, and a reservoir is fashioned from the ileum, which is drawn through the sleeve of muscle of the rectal stump and anastomosed to the anal canal. This procedure is cosmetically acceptable to patients and mimics the normal anatomy and defecation process. However, experience with this procedure is limited, and complications have been relatively common, including leakage from the anastomosis, "pouchitis," and partial incontinence.

In emergency situations the conventional ileostomy is the procedure of choice. In the elective situation the timing and type of surgical procedure should be individualized. Careful consideration should be given to the skill and experience of the local surgical team and also to the patient's emotional stability and potential ability to adjust psychosocially to stoma care. The patient should be counseled well in advance and the complications of each procedure should be outlined; postoperative care and stoma care are explained by an enterostomal therapist. It is important that the patient understand that

the continent procedures may fail and require repeat surgery; complications may necessitate complete surgical revision, possibly requiring a standard ileostomy.

MANAGEMENT OF CROHN'S DISEASE

Since ulcerative colitis and Crohn's disease have several features in common, the management of Crohn's disease is similar to that of ulcerative colitis in many respects. This is particularly true when clinically active disease is limited to the colon. However, certain features of the inflammatory process in Crohn's disease raise additional and often difficult management issues:

Distinction Between Disease Activity and Septic Complications

The transmural inflammatory process of Crohn's disease is frequently complicated by the occurrence of intra-abdominal and perineal sepsis. Since steroids and immunosuppressive therapy may have detrimental effects in the presence of sepsis, the distinction between disease activity and septic complications is a problem that requires constant vigilance.

Pain Management

Transmural inflammation and cicatrization commonly lead to severe cramping abdominal pain in patients with Crohn's disease. Iatrogenic analgesic drug addiction unfortunately has become a common problem. This complicates treatment and is a heavy burden for these already handicapped patients to bear. It is important to note that the treatment of pain in Crohn's is control of the inflammatory process or surgical removal of fibrosing strictures. Patients should never be given opiates on a long term basis.

Intestinal Obstruction—Adhesion, Scar, or Inflammation?

Unlike ulcerative colitis, episodes of intestinal obstruction are a frequent component of the life history of a patient with Crohn's disease. The obstruction is usually incomplete, but deciding whether it is due to the inflammatory process and therefore potentially amenable to anti-inflammatory therapy or due to fibrosis or adhesions from previous surgery poses a difficult clinical problem often resolved by a trial of medical therapy. This includes intravenous fluid and electrolyte replacement, nasogastric suction, steroids, and broad spectrum anti-biotics.

Drug Therapy—Limited Efficacy

Drug therapy for the inflammatory process appears to be less effective in Crohn's disease than in ulcerative colitis. One of the major difficulties in judging the efficacy of any drug in Crohn's disease is the lack of useful parameters for assessing disease activity. Sulfa-salazine is the drug most commonly employed initially for the colonic manifestations of the disease. The role of sulfasalazine in Crohn's disease limited to the small intestine is unproven. Theoretically the drug should not have any efficacy in the small intestine, but since patients with Crohn's disease frequently have an increase in the small bowel bacterial count, sufficient amounts of the active metabolite, 5-ASA, may be released.

Systemic steroid therapy is used on a short term basis for acute flares of disease activity provided there is no evidence of intercurrent abdominal sepsis. The use of immunosuppressive drugs such as azathioprine and its active metabolite, 6-mercaptopurine, in inflammatory bowel disease is a controversial issue. However, recent studies indicate that these drugs are effective in many patients with disease that is unresponsive to steroids. Fistulas have been surprisingly responsive to these drugs, although recurrences are frequent after the completion of therapy. Immunosuppressive drugs also should be considered when a steroid sparing effect is desirable. However, it should be remembered that the clinical response to these drugs is delayed—on the average, up to 3 months. During this induction period steroid therapy therefore must be continued.

Nutrition

As with ulcerative colitis, specific dietary recommendations have little role as primary therapy. The general recommendations outlined earlier are discussed with all patients, but the emphasis is on the prevention and treatment of specific and global nutrient deficits, which are more commonly encountered in patients with extensive Crohn's disease than in ulcerative colitis. Nutritional deficits may arise because of anorexia, malab-sorption, short bowel syndrome, or protein loss from the bowel. In addition, there are often increased requirements because of increased catabolism associated with sepsis, fever, and fistulas. Home parenteral nutrition programs have been a major advance in the management of the short bowel syndrome in the patients who have undergone extensive bowel resection. For hospitalized patients with extensive and severely active disease, bowel rest with parenteral nutrition may help reduce disease

activity and occasionally even leads to closure of fistu-las. This should be regarded as an adjunct to anti-inflammatory medication, not simply as a primary treatment.

Surgery Is Never Curative

Crohn's disease has a propensity to occur and recur in any segment of the gastrointestinal tract and therefore, unlike the situation in ulcerative colitis, surgery is never curative. With long term postoperative follow-up the incidence of recurrence approaches 100 percent. Unfortunately, although surgery is deferred for as long as possible, up to 50 percent of the patients at some stage of the illness require one or more operative procedures. The indications for surgery in Crohn's disease are mainly the complications of the disease. Thus, absolute indications include life threatening situations such as free perforation, massive hemorrhage, and carcinoma. In addition, suspected appendicitis is a surgical problem and must be treated as it is in patients without Crohn's disease. Less urgent complications such as intestinal obstruction (if not fixed owing to scarring) and fistulas may be treated with a trial of medical therapy first. "Intractable disease," although usually listed as a surgical indication, is difficult to define and probably implies a complication, such as a fixed stricture. Surgery should be directed to the lesion responsible for the symptoms, and only a limited intestinal resection should be performed with preservation of as much macroscopically normal bowel as possible. Thus, it is not necessary to excise all diseased bowel—only the segment involved by complications. An end to end anastomosis should be performed. Wide margins at the time of resection do not reduce the incidence of recurrence, and disease at the margin of resection does not confer an adverse prognosis or higher recurrence incidence. Intestinal by-pass procedures are avoided because of persistent inflammation and the risk of bacterial overgrowth, malabsorption, and intestinal cancer. The Kock continent ileostomy is contraindicated in Crohn's disease.

Fistula Formation and Perianal Disease

Fistula formation is an important complication of Crohn's disease, which requires special consideration. In addition, perianal lesions (including fistulas, fissures, and abscesses) are a particularly distressing feature of Crohn's disease for many patients. They occur at some stage in the course of Crohn's disease in up to 50 percent of the patients and may precede other manifestations. In contrast, in ulcerative colitis fistulas are rare and perianal problems are uncommon—usually nonspecific, superficial, and secondary to diarrhea.

The management of fistulas in Crohn's disease includes aggressive treatment of the underlying inflammatory process and control of nutritional and septic complications. There is some evidence that 6-mercaptopurine is useful in promoting closure of fistulas and our clinical experience concurs with this. Unfortunately fistulas frequently recur after therapy with the drug is halted. Total parenteral nutrition with bowel rest in some cases may lead to fistula closure and is often a necessary adjunct to surgery. For enteroperineal fistulas, metronidazole reportedly has been beneficial. Although we have not been impressed in our own experience using this drug, we believe that a trial of therapy is reasonable in most patients. However, when perineal fistulas persist despite medical therapy and are a source of pain and discomfort, surgery is indicated. Surgical intervention for a perineal fistula usually implies more than simple fistulectomy. To be maximally effective, it should involve resection of the involved bowel from which the fistula track arises. A full assessment of the underlying bowel disease and the extent of fistula tracks is therefore required. Fistula formation between the bowel and the bladder poses special problems because of their resistance to anti-inflammatory and immunosuppressant therapy and the risk of recurrent urinary tract infection and chronic renal disease. Surgery is the treatment of choice.

SPECIAL THERAPEUTIC CONSIDERATIONS IN INFLAMMATORY BOWEL DISEASE

Extragastrointestinal Disorders

The management of the extraintestinal immunologic disorders associated with ulcerative colitis and Crohn's disease is reviewed elsewhere in this volume and is beyond the scope of this article. However, it is important that both physician and patient be aware of the relationship between intestinal disease activity and the activity of any given associated disease. In general uveitis, erythema nodosum, and peripheral arthritis respond to treatment of the bowel disease. In contrast, the clinical activity of ankylosing spondylitis tends to be independent of the bowel disease and does not improve after colectomy in patients with ulcerative colitis. The responsiveness of pyoderma gangrenosum to treatment of the bowel disease is variable. The clinical course of sclerosing cholangitis is difficult to assess but in most instances appears to be independent of the intestinal disease.

Pregnancy

Since inflammatory bowel disease is so frequently a disease of young adults in the reproductive phase of life, the issue of pregnancy is a relatively common one and should be discussed with patients so that misconceptions and unnecessary fears may be dispelled. Although the literature is somewhat contradictory, we believe that the following generalizations may be made.

Inflammatory bowel disease does not adversely affect fertility. An exception, which should seldom be seen today, is the patient with extreme weight loss and malnutrition. Male patients should be informed that sulfasalazine may cause a reversible inhibition of spermatogenesis. We do not discourage patients from becoming pregnant. We, however, do advise them to postpone pregnancy until remission of inflammatory bowel disease is achieved. Unless the life of the mother is threatened (a situation almost never encountered), pregnancy with inflammatory bowel disease is not an indication for therapeutic abortion. The weight of evidence suggests that for the majority of patients, pregnancy does not adversely affect the course of either Crohn's disease or ulcerative colitis. Likewise most studies indicate that the outcome of pregnancy should not be adversely affected by inflammatory bowel disease if well managed.

The management of inflammatory bowel disease in pregnancy is similar to that in the nonpregnant individual. However, two patients are involved—the mother and the unborn child—and follow-up must be frequent with close attention to detail. Investigative endoscopic studies should be performed during pregnancy for diagnostic purposes only but never for assessing the clinical course. Experience with steroids and sulfasalazine in pregnancy is extensive, and if used judiciously, these drugs do not appear to adversely affect the fetus. Metronidazole and nonsteroid immunosuppressants should not be used in pregnant patients, and such therapy should be discontinued in patients who wish to become pregnant. Physicians using such drugs clearly need to know their patients well, and a discussion of family planning is an important part of the long term management of inflammatory bowel disease.

Childhood and Adolescence

The clinical manifestations of inflammatory bowel disease in childhood and adolescence are similar to those seen in the adult patient. One major additional management problem, however, is growth retardation. This is significantly more common in Crohn's disease and may occur in patients with apparently quiescent disease. Growth failure occasionally may be the presenting feature of inflammatory bowel disease. Malnutrition appears to be the chief cause of growth failure. Corticosteroids adversely affect growth when used in high dosages over prolonged periods, but if used on a short term basis to suppress disease activity, they actually may promote growth. Surgical removal of inflamed intestine in pre-pubertal patients is occasionally associated with post-operative catch-up growth, but the usefulness of this approach unfortunately is limited by the high incidence of recurrence. Nutritional supplementation must be vigorously pursued with frequent counseling and clinical assessment. Success often depends on the motivation of the young patient and his family. A well balanced nutritious diet is encouraged at each outpatient visit; this may require the addition of a commercially prepared liquid formula. Night-time nasogastric infusions and even home parenteral nutrition may be required in patients who are not gaining weight or growing satisfactorily.

SUGGESTED READING

Holdsworth CD. Sulfasalazine desensitization. Br Med J 1981; 282:110.
Korelitz BI, Present DH. Favorable effect of 6-mercaptopurine on fistulae in Crohn's disease. Dig Dis Sci 1985; 30:58–64.
Meyers S, Sacher DB, Goldberg JD, Janowitz HD. Corticotropin versus hydrocortisone in the intravenous treatment of ulcerative colitis. A prospective, randomized, double blind clinical trial. Gastroenterology 1983; 85:351–357.
Purdy BH, Philips DM, Summers RW. Desensitization to sulfasalazine skin rash. Ann Intern Med 1984; 100:512–514.
Ridell RH, Goldman H, Ransohoff DF, Appelman HD, Fenoglio CM, Haggitt RC, Ahren C, Correa P, Hamilton SR, Morson BC, Sommers SC, Yardley JH. Dysplasia in inflammatory bowel disease: standardized classification with provisional clinical application. Hum Pathol 1983; 14:931–968.
Taffet SL, Das KM. Desensitization of patients with inflammatory bowel disease to sulfasalazine. Am J Med 1982; 73:520–524.

CHRONIC ACTIVE HEPATITIS

H. FRANKLIN HERLONG, M.D.

Autoimmune chronic active hepatitis is a form of chronic liver disease in which alterations in host immunity result in progressive hepatocellular necrosis. Several terms have been used to describe this disorder, including "idiopathic" and "lupoid" hepatitis. This subset of chronic hepatitis occurs in the absence of recognizable causes of liver disease, including viruses, drugs, or metabolic disorders. There is a striking predominance in women, both adolescent and menopausal. Typically the onset is insidious, but occasionally the disease develops abruptly with clinical features similar to those of viral hepatitis. Chronic active hepatitis is associated with a high incidence of autoantibodies and other autoimmune diseases. Eighty percent of the patients have an antinuclear antibody, smooth muscle antibody, or LE cells. Occasionally other autoimmune phenomena, such as fibrosing alveolitis or hemolytic anemia, may dominate the clinical picture. Elevations in the serum aminotransferase and globulin levels are characteristic biochemical features. The gamma globulin elevation is characterized by a polyclonal increase in the IgG class.

A liver biopsy is essential in the management of patients with chronic active hepatitis. Accurate interpretation of histologic changes in the liver by an experienced pathologist is the single most important factor in the treatment of these patients. The decision to institute immunosuppressive therapy is based on clinical, biochemical, and histologic data. Patients with mild non-progressive liver disease should not be exposed to the risk of prolonged immunosuppressive therapy. However, prompt institution of therapy in patients with severe disease who are symptomatic and have marked elevation of the aminotransferase level with extensive inflammation on liver biopsy significantly reduces morbidity and mortality.

The indications for immunosuppressive therapy in patients with idiopathic chronic active hepatitis are summarized in Table 1. Any one of these criteria justifies initiating therapy.

TREATMENT OPTIONS FOR IDIOPATHIC CHRONIC ACTIVE HEPATITIS

Two treatment regimens have been used to treat idiopathic chronic active hepatitis. Each has similar efficacy (Table 2).

1. Therapy with prednisone alone is started at a daily dosage of 60 mg and tapered to a maintenance dosage of 20 mg over 1 month. There is no advantage

TABLE 1   Indications for Treatment of Idiopathic Chronic Active Hepatitis

Alanine aminotransferase >10× normal

Alanine aminotransferase >5× normal and gamma globulin >2× normal

Bridging or multilobular necrosis on liver biopsy

Progressive hepatocellular failure (ascites, encephalopathy, or coagulopathy)

TABLE 2 Treatment Regimens for Idiopathic Chronic Active Hepatitis

Combination therapy*		Prednisone Only
Prednisone 30 mg qd + azathioprine 50 mg qd (week 1)		60 mg qd × 1 week
Prednisone 20 mg qd + azathioprine 50 mg qd (week 2)	OR	40 mg qd × 1 week
Prednisone 15 mg qd + azathioprine 50 mg qd (week 3)		30 mg qd × 2 weeks
Prednisone 10 mg qd + azathioprine 50 mg qd (maintenance)		20 mg qd (maintenance)
Special indications		
Postmenopausal women		Cytopenia
Osteoporosis		Pregnancy
Diabetes		
Hypertension		
Steroid side effects		

* Preferred treatment.

of prednisolone over prednisone, since hepatic conversion of prednisone to prednisolone is not impaired in chronic active hepatitis.

2. Combination therapy with prednisone and azathioprine. Several clinical trials have confirmed the efficacy of the concurrent use of azathioprine with prednisone in the management of chronic active hepatitis. This regimen reduces the likelihood of serious corticosteroid induced side effects. As with single agent therapy, the dosage of prednisone is tapered over a 1 month period to a maintenance dosage.

The choice of the regimen to use is based primarily on the potential side effects. For patients with severe chronic active hepatitis, who will likely need prolonged therapy, a lower dosage of prednisone in combination with azathioprine is preferred.

Similarly patients with disorders that predispose to steroid induced complications (diabetes, hypertension, or postmenopausal osteoporosis) should receive combination therapy. Prednisone alone is recommended only for those few patients who have significant cytopenia or previous sensitivity to azathioprine.

In general, alternate day prednisone therapy should not be used in this disease. The potential advantage of a reduction in steroid side effects has not proven to be the case here. In addition, alternate day steroid therapy is less effective in inducing histologic evidence of remission.

TREATMENT OUTCOMES

The objectives of therapy in idiopathic chronic active hepatitis are to control symptoms, decrease the likelihood of developing cirrhosis, and increase survival. Relief of symptoms is usually the first response. In most patients fatigue, malaise, and arthralgias resolve within 3 months after initiating therapy. Relief of symptoms alone, however, should not imply resolution of disease.

The conventional way to assess the response to treatment is by measurement of the serum aminotrans-

ferase level. The aspartate aminotransferase (AST, SGOT) and alanine aminotransferase (ALT, SGPT) levels should be measured monthly for the first 6 months. After 3 months of treatment the serum aminotransferase levels return to normal or are less than twice the upper limit of normal in most patients. Unfortunately histologic evidence of resolution does not always parallel improvement indicated in biochemical test results. For this reason it may be useful to repeat the liver biopsy after 6 months of therapy to ensure that there has been a histologic response. Therapy should be continued until remission of the disease occurs.

Arbitrary criteria used to define a remission include an absence of symptoms, normalization or reduction in the alanine aminotransferase concentration to less than twice normal, and histologic evidence of improvement (Table 3). Most patients should receive at least 6 months of therapy, although some may require 2 years of therapy to obtain a remission. A sustained remission justifies the gradual withdrawal of steroid therapy. The prednisone dosage is tapered over a 6 week period according to a

TABLE 3 Treatment End Points

Remission	Absence of symptoms
	Serum aminotransferase <2× normal
	Gamma globulin and bilirubin normal
	Liver biopsy: normal or portal inflammation only with or without inactive cirrhosis
Relapse	Return of symptoms
	Elevation of aminotransferase level to >3× normal
	Liver biopsy: return of periportal necrosis
Treatment failure	Elevation of aminotransferase or bilirubin level by >67% or development of ascites or hepatic encephalopathy during treatment
Nonresponse	Lack of remission or treatment failure

TABLE 4   Schedule for Discontinuation of Treatment in Idiopathic Chronic Active Hepatitis

	Combination	Prednisone Only
Prednisone	7.5 qd × 2 weeks	15 mg qd × 1 week
	5 mg qd × 2 weeks	10 mg qd × 1 week
	2.5 mg qd × 2 weeks	5 mg qd × 2 weeks
	Then 0	2.5 mg qd × 2 weeks
		Then 0
Azathioprine	50 mg qd × 3 weeks	
	25 mg qd × 3 weeks	
	Then 0	

TABLE 5   Management of Treatment Failure

Medication	Daily Dosages	
	Drug Combination	Prednisone Only
Prednisone	30 mg	60 mg
Azathioprine*	150 mg	None
If alanine aminotransferase level decreases by 33 percent or becomes normal, taper prednisone dosage by 10 mg/month and azathioprine by 50 mg/month		
Maintenance therapy for at least 6 months		
Prednisone	10 mg/day	20 mg/day
Azathioprine	50 mg/day	

* Requires determination of leukocyte and platelet counts each week of treatment.

schedule in Table 4. After discontinuing treatment, the patient should be carefully monitored for at least 12 months. At monthly intervals for the first 6 months symptoms are recorded and aminotransferase levels are determined with careful documentation of signs of chronic liver disease or portal hypertension.

Relapse after the discontinuation of therapy is defined by an increase in the serum aminotransferase level with or without symptoms. This occurs in about 50 percent of the patients during the first year after therapy is stopped. A relapse should prompt reinstitution of the original therapeutic regimen that initially induced a remission.

Unfortunately some patients with severe chronic active hepatitis deteriorate during therapy. These patients have persistent fatigue, malaise, progressive elevations of the aminotransferase levels, and worsening as evidenced by histologic activity. Some go on to develop ascites, encephalopathy, or spontaneous bleeding. It is important to recognize these treatment failures, since higher than conventional dosages of immunosuppressive therapy can reverse the signs of progressive liver failure. Thirty milligrams of prednisone and 150 mg of azathioprine are given daily. If single agent prednisone must be used, 60 mg is administered daily. Aminotransferase levels are determined biweekly. Once the aminotransferase level has decreased by one third, dosages can be tapered to maintenance levels. If combination therapy is used, the dosage of prednisone is tapered by 10 mg a month down to a maintenance level of 10 mg. The dosage of azathioprine is tapered by 50 mg each month to a maintenance level of 50 mg. If prednisone alone is used, the dosage is tapered by 10 mg a month to a maintenance dosage of 20 mg (Table 5).

Some patients with autoimmune chronic active hepatitis fail to improve and yet do not deteriorate despite protracted periods of immunosuppressive therapy (nonresponse). Continuation of immunosuppressive therapy beyond 2 years is not justified in such patients, since the likelihood of a favorable response is remote and the prospect for steroid induced side effects is significant. After treatment has been discontinued, apparent nonre-

sponders should continue to be monitored closely. Reinstitution of treatment is justified should the disease worsen after therapy has been discontinued.

COMPLICATIONS OF THERAPY

The risk of developing serious side effects from immunosuppressive therapy depends on the dosage of medication and the duration of therapy. Since most patients with severe chronic active hepatitis may be treated for up to 2 years, many develop side effects. Cushingoid features such as acne, hirsutism, and obesity develop in most patients regardless of the regimen used. However, they are less severe in patients who are treated with combination therapy. Serious complications such as aseptic necrosis, vertebral collapse, diabetes, hypertension, and cataract formation occur in fewer than 10 percent of the patients with the two drug regimen. Side effects can be minimized by continuing the appropriate treatment regimens for the minimal time necessary to establish a remission.

Special attention should be directed toward reducing the likelihood of progressive osteoporosis, particularly in postmenopausal women. Supplementation with oral doses of calcium and vitamin D may help to reduce this risk. Since estrogen supplementation may adversely affect the course of the underlying liver disease, adjuvant therapy with these compounds is not recommended. Patients receiving azathioprine must be monitored for evidence of bone marrow suppression or gastrointestinal upset. In treatment regimens including azathioprine, a complete blood count determination should be performed every week for the first 3 months and at least every month thereafter. Uncommonly azathioprine causes arthralgias, skin rash, or pancreatitis. Rarely a hepatotoxic reaction to azathioprine results in elevation of the alkaline phosphatase level, which resolves on discontinuing the medication.

SUGGESTED READING

Czaja AJ, et al. Clinical features and prognosis of severe chronic active liver disease (CALD) after corticosteroid-induced remission. Gastroenterology 1980; 78:518–523.

Gurwin LE, et al. Immunologic diagnosis of chronic active "autoimmune" hepatitis. Hepatology 1985; 5:397–402.

McCullough AJ, Czaja AJ. Relapse following treatment withdrawal in autoimmune chronic active hepatitis. Hepatology 1984; 4:747–748.

Mistilis SP, et al. Natural history of active chronic hepatitis. I. Clinical features, course, diagnostic criteria, morbidity, mortality, and survival. Aust Ann Med 1968; 17:214–223.

Murray-Lyon IM, et al. Controlled trial of prednisone and azathioprine in active chronic hepatitis. Lancet 1973; 2:735–736.

PRIMARY BILIARY CIRRHOSIS

WILLIS C. MADDREY, M.D.

Primary biliary cirrhosis is a chronic, usually progressive liver disease of unknown etiology characterized histologically by destruction and subsequent disappearance of small intralobular hepatic ducts. Extrahepatic bile ducts are not affected. Primary biliary cirrhosis is predominantly a disease of women (90 percent) and most often is diagnosed between the ages of 20 and 60 years. The disorder is rarely found in patients younger than 20 years of age. There is no evidence that primary biliary cirrhosis occurring in men differs from that found in women. Most patients at the time of diagnosis have evidence of chronic cholangitis with variable amounts of portal fibrosis. Frank cirrhosis is a late manifestation.

The etiology of primary biliary cirrhosis is unknown. A number of characteristics of the disorder suggest that the injury is mediated by immunologic mechanisms. These features include the presence of lymphoid aggregates and granulomas in the liver, the presence of antimitochondrial and other autoantibodies, increased serum IgM levels, the frequent finding of skin test anergy, and the association with many other disorders thought to be caused by immunologic mechanisms.

CLINICAL AND LABORATORY FEATURES

The major clinical manifestations of primary biliary cirrhosis relate to cholestasis with a gradual, often insidious onset of pruritus, fatigue, and darkening of the skin followed by the appearance of jaundice with dark urine and pale stools. Once symptoms and signs of liver disease develop, the course is usually one of progressive deterioration and death over 1 to 12 years. Earlier series of cases of primary biliary cirrhosis emphasized the late, progressive, and often rapidly fatal form of the disorder characterized by deep jaundice, severe pruritus, hyper-

lipidemia with xanthomas and xanthomatous neuropathy, bone pain and fractures, and the development of hepatocellular failure, ascites, portal hypertension, and hepatic encephalopathy. Increased awareness of primary biliary cirrhosis and the widespread availability of percutaneous liver biopsy and determination of antimitochondrial antibodies have allowed the diagnosis of primary biliary cirrhosis to be established in many asymptomatic patients who are evaluated following detection of an elevated serum alkaline phosphatase level. Many of these asymptomatic patients have a benign nonprogressive illness with an excellent prognosis and no evidence of a decrease in life expectancy.

Almost all patients with primary biliary cirrhosis have an elevation in the serum alkaline phosphatase level reflecting obstruction of bile flow. 5-Nucleotidase and gamma glutamyl transpeptidase levels are increased to a similar extent with the serum alkaline phosphatase level. The serum cholesterol level is elevated in the majority of patients with symptomatic disease. In patients with xanthomas and xanthomatous neuropathy, cholesterol levels may exceed 1000 mg per dl. Serum aminotransferase levels are usually only minimally increased. The serum bilirubin level is normal or only slightly elevated in asymptomatic patients and early in the course in patients who develop progressive disease. A progressive rise in the serum bilirubin level is an ominous prognostic sign.

The detection of antimitochondrial antibodies and serum IgM is of considerable value in the diagnosis of primary biliary cirrhosis. The antimitochondrial antibody test is positive in more than 90 percent of the patients with the disorder. Antimitochondrial antibody is rarely found (in less than 2 percent) in patients with mechanical obstruction of the biliary tract and therefore is most useful in differentiating mechanical obstruction of the bile duct from primary biliary cirrhosis. Antimitochondrial antibody is found in 5 to 15 percent of the patients with idiopathic chronic active hepatitis, and in some patients a clear distinction between primary biliary cirrhosis and chronic active hepatitis is not possible. The serum IgM level is increased in approximately 75 percent of the patients.

Many disorders with features suggesting an immunologically mediated mechanism of damage are found in association with primary biliary cirrhosis. These include Sjögren's syndrome, polymyositis, polyarthritis, renal tubular acidosis, Hashimoto's thyroiditis, and interstitial pneumonitis. Non-Hodgkin lymphomas and breast cancer are found more frequently in patients with primary biliary cirrhosis. Of particular note are patients with primary biliary cirrhosis and the CREST syndrome (calcinosis, Raynaud's phenomenon, esophageal motility disorders, sclerodactyly, and telangiectasia). Occasionally clinical and laboratory manifestations suggest primary biliary cirrhosis, sarcoidosis, or both disorders.

The principal early lesion of primary biliary cirrhosis is cholangitis involving small interlobular bile ducts. The bile duct lesions are often focal and may involve only a segment of the duct wall. Granulomas are often found, especially around the bile ducts. The predominant inflammatory cells are lymphocytes and plasma cells, which accumulate in the portal triads. Plasma cells in the portal triads in patients with primary biliary cirrhosis have been shown to produce IgM. The histologic features of lesions of primary biliary cirrhosis are similar to those found in graft versus host reactions.

Liver biopsy findings in patients with primary biliary cirrhosis have led to a histologic classification of the disorder into four broad stages. The classification is arbitrary and features of several stages may coexist. There is often poor correlation between clinical and histologic manifestations of the disease:

Stage I: Florid duct lesions with damage to the small interlobular bile ducts, which are often surrounded by a dense infiltrate of lymphocytes and plasma cells. Granulomas are found near the damaged ducts in 40 percent of the patients.

Stage II: Ductular proliferation with continued inflammation, early fibrosis, and occasional deposits of Mallory's hyaline. Periportal inflammation and destruction may be prominent.

Stage III: Scarring with fibrosis bridging between portal areas.

Stage IV: Cirrhosis with regenerative nodules is an end stage finding. Often at this phase of the illness the more characteristic earlier features have disappeared.

DIAGNOSIS OF PRIMARY BILIARY CIRRHOSIS

Primary biliary cirrhosis should be suspected in a middle aged woman with fatigue, pruritus, and an elevated serum alkaline phosphatase level. The diagnosis is established by a positive antimitochondrial antibody test and compatible liver biopsy findings. If there is doubt regarding possible obstruction in the extrahepatic bile ducts, endoscopic retrograde cholangiography is indicated. The major alternative diagnoses to be considered include chronic drug induced cholestasis (especially that induced by phenothiazines), sclerosing cholangitis, chronic active hepatitis, and bile duct carcinoma.

PROGNOSIS OF PRIMARY BILIARY CIRRHOSIS

The course of primary biliary cirrhosis is variable, and the disorder often pursues a progressive downhill course in symptomatic patients. However, many patients with clinically apparent symptomatic disease survive for more than a decade. In one series the presence of granulomas on liver biopsy was reported to be a good prognostic sign. However, in a large multicenter study granulomas were found at all stages of primary biliary cirrhosis and were not indicative of early disease. An increasing serum bilirubin level is a sign of poor prognosis. The presence of associated autoimmune disorders, including thyroiditis, the CREST syndrome, and Raynaud's phenomenon, correlates with decreased survival.

MANAGEMENT OF COMPLICATIONS OF PRIMARY BILIARY CIRRHOSIS

The management of primary biliary cirrhosis must emphasize general support of the patient and the institution of measures designed to minimize the effects of complications, especially those that result from cholestasis. There is as yet no satisfactory treatment for the underlying disease.

Pruritus is often a major disabling feature of primary biliary cirrhosis. The use of the nonabsorbed quaternary ammonium exchange resin cholestyramine (4 to 24 g per day) may be effective in the management of pruritus, especially in patients who have only slight elevations of the serum bilirubin level. It is assumed that one or more pruritogens are bound and excreted in the feces. The precise pruritogen bound by cholestyramine has not been established. Cholestyramine stimulates the hepatic synthesis of bile acids by decreasing the enterohepatic circulation of bile salts and may thereby promote choleresis. There is probably an advantage in giving a large part of the daily dosage of cholestyramine early in the morning when presumably there is the greatest concentration of pruritogen in the bowel following emptying of the gallbladder after an overnight accumulation of bile. Cholestyramine is not effective when the bilirubin level is markedly elevated (greater than 5 to 10 mg per dl), indicating a reduction in bile flow. Cholestyramine is taken with meals and may be made more palatable by mixing with applesauce or undiluted grape juice. No other orally administered drugs should be given for 2 hours before or after cholestyramine is taken in order to avoid binding of the drug by the resin. Colestipol is an alternative nonabsorbed anion exchange resin that may be used (approximately 15 g per day) instead of cholestyramine and is found to be more palatable by some patients.

Occasionally addition of an antihistaminic compound is helpful. Phenobarbital may be a useful adjunctive therapy for pruritus through its choleretic effects, but the dosage initially should be low (16 to 32 mg) and gradually increased to avoid excessive sedation or promotion of encephalopathy. Phototherapy is an experimental mode of therapy for pruritus that has proven of limited (if any) value. In intractable pruritus, plasmapheresis may be useful with 500 to 2000 ml of plasma removed in one treatment and replaced by saline and albumin or fresh frozen plasma. However, plasmapheresis is expensive, has to be repeated frequently, and has not been shown to have any effect on the progression of the underlying disorder.

Administration of the fat soluble vitamins A, D, and K is often required in patients with primary biliary cirrhosis, with deficiencies of these vitamins resulting from steatorrhea and malabsorption. Vitamin A deficiency with decreased serum levels and impaired dark adaptation is frequent. Overt symptoms of night blindness are unusual. Oral doses of vitamin A (25,000 to 50,000 units per day) may be required to correct the deficit. In some patients with vitamin A deficiency there is the coexistence of zinc deficiency, which also must be corrected in order to reverse abnormal dark adaptation. Serum vitamin A levels should be monitored to prevent overdosage.

Vitamin D deficiency is regularly found in patients with primary biliary cirrhosis. Serum 25-hydroxy vitamin D levels are usually decreased. Hepatic osteodystrophy is a major problem in patients with primary biliary cirrhosis and there is no satisfactory therapy. Bone fractures are frequent, especially in more advanced disease. The etiology of hepatic osteodystrophy remains unknown.

The major bone disease in primary biliary cirrhosis is osteoporosis with a loss of bone matrix. It is important for the patient to avoid prolonged immobilization. The patient should be encouraged to be exposed to sunlight. There are no convincing studies that administration of vitamin D to these patients leads to reversal of the bone disease, but the rate of progression of osteoporosis may be slowed. 25-Hydroxycholecalciferol (50 to 100 μg orally daily) usually leads to a normal serum vitamin D level. Serum 25-hydroxycholecalciferol levels should be monitored. In addition, we administer approximately 1 g of calcium orally each day. Fluoride supplementation as a treatment for the hepatic osteodystrophy is being evaluated.

Vitamin K deficiency as indicated by a prolonged prothrombin time may respond to daily oral doses of vitamin K (5 to 10 mg per day), or in patients with advanced cholestasis the parenteral administration of vitamin K may be required. It is not established whether vitamin E replacement is necessary in patients with primary biliary cirrhosis even though some individuals have low serum vitamin E levels. The presence of peripheral neuropathy related to vitamin E deficiency has been suggested but not fully established in adults with primary biliary cirrhosis. Folic acid (1 mg per day) and a general multivitamin may be useful to ensure that no additional deficiencies develop. Iron deficiency anemia may develop, in part related to iron malabsorption or unrecognized gastrointestinal blood loss.

In patients with severe steatorrhea and weight loss, medium chain triglyceride oil (up to 60 ml) may be administered as a high caloric, well absorbed dietary supplement. Some restriction in dietary fat may reduce steatorrhea.

The extraordinarily high serum levels of lipids in primary biliary cirrhosis may lead to xanthoma formation and xanthomatous neuropathy. Administration of clofibrate has been disastrous, with a paradoxic increase in the serum cholesterol level. Serum lipid levels may be lowered by repeated plasmapheresis with resolution of the xanthomas and xanthomatous neuropathy. Such therapy although temporarily effective is time consuming and expensive.

If a patient with primary biliary cirrhosis develops bleeding esophagogastric varices, ascites, or hepatic encephalopathy, the usual measures to manage these complications should be instituted, and if the patient is a fit candidate, hepatic transplantation should be performed.

TREATMENTS DIRECTED TOWARDS THE UNDERLYING PROCESS

There is no proven effective treatment in patients with primary biliary cirrhosis once progressive bile duct inflammation and obliteration have begun. A number of anti-inflammatory and antifibrotic drugs have been evaluated with the most promising results from the use of colchicine and azathioprine.

Corticosteroids

There is scant enthusiasm for conducting a trial of corticosteroid therapy in patients with primary biliary cirrhosis despite the well established anti-inflammatory activity of these drugs. Corticosteroids are not recommended in patients with advanced primary biliary cirrhosis because of possible (even probable) acceleration of osteoporosis and skeletal collapse. Whether corticosteroid therapy would be useful early in the course of primary biliary cirrhosis is unknown.

Azathioprine

The immunosuppressive drug azathioprine in a dosage of 50 to 100 mg a day was reported to prolong survival significantly in patients with primary biliary cirrhosis in a randomized multinational trial. Azathioprine treated patients had an improved survival with an estimated average 20 additional months of life. Effects of azathioprine on biochemical test results and histologic changes were not described. Side effects from azathioprine were few and included rash, nausea, vomiting, and occasionally marrow depression. Earlier trials involving fewer patients had not demonstrated any effect of the drug. Undoubtedly the favorable effects of azathioprine on survival in patients with primary biliary cirrhosis will lead to further evaluation.

Chlorambucil

Chlorambucil is an alkylating drug with immunosuppressive properties, which have been reported to be beneficial in several disorders with presumed autoimmune etiologies, including systemic lupus erythematosus and Wegener's granulomatosis. Chlorambucil has been evaluated in the treatment of patients with primary biliary cirrhosis in a small prospective randomized trial. Patients received chlorambucil (0.5 to 4 mg per day) or placebo and were followed for 2 to 6 years. The dosage was adjusted on the basis of blood counts. Serum bilirubin, aminotransferase, and albumin levels remained unchanged in chlorambucil treated patients but worsened in controls. The serum IgM level decreased to normal in all treated patients. There was a decrease in hepatic inflammatory infiltrates in chlorambucil treated patients, but no effects on fibrosis or the histologic stage of primary biliary cirrhosis were noted. No significant effects on mortality were noted, but the number of patients was small. Side effects of chlorambucil, including bone marrow suppression and the development of bacterial and viral infection, led to discontinuation of the drug in approximately one third of the treated patients. Therefore, although chlorambucil appears to show some therapeutic promise, the frequent and occasionally important side effects will probably limit its use.

d-Penicillamine

d-Penicillamine has been extensively evaluated as a treatment for primary biliary cirrhosis. Potentially favorable actions of d-penicillamine that led to the evaluations included a reduction of elevated hepatic copper levels, an established antifibrotic effect, and a favorable effect on reduction of circulating immune complexes. Side effects from the drug are frequent and include neutropenia, optic neuritis, and renal tubular damage.

A large randomized double blind trial of d-penicillamine therapy at the Mayo Clinic initially indicated increased survival in treated patients who entered the study with early (stage 1 or 2) histologic lesions. Furthermore, an early trend toward improved survival, which

did not achieve statistical significance, was noted in patients entering the trial with more severe disease. Significant improvement in SGOT, alkaline phosphatase, and IgM levels and in the sedimentation rate occurred in the treated group. The hepatic copper concentration decreased significantly. However, with longer follow-up the Mayo Clinic group concluded that use of the drug did not result in any improvement in survival. Moreover, no differences were found in the 10 year study in the rate of progression of primary biliary cirrhosis or in morphologic changes on sequential liver biopsy. Major side effects of d-penicillamine led to permanent discontinuation of the drug in 22 percent of those receiving it. Therefore, despite early enthusiasm for the use of d-penicillamine in the therapy of primary biliary cirrhosis, there is now scant evidence or hope that the drug should be used.

Colchicine

Colchicine has been reported to produce significant improvement in survival as well as having favorable effects on serum bilirubin, alkaline phosphatase, and aminotransferase levels in patients with primary biliary cirrhosis. In a randomized double blind prospective trial of colchicine therapy in primary biliary cirrhosis in Boston, 30 patients with early disease (stages 1 and 2) and 30 patients with advanced disease were studied. Favorable therapeutic results were obtained in patients with early and advanced disease who received 0.6 mg of colchicine twice a day. Patients receiving colchicine had improvement in serum albumin, serum bilirubin, alkaline phosphatase, and aminotransferase levels. There were no decreases in symptoms or physical findings nor were significant differences found in the histologic extent of injury in follow-up liver biopsies. Four years after entry there was a cumulative 21 percent mortality in patients receiving colchicine as compared to 47 percent in those receiving placebo. Colchicine is a safe drug, dose related diarrhea being the only frequent side effect reported.

The mechanism of action of colchicine in patients with primary biliary cirrhosis is unknown. The drug inhibits intracellular microtubular assembly, stimulates collagenase synthesis, and interferes with collagen secretion as well as having anti-inflammatory effects. The encouraging results from the use of colchicine and its excellent safety profile will undoubtedly stimulate further use and study of this drug.

Hepatic Transplantation

Patients with primary biliary cirrhosis are considered especially good candidates for hepatic transplantation. Indications include advanced symptomatic disease, a rising serum bilirubin level (especially after the level passes 10 mg per dl), bleeding from gastroesophageal varices, severe metabolic bone disease, intractable pruritus, and advanced muscle wasting. Whether liver transplantation will favorably affect the course of advanced hepatic osteodystrophy remains to be established. Apparent recurrence of primary biliary cirrhosis in the transplanted liver has been reported, but the similarities between the histologic findings in primary biliary cirrhosis and those found in graft versus host disease make assessment of recurrence especially difficult. The excellent results with liver transplantation have led to consideration and recommendation of transplantation in patients earlier in the course of the illness before major life threatening complications, including wasting and malnutrition, occur.

SUGGESTED READING

Christensen E, Neuberger J, Crowe J, Altman DG, Popper H, Portmann B, Doniach D, Ranek L, Tygstrup N, Williams R. Beneficial effect of azathioprine and prediction of prognosis in primary biliary cirrhosis. Gastroenterology 1985; 89:1084–1091.

Kaplan M. Primary biliary cirrhosis. N Engl J Med 1987; 316:521–528.

Herlong FH, Russell RM, Maddrey WC. Vitamin A and zinc therapy in primary biliary cirrhosis. Hepatology 1981; 1:348–351.

Herlong FH, Recker RR, Maddrey WC: Bone disease in primary biliary cirrhosis: histologic features and response to 25-hyroxyvitamin D. Gastroenterology 1982; 83:103–108.

Hoofnagle JH, Davis GL, Schafer DF, Peters M, Avigan MI, Pappas C, Hanson RG, Minuk GY, Dusheiko GM, Campbell G, MacSween RNM, Jones EA. Randomized trial of chlorambucil for primary biliary cirrhosis. Gastroenterology 1986; 91:1327–1334.

Kaplan MM, et al. A prospective trial of colchicine for primary biliary cirrhosis. N Engl J Med 1986; 315:1448–1454.

ACUTE RHEUMATIC FEVER

GIANNI MARONE, M.D.
MARIO CONDORELLI, M.D.

Acute rheumatic fever is an autoimmune disease whose etiologic agent is the group A beta-hemolytic streptococcus. Although the etiology of this disease is well established, its pathogenesis is largely unknown. The incidence of rheumatic fever has markedly decreased over the last 3 decades in most of the industrialized world. However, this disease continues to be a major public health problem in some areas of the world, and a recent resurgence of the disease in a region of Utah indicates that it remains a threat even in the most advanced nations. Fifteen to 20 million new cases appear each year in the "developing" or third world countries. The incidence may be even higher, since many of the cases remain undiagnosed and only appear later as chronic rheumatic heart disease. Furthermore, most patients survive the acute carditis and then develop chronic rheumatic valvular disease.

PRIMARY PREVENTION

Primary prevention of rheumatic fever consists of prompt eradication of acute streptococcal infection, which might lead to the disease. Patients with fever, a fiery red throat with exudate, and tender anterior cervical lymph nodes are more likely than others to have streptococcal pharyngitis, but even this "classic" picture may be caused by viruses. Conversely, some mild sore throats may be of streptococcal origin and may be followed by rheumatic fever or glomerulonephritis. Therefore, a throat culture should be done in all patients with acute pharyngitis, and all those with a positive culture should be treated with antibiotics.

When and whether to start treatment without a throat culture depend on how sick the patient is. Treatment may be started at once in a febrile patient with exudative pharyngitis, whereas the milder the symptoms and signs, the safer it is to delay treatment until an etiologic diagnosis is made. A few days' delay in initiating treatment is not harmful in terms of rheumatic fever prevention.

If treatment is started with oral therapy before the culture results are known, the option remains open to discontinue medication the morning after if the throat culture is negative for beta-hemolytic streptococci.

In military populations with a high frequency of severe streptococcal pharyngitis, penicillin therapy has reduced the incidence of rheumatic fever from 3.0 to 0.3 per cent. Primary prevention in civilian populations, particularly in children with sporadic or endemic streptococcal infections, is more difficult. There is the problem of differentiating viral pharyngitis in carriers of group A streptococci from those with current streptococcal infection; in addition frequent streptococcal exposure in children tends to keep streptococcal antibody titers elevated. Thus, throat cultures are helpful in avoiding the use of penicillin therapy in patients with nonstreptococcal infection.

When cultures are positive for group A streptococci in a patient with a sore throat, the appropriate treatment should be given. Penicillin is the drug of choice. Group

A streptococci are highly susceptible to penicillin, and thus high serum levels of this antibiotic are not required. Prevention of acute rheumatic fever depends upon eradication of the infecting organisms from the pharynx, an effect that requires prolonged exposure to the antibiotic. A single intramuscular injection of benzathine penicillin G (600,000 units for patients weighing less than 27 kg [60 lb] and 1,200,000 units for all others) provides the necessary therapeutic dose of penicillin and is the most effective means of primary prevention. If a combination of procaine penicillin and benzathine penicillin is used, the latter should still be given in the amounts just noted. If oral penicillin therapy is elected, penicillin G in a dosage of 250,000 units three or four times daily should be administered 30 minutes before or 1 hour after meals. This therapy must be continued for a full 10 days; however, patient compliance becomes difficult once the acute symptoms have abated.

Penicillin allergy is a cause for genuine concern. Care should be taken to obtain a good history and to keep epinephrine (adrenaline) at hand. Penicillin allergic individuals should be treated with erythromycin (250 mg four times a day or 40 mg per kg per day in younger children in divided doses for 10 days). Tetracyclines are not recommended, because streptococci resistant to them are prevalent in certain geographic regions. Sulfonamides, which are effective in the prophylaxis of acute rheumatic fever, do not eradicate streptococci from the pharynx and therefore should not be used for treatment.*

Family members of a patient with symptomatic streptococcal pharyngitis are at a high risk of being infected. Some therefore advise the culture of all family contacts with recent upper respiratory symptoms and the treatment of those with positive cultures.

Follow-up visits are necessary to ascertain whether the infection has cleared, to stimulate compliance in patients taking medication orally, and to investigate for streptococcal sequelae.

Streptococcal relapses can be clinical and bacteriologic (sore throat with a positive throat culture) or bacteriologic only (a positive throat culture without sore throat). The recommended practice is to treat both kinds of recurrence with a second course of penicillin therapy (preferably benzathine penicillin injections) or oral doses of erythromycin.

SECONDARY PREVENTION

The extreme susceptibility of rheumatic hosts to recurrent attacks of acute rheumatic fever makes it vitally important to protect such individuals from streptococcal infections (''secondary prevention''). This is

*See the discussions by Markowitz and Gordis and by Stollerman for explanations of specific issues concerning primary prevention, e.g., management of treatment failures, streptococcal carriers, family contacts, and epidemic situations.

accomplished by continuous antimicrobial prophylaxis.

As in the treatment of streptococcal pharyngitis, the most effective regimen is benzathine penicillin G, which should be administered in a single intramuscular dose of 1,200,000 units every 4 weeks. Oral regimens endorsed by the American Heart Association include: (1) sulfadiazine, 1 g once daily for those patients over 27 kg (60 lb) and 0.5 g once daily for those under 27 kg (60 lb); (2) penicillin G, 200,000 or 250,000 units twice a day; and (3) erythromycin, 250 mg twice daily for patients who are allergic to both penicillin and sulfonamides. Patients taking sulfadiazine should have a blood count after 2 weeks and also if they develop a rash in association with fever or sore throat. Therapy with the drug should be stopped if the white count falls below 4,000 and the neutrophil level falls below 35 percent.

It should be recognized that the oral regimens are clearly inferior to benzathine penicillin G in protecting against intercurrent streptococcal infections and acute rheumatic fever recurrences. The overall incidences of rheumatic fever recurrence per 100 patient-years in the Irvington House studies were as follows: benzathine penicillin G group, 0.5; oral penicillin, 5.5; oral sulfadiazine, 2.8. Reaction incidences are low with both oral medications and are rare after the first months of prophylaxis. Oral prophylaxis should be given only in patients with no or with minimal residual cardiac disease who have had a single rheumatic attack and who have a relatively low risk of exposure to streptococcal infection.

The duration of rheumatic prophylaxis has yet to be established. Some physicians suggest continuous lifelong antibiotic prophylaxis. However, the risk of rheumatic fever recurrence is known to decline with age and increasing interval since the previous attack. Patients who did not have carditis during the initial attack are less likely to develop carditis if they suffer a recurrence of acute rheumatic fever. These facts, coupled with the relative rarity of severe forms of streptococcal pharyngitis and of acute rheumatic fever in many areas, suggest that rheumatic prophylaxis might be safely discontinued in certain subgroups of patients. However, there are no guidelines for selecting such patients.

The American Heart Association states that ''in making such decisions—to suspend continuous prophylaxis—the physician must carefully weigh a number of factors, including the patient's risk of acquiring a streptococcal infection, the anticipated recurrence rate per infection, and the consequences of recurrence.'' Adults with a high risk of exposure to streptococcal infection include parents of young children, school teachers, physicians, nurses and allied medical personnel, and those in military service. High risk patients are those with a recent previous attack (3 years or less) or with multiple attacks, or those unlikely to take diligently a daily medication. Additional risk factors are young age (childhood and adolescence), exposure to young people, and crowding in the home. Exceptions to instituting or maintaining prophylaxis should be made only in patients who do not fall into the aforementioned categories.

Patients with rheumatic valvular disease must be protected from bacterial endocarditis whenever they undergo dental or surgical procedures likely to evoke bacteremia. Rheumatic heart disease predisposes to infective endocarditis. The antibiotic regimens suggested for endocarditis prophylaxis are entirely different from those required for the prophylaxis of acute rheumatic fever. The two types of prophylaxis are frequently confused by physicians and dentists. Revised recommendations for antimicrobial prophylaxis of bacterial endocarditis have been published by the American Heart Association.

GENERAL MANAGEMENT

The management of acute rheumatic fever depends upon the manifestations and severity of the attack. Patients should remain in bed until clinical and laboratory evidence of inflammation subsides. The pulse rate, particularly the sleeping pulse rate, should be carefully noted. In afebrile patients the presence of tachycardia during sleep is usually indicative of carditis. Initial laboratory studies should include a hematocrit determination, white blood cell count, C reactive protein level, erythrocyte sedimentation rate, throat cultures (one or more taken before the onset of penicillin treatment, since the numbers of group A streptococci remaining in the throat may be small), streptococcal antibody titers (e.g., ASO or anti-DNase B), a roentgenogram of the chest, and then an electrocardiogram. Echocardiograms may be useful in detecting pericardial effusion and valvular dysfunction.

It is important not to administer anti-inflammatory drugs until the disease process is clearly expressed. Aspirin or corticosteroids administered prematurely to a patient with arthralgia or early monoarticular arthritis and fever may mask the disease process and cause diagnostic confusion.

Once the diagnosis of acute rheumatic fever is established, penicillin therapy in doses sufficient to eradicate residual group A streptococci should be initiated. Although prompt treatment of streptococcal pharyngitis prevents initial attacks of acute rheumatic fever (primary prophylaxis), several studies have shown that administration of antibiotics after the onset of rheumatic fever does not influence the course of the disease. Nevertheless the current recommendation is for the administration of a course of antibiotics that can eradicate streptococci that may be present in pharyngeal and tonsillar tissue, even though throat cultures may be negative.

The recommended course of antibiotics is that used for the treatment of streptococcal pharyngitis. The preferred therapy consists of an intramuscular injection of 1,200,000 units of benzathine penicillin G. The advantage of this form of therapy is that it will set the course

for subsequent prophylaxis using the same dose at monthly intervals. An alternative regimen is to give oral doses of penicillin, 250 mg four times daily for 10 days. Patients with a history of allergy to penicillin should receive erythromycin, 40 mg per kg (maximal dosage, 1 g) per day divided into four doses for 10 days. The initial course of therapy should be followed by a regimen for prophylaxis against subsequent streptococcal infections (secondary prophylaxis).

ANTIRHEUMATIC THERAPY

It is now almost unanimously agreed that selection of an antirheumatic drug is not critical to the outcome of most attacks of rheumatic fever. Corticosteroids and salicylates are valuable anti-inflammatory drugs; neither is curative. However, both corticosteroids and salicylates control the toxic manifestations of the disease, contribute to the comfort of the patient, and combat anemia, anorexia, and other symptoms. In severe rheumatic carditis associated with heart failure, corticosteroids may reduce the burden on the heart and occasionally may tilt the balance in favor of the survival of a critically ill patient. Corticosteroids are often more potent than salicylates in suppressing acute inflammation, and some patients in whom salicylates fail to control the disease respond quickly to relatively large doses of corticosteroids. The effect of such doses on the course of chronic rheumatic carditis is disappointing, however, and their use in cases of occult carditis does not decrease residual heart disease. Prolonged use of large doses beyond the period of time required to control acute manifestations is not justified.

Patients with mild arthritis or arthralgia and no carditis may be treated with an analgesic, such as codeine, as needed. The advantage of this approach is that the diagnosis may be made more certain by the appearance of definite arthritis in some of the initially questionable cases.

The arthritis of acute rheumatic fever, unlike other collagen diseases, is very responsive to salicylate therapy. Patients with frank arthritis only should be treated initially with 75 to 80 mg per kg per day of aspirin, divided into four doses. Taking aspirin with a meal or with milk reduces gastric irritation. Large doses of sodium bicarbonate enhance renal excretion of salicylates and should be avoided. Most patients with rheumatic polyarthritis respond to this dosage in less than 72 hours. If a response is not evident, the dosage may be increased; however, it should not exceed 100 mg per kg per day nor should the serum salicylate level rise beyond 30 mg per dl. A lack of response to this dosage of salicylates should raise questions about the diagnosis of acute rheumatic fever. The therapeutic dosage is continued for 2 to 4 weeks and gradually reduced over the next 4 to 6 weeks. Determinations of the acute phase reactants (i.e., the erythrocyte sedimentation rate and C reactive protein level), twice weekly initially and then once weekly, are helpful in gauging the response to therapy. Corticosteroids are not needed nor should they be used in patients with arthritis without carditis.

Toxic manifestations are common with the use of larger dosages of salicylates, and hence the dosage may have to be reduced before the response is adequate. If control of the inflammatory state is not adequate with lower subtoxic dosages, substitution or addition of another drug should be considered. Since the absorption of salicylate varies considerably from patient to patient, determination of salicylate blood levels is useful if the patient does not appear to respond well to treatment. The serum level at which patients respond best is between 20 and 30 mg per dl.

Confinement to bed is limited to the duration of the acute arthritis. Once the arthritis subsides, ambulation should be allowed, with a gradual return to full activity at the end of salicylate therapy. Despite the form of therapy used, about 5 percent of the attacks of rheumatic fever persist with clinically overt rheumatic manifestations for more than 6 months. The duration of treatment therefore depends on the severity of the illness. For example, a mild attack may be treated for 2 to 4 weeks, tapering the dosage of the antirheumatic drug during the ensuing 4 to 6 weeks.

The management of carditis is related to the severity of cardiac involvement. Many physicians believe that corticosteroids should be used whenever a patient has acute rheumatic carditis. However, the majority reserve this form of therapy for patients with severe carditis with congestive failure. Despite the lack of definitive evidence, clinical experience suggests that the use of corticosteroids in patients with pancarditis may be lifesaving. Patients with mild carditis without significant cardiomegaly can be given salicylate therapy according to the regimen already outlined. Many physicians prefer a treatment period of 9 to 12 weeks. Should a good clinical response and a return of acute phase reactant levels toward normal be obtained, anti-inflammatory therapy may be gradually withdrawn.

In patients with severe carditis with marked cardiomegaly with or without congestive failure, and particularly in those with pancarditis as manifested by the presence of pericarditis, corticosteroids are the drugs of choice. Prednisone at a dosage of 40 to 60 mg per day for adults and children alike should be administered for 2 to 4 weeks, depending on the clinical response, followed by gradual withdrawal over 2 to 3 weeks. Corticosteroids can be administered initially in divided doses to obtain the maximal immunosuppressive effect, and after the initial clinical response, they can be administered in a single morning dose. One week prior to withdrawing corticosteroids a salicylate regimen should be started, as already described. This regimen minimizes the occurrence of rebound episodes.

Digitalis should be reserved for patients with severe carditis or congestive failure. Digoxin is preferred for children. A total digitalizing dosage of 0.02 to 0.03 mg

per kg should be given (maximal dosage 1.5 mg). Some patients with rheumatic myocarditis appear to be sensitive to digitalis. It is preferable to start at a lower dosage and then increase the dosage as needed in order to avoid digitalis toxicity. The daily maintenance dosage is about one fourth of the total digitalizing dosage, given in two equal doses. Therapy with other cardiac drugs should be instituted if digoxin alone does not control the congestive failure.

Bed rest for patients with severe carditis is usually dictated by the condition of the patient. Bed rest may be advisable during the first 2 to 4 weeks, with gradual ambulation thereafter. Although it is agreed that bed rest should be adhered to, it is difficult to provide convincing evidence that this alters the course of the disease. It is advisable to restore gradual ambulation as soon as the carditis stabilizes or disappears. It is important to avoid extreme measures that could be detrimental, such as rapid resumption of full activity in a patient recovering from severe carditis, or to completely restrict to bed a patient with minimal or no carditis.

The manifestations of Sydenham's chorea are self-limited in the majority of patients. In mild cases treatment may be not necessary. In more severe cases bed rest in a quiet room and avoidance of stress are helpful. There is no unanimity as to the value of sedatives. Some patients appear to benefit from phenobarbital given in doses of 15 to 30 mg every 6 to 8 hours. Recent experience with haloperidol suggests that it may be effective in controlling choreiform activity. The dose required varies greatly from patient to patient; a low dose (0.5 mg) given every 8 hours may be initiated and increased to 2.0 mg every 8 hours. Thus, the therapy for Sydenham's chorea should be individualized. Corticosteroids and anti-inflammatory drugs have no role in the treatment of isolated Sydenham's chorea.

REBOUNDS OF RHEUMATIC ACTIVITY

Clinical or laboratory evidence of rheumatic activity may reappear when antirheumatic therapy is discontinued. Such reactivation has been termed a "rebound" and should clearly be distinguished from a recurrence. Spontaneous rebounds do not occur more than 5 weeks after complete cessation of all antirheumatic therapy; the majority occur within 2 weeks, but most occur within a few days or while the dosage is being reduced. Mild rebound episodes can be characterized only by fever, arthralgia, or mild arthritis. Some patients may have only laboratory evidence of relapse, such as re-elevation of the C reactive protein level and the erythrocyte sedimentation rate. Murmurs may reappear. In patients with carditis, rebounds may be severe, and a flare-up of pericarditis or congestive heart failure may occur and on occasion may be more severe than during the initial period of treatment. Mild rebounds subside spontaneously within 1 or 2 weeks and do not require medication. If treatment is necessary, salicylates are preferred. Severe rebound episodes often can be prevented or minimized by giving salicylates as the corticosteroid dosage is tapered.

CONTINUING MANAGEMENT

The responsibility of the physician to the patient with acute rheumatic fever does not cease with treatment of the acute disease. The first responsibility is to insure that the patient is started and continues on antistreptococcal prophylaxis. Secondary prophylaxis offers the only hope for healing and recovery from cardiac disease. For the patient with residual cardiac involvement, monitoring of the cardiac disease and its management (both medical and if necessary surgical) should be continued. Patients should be seen at frequent intervals initially, later at monthly and bimonthly intervals, and then at a half yearly or yearly intervals, to insure that prophylaxis is being complied with. Testing of the urine for antibiotics and determination of streptococcal antibody titers are useful monitors to insure adherence to prophylaxis. Education of the patient should continue through adolescence. Part of the continued care includes emphasis on dental hygiene and increasing the patient's awareness regarding the need for prophylaxis against bacterial endocarditis as recommended by the Committee of the American Heart Association. The patient should be encouraged and informed that these efforts will result in good control of the cardiac disease and return to a normal way of life.

PROGNOSIS

As has been emphasized, except for cardiac involvement, the other major manifestations of rheumatic fever are self-limited. Carditis carries a risk of prolonged morbidity if not mortality. The greatest risk for mortality occurs during the acute phase of severe myocarditis and pancarditis, or later with progressive valvular disease. Mortality may also result from attempts at surgical repair or from bacterial endocarditis. Although in the United States death from acute carditis is now rare, progressive valvular disease is still encountered elsewhere.

The long term prognosis in rheumatic fever has been carefully investigated and found to be closely correlated with the cardiac status during the acute attack. Thus, as a general rule, patients who do not experience carditis during an initial attack of rheumatic fever and who are protected from recurrent rheumatic attacks do not develop rheumatic heart disease. Individuals with "pure" chorea represent an exception to this rule, because 25 per cent of them may develop rheumatic heart

disease. It is possible in such cases that evidence of carditis may have been present earlier but had subsided by the time chorea made its appearance.

ANTISTREPTOCOCCAL VACCINE

Despite the efficacy of antibiotics and chemotherapeutic drugs, infectious diseases have been eradicated only by vaccines (or improved environmental sanitation). Attempts to develop a streptococcal vaccine are based on studies of M proteins, the only streptococcal components that elicit protective antibodies. These efforts have been hampered by the lack of preparations that are highly antigenic and well tolerated. Until recently even "highly purified" M protein preparations elicited delayed hypersensitivity reactions, which were not directed to the type specific determinant. There is now evidence that preparations of M proteins are highly immunogenic in man and relatively free of side effects. However, because even highly purified M proteins contain epitopes cross reacting with heart antigens, it is unlikely that they can be used for in vivo immunization. Two possible solutions are now under investigation. One is to isolate the immunogen portion of M protein from the part containing the epitopes cross reacting with the human heart. Alternatively it will be possible to synthesize the immunogen fragment of M proteins. However, multivalent nontoxic streptococcal vaccines for human use are still far from our reach.

SUGGESTED READING

Ayoub EM, Barrett DJ. Immune mechanisms in rheumatic heart disease. In: Condorelli M, Marone G, Lichtenstein LM, eds. Advances in clinical immunology. The role of chemical mediators in pulmonary and cardiac diseases. Florence: O.I.C. Medical Press, 1984:147.

Committee on Prevention of Rheumatic Fever and Bacterial Endocarditis of the American Heart Association. Prevention of bacterial endocarditis. Circulation 1977; 56:139A–143A.

Committee on Prevention of Rheumatic Fever and Bacterial Endocarditis of the American Heart Association. Prevention of rheumatic fever. Circulation 1977; 55:1–4.

Dale JB, Beachey EH. Multiple, heart-cross-reactive epitopes of streptococcal M protein. J Exp Med 1985; 161:113–122.

Markowitz M, Gordis L. Rheumatic fever. 2nd ed. Philadelphia: WB Saunders, 1972:71.

Stollerman GH. Rheumatic fever and streptococcal infection. New York: Grune & Stratton, 1975:66.

Veasy LG, Wiedmeier SE, Orsmond GS, Ruttenberg HD, Boucek MM, Roth SJ, Tait VF, Thompson JA, Daly JA, Kaplan EL, Hill HR. Resurgence of acute rheumatic fever in the intermountain area of the United States. N Engl J Med 1987; 316:421–427.

Wood HF, Simpson R, Feinstein AR, et al. Rheumatic fever in children and adolescents. I. Description of the investigative techniques and the population studied. Ann Intern Med 1964; 60 (Suppl 5): 6–17.

POSTCARDIAC INJURY SYNDROME

JOSEPH E. PARRILLO, M.D.

Three historically distinct but clinically similar syndromes—the postpericardiotomy syndrome, the postmyocardial infarction (Dressler's) syndrome, and the postcardiac trauma syndrome—occur following injury to the pericardium or to the pericardium and the heart. Because of their similar clinical manifestations, probably similar pathogeneses, and analogous treatment regimens, it is preferred to combine these three syndromes into one entity, termed the postcardiac injury syndrome. Table 1 summarizes the clinical and laboratory manifestations of these syndromes. Although the pathogenesis of the postcardiac injury syndrome has not been fully elucidated, clinical and laboratory evidence strongly suggests an immune pathogenesis. In the postpericardi-

otomy syndrome there is evidence that viral infection also may play a pathogenic role. One hypothesis argues that a viral infection temporally associated with cardiac surgery results in an immunologic reaction that is much more likely to sensitize a patient to his own cardiac antigens.

GENERAL CONSIDERATIONS

Several points are worthy of emphasis with regard to the optimal treatment plan for patients with this syndrome. First, it always occurs after some form of cardiac injury. It is important to evaluate the patient's chest pain clinically to be sure that one is not dealing with a recurrence of the original injury (for example, myocardial infarction) rather than the postcardiac injury syndrome. Furthermore, the echocardiogram is a sensitive method of detecting pericardial fluid, and echocardiographic evidence of pericardial effusion is seen frequently after cardiac injury. The presence of a pericardial effusion alone does not justify the diagnosis of postcardiac injury syndrome. Rather, given the appropriate symptom complex and laboratory evidence of systemic

TABLE 1   The Three Historical Syndromes That Constitute the Postcardiac Injury Syndrome

Syndrome	Clinical Setting	Clinical Manifestations*	Onset	Incidence	Differential Diagnosis	Laboratory Findings†
Postpericardiotomy syndrome	Occurs after cardiac surgery that involves pericardium or pericardium and heart	Chest pain, fever, pericarditis, pericardial effusion, pleural effusion, pneumonitis	Usually 7 days to 4 weeks; may occur up to 6 to 12 months after surgery	Range, 10 to 63 percent; most series show 25 to 30 percent incidence	Must differentiate from incisional chest pain, post-pump syndrome (caused by cytomegalovirus or toxoplasmosis 6 to 8 weeks after surgery), and pulmonary embolism	Elevated ESR; elevated WBC count; chest x-ray view shows pericardial or pleural effusions, rarely pneumonitis; EKG sometimes shows pericarditis
Postmyocardial infarction syndrome	Occurs after both transmural or subendocardial myocardial infarction	Chest pain, fever, pericarditis, pericardial effusion, pleuritis, pleural effusion, pneumonitis	Usually 7 days to 3 weeks; may occur up to 3 months after infarction	From 1 to 4% of myocardial infarctions	Must differentiate from recurrent coronary ischemic pain, early (irritative) post-transmural infarction pericarditis (1 to 4 days after infarction), and pulmonary embolism	Elevated ESR or WBC; chest x-ray examination shows pericardial or pleural effusions and rarely pneumonitis; EKG shows pericarditis in about 50 percent of cases
Postcardiac trauma syndrome	Reported after sharp and blunt chest trauma; also reported after left ventricular puncture, cardiac perforation with a catheter, and pacemaker implantation	Chest pain, pericarditis, pericardial effusion, fever, pleural effusion	4 days to 8 weeks after trauma	Poorly documented; probably about 8 percent of post-left ventricular puncture; post-trauma, hemopericardium incidence may be 20 to 30 percent	Chest pain secondary to trauma or coronary artery injury; pulmonary embolism	Elevated ESR or WBC; chest x-ray examination shows pericardial or pleural effusions; EKG may show pericarditis

* Most common manifestations are listed first; less common ones are listed last.
† Echocardiogram demonstrates pericardial effusion in most patients with postcardiac injury syndrome.

inflammation, determining the presence of a pericardial effusion is a useful confirmatory test.

Second, once a patient has suffered one bout of this disease, he is susceptible to recurrences. In the postmyocardial infarction syndrome recurrences occur in as many as 50 percent of the patients. Recurrences usually occur 2 to 4 months after the original bout but may recur as late as 2 years after the first episode. Furthermore, many patients have more than two episodes: As many as six or seven relapses have been reported over a 2 or 3 year period. Thus, when treating the first episode, one must consider the issue of recurrent episodes and also educate the patient about the likelihood of recurrence of symptoms. A recurrence after 2 years without symptoms of the disease would be very unusual; this should arouse suspicion that a new bout of the postcardiac injury syndrome or a new disease process has intervened.

Third, the postcardiac injury syndrome is generally regarded as a "benign" syndrome without serious consequences. Although it is a benign (although uncomfortable) disease in most patients, it does have several important complications or sequelae that must be carefully monitored—cardiac tamponade, severe pneumonitis, severe incapacitating chest pain, and the late development of constrictive pericarditis.

PHARMACOLOGIC THERAPY WITH ASPIRIN

A major consideration in designing appropriate treatment for the patient with the postcardiac injury syndrome is the severity of the illness (Table 2). Patients who present with mild to moderate chest pain along with evidence of pericarditis on examination or electrocardiography should undergo laboratory evaluations (erythrocyte sedimentation rate and white blood cell count), chest x-ray examination, and echocardiography. Most patients demonstrate a modest increase in the sedimentation rate and leukocyte count along with small pleural effusions and a small to moderate pericardial effusion evident on the echocardiogram. If the chest pain is not severe, if no evidence of cardiac tamponade is found on physical examination, and if no pulmonary infiltrates are seen on chest x-ray views, one should begin therapy with aspirin. The initial dosage should be 600 mg orally every 4 hours. This commonly results in a symptomatic response within the first few doses, with a decrease in fever to a normal or nearly normal temperature, a substantial diminution in chest pain, and an increase in the sense of general well-being. Although aspirin results in a decrease in symptoms in the majority of patients with mild to moderate postcardiac injury syndrome, it usually does not reduce the size of pleural or pericardial effusions, and the sedimentation rate and leukocyte count usually are unaffected also. However, because the postcardiac injury syndrome is a self-limited disease in most cases, providing symptomatic relief is all that is necessary. In evaluating the response to therapy, one should consider a variety of symptoms, signs, and laboratory findings. The most useful parameters for following the clinical course are listed in Table 3.

In some patients who respond to aspirin therapy, mild chest pain may remain and small occasional intermittent doses of codeine (60 mg orally every 4 hours as needed) usually eliminate the remaining discomfort. If aspirin therapy is effective, it is generally useful to give

TABLE 2 Treatment Regimens for the Postcardiac Injury Syndrome

Clinical Stage	Treatment Regimen
Mild to moderate chest pain	Aspirin, 600 mg orally every 4 hours for 2 days. If effective, continue for 2 to 3 weeks.
Pericarditis on examination or electrocardiography	
Mild to moderate pericardial effusion	
Mild to moderate pleural effusion	
Elevated ESR and WBC	If aspirin is ineffective after 2 days and symptoms are modest, begin ibuprofen, 400 mg orally t.i.d. for 3 days. If effective, continue for 3 weeks. If ibuprofen is ineffective, begin indomethacin, 25 mg t.i.d., and increase to 50 mg t.i.d.
Severe chest pain	Indomethacin, 25 then 50 mg t.i.d. for 3 days. If ineffective and chest pain is limiting and difficult to control with narcotic analgesics, begin prednisone, 60 mg daily for 5 to 7 days; then taper off or to alternate day regimen. Discontinue at 2 to 3 weeks. If indomethacin is effective, give a 2 to 3 week course.
Penumonitis on chest x-ray views	Methylprednisolone, 60 mg IV, then 20 mg IV every 8 hours for 1 to 2 weeks. Convert to prednisone, 60 mg daily. Slowly taper to an alternate day regimen.
Nonemergency cardiac tamponade	
Emergency cardiac tamponade	Pericardiocentesis. Methylprednisolone, 20 mg IV every 8 hours for 2 to 3 weeks; then prednisone, 60 mg daily. For tapering see text.
Recurrent cardiac tamponade despite appropriate therapy	Pericardiectomy
Constrictive pericarditis	Pericardial stripping

TABLE 3 Useful Parameters to Follow When Therapeutically Managing Postcardiac Injury Syndrome

Fever

Symptoms: chest pain, general well-being

Erythrocyte sedimentation rate

Size of pericardial effusion on echocardiogram and on chest x-ray views

Pleural effusions (chest x-ray views)

Resolution of pneumonitis or pericardial tamponade

a 2 to 3 week course of therapy (2.4 to 3.6 g per day in four divided doses with meals) to prevent a recurrence of symptoms.

Aspirin's mechanism of action in the postcardiac injury syndrome relates to its analgesic and anti-inflammatory properties. Some, perhaps most, of these properties are mediated through aspirin's inhibition of prostaglandin production and release from cells. The major side effects of aspirin are gastrointestinal bleeding and erosions, platelet dysfunction causing a prolonged bleeding time, mild liver function test abnormalities, and, when taken in high prolonged dosages, nephropathy. In general, aspirin should be taken with antacids or meals, since this mode of administration may lessen the gastrointestinal side effects.

USE OF PLATELET ACTIVE DRUGS IN ANTICOAGULATED PATIENTS

The question of whether to use a platelet inhibiting drug (such as aspirin or a nonsteroidal anti-inflammatory drug) in a patient with the postcardiac injury syndrome who is taking anticoagulant therapy is a recurring problem. Hemorrhagic pericarditis leading to cardiac tamponade can occur in the postcardiac injury syndrome, and there is little doubt that use of warfarin anticoagulants in this disorder increases the likelihood of pericardial hemorrhage. Therefore patients with the postcardiac injury syndrome must have strong indications for anticoagulant therapy, or the warfarin should be discontinued. Therapy with aspirin or most other nonsteroidal anti-inflammatory drugs probably increases the chance of developing hemorrhagic pericarditis if the patient is taking oral anticoagulant therapy. However, the increased risk of pericardial hemorrhage is exceedingly small. Thus, although the threshold for using aspirin in an anticoagulated patient with the postcardiac injury syndrome should be somewhat higher than in the nonanticoagulated patient, aspirin frequently has been used in this setting without any complications.

As in all patients taking warfarin anticoagulant therapy, the prothrombin time must be evaluated every 2 to 4 weeks. Early in therapy with both warfarin and aspirin, the prothrombin time should be determined more frequently (approximately twice a week) and the value should be kept slightly lower than usual, e.g., 17 to 20 seconds (with a 12 second control) rather than 20 to 24 seconds, the usual prothrombin time prolongation. Keeping the prothrombin time in a lower range is believed to reduce the chance of pericardial hemorrhage during therapy with aspirin and warfarin.

IBUPROFEN

A substantial number of patients with mild to moderate symptoms that are unresponsive to aspirin respond to one of the newer nonsteroidal anti-inflammatory drugs. Ibuprofen (Motrin), 400 mg orally three times daily, is useful in relieving symptoms in the postcardiac injury syndrome. As with aspirin, it usually does not reduce pericardial or pleural effusion, although it does reduce fever and decrease chest discomfort. Side effects are similar to those with aspirin: gastrointestinal upset and erosion and platelet dysfunction. Visual disturbances, including blurred vision and toxic amblyopia, have been seen infrequently; if visual disturbances occur, ibuprofen therapy should be discontinued.

INDOMETHACIN

In patients who have failed to improve during therapy with aspirin, ibuprofen, or both, and in those presenting with severe chest pain, indomethacin is the drug of choice. Therapy begins with 25 mg three times daily, and the dosage should be increased to 50 mg three times daily if the lower dosage is well tolerated. In many patients indomethacin provides prompt relief of even severe debilitating chest pain resulting from the postcardiac injury syndrome. Patients usually obtain relief after several doses, but it may take 2 or 3 days of therapy to obtain maximal efficacy. Indomethacin has powerful analgesic and anti-inflammatory effects. It reduces fever, relieves chest pain and in some patients decreases sedimentation rate and leukocyte count elevations and reduces pleural and pericardial effusions. If therapy is effective, it should be continued for 2 to 3 weeks to prevent a return of symptoms.

Indomethacin is a powerful inhibitor of the prostaglandin forming cyclo-oxygenase, and it is likely that much of the drug's anti-inflammatory and analgesic efficacy is mediated via prostaglandin synthesis inhibition. The major side effect of indomethacin is gastrointestinal upset: as many as 15 to 30 percent of the patients are not able to take the drug because of gastric distress. The abdominal pain and epigastric distress can be decreased by taking indomethacin with an antacid or food. Indomethacin also can cause gastritis and gastric ulceration with upper gastrointestinal bleeding. As with aspirin, platelet dysfunction occurs and must be considered in patients taking anticoagulants.

An important side effect of indomethacin is its tendency to cause salt and water retention. This fluid accumulation can precipitate congestive heart failure in patients with poorly compensated ventricles. This side effect should be treated with concomitant diuretic administration. Some patients develop headaches with indomethacin, which usually abate with continued therapy. However, an occasional patient cannot tolerate the drug because of persistent headache.

CORTICOSTEROIDS

Corticosteroids are highly effective in treating both the symptoms and the manifestations of the postcardiac injury syndrome. Because of the potentially serious side effects of corticosteroids, and because of the tendency for the syndrome to flare after discontinuation of corticosteroid treatment, this mode of therapy is reserved for severe disease or disease unresponsive to other modes of therapy (see Table 2).

In patients with severe incapacitating chest pain or chest pain that has been unresponsive to therapy with salicylates and nonsteroidal anti-inflammatory drugs (including indomethacin), corticosteroids become the drugs of choice. Therapy should be started with prednisone, 60 mg orally daily. Most patients respond dramatically to prednisone administration with rapid defervescence, relief of chest pain, and an increased sense of well-being. In addition, prednisone usually causes a dramatic decrease in the sedimentation rate and the leukocyte count, and one usually sees a decrease in pleural and pericardial effusions. After 5 to 7 days of prednisone therapy, one must make a clinical judgment as to how long the patient will require corticosteroid therapy. If the patient has manifested a rapid disappearance of all symptoms and signs of postcardiac injury syndrome, many patients can be tapered off prednisone therapy by decrements of 10 mg per day and complete a 10 day course. Ten days' therapy with prednisone has been shown not to cause any long term suppression of adrenal pituitary-hypothalamic axis function. Therefore, terminating therapy at 10 days has the advantage of avoiding a need for steroid coverage for "stress" situations.

Patients who have recurrences of symptoms or signs of the postcardiac injury syndrome during the period of steroid tapering can be treated in two ways. First, one can institute therapy with indomethacin during the tapering to control symptoms. This is usually effective only in patients with a mild flare of symptoms. Second, in more severe cases one can reinstitute prednisone therapy at 60 mg every day and then slowly convert to alternate day therapy by gradually decreasing the "off" prednisone dosage by 5 mg every other day; a reasonable sequence would be 60, 55, 60, 50, 60, 45, 60, 40 mg, and so on. When one reaches a level of 60 mg alternating

with 20 mg, the alternate day tapering should be slowed and the "off" day dosage decreased by 2.5 mg every other day. With this alternate day tapering regimen, a patient can be converted to 60 mg orally every other day in several weeks.

On alternate day prednisone therapy, the side effects of long term prednisone administration are markedly diminished (to be discussed). The dosage then can be slowly tapered (over 2 to 6 weeks) from the alternate day prednisone regimen. Most patients do not experience a flare of the disease with this tapering schedule. Patients in whom flares occur with the alternate day tapering regimen should have the alternate day dosage increased to control the postcardiac injury syndrome manifestations; then a slower tapering of the alternate day prednisone dosage should be initiated. Some patients who are difficult to taper off prednisone benefit from the addition of indomethacin to an alternate day prednisone regimen.

In general, when using prednisone in this (and most) diseases, one does best to begin with a high daily dosage to control the inflammatory disease process. One then can slowly taper off or to an alternate day regimen. If a significant flare occurs during the tapering, one has to increase the prednisone dosage substantially to reestablish control over the inflammatory process. Then tapering can begin again—this time at a slower rate.

The side effects of long term daily prednisone therapy are glucose intolerance, cataract formation, cushingoid features, weight gain and edema, hypertension, acne, and an increased susceptibility to infection. Most of these side effects can be substantially or completely avoided by employing an alternate day prednisone regimen. Long acting steroid preparations, such as dexamethasone, are not useful for alternate day regimens because their long half-lives do not allow a steroid free period with an alternate day dosage schedule.

TREATMENT OF SERIOUS COMPLICATIONS OF THE POSTCARDIAC INJURY SYNDROME

Patients who present with one of the serious complications of the postcardiac injury syndrome (pericardial tamponade or pneumonitis) should be hospitalized immediately. With pericardial tamponade, one must make an immediate assessment of the severity of hemodynamic compromise. Patients with a systolic blood pressure of 85 mm Hg or less and with evidence of poor organ perfusion (mental confusion, oliguria, cold skin) coupled with other signs of tamponade (elevated jugular venous pressure, engorged liver, and pulsus paradoxus) should be considered candidates for immediate needle pericardiocentesis. While the equipment for needle pericardiocentesis is being set up, the patient should be given fluids intravenously (300 to 500 cc per hour) to increase cardiac output transiently. If time permits, it is useful to perform echocardiography to confirm the presence of anterior and posterior pericardial fluid and right sided heart catheterization to confirm the diagnosis of pericardial tamponade. One looks for pulsus paradoxus (decreased systolic blood pressure during inspiration) and an elevation and equilibration of right sided heart pressures: The right atrial mean, the right ventricular end diastolic, the pulmonary artery end diastolic, and the pulmonary capillary wedge mean pressures are usually identical in cardiac tamponade, but always are all within 5 mm Hg of one another.

Needle pericardiocentesis should be performed from the subxiphoid approach with the needle attached to the V lead of an electrocardiogram to avoid cardiac puncture. An injury current on the electrocardiogram indicates contact of the needle with the epicardium, and the needle should be withdrawn. Entrance into the pericardial space is signaled by the return of serous or hemorrhagic fluid; the latter should not clot if it is from the pericardial space. Removal of even a small amount of fluid (10 to 20 ml) usually results in a profound improvement in the hemodynamic state. It is generally wise to advance a soft plastic catheter (to prevent cardiac trauma) over the pericardiocentesis needle into the pericardial space and drain off as much fluid as one can over a several hour period. The pericardial catheter then should be removed.

At the time of pericardiocentesis for postcardiac injury syndrome induced tamponade, the patient should be given methylprednisolone, 60 mg intravenously and then 20 mg intravenously every 8 hours for 1 to 2 weeks, to obtain the maximal anti-inflammatory effect and prevent a recurrence of tamponade. The intravenous route is employed in this situation because cardiac tamponade can cause decreased gastrointestinal absorption owing to venous engorgement and poor arterial flow to the gut. The patient then should be given prednisone, 60 mg orally daily, and the dosage slowly tapered (see foregoing discussion) to an alternate day prednisone regimen. Most patients do not have a recurrence of tamponade after adequate pericardiocentesis and prednisone therapy. In these patients alternate day prednisone therapy should be continued for 2 to 3 months and then slowly tapered off.

In patients who have postcardiac injury syndrome induced pneumonitis or pericardial tamponade without signs of imminent hemodynamic compromise, therapy with methylprednisolone, 60 mg intravenously and then 20 mg intravenously every 8 hours, should be instituted. In many patients the tamponade disappears following the use of parenteral steroid therapy without the need for pericardiocentesis. Pneumonitis almost always resolves rapidly following corticosteroid therapy. Parenteral corticosteroid therapy should be continued for 1 to 2 weeks; then oral therapy with prednisone should be instituted and the dosage slowly tapered as already outlined for the treatment of pericardial tamponade after pericardiocentesis.

In patients showing grossly hemorrhagic pericarditis secondary to the postcardiac injury syndrome, se-

rious consideration should be given to discontinuation of anticoagulants unless they are absolutely necessary. Aspirin and nonsteroidal anti-inflammatory drugs should be avoided because they can cause platelet dysfunction. Most patients with postcardiac injury syndrome-induced hemorrhagic pericarditis respond to corticosteroid therapy; however, if hemorrhagic pericarditis recurs after steroid tapering, one should consider pericardiectomy (see next section).

RECURRENCES OF THE POSTCARDIAC INJURY SYNDROME

Recurrences of the postcardiac injury syndrome generally should be treated the same as first episodes (see Table 2). However, it is useful to remember that drugs that have failed to benefit a given patient usually fail if used again. Reinstitution of the previously successful therapy is therefore generally indicated. The only notable exception to this rule is the patient with unrelenting or severe chest pain (but no other major symptoms or signs) finally requiring prednisone therapy. It is usually best to try indomethacin again in these patients before being compelled to reinstitute prednisone therapy.

Patients who have had an episode of postcardiac injury syndrome-induced pericardial tamponade and who redevelop tamponade after an adequate course of corticosteroids should be considered candidates for pericardiectomy. This surgical procedure essentially eliminates the chance of recurrent tamponade, and it reduces chest pain in most patients. However, in a subpopulation of patients chest pain may remain a problem even after pericardiectomy, and long term alternate day prednisone therapy may have to be used to control recurrent debilitating symptoms. As already mentioned, recurrence of hemorrhagic pericarditis is a strong indication for pericardiectomy.

PROBLEM PATIENTS

On rare occasions a patient may have recurrent severe symptoms despite long courses of therapy with corticosteroids. Another type of problem patient is one with recurrent pericardial tamponade who is unable to undergo surgical pericardiectomy because of other serious medical problems. A small number of these patients have been treated successfully with cytotoxic therapy (azathioprine, 2 mg per kg per day, or cyclophosphamide, 1 to 2 mg per kg per day), along with alternate day prednisone therapy. Use of the cytotoxic drug has effected control of symptoms and recurrent tamponade and also facilitated corticosteroid tapering. Patients must be closely monitored for signs of leukopenia, bone marrow suppression, hepatitis (azathioprine), hemorrhagic cystitis (cyclophosphamide), and sterility (cyclophosphamide). After 1 to 2 years of cytotoxic therapy, all anti-inflammatory therapy has been discontinued in several patients without recurrence of postcardiac injury syndrome. Fortunately patients with the syndrome who require this form of therapy are rare.

CONSTRICTIVE PERICARDITIS

A small percentage of patients with the postcardiac injury syndrome develop constrictive pericarditis. It is not known whether any form of anti-inflammatory therapy prevents this late complication. Patients who develop symptoms of constrictive pericarditis require car-

diac catheterization to establish the diagnosis and then pericardial stripping to cure the disease.

SUGGESTED READING

Dressler W. Idiopathic recurrent pericarditis: comparison with the post-commissurotomy syndrome, consideration of etiology and treatment. Am J Med 1955; 18:591–601.
Engle MA, Zabriskie JB, Senterfit LB, Ebert PA. Postpericardiotomy syndrome: a new look at an old condition. Mod Concepts Cardiovasc Dis 1975a; 44:59–64.
Engle MA, Zabriskie JB, Senterfit LB, Gay WA Jr, O'Loughlin JE Jr, Ehlers KH. Viral illness and the postpericardiotomy syndrome: a prospective study in children. Circulation 1980; 62:1151–1158.
Parrillo JE, Fauci AS. Immunologic diseases of the cardiovascular system. In: Lockey A, Bukantz S, eds. Principles of immunology and allergy. Philadelphia: WB Saunders, 1987: 271–287.

INFLAMMATORY MYOPERICARDITIS

JOSEPH E. PARRILLO, M.D.

Inflammation of the pericardium or myocardium can be caused by a wide variety of pathogenic mechanisms: infections, neoplasms, uremia, trauma, the postcardiac injury syndrome, collagen vascular diseases, drug hypersensitivity, and idiopathic agents. In a number of these specific myopericarditides it is important to establish the precise diagnosis because specific therapy is available, for example, in bacterial pericarditis, tuberculous pericarditis, uremic pericarditis, and the myopericarditis seen with certain collagen vascular diseases or caused by drug hypersensitivity. The therapy of the postcardiac injury syndrome (which includes the postmyocardial infarction syndrome, the postpericardiotomy syndrome, and the postcardiac trauma syndrome) is discussed in the chapter *Postcardiac Injury Syndrome*.

In many cases of myopericarditis no etiologic agent is discovered with certainty despite an exhaustive workup to rule out the aforementioned causes. Most of these undiagnosed bouts of myopericarditis are ascribed to an idiopathic cause and many are presumed to be of viral origin, although there usually are no convincing diagnostic studies, i.e., viral isolation or a fourfold rise in antibody titer to a specific viral agent. Many authors have ascribed an immune pathogenesis to these large numbers of undiagnosed bouts of myopericarditis be-

cause the following characteristics suggest immune mediation: Myopericarditis is commonly associated with inflammatory or immune abnormalities or both (elevations in the erythrocyte sedimentation rate and peripheral white blood cell count, and positive results in antinuclear antibody tests); bouts of myopericarditis recur in many patients, suggesting recrudescence of a hypersensitivity phenomenon; a number of patients with this disease have circulating antibodies to heart tissue; and treatment of these bouts with anti-inflammatory therapy affords most patients symptomatic relief and may hasten resolution of the syndrome.

When considering the best treatment regimen for a patient with myopericarditis, it is useful to decide whether the patient has predominantly pericarditis or myocarditis or a combination of the two (Table 1). Patients with pericarditis alone manifest fever, pleuritic chest pain, an elevated sedimentation rate, and a pericardial rub; commonly a pericardial effusion is demonstrable on the echocardiogram or chest x-ray view. Patients with pericarditis and superficial myocarditis (epicarditis) demonstrate electrocardiographic changes (ST segment elevation or depression, T wave inversion) or rhythm disturbances along with the manifestations of pericarditis. Patients with myocarditis may or may not demonstrate signs of concomitant pericarditis. Most important, patients with moderate to severe diffuse myocarditis demonstrate compromise of cardiac muscle function resulting in symptoms and signs of congestive heart failure, rhythm disturbances, or both. Evaluation of cardiac function with echocardiography, nuclear scanning, or cardiac catheterization demonstrates a reduction in myocardial systolic function due to myocardial inflammation. Patients who demonstrate diffuse myocarditis have a much more serious disease than those with pericarditis

TABLE 1 Differentiation of Pericarditis from Myocarditis

Diagnostic Category	Diagnostic Criteria
Pericarditis	Fever
	Chest pain
	Pericardial rub
	Elevated ESR
	Pericardial effusion on chest x-ray view or echocardiogram
Pericarditis and superficial myocarditis (that is, epicarditis)	All the above plus:
	Electrocardiographic abnormalities (ST segment changes)
	Arrhythmias (especially atrial)
Pericarditis with diffuse myocarditis	All the above may or may not be present plus:
	Congestive heart failure
	Atrial and ventricular arrhythmias
	Evidence of reduced ventricular systolic function (by echocardiography, nuclear scan, or cardiac catheterization with angiography)

or pericarditis with epicarditis. Therefore the treatment regimens for patients suffering from pericarditis and those who have predominantly myocarditis are different (Tables 2, 3).

In general, idiopathic inflammatory pericarditis is a benign self-limited disease process. However, several serious complications should be kept in mind when managing patients with pericarditis: cardiac tamponade, severe debilitating chest pain, and the late development of constrictive pericarditis. The latter condition is a relatively rare sequela of a single bout of inflammatory pericarditis; however, constriction becomes much more likely in patients with recurrent bouts of pericardial inflammation.

THERAPY OF PERICARDITIS

The general approach to the treatment of pericarditis is summarized in Table 2. Initial therapy depends on the clinical stage of the disease and the severity of symptomatology. Many patients with acute pericarditis have a 1 to 3 day bout of moderately severe chest pain. In these very mild episodes it is reasonable to give no therapy and allow the process to subside by itself.

Aspirin and Ibuprofen

In patients with prolonged mild to moderate symptomatology, aspirin, 600 mg orally every 4 hours, commonly decreases fever and relieves chest pain. One may increase the aspirin dosage to 3 to 6 g per day in four divided doses to obtain therapeutic levels of 20 to 40 mg per 100 ml. In some patients the fever and chest pain are not completely relieved but are decreased to a tolerable level. Most patients respond to aspirin within 3 days if they are going to respond at all. Therefore, patients not deriving benefit from 3 days of treatment should be given one of the newer nonsteroidal anti-inflammatory drugs. Ibuprofen, 400 mg orally three times daily, provides analgesic and anti-inflammatory

TABLE 2 Treatment Regimen for Inflammatory Pericarditis

Clinical Stage	Treatment Regimen
Fever, chest pain Pericardial rub Elevated ESR Pericardial effusion EKG changes (ST or T wave abnormalities)	Aspirin, 650 mg orally every 4 hours (up to 3–6 g/per day in four divided doses) for 3 days; if effective, continue for 2 weeks; if ineffective, after 3 days begin:
	Ibuprofen, 400 mg orally t.i.d. for 3 days
	If symptoms continue, begin indomethacin, 25 then 50 mg orally t.i.d.
Atrial arrhythmias with above manifestations	Antiarrhythmics (digoxin, verapamil, propranolol, quinidine)
	Indomethacin, 25 then 50 mg orally t.i.d.
	If atrial arrhythmias are refractory to above regimen, begin prednisone, 20 mg orally every 8 hours for 5 to 7 days; then taper off or to alternate day regimen
Severe unresponsive chest pain	Prednisone, 60 mg orally every day for 5 to 7 days; then taper off or to alternate day regimen
Pericardial tamponade	Pericardiocentesis
	Methylprednisolone, 60 mg IV; then 20 mg IV every 8 hours for 2 weeks; then convert to prednisone, 60 mg orally every day and taper to alternate day regimen
Recurrent pericardial tamponade	Pericardiectomy
Constrictive pericarditis	Pericardial stripping

TABLE 3   Treatment Regimen for Inflammatory Myocarditis

Clinical Stages		Treatment Regimen
Fever, chest pain Pericardial rub Elevated ESR Pericardial effusion EKG changes (ST and T wave abnormalities)	May or may not be present	
Congestive heart failure		Treat congestive failure with digoxin, diuretics, and afterload reduction
Atrial and/or ventricular arrhythmias		Treat rhythm disturbances with antiarrhythmics (quinidine, procainamide, digoxin, verapamil, propranolol, disopyramide)
Reduced ventricular systolic function (by echocardiography, nuclear scan, or cardiac catheterization with angiography)		Prednisone, 20 mg orally every 8 hours; carefully follow measures of ventricular function and cardiac inflammation to determine whether therapy is effective in improving ventricular function and decreasing inflammation
		If prednisone is ineffective after 2 to 3 weeks, consider therapy with cyclophosphamide, 2 mg/kg/day, or azathioprine, 2 mg/kg/day; follow symptoms, ventricular function, and measures of cardiac inflammation to determine efficacy

properties similar to those of aspirin. However, a substantial number of patients derive symptomatic relief from ibuprofen and not from aspirin—enough so that a trial of this drug is worthwhile. Again most patients respond to ibuprofen within 3 days if they are going to derive benefit from this medication. If therapy with either aspirin or ibuprofen is successful, a 2 week course of therapy should be given to minimize the chance of recurrence of symptoms when therapy with the drug is stopped.

Aspirin and ibuprofen have similar modes of action (inhibiting the prostaglandin forming cyclo-oxygenase) and have largely gastrointestinal side effects. Both drugs can be associated with gastric erosion, gastritis, and gastrointestinal hemorrhage. Ibuprofen is promoted as causing less gastrointestinal toxicity than aspirin, and the incidence of gut side effects is probably slightly less with ibuprofen. In patients with a history of upper gastrointestinal problems, I usually begin therapy with ibuprofen rather than aspirin.

Both aspirin and ibuprofen cause a platelet defect that prolongs the bleeding time. This could be of considerable theoretic importance in patients already taking heparin or warfarin anticoagulation, since causing a platelet defect in these anticoagulated patients could cause generalized bleeding or bleeding into the inflamed pericardial space (hemorrhagic pericarditis). Although the risk of this complication is quite small, it is nonetheless possible. In general, idiopathic pericarditis is a relative contraindication to anticoagulation, and aspirin or ibuprofen may theoretically make bleeding even more likely by inhibiting platelet function. Patients who develop pericarditis should continue to receive anticoagulation only if the indication is very strong, for example, the need to anticoagulate a patient with a mechanical prosthetic valve. In patients who have idiopathic pericarditis and are not anticoagulated, aspirin and ibuprofen

do not appear to increase the incidence of hemorrhagic pericarditis. In general, aspirin and ibuprofen can be used in anticoagulated patients, but such therapy should be undertaken with considerable caution and very frequent follow-up. Furthermore, when forced to combine antiplatelet drugs with warfarin therapy, I try to keep the prothrombin time in patients given warfarin anticoagulation in the low therapeutic range (18 to 20 seconds).

Other side effects of these medications include aspirin's capacity to produce hepatitis and ibuprofen's to produce visual disturbances. Appearance of the latter complication necessitates discontinuation of the drug.

Indomethacin

Indomethacin is a powerful inhibitor of prostaglandin synthesis and release, and it is likely that this mechanism accounts for many of the drug's strong analgesic and anti-inflammatory properties. Although it causes more side effects than aspirin, indomethacin is clearly more efficacious in treating patients with inflammatory pericarditis. In addition to its capacity to decrease the fever and chest pain of pericarditis, indomethacin causes a decrease in the sedimentation rate and reduces the volume of pericardial fluid in many patients.

Indomethacin therapy is indicated in patients who have failed to improve following therapy with aspirin or ibuprofen and in those who have pericarditis and superficial myocarditis with arrhythmias (usually atrial). In the latter clinical setting indomethacin's anti-inflammatory capability helps prevent further atrial arrhythmias. The atrial arrhythmias should also be treated with antiarrhythmic therapy, which usually includes digitalis and may include verapamil, quinidine, or propranolol.

An important side effect of indomethacin is that it causes most patients to retain salt and water. In patients with underlying heart disease this fluid accumulation may precipitate or worsen congestive heart failure. Patients should have frequent cardiac examinations and should be weighed daily to follow this fluid retention. If the patient has a weight increase of more than 1 to 2 kg, a diuretic should be given (or the diuretic dose increased) during indomethacin therapy. Another side effect of indomethacin is headaches, which can be severe. Indomethacin also produces platelet dysfunction, and this should be considered in patients taking anticoagulants (see foregoing discussion).

Indomethacin therapy should be started at a dosage of 25 mg orally three times daily and increased to 50 mg three times daily if the lower dosage is well tolerated. Many patients obtain a therapeutic response after a few doses, but it may take 2 to 3 days of therapy to obtain maximal efficacy. If therapy is effective, it should be continued for about 2 weeks to prevent recurrences. Indomethacin should be taken with food, antacids, or both to prevent gastrointestinal side effects.

Corticosteroid Therapy

Corticosteroids have powerful anti-inflammatory and immunosuppressive properties, and corticosteroid administration is highly effective in controlling the signs and symptoms of pericarditis. However, corticosteroids have potentially serious side effects and therefore should be reserved for the following indications (see Table 2): severe persistent debilitating chest pain that has been unresponsive to aspirin, ibuprofen, and indomethacin therapy; arrhythmias that are refractory to indomethacin and antiarrhythmic therapy; and pericarditis with pericardial tamponade.

Corticosteroid therapy usually produces rapid relief of even severe debilitating chest pain from pericarditis. Corticosteroids also reduce fever, decrease the sedimentation rate, and hasten the resorption of pericardial fluid. They also commonly halt arrhythmias refractory to antiarrhythmic drugs and other less potent anti-inflammatory drugs. This presumably occurs owing to abolition of the inflammatory foci in the epicardium of the heart.

Patients should be started on prednisone therapy, 60 mg orally every day, and continued on this daily dosage for 5 to 7 days. If rapid relief of symptoms occurs, the prednisone dosage can be tapered by 5 to 10 mg per day with a 10 to 14 day course of therapy. This short course of prednisone has the advantage of not producing adrenal-pituitary-hypothalamic axis suppression so that the patient will not have to receive corticosteroids for future episodes of "stress." However, a 10 day course is frequently not sufficient to control pericarditis, and disease manifestations may recur during the tapering. If these manifestations are mild, they may be controlled with indomethacin. However, a significant flare of symptoms during prednisone tapering necessitates reinstitution of higher dosage daily prednisone therapy to control symptoms.

Under these circumstances the dosage should be slowly tapered to an alternate day prednisone regimen. This can be accomplished by decreasing the "off" day of prednisone therapy by 5 mg per day, that is, 60, 55, 60, 50, 60, 45, 60, 40 mg, and so on, down to 60 alternating with 20 mg. At this point one should decrease the dosage more slowly on the "off" day because flares are more common at this dosage range. Once a dosage of 60 mg of prednisone every other day is achieved, one can maintain this alternate day regimen for several months if necessary, with the side effects of daily corticosteroid therapy greatly reduced by the alternate day dosage schedule (to be discussed). One then can slowly taper the alternate day regimen by 5 mg every other day, watching carefully for evidence of disease flare.

In general, when using prednisone in this (and most) diseases, one does best to begin with a high daily dosage to control the inflammatory disease process. Then one can slowly taper the daily dosage to the point of discontinuation or convert to an alternate day regimen. If a significant flare occurs during the tapering, one must increase the prednisone dosage substantially to re-establish control over the inflammatory process. Prednisone tapering then can be started again, this time at a slower rate. Long acting steroid preparations such as dexamethasone are not useful for an alternate day regimen because their long half-lifes do not allow a significant steroid free interval between doses on an alternate day schedule.

The side effects of long term daily corticosteroid administration are many and well known. They include glucose intolerance, cushingoid facies, acne, cataract formation, weight gain and edema, hypertension, and an increased incidence of infection. Most of these side effects are substantially reduced by using an alternate day prednisone regimen. The serious potential complication of increased infection in patients receiving daily corticosteroid therapy appears not to be a problem with an alternate day regimen. It is important to monitor patients for corticosteroid induced side effects so that they may be treated if these occur.

TREATMENT OF PERICARDITIS AND PERICARDIAL TAMPONADE

When pericardial tamponade is present, the tempo of the treatment regimen depends upon the degree of hemodynamic compromise in the patient. In a patient with severe cardiac tamponade demonstrating a systolic blood pressure of less than 85 mm Hg, engorged neck veins, and signs of poor organ perfusion (mental confusion, oliguria, cold clammy skin), a medical emergency exists that requires prompt therapy. While arranging to perform emergency needle pericardiocentesis, one can administer fluids intravenously at a rapid rate (500 to 1000 cc per hour) to try to increase the stroke volume; pressors such as isoproterenol may also assist transiently in enhancing the stroke volume and thus the cardiac output. Pericardiocentesis should be rapidly performed from the subxiphoid approach using electrocardiographic V lead monitoring to avoid cardiac laceration. Serous or hemorrhagic pericardial fluid is aspirated through the needle once the pericardium is entered. Removal of a small amount of fluid (50 to 100 cc) usually results in dramatic hemodynamic improvement. A plastic catheter should be advanced over the needle into the pericardial sac to drain pericardial fluid over a several hour period; the catheter can then be removed when appropriate.

In pericarditis with pericardial tamponade, following removal of pericardial fluid, which may be hemorrhagic, exudative, or both, corticosteroid therapy can be used to prevent recurrence of pericardial fluid accumulation. In patients with nonemergency pericardial tamponade, one can first perform echocardiography to confirm the presence of anterior and posterior pericardial fluid, and also perform a right sided heart catheterization to confirm the presence of a tamponade type of physiology, that is, pulsus paradoxicus (decreases in systolic blood pressure greater than 8 mm Hg with inspiration) and diastolic equalization of all the pressures in the right side of the heart. Thus in emergency tamponade one performs pericardiocentesis and gives corticosteroids, whereas in nonemergency cases one confirms the diagnosis (with echocardiography and right heart catheterization) and gives corticosteroids.

In pericardial tamponade with an inflammatory etiology, I use methylprednisolone, 60 mg intravenously and then 20 mg intravenously every 8 hours for 1 to 2 weeks. Intravenous corticosteroid therapy is employed because gastrointestinal tract absorption may have been compromised by the tamponade. Divided doses are employed to render a maximal anti-inflammatory effect. After several weeks prednisone therapy, 60 mg orally every day, can be instituted, and this can be slowly converted to an alternate day regimen.

Corticosteroid therapy commonly prevents nonemergency tamponade from recurring. However, if tamponade recurs, pericardiocentesis should be repeated and the patient should be considered for surgical pericardiectomy. Pericardial tamponade is too dangerous to allow it to occur repeatedly.

Pericardiectomy eliminates the problem of recurrent tamponade and usually controls the symptoms of recurrent pericarditis, although some patients continue to have recurrent chest pain, presumably secondary to continuing epicarditis. Recurring symptoms can be treated as outlined in Table 2.

CONSTRICTIVE PERICARDITIS

This serious complication usually occurs years (occasionally months) after pericarditis—most often in pa-

tients who have had recurrent episodes of pericarditis. The diagnosis is established by cardiac catheterization, and surgical pericardial stripping generally cures it.

RECURRENT PERICARDITIS

Recurrences of idiopathic inflammatory pericarditis should be treated the same as first episodes (see Table 2). In general, therapies that have been successful in the past should be reinstituted. However, if one can substitute aspirin or indomethacin for prednisone therapy, one saves the patient from the side effects of corticosteroids.

Occasionally one is confronted with a "problem patient" who has recurrent bouts of pericarditis that are poorly responsive or unresponsive to long courses of corticosteroids. A small number of these patients have been successfully controlled with immunosuppressive cytotoxic therapy, such as azathioprine or cyclophosphamide (both at low dosages of 1 to 2 mg per kg per day). (Use of these drugs is summarized in the chapter *Postcardiac Injury Syndrome*.) If symptoms are severe and recurrent, one can consider surgical pericardiectomy as a last resort for such "problem patients." Pericardiectomy prevents tamponade and usually prevents severe chest pain, although in rare cases the pain does not remit even with pericardiectomy.

THERAPY OF MYOCARDITIS OR MYOPERICARDITIS

The treatment of myocarditis is not so well defined as that of pericarditis, and there are several reasons for this. First, until recently most cases of myocarditis were assumed to be secondary to a viral infection, and experimental evidence suggested that corticosteroid therapy could worsen viral myocarditis. Recent observations suggest that although the initiating event and first few days of myocardial inflammation in some cases may be a result of viral infection, prolonged myocarditis (longer than 2 to 7 days) is almost certainly due to an inflammatory or immunologically mediated mechanism. Second, until the recent development of transvenous myocardial biopsy as a safe diagnostic procedure, the diagnosis of myocarditis was always presumed but not definitively established until postmortem examination. Therefore the efficacy of drug regimens was difficult to evaluate because one did not have a measure of the degree of inflammation nor did one know whether it was changed by therapy. Third, myocarditis was believed to be a rare disease, and no single institution had enough experience to make statements regarding the relative merits of various medication regimens.

In the past few years the use of transvenous myocardial biopsy has revealed that up to 20 percent of the patients with congestive idiopathic cardiomyopathy have myocarditis. Therefore myocarditis is probably much more common than previously appreciated. Furthermore a number of small series have shown that corticosteroids alone, or corticosteroids with a cytotoxic drug, can decrease signs of myocardial inflammation and improve ventricular function in some patients.

On the basis of current evidence, an anti-inflammatory regimen is likely to be efficacious in a significant number of patients with myocarditis. The extent and severity of myocardial inflammation should be evaluated with measures of ventricular function (echocardiography, nuclear scanning of the heart, and cardiac catheterization and angiography) to confirm the presence of decreased systolic ventricular performance. Echocardiographically determined fractional shortening or nuclear scanning determined ejection fractions should allow the categorization of ventricular function as mild, moderate, or severely reduced. Furthermore, one should evaluate each patient for evidence of an inflammation elevated sedimentation rate or leukocyte count, or a positive gallium scan uptake in the heart (gallium localizes in inflammatory sites). If available, transvenous myocardial biopsy should be performed with light microscopy to detect inflammation, and tissue immunofluorescence should be used to identify immunoglobulin or complement component deposition in the heart. In general, it is useful to perform these tests of ventricular function and myocardial inflammation serially to determine whether there has been a good response to therapy, that is, an improvement in cardiac ventricular function and a decrease in measures of cardiac inflammation.

Restriction of Activity

Patients with myocarditis should be at bed rest during the acute phase of the illness. Experimental evidence suggests that exercise worsens myocardial inflammation. Therefore any strenuous exercise should be avoided. Patients also should receive an optimal cardiac regimen for congestive heart failure (digoxin, diuretics, and afterload reducing drugs) and rhythm disturbances (quinidine, procainamide, lidocaine, digoxin, verapamil, propranolol, or disopyramide). Prolonged bed rest and heart failure predispose to pulmonary and systemic emboli. However, pericarditis is a relative contraindication to long term anticoagulation. One must weigh the risks and benefits of anticoagulation in this situation. In general, I use warfarin to provide anticoagulation in most patients with significant heart failure resulting from myocarditis.

Corticosteroid Therapy of Myocarditis

Presently only retrospective and anecdotal studies are available to suggest that corticosteroid therapy is efficacious in some myocarditis patients. Patients with decreasing ventricular function are the major candidates

for this treatment regimen (Table 3). Therapy should be started with prednisone, 20 mg orally every 8 hours for several weeks, while clinical symptoms and signs, tests of ventricular function, and measures of myocardial inflammation are followed serially. Corticosteroids commonly produce a salutary response within a few days; however, it may take several weeks to reach maximal efficacy. I usually repeat tests of ventricular function and myocardial inflammation 1 to 2 months into therapy. If there are signs of significant improvement, the prednisone dosage is tapered to 60 mg orally every morning. After 2 to 3 months of therapy, the prednisone dosage is slowly tapered to an alternate day regimen. Repeated assays of cardiac performance and inflammation are done at approximately 3 month intervals. Alternate day prednisone therapy is continued for 6 to 12 months and then slowly tapered again following serial testing. A significant proportion of patients have a flare of myocarditis with tapering and require reinstitution of a higher dosage and slower tapering. (The method of tapering to alternate day prednisone has been outlined in the section on pericarditis therapy.) If there is no evidence of improvement after 2 months of prednisone therapy, prednisone is considered ineffective and the dosage should be tapered and discontinued.

Immunosuppressive Therapy with Cytotoxic Drugs

If prednisone is ineffective, or if one is unable to taper the patient off a high daily dosage of prednisone, daily low dosage cytotoxic therapy can be used, which has been shown to be efficacious in a few studies of myocarditis. Cyclophosphamide, 1 to 2 mg per kg per day, or azathioprine, 1 to 2 mg per kg per day, should be added to the prednisone regimen. These drugs do not produce any effect prior to 7 to 10 days of therapy and several months may be necessary for a maximal effect to be evident. Again serial measure of cardiac function and inflammation should be performed to determine whether the therapy is efficacious. If at 3 months no improvement is noted, the drugs should be discontinued. The cytotoxic drugs can be discontinued at once, but the corticosteroid dosage must be slowly tapered. If these drugs do improve cardiac performance and decrease cardiac inflammation, they should be continued for 6 to 12 months and then slowly tapered using serial measures of ventricular function and myocardial inflammation as guides to continued therapy.

The side effects of cyclophosphamide are bone marrow suppression with leukopenia and rarely thrombocytopenia, hemorrhagic cystitis, mild alopecia, rare tumorigenesis, and a significant chance of producing sterility. Azathioprine also produces leukopenia and can produce hepatitis, but there is a very low incidence of sterility. Azathioprine is probably not as powerful (on a milligram basis) an immunosuppressant drug as cyclophosphamide.

Successful safe therapy with these drugs depends upon frequent evaluation for the aforementioned side effects. Specifically, at 7 to 10 days into therapy with these drugs, leukopenia may result, which may necessitate lowering the dosage to prevent the absolute leukocyte count from falling below 3000 cells per cu mm. Therefore daily leukocyte counts are performed during the first several weeks of therapy, and weekly or biweekly counts are performed thereafter with appropriate lowering of the dosage (to maintain the blood leukocyte count higher than 3000 cells per cu mm) if necessary.

Controlled trials now under way should define the subpopulations of patients with myocarditis who are most responsive to therapy with corticosteroids or corticosteroids and cytotoxic drugs. Preliminary data from these studies have revealed that prednisone therapy is capable of increasing ventricular function in patients with evidence of a reactive myocardial process at the 3 month follow-up. However, longer follow-up will be necessary before one can recommend routine treatment of such patients. Currently therapy with these drugs should be undertaken carefully in patients with myocarditis; it should be continued if efficacious, but discontinued if no objective salutary response is demonstrated.

SUGGESTED READING

Fuster V, Gersh BJ, Giuliani ER, Tajik AJ, Brandenburg RO, Grye RL. The natural history of idiopathic dilated cardiomyopathy. Am J Cardiol 1981; 47:525–531.

Johnson RA, Palacios I. Dilated cardiomyopathy of the adult. N Engl J Med 1982; 307:1051–1126.

Mason JW, Billingham ME, Ricci DR. Treatment of acute inflammatory myocarditis assisted by endomyocardial biopsy. Mod Concepts Cardiovasc Dis 1975; 44:65.

Parrillo JE, Aretz HT, Palacios I, Fallon JT, Block PC. The results of transvenous endomyocardial biopsy can frequently be used to diagnose myocardial diseases in patients with idiopathic heart failure: endomyocardial biopsy in 100 consecutive patients revealed a substantial incidence of myocarditis. Circulation 1984; 69:93–101.

IDIOPATHIC THROMBOCYTOPENIC PURPURA

N. RAPHAEL SHULMAN, M.D.

Idiopathic thrombocytopenic purpura is characterized by a low platelet count, a normal or increased number of megakaryocytes in the bone marrow, and no concurrent abnormality or disease process that may account for these findings. There are acute and chronic forms of the disease. It is the most common symptomatic thrombocytopenia.

Early studies showed that plasma from some patients with idiopathic thrombocytopenic purpura contained a gamma globulin that could depress platelet counts when transfused into normal recipients or when autoinfused into a patient after remission. However, even current sensitive in vitro tests cannot detect serum antiplatelet antibodies in most cases (see section on serology). Antibodies that have been detected react via the Fab domain with autologous as well as homologous platelets, and some studies, but not all, indicate that patients with chronic idiopathic thrombocytopenic purpura are more likely to have HLA phenotypes predisposing to autoimmunity (HLA-B8 and HLA-B12 or HLA-DRw2). Although autoimmunity is generally assumed to be the basis for chronic idiopathic thrombocytopenic purpura, other mechanisms such as platelet adsorption of immune complexes, or of foreign antigens followed by antibody, may be responsible in different cases. The latter possibilities may be more common in acute idiopathic thrombocytopenic purpura.

SYMPTOMATOLOGY

Acute idiopathic thrombocytopenic purpura occurs chiefly in children before the age of 10, affecting both sexes with equal frequency. It is self-limited to a period of weeks or months. It most often follows a nonspecific viral infection or one of the various childhood exanthems and responds to certain forms of therapy differently from the chronic form. If the disease lasts for more than approximately 1 year, it should be considered chronic.

Chronic idiopathic thrombocytopenic purpura may have an onset at any age but is rare in childhood, the highest incidence being between the ages of 20 and 50 years; females are affected two to three times more frequently than males. There is no antecedent event related to development of the chronic disease. Most patients with chronic idiopathic thrombocytopenic purpura, if untreated, maintain a subnormal platelet level, which may not significantly vary for long periods of time (years), although temporary (weeks to months) exacerbations may occur, sometimes in association with stress or infections. Spontaneous partial remissions, sometimes lasting for many months, are not unusual in milder cases of the disease. However, spontaneous complete and permanent remissions are rare, even though the course of the disease often tends to ameliorate several months to years after onset. The unpredictable course of idiopathic thrombocytopenic purpura makes evaluation of newer forms of therapy difficult.

Manifestations are variable. Mild idiopathic thrombocytopenic purpura with platelet levels of 20,000 to 30,000 per μl or higher is essentially asymptomatic. When platelet levels are in the range of 10,000 to 20,000 per μl, hemorrhagic symptoms may be trivial. At levels below 5000 per μl, symptoms often become generalized but usually are not severe or life threatening unless levels are below 2000 per μl. Circulating platelets in idiopathic thrombocytopenic purpura are much younger than normal owing to rapid turnover and appear to be more effective hemostatically in that less hemorrhage occurs at a given platelet level in idiopathic thrombocytopenic purpura than in disorders of platelet production, such as marrow aplasia or leukemia. Severe symptoms consisting of confluent elevated petechiae, hemorrhagic bullae in mucous membranes, periodontal bleeding, and retinal hemorrhage usually do not occur unless platelet counts are below 2000 per μl. These ominous occurrences usually precede life threatening massive internal bleeding or intracranial hemorrhage. Intracranial hemorrhage accounts for the 1 to 2 percent overall mortality, and for the 30 to 50 percent mortality in patients with the severest symptoms.

DIAGNOSIS

Idiopathic thrombocytopenic purpura is essentially a diagnosis of exclusion. When the onset of thrombocytopenia is fulminant, drug purpura is the principal disorder to be differentiated from idiopathic thrombocytopenic purpura. If after discontinuing therapy with possible causative drugs, symptoms cease within a few days and the platelets return to normal within 10 days, drug purpura is likely and often can be confirmed by appropriate tests for drug dependent antibodies. Posttransfusion purpura should be considered in adults if blood products were received 5 to 10 days prior to the onset of precipitous thrombocytopenia; there are reliable serologic tests to diagnose this disease. Causes of thrombocytopenia such as septicemia, disseminated intravascular clotting, thrombotic thrombocytopenic purpura, hypersplenism, and a platelet production defect usually are recognized by other associated clinical and laboratory findings. The bone marrow in idiopathic thrombocytopenic purpura characteristically contains normal to greatly increased numbers of megakaryocytes and is an essential examination to rule out hematologic or metastatic malignant disease and aplastic anemia. Differentiation of idiopathic thrombocytopenic purpura from the similar syndrome associated with lupus erythematosus or occult lymphomas may not be possible for months or years if thrombocytopenia is the presenting manifestation of these disorders. An antinuclear antibody test should be carried out.

Because most cases of chronic idiopathic thrombocytopenic purpura respond rapidly to adrenocorticosteroid therapy (see later discussion), a trial with this drug may help differentiate idiopathic thrombocytopenic purpura from an obscure platelet production defect. Platelet survival studies with radiolabeled platelets are rarely necessary to differentiate between the increased platelet destruction of idiopathic thrombocytopenic purpura and disorders of decreased production or hypersplenism.

PATHOPHYSIOLOGY

When radiolabeled platelets are infused into patients with idiopathic thrombocytopenic purpura and disappear from the circulation, they localize primarily in the spleen in patients with mild disease and in the liver in patients with severe disease. Macrophages in these organs (the reticuloendothelial system) and also in bone marrow and blood have been found to contain phagocytized platelets. The long transit time of platelets in the spleen and the unique splenic anatomy that permits close interaction between blood cells and macrophages most likely account for the effectiveness of this organ in sequestering platelets that are lightly sensitized by antibody. The liver, which is less effective in removing lightly sensitized platelets, becomes the predominant organ of sequestration if platelets are heavily sensitized. Heavily sensitized platelets apparently are phagocytosed so efficiently that conditions of interaction between immunologically altered cells and macrophages are less critical; and the liver, by virtue of its size, has more macrophages and a greater blood flow than the spleen. Because platelets in idiopathic thrombocytopenic purpura appear to be destroyed primarily by an indirect process of phagocytosis rather than by direct lysis in the circulation, the most successful forms of therapy are those that interfere with phagocytic function of the reticuloendothelial system.

Platelet survival in idiopathic thrombocytopenic purpura is shortened in proportion to the degree of decrease in the platelet count and becomes normal when patients are in remission. During thrombocytopenia, platelet production is usually normal or, at most, increased two- to threefold. However, spontaneous or therapeutic remissions are rarely, if ever, attributable to a "compensated thrombolytic state" based on increased platelet production. Although some investigators have suggested that the relative amount of sequestered radioactivity in the spleen and liver at the end of platelet survival is predictive of the response to therapy, most studies indicate that such measurements are not helpful in assessing the degree of benefit that may result from splenectomy or any other treatment.

SEROLOGY

The IgG level associated with circulating platelets (platelet associated IgG) is often elevated when platelet levels in idiopathic thrombocytopenic purpura are below approximately 50,000 per μl, and the degree of elevation is roughly inversely proportional to the platelet count. Platelet associated IgG elevations were initially interpreted by most investigators as representing antiplatelet antibody responsible for idiopathic thrombocytopenic purpura and were considered to have the same significance as the direct antiglobulin test in acquired hemolytic anemia. However, in the past few years it has become evident that elevation of the platelet associated IgG level is a nonspecific phenomenon associated with thrombocytopenic states generally, regardless of whether caused by immune mechanisms. It is probably in large part due to the association of various plasma proteins (including albumin) with debris from injured cells. The platelet associated IgG value has no diagnostic or prognostic import.

Techniques applied most recently to measure serum antibody levels in patients with idiopathic thrombocytopenic purpura utilize microtiter wells coated with intact or solubilized normal platelets or Western blots (nitrocellulose transfer) of electrophoresed solubilized platelets as target antigens. The indicator system used to detect antibodies attached to platelets or their components is antihuman globulin labeled with ^{125}I (RIA), an enzyme (ELISA) such as peroxidase, or fluorescein.

Different workers report variable degrees of success in detecting serum antibodies in idiopathic thrombocytopenic purpura, the frequencies of positive results varying from approximately 5 percent to a high of 90 percent. Some idiopathic thrombocytopenic purpura sera react with well defined platelet membrane glycoproteins (GP-Ib, GP-IIb, GP-IIIa) and some with other less well characterized membrane proteins and lipids. As yet, antibodies detected in idiopathic thrombocytopenic purpura provide no predictive value in management. Widespread interest in further analyzing immune reactions in idiopathic thrombocytopenic purpura promise further insight into the nature of the disease and possible approaches to diagnosis and therapy.

TREATMENT

Symptoms rather than the platelet count should dictate therapy. Patients can be harmed by overtreatment in attempts to keep the platelet level closer to normal when much lower levels may effect adequate hemostasis (see discussion of symptomatology).

The acute and chronic forms of idiopathic thrombocytopenic purpura differ in their responses to treatment, which may reflect differences in etiology or differences between the physiologic effects of therapy on the reticuloendothelial system in children and adults.

Acute (Childhood) Idiopathic Thrombocytopenic Purpura

Most patients (over 80 percent) with acute idiopathic thrombocytopenic purpura have mild symptoms and recover spontaneously within a few weeks to months. Treatment is reserved only for serious hemorrhagic manifestations.

Corticosteroids

Corticosteroids are relatively ineffective in the treatment of acute idiopathic thrombocytopenic purpura. Although platelet increases do not occur promptly in most patients given corticosteroids, platelet levels appear to increase sooner, on the average, in groups so treated, compared to untreated patients. A short course (1 to 3 weeks) of high dose prednisone (1.5 to 2 mg per kg per day) along with other treatment (to be discussed) may be advisable if symptoms are pronounced at the onset, since the most serious complication, intracranial hemorrhage, occurs chiefly during the first few weeks of illness. If the acute disease persists longer than 1 month, symptoms usually abate, even if the platelet count does not rise more than 2000 to 5000 per μl above initial levels. When responses to prednisone occur, the drug dosage can be tapered rapidly (approximately 10 percent of the dosage every other day) to find the lowest dosage that prevents symptoms. Children with acute idiopathic thrombocytopenic purpura and platelet counts above 10,000 per μl, if asymptomatic, do not require special restrictions at school or home other than care to avoid vigorous activities that might lead to bruising or head trauma.

Gamma Globulin Therapy

Intravenous gamma globulin therapy has been found to be particularly effective in treating acute idiopathic thrombocytopenic purpura of childhood and has replaced corticosteroids as the treatment of choice. Most studies suggest that the intravenous administration of IgG causes "blockade" of the reticuloendothelial system, perhaps by saturating Fc receptors. IgG in intravenous dosages of 0.4 g per kg given for 5 consecutive days (a total of 2 g per kg, or a total of 1 to 1.5 g per kg given over 4 to 5 days) usually increases depressed platelet levels to safe hemostatic levels within 5 days. Initial rises may occur during the first day of treatment in some cases. Beneficial effects last for periods of several days to several months following one course of infusions, and in some cases thrombocytopenia does not recur. If further treatment is necessary, adequate responses often can be obtained by single doses of 0.4 to 1.0 g per kg. Little or no toxicity is associated with intravenous therapy. Experience is insufficient for us to know the expected frequency of response with respect to the severity of disease or the optimal dose under different clinical circumstances. However, all evidence indicates that intravenous IgG therapy is effective in acute idiopathic thrombocytopenic purpura when hemorrhagic symptoms are severe. Prior infusion of IgG does not interfere with, and may act synergistically with, any other form of treatment. The major drawback to intravenous IgG therapy is the high cost.

If the history and peripheral blood examination in a young child are strongly suggestive of acute idiopathic thrombocytopenic purpura, a rapid response to intravenous IgG therapy would be confirmatory and make a bone marrow examination unnecessary.

Splenectomy

Splenectomy for acute idiopathic thrombocytopenic purpura is done only as an emergency procedure for life threatening hemorrhage. It removes a major organ of platelet sequestration. The decision to perform splenectomy is most often precipitated by symptoms of intracranial hemorrhage, either in association with other severe hemorrhagic symptoms or following trauma in milder forms of the disease. A single intravenous infusion of 0.4 to 1.0 g per kg of IgG combined with, or followed by, platelet transfusions may result in a sufficiently high level of circulating platelets to vitiate indication for splenectomy or may promote better survival of platelets during and after operation.

In an emergency, splenectomy may have to be performed when the platelet count is less than 2000 per μl. Although postoperative morbidity due to intraperitoneal or incisional bleeding is increased under these circumstances, the amount of hemorrhage is usually surprisingly scant. Peritoneal drainage usually prevents serious abdominal complications from hemorrhage if the platelet level fails to increase after splenectomy.

The mortality from emergency splenectomy in idiopathic thrombocytopenic purpura has been reported to vary from 1.4 to 4.9 percent and the subsequent postsplenectomy fatality due to sepsis in childhood cases is approximately 1 to 3 percent. However, the mortality in patients with idiopathic thrombocytopenic purpura and intracranial hemorrhage approaches 100 percent. Splenectomy may reduce the incidence of fatal outcome of this complication to less than 50 percent, and use of intravenous IgG and platelet transfusion combined with splenectomy may further improve survival. All splenectomized patients should be given pneumococcal vaccine, and *Haemophilus influenzae* type b vaccine also should be considered. Some recommend that children less than

6 years old, the group with the greatest susceptibility to infection, should be given prophylactic penicillin therapy.

Platelet Transfusion

Platelet transfusions are often used as a temporizing measure in attempts to prevent rapid progression of life threatening hemorrhage, but the markedly short survival of transfused platelets in severely thrombocytopenic patients usually nullifies their utility. The effectiveness of platelet transfusions may be enhanced by prior intravenous treatment with IgG or splenectomy. If the platelet count cannot be elevated by medication prior to splenectomy, platelet transfusions will not be of significant benefit. If the physician feels compelled to transfuse platelets in association with surgery, transfusion should at least be reserved until the splenic pedicle is clamped, rather than given preoperatively.

Plasma Exchange

Plasma exchange to decrease the titer of antiplatelet antibody has received limited evaluation as treatment for acute idiopathic thrombocytopenic purpura chiefly in adults. Among those with severe thrombocytopenia who have had favorable responses, marked elevation of the platelet level occurred within 1 to several days. The beneficial effect of plasma exchange may have been due to a factor in the infused plasma, perhaps IgG, rather than to the modest decreases in circulating antibody or immune complexes.

Chronic Idiopathic Thrombocytopenic Purpura

The initial therapy in chronic idiopathic thrombocytopenic purpura is corticosteroids followed, if necessary, by splenectomy. Patients not responding satisfactorily to these measures are considered refractory and are candidates for one or another of the newer, less predictable methods of treatment.

Corticosteroids

Corticosteroids act primarily by immediately inhibiting the reticuloendothelial system and, when given over long periods, may decrease antibody production slightly. Steroids do not interfere with antibody reactions and apparently do not enhance capillary resistance directly without a concomitant, albeit slight, rise in the platelet level.

An initial dosage sufficient to cause maximal inhibition of platelet sequestration is given (1 to 1.5 mg per kg per day). Rarely dosages as high as 4 mg per kg per day may be effective for short periods (5 to 10 days) in elevating the platelet count in otherwise refractory patients. No adrenocorticosteroid is more advantageous than prednisone, provided equivalent dosages are given. A favorable clinical response to steroids (with at least partial correction of the platelet count) is obtained in 70 to 90 percent of the patients. If a response occurs, some elevation of the platelet count or amelioration of symptomatology usually is evident within 1 to 3 days, a maximal response usually occurring within 5 to 10 days. High dosages of steroids should not be given for more than approximately 10 days if the response is poor, since improvement is unlikely to occur with prolonged administration of the drug and toxicity may be considerable. To minimize the toxic side effects of steroids, the initial high dosage should be tapered to determine the amount that will maintain the platelet count in the range of 25,000 to 50,000 per μl. This platelet level may be associated with an increased tendency to bruise following trauma and rarely is associated with spontaneous hemorrhage such as petechiae or menorrhagia but, in our experience and that of others, never with serious hemorrhage.

In tapering the corticosteroid dosage, a reasonable incremental decrease for prednisone is 10 mg every other day until a dosage of 40 mg per day is reached, followed by a decrease of 2.5 to 5 mg every third day. This regimen permits assessment of the minimal effective steroid dosage, provided platelet counts are determined two to three times a week. If the platelet count falls to an unsafe level, the dosage is increased to the amount given prior to the fall, and this dosage is usually satisfactory for maintenance.

Platelet sequestration appears to be very sensitive to the in vivo steroid level. A regimen in which the same total dosage per day is given twice daily may be more effective than a single dose, but twice the daily dosage given every other day is usually much less effective. In the initial course of treatment, a maintenance dosage of steroids is usually given for about 4 weeks. Since steroids do not alter the underlying disorder, this form of treatment is expedient in anticipation of possible spontaneous amelioration. If results are not satisfactory when the drug is discontinued, the maintenance steroid dosage that had been given previously usually has the same effectiveness when reinstituted. Several courses of steroids may be tried, depending on the patient's acceptance of splenectomy, but in most cases of chronic idiopathic thrombocytopenic purpura, continued symptomatology or recurrence after steroid induced remissions eventually leads to splenectomy after 6 months to 1 year.

The probability of responsiveness to therapy cannot be judged by the platelet count or the symptomatology at presentation. However, patients whose platelet counts rise to levels of 50,000 per μl or higher within 1 week after corticosteroid administration have a much more favorable prognosis for an effective response to contin-

ued corticosteroid therapy or to splenectomy than do those who are initially refractory to this medication.

Splenectomy

Significant improvement is obtained in 70 to 90 percent of the patients and permanent complete remission occurs in 45 to 60 percent following splenectomy. Even if splenectomy does not prevent the recurrence of symptoms in more severe cases, absence of the spleen usually facilitates management by decreasing the steroid requirement. Corticosteroids are used preoperatively to bring the platelet count to a safe hemostatic level if possible (more than 30,000 per μl), and the dosages are tapered postoperatively as soon as it is evident that a satisfactory platelet response has occurred. Other forms of treatment may be tried preoperatively if steroids are ineffective (e.g., see discussion of acute idiopathic thrombocytopenic purpura).

The rate of platelet rise in those who attain a good response is usually at least 20,000 per μl per day and may be several times this rate, reaching a peak in 7 to 12 days. A favorable long term response is likely if the peak value is greater than 500,000 per μl. A peak of 1 million per μl is not uncommon and values of 2 million or more per μl are observed occasionally. Thereafter the platelet count returns to a normal value over a period of weeks. If the count exceeds 1 million per μl, aspirin, 300 mg per day, or low dose heparin therapy is sometimes instituted as prophylaxis against thrombosis, although no controlled study has suggested that this therapy is necessary.

Other Measures

Pneumococcal vaccine should be given at least 2 weeks preoperatively, if possible, because the immune response is impaired after splenectomy (also see the discussion of acute idiopathic thrombocytopenic purpura).

Accessory spleens not apparent at splenectomy may cause a failure to respond immediately postoperatively or months to years after an initial good response. Accessory spleens can be detected by external scanning or intraoperatively after injecting ^{111}In labeled platelets or heated ^{51}Cr labeled red cells. However, accessory splenectomy usually is not beneficial.

Platelet transfusions are used as in acute idiopathic thrombocytopenic purpura (see foregoing discussion).

The following therapeutic modalities are effective in some cases of refractory idiopathic thrombocytopenic purpura. The more toxic drugs (vinca alkaloids and immunosuppressives) should not be used unless splenectomy and steroid therapy prove to be inadequate or unacceptable.

Danazol, an attenuated androgen, may act by downgrading macrophage Fc receptors. In different reports 10 to 50 percent of patients with refractory idiopathic thrombocytopenic purpura sustained partial to complete remissions while taking danazol. The dosage used was 400 to 600 mg daily in divided doses. Increases in platelet counts occurred after 2 to 6 weeks of therapy, with maximal rises occurring as late as 10 weeks. Corticosteroid dosages often could be tapered or discontinued during danazol treatment. A masculinizing effect in females occasionally was a distressing side effect.

Vincristine inhibits phagocytes and with long term treatment, possibly antibody production. It stimulates the release of platelets but probably does not increase overall production. Given as an intravenous bolus at 1 to 2 mg per sq in, it can produce elevations of platelet counts beginning within 2 or 3 days and peaking in 4 to 7 days. However, platelet levels usually fall to pretreatment levels by 1 to 2 weeks. Repeated doses can be given at 1 to 2 week intervals. Rarely a sustained response is obtained for several weeks to months. If there is no response to three doses, further therapy is unlikely to produce benefit. Toxic effects, including severe paresthesias, neuropathies, constipation, and hair loss, can be cumulative and progressively severe, particularly in adults after age 50, but usually are reversed after discontinuation of the drug. This drug is too toxic for use in any but the most severe cases of idiopathic thrombocytopenic purpura.

Vinblastine given by slow infusion or vinblastine preincubated with platelets has essentially the same therapeutic and toxic effects as vincristine.

The intravenous administration of gamma globulin appears to have beneficial effects in children with chronic idiopathic thrombocytopenic purpura, although less frequently than in children with acute disease, and the effects are more transient. The intravenous administration of IgG is rarely effective in refractory cases in adults and because of its expense is not useful in the routine treatment of adult cases. However, in idiopathic thrombocytopenic purpura in all age groups, IgG given intravenously appears to have a place in the management of emergency hemorrhagic events and in preparation for splenectomy when the platelet count is severely depressed and unresponsive to corticosteroids.

Immunosuppressive therapy with azathioprine or cyclophosphamide has been reported to produce responses in refractory cases of idiopathic thrombocytopenic purpura if given daily for a minimum of 1 to 2 months. Results are difficult to interpret, because the best responders have been those who have had the disease for less than 1 year, a time during which spontaneous amelioration of symptoms is frequent; moreover, no control studies have been done to verify the initial optimistic reports. A major immediate potential toxic effect of these drugs is suppression of thrombopoiesis, leading to exacerbation of hemorrhagic symptoms. Other toxic effects include leukopenia, gonadal dysfunction, and increased carcinogenic risk. We have never observed a clearly beneficial response to either drug in refractory idiopathic thrombocytopenic purpura and believe that the risks of such treatment outweigh the unknown potential advantage. Bolus intravenous cytoxan therapy, 1 g per sq m given monthly, appears to be as effective as daily oral doses and is less toxic.

Other drugs that have been reported to benefit patients with refractory idiopathic thrombocytopenic purpura, but for which evidence is meager and toxicity considerable, are frentizol, colchicine, bleomycin, and cyclosporine.

IDIOPATHIC THROMBOCYTOPENIC PURPURA AND PREGNANCY

The overall fetal mortality associated with maternal idiopathic thrombocytopenic purpura is approximately 2 percent due to hemorrhage in live births, approximately 5 percent due to hemorrhage in stillbirths, and approximately 8 percent due to other causes.

The incidence of passively transferred neonatal idiopathic thrombocytopenic purpura correlates somewhat with the maternal platelet count of mothers who are not taking steroids. In nonsplenectomized mothers with platelet counts over 100,000 per μl, approximately 30 percent of the infants are affected, and with counts that are less than 100,000 platelets per μl, approximately 75 percent are affected. At a given platelet level splenectomized mothers are more likely to have thrombocytopenic infants than nonsplenectomized mothers. During pregnancy mothers with idiopathic thrombocytopenic purpura should be given corticosteroids for the same indications as other patients. However, splenectomy should not be performed, except for uncontrollable hemorrhage, because the operative morbidity is high, particularly late in pregnancy, and the incidence of abortion postoperatively is approximately 25 percent. Postpartum hemorrhage may be excessive from lacerations or episiotomy but usually not from the placental site. There has been no report of maternal death due to idiopathic thrombocytopenic purpura in the past 30 years.

Mothers with idiopathic thrombocytopenic purpura in remission who take high doses of prednisone often give birth to thrombocytopenic infants because the fetal concentration of the active metabolite of this corticosteroid is too low to be protective. The use of high dose dexamethasone or betamethasone therapy in mothers to provide an effective fetal level of active corticosteroid would be more likely to ameliorate antenatal thrombocytopenia. The use of high intravenous doses of IgG in mothers in attempts to increase the fetal IgG level or to competitively interfere with placental transfer of idiopathic thrombocytopenic purpura antibody is under investigation. Cesarean section has been recommended to decrease birth trauma when the maternal platelet count is less than 10^5 per μl. However, intrauterine intracranial hemorrhage and porencephaly can occur in thrombocytopenic fetus. There are no data establishing the value of cesarean section for prevention of neonatal intracranial hemorrhage.

In neonatal idiopathic thrombocytopenic purpura, the infant's platelet count may be normal at birth and fall gradually during the first week, or be depressed at birth but reach a nadir in approximately 1 week.

Prednisone, 1 to 2 mg per kg, should be given to newborn infants with symptomatic thrombocytopenia, and after a response the dosage can be tapered to the lowest level capable of maintaining a hemostatically effective platelet level. The intravenous administration of IgG, 0.4 g per kg appears to be as effective as steroids, and the two medications can be given together because of their synergistic effect in severe cases. In rare instances of poor response to medication, exchange transfusion should be instituted; repeated exchanges of one blood volume may be necessary. In addition, platelet transfusion may be necessary if serious hemorrhage occurs. Splenectomy should not be done.

SUGGESTED READING

Harrington WJ, Minnich V, Arimura G. The autoimmune thrombocytopenias. Prog Hematol 1956; 1:166–192.
Karpatkin S. Autoimmune thrombocytopenic purpura. Blood 1980; 56:329–343.
McMillan R. Chronic idiopathic thrombocytopenic purpura. N Engl J Med 1981; 304:1135–1147.
Shulman NR, Jordan JV. Platelet immunology. In: Coleman RW, Marder VJ, Salzman EW, eds. Hemostasis and thrombosis. 2nd ed. Philadelphia: JB Lippincott, 1987; 452.
Shulman NR, Jordan JV. Platelet kinetics. In: Coleman RW, Marder VJ, Salzman EW. eds. Hemostasis and thrombosis. 2nd ed. Philadelphia: JB Lippincott, 1987; 431.
Shulman NR, Marder VJ, Weinrach RS. Similarities between known antiplatelet antibodies and the factor responsible for thrombocytopenia in idiopathic thrombocytopenic purpura: physiologic, serologic, and isotopic studies. Ann NY Acad Sci 1965; 124:499–542.

AUTOIMMUNE HEMOLYTIC ANEMIA

ALAN D. SCHREIBER, M.D.

The autoimmune hemolytic anemias represent a group of disorders in which individuals produce antibodies directed toward one or more of their own erythrocyte membrane antigens. This in turn leads to destruction of the erythrocytes. An effective manner of approaching autoimmune hemolytic anemia is to determine which class of antibody is responsible for the hemolysis. In general, there are two major classes of antierythrocyte antibodies that produce hemolysis in man: IgG and IgM. The pattern of red blood cell clearance, the site of organ sequestration, the response to therapy, and the prognosis all relate to the class of antierythrocyte antibody involved.

This article deals only with immune hemolytic anemia caused by antierythrocyte antibodies. Paroxysmal nocturnal hemoglobinuria is a disease in which immune hemolysis is probably often antibody independent. In this chronic hemolytic disorder, complement activation, occurring in either the presence or absence of antibody, results in excessive binding of individual complement components onto the abnormal erythrocyte membrane present in this disorder. This results in excessive intravascular lysis of these erythrocytes. The excessive complement activation appears to be largely due to the absence of membrane derived complement regulatory proteins on the erythrocytes of patients with paroxysmal nocturnal hemoglobulinemia, favoring activation of the terminal complement components.

IgM INDUCED IMMUNE HEMOLYTIC ANEMIA

Autoimmune hemolytic anemia caused by IgM antibody in humans is generally restricted to the clinical entity of cold hemagglutinin disease. The most common form of chronic cold hemagglutinin disease is the primary or idiopathic form caused by an IgM antibody. This is a clonal disorder and is associated with the presence of a monoclonal IgM antibody, which usually has a high cold agglutinin titer. The IgM antibody is usually directed against the I antigen or related antigens on the human erythrocyte membrane. As with all IgM antibodies, agglutinating activity is particularly efficient because of the multiple antigen combining sites on the IgM molecule. The cold agglutinin titer represents the least dilution of patient plasma or serum capable of agglutinating human red blood cells in the cold. In most patients with hemolysis the cold agglutinin titer is greater than 1:1000.

Secondary cold hemagglutinin disease is most commonly associated with an underlying Mycoplasma infection, particularly *Mycoplasma pneumoniae*. It also may occur with other infections, such as infectious mononucleosis and cytomegalovirus. Cold hemagglutinin disease (IgM induced immune hemolytic anemia) also can be seen with an underlying immunoproliferative disorder, such as chronic lymphocytic leukemia, non-Hodgkin's lymphoma, or systemic lupus erythematosus. The disease may be chronic, and the IgM protein may be of restricted heterogeneity (oligoclonal) or may even be monoclonal. When this is the case, one should suspect an underlying malignant immunoproliferative disorder and the prognosis is adversely affected.

As in all patients with autoimmune hemolytic anemia, erythrocyte survival is generally proportional to the amount of antibody on the erythrocyte surface. In cold hemagglutinin disease the extent of hemolysis is a function of the titer of the antibody (cold agglutinin titer), the thermal amplitude of the IgM antibody (the highest temperature at which the antibody is active), and the level of the circulating control proteins of the C3b inactivator system. Hemolysis is complement dependent, and the IgM coated erythrocytes become coated with C3b by classic complement pathway activation. These C3b coated erythrocytes are cleared primarily by the macrophage C3b receptors in the liver. Two uncommon variants of cold hemagglutinin disease, low IgM titer cold hemagglutinin disease and cold hemagglutinin disease mediated by IgG antibody, are more responsive to therapy.

IgG INDUCED IMMUNE HEMOLYTIC ANEMIA

In IgG induced immune hemolytic anemia, the antibodies are of the IgG class and the antigen to which the antibody is directed is usually an Rh erythrocyte antigen. The antibody exerts its maximal activity at 37°C, and thus this entity has been termed warm antibody induced hemolytic anemia. IgG induced immune hemolytic anemia may occur without an apparent underlying disease (idiopathic type); however, it may also occur with an underlying immunoproliferative disorder, such as chronic lymphocytic leukemia, non-Hodgkin's lymphoma, or systemic lupus erythematosus. The signs and symptoms are those of anemia, in general. The diagnosis is established by directly examining the erythrocyte surface for the presence of cell surface proteins (IgG and C3b).

In addition to C3b receptors, macrophages within the reticuloendothelial system have receptors for the Fc fragment of IgG, called Fcγ receptors. The macrophage Fcγ receptors can detect IgG coated erythrocytes, bind them, make them spherical, or phagocytose them in the absence of C3b. However, once C3b is placed on the erythrocyte surface, through complement activation, erythrocyte clearance is further accelerated. Thus, IgG coated erythrocytes are progressively cleared from the circulation by macrophages possessing an Fcγ receptor. Hemolysis is almost always extravascular, and these IgG coated cells are cleared predominantly in the spleen.

DRUG INDUCED IMMUNE HEMOLYTIC ANEMIA

Drug induced immune hemolytic anemia can be divided into four major pathophysiologic groups. The clinical signs and symptoms are identical to those of the other autoimmune hemolytic anemias. The diagnosis is established primarily by the history.

Hapten Type

This type of drug induced immune hemolytic anemia classically develops in patients exposed to high doses of penicillin. A portion of the penicillin molecule or its active metabolites combines with the erythrocyte surface, acting as a hapten. This induces an antibody response directed against the penicillin coated erythrocyte membrane. This is usually an IgG response, and complement activation is common. The patient's erythrocytes become coated with IgG and often with C3. Patients rarely develop this syndrome unless they have received 10 to 20 million units of penicillin a day. The diagnosis can be established by incubating the patient's serum with donor erythrocytes preincubated with penicillin. The deposition of IgG antibody occurs only in the presence of penicillin and can be detected with the Coombs' test.

Quinidine Type

This type of autoimmune hemolytic anemia most commonly occurs with the use of quinidine or its derivatives. Commonly called an innocent bystander reaction, it is believed to be due to an antibody directed against quinidine bound to a plasma protein acting as a hapten. This interaction results in activation of the classic complement pathway and deposition of C3 on the erythrocyte surface. With quinidine it is commonly caused by IgM antiquinidine antibody. The diagnosis can be established in vitro by examining for complement deposition on donor erythrocytes by patient serum, which occurs only in the presence of the drug, e.g., quinidine.

α-Methyldopa Type

α-Methyldopa and its derivatives produce a clinical syndrome virtually identical to IgG induced immune hemolytic anemia. The mechanism of the IgG antibody formation is poorly understood. Many patients (up to 25 percent) exposed to α-methyldopa develop a positive Coombs' test for IgG. These IgG antibodies have specificity for the Rh locus. Most patients do not develop sufficient IgG coating for hemolysis; however, hemolysis is observed in approximately 0.8 percent of the patients exposed to α-methyldopa. The diagnosis can be made by examining the patient's red blood cells and plasma. In vitro it is not necessary for the drug to be present for the patient's plasma to deposit IgG antibody on donor erythrocytes. A similar syndrome has been reported with mefenamic acid.

Nonspecific Coating

Nonspecific coating of the erythrocyte surface has been observed with the antibiotic cephalothin, in which cephalothin becomes bound to the erythrocyte membrane and causes the red blood cells to be coated by many plasma proteins. The Coombs' test is positive, but hemolytic anemia is rare. Cephalothin, however, can cause hemolytic anemia by acting as a hapten by a mechanism similar to that of penicillin.

In all these types the patients respond to withdrawal of the offending drug. If necessary, a brief course of glucocorticoid therapy can be effectively administered.

THERAPEUTIC MEASURES

In many patients with IgG or IgM induced immune hemolytic anemia, no therapeutic invention is necessary, since the hemolysis may be mild. If an underlying disease is present, control of this disease often brings the hemolytic anemia under control as well. However, if the patient is having significant anemia secondary to hemolysis, therapeutic intervention is in order.

Glucocorticoids

Patients with IgG induced immune hemolytic anemia usually respond to glucocorticoid therapy in dosages equivalent to 40 to 120 mg of prednisone a day. Glucocorticoids work in IgG induced hemolytic anemia by three primary mechanisms. First, they decrease the production of the abnormal IgG antibody; this is the most common effect and produces a gradual increase in the hemoglobin level within 2 to 6 weeks. Second, glucocorticoids in several cases have been demonstrated to cause the elution of IgG antibody from the erythrocyte surface, improving red blood cell survival; this is probably an uncommon effect of therapy. Third, glucocorticoids have been shown in vitro and in vivo to interfere with the macrophage Fcγ and to a lesser extent C3b receptors responsible for the erythrocyte destruction in this disease. This effect may be rapid and is probably responsible for the rise in the hemoglobin level that occurs in some patients within 1 to 4 days of therapy.

This action of glucocorticoids causes an improvement in erythrocyte survival despite the continued presence of IgG and C3b on the erythrocyte surface.

Once a therapeutic response is achieved, tapering of the glucocorticoid dosage should be initiated. This may take several months. Alternate day glucocorticoid therapy may be utilized during this time, or until the patient's hematologic picture stabilizes.

Since glucocorticoids may improve erythrocyte survival by interfering with macrophage detection of IgG coated erythrocytes, the Coombs' test may remain positive in the face of improved erythrocyte survival. Thus, some patients may continue to improve hematologically despite a persistently positive Coombs' test.

Approximately 80 percent of the patients have an initial response to high dose glucocorticoid therapy. Nevertheless only 20 to 30 percent have a sustained response following discontinuation of therapy. Several patients maintain control of the hemolytic process with low or medium dose glucocorticoid therapy. For the patients who are steroid dependent, the initial and long term side effects of steroids must be considered. These include gastritis, peptic ulcer disease, emotional lability, exacerbation of diabetes and hypertension, electrolyte imbalance, increased appetite and weight gain, a moon-like facies, osteoporosis, myopathy, and increased susceptibility to infection. The severity of these side effects relates to both dosage and duration of therapy. We recommend splenectomy for patients who are unresponsive to steroids or who require more than 10 to 20 mg of prednisone equivalent per day or 20 to 25 mg every other day for maintenance.

Each patient requires individual evaluation of the underlying disease, surgical risk, extent of anemia, and steroid intolerance. In some patients the presence of a mild hemolytic anemia may be preferable to splenectomy or other treatment options. The initial goal of therapy is to return the hematologic values to normal with nontoxic levels of glucocorticoid therapy. However, in some patients a secondary goal of achieving a decrease in hemolysis to a clinically asymptomatic state with minimal glucocorticoid side effects is more realistic. Alternate day glucocorticoid therapy is worthy of consideration in many patients. Its efficacy is not generally appreciated.

Glucocorticoids are not usually effective in cold hemagglutinin disease, probably because these patients generally have large amounts of IgM antierythrocyte antibody and large amounts of C3b on the erythrocyte surface. In addition, some of the hemolysis may be intravascular. The few patients with a low titer cold hemagglutinin disease syndrome, in which the IgM antierythrocyte antibody is active at temperatures approaching 37° C, and patients with cold hemagglutinin disease mediated by IgG antibodies do respond to glucocorticoid therapy. Patients with cold hemagglutinin disease respond best to the avoidance of cold and control of the underlying disease. Fortunately, in many patients hemolytic anemia is mild.

Splenectomy

The reticuloendothelial system of the spleen with its resident macrophages is the major site for sequestration of IgG coated blood cells. This appears to be the result of the unique circulatory pathways in the spleen whereby hemoconcentration occurs in the splenic cords. This in turn results in intimate contact between macrophages (with their membrane Fcγ receptors) and IgG coated blood cells in the presence of a minimal amount of plasma IgG; plasma IgG competitively inhibits the macrophage Fcγ receptor binding of IgG coated cells. Thus, the spleen is usually the major site of red cell sequestration in autoimmune hemolytic anemia, with the liver accounting for a variable degree of sequestration.

Removal of the major site of red cell destruction is an effective therapeutic strategy in IgG induced immune hemolytic anemia. The incidence of response to splenectomy is approximately 50 to 70 percent; however, the majority of the responses are partial remissions. The partial remissions are often helpful in that they result in a lessening of the rate of hemolysis, with a rise in the hemoglobin value, or allow for a reduction in the amount of glucocorticoids needed to control the hemolytic anemia. Patients who are unresponsive to glucocorticoids, who require moderate to high maintenance doses of glucocorticoids, or who have developed glucocorticoid intolerance are generally candidates for splenectomy. ^{51}Cr labeled red cell kinetic studies are probably not beneficial, since the procedure is time consuming, expensive, and not a reliable indicator of the response to splenectomy.

Splenectomy is effective in IgG induced hemolytic anemia because the cells are cleared primarily in the spleen. In addition, it has been shown that splenectomy can decrease the production of the IgG antierythrocyte antibodies, as the spleen contains a large B cell pool. The patients in whom splenectomy fails are probably those with very high concentrations of IgG on the erythrocyte surface; in such patients the liver plays a more prominent role in clearance.

Splenectomy is not effective in patients with traditional cold hemagglutinin disease because IgM coated erythrocytes are cleared predominantly in the liver, not in the spleen. An occasional case in which a patient with apparent IgM induced hemolytic anemia responded to splenectomy has been reported. This may be due to decreased production of IgM antibody by the spleen in these patients. However, patients with the uncommon IgG induced cold hemagglutinin disease syndrome do respond to splenectomy.

The side effects of splenectomy vary greatly from institution to institution. We generally have attempted to identify one or two surgical colleagues who carry out most of the splenectomies in our patient population. This experience enhances both the surgical procedures (speed and safety) and the postoperative follow-up. Postoperative thromboses and infection can occur both above and below the diaphragm. The risk of morbidity and mortality is greater in older patients, in those with related underlying disease (benign or malignant immunoproliferative disorder), and in those with unrelated medical problems, and to some extent is influenced by the intensity of glucocorticoid side effects. Thus, a thoughtful analysis of the benefit-versus-risk factors needs to be undertaken for each patient. A final consideration is that adults who undergo splenectomy in rare instances may have a susceptibility to life threatening infection, particularly with pneumococcus. For this reason we generally immunize patients with Pneumovax some weeks prior to elective splenectomy in an effort to reduce this long term complication.

Immunosuppressive Drugs

Several chemotherapeutic drugs with known immunosuppressive effects have been used to treat immune hemolytic anemia. The drugs most commonly used include the thiopurines (6-mercaptopurine, azathioprine, and thioguanine) and alkylating drugs (cyclophosphamide and chlorambucil). Immunosuppressive therapy may be effective for treating IgG induced immune hemolytic anemia when the patient is refractory to steroids or splenectomy. Immunosuppressive drugs work by decreasing the production of antibody, and, therefore, it generally takes at least 2 weeks before any therapeutic result is observed.

Patients are selected for immunosuppressive therapy because they have a clinically unacceptable degree of hemolytic anemia resistant to glucocorticoid and splenectomy treatment. Alternatively, they may be intolerant of or resistant to glucocorticoids and poor surgical risks for splenectomy. Clinical benefit has been noted in about 50 percent of the patients. A reasonable trial of this drug is about 3 to 4 months, and if no beneficial effect is noted, therapy is discontinued. If clinical benefit occurs, one can maintain the dosage level for a total of 6 months and then taper over several months. During therapy, patients are instructed to maintain a high fluid intake to reduce the incidence of chemical cystitis seen with cyclophosphamide. In addition, weekly blood counts are required to monitor bone marrow suppression, which can occur with any of these immunosuppressive drugs. The dosage should be adjusted to maintain the leukocyte count higher than 2000, the granulocyte count higher than 1000, and the platelet count higher than 50,000 to 100,000 per cubic mm.

Cyclophosphamide is usually well tolerated, but a variety of side effects may occur, including bone marrow suppression (primarily leukopenia), hemorrhagic cystitis, nausea, partial alopecia, amenorrhea, and impaired spermatogenesis. The use of alkylating agents may also have long term potential for increasing the incidence of malignant disease, particularly acute leukemia. These side effects require that the clinical indications for immunosuppressive therapy be strong and that patient exposure to the drug be limited.

Aside from supportive measures, immunosuppressive therapy has been the major therapy in traditional high titer IgM induced cold hemagglutinin disease. Alkylating drugs (cyclophosphamide or chlorambucil) have been the primary drugs used and appear to have a beneficial effect in up to 50 to 60 percent of the cases. Unresponsiveness is seen probably because so little antibody is necessary for significant hemolysis to occur.

Miscellaneous Therapy

Plasmapheresis has been used in patients with severe IgG induced immune hemolytic anemia, but has met with limited success, possibly because more than half the IgG is extravascular and the plasma contains only small amounts of the antibody (most of the antibody being on the red blood cell surface). However, plasmapheresis has been effective in IgM induced hemolytic anemia. This is only a short term benefit, but has reduced the level of cold agglutinins by virtue of the fact that IgM is a high molecular weight molecule that remains predominantly within the intravascular space.

Other measures that have been used effectively in IgG induced hemolysis are vincristine and vinblastine infusions, gamma globulin infusion, and hormonal therapy. Gamma globulin infusion is effective in IgG induced immune hemolytic anemia, probably primarily by inhibiting clearance of the IgG coated cells. In hormonal therapy the synthetic androgen danazol has been effective in several patients. Because of the limited side effects (limited masculinizing effects, mild weight gain), danazol or a similar drug may become an attractive alternative to glucocorticoid therapy in some patients with IgG induced immune hemolytic anemia. However, danazol does not appear to be effective in IgM induced hemolytic anemia. The data suggest that one mechanism of danazol's effect is through modulation (inhibition) of macrophage Fcγ receptor expression. Hormonal influence of macrophage Fcγ expression probably explains, at least in part, the increased clinical activity of IgG induced immune hemolytic anemia during pregnancy. During pregnancy, blood estrogen levels increase to an extent that they enhance splenic macrophage Fcγ receptor expression and thereby accelerate the clearance of IgG coated cells.

Supportive Transfusion Therapy

The majority of patients with autoimmune hemolytic anemia do not require transfusion therapy because the anemia has occurred gradually and there has been physiologic compensation. However, occasionally patients experience acute or severe anemia and require transfusions for support until other treatment modalities reduce the hemolysis. Transfusion therapy is complicated by the fact that the blood bank may be unable to find any "compatible" blood. This is because the autoantibody is directed to a component of the Rh locus that is present on the erythrocytes of essentially all potential donors, regardless of Rh subtype. The usual recommendation is for the blood bank to identify the most compatible units of blood of the patient's own major blood group and Rh type. With this approach it is unlikely that the donor blood will have a dramatically shortened red blood cell survival.

The indication for transfusion therapy is prevention of any serious complications due to the anemia. These include angina, congestive heart failure, and central nervous system symptoms of hypoxia (for example, syncope, lightheadedness, impairment of mental acuity). In addition, if the patient is experiencing blood loss, transfusion is required. The slow infusion of 1 to 2 units of packed red cells usually improves the clinical status of the patient. Elderly patients especially need to be monitored for circulatory overload and for transfusion reactions. The latter are unlikely to be serious since hemolysis is usually extravascular. In the rare patient with little or no response to steroids and a continuing need for transfusions because of serious side effects of anemia over the first 4 to 6 days of therapy, an early decision to carry out splenectomy may be necessary.

In cold agglutinin disease it is important to prewarm all intravenous infusions, including whole blood, to 37° C, since a decrease in temperature locally in a vein can enhance binding of the IgM antibody to red cells and accelerate the hemolytic process. In addition, erythrocyte agglutination in a small blood vessel can result in vascular compromise and ischemia of an extremity.

SUGGESTED READING

Friedman D, Nettl F, Schreiber AD. Effect of estradiol and steroid analogues on the clearance of IgG coated erythrocytes. J Clin Invest 1985; 75:162–167.
LoBuglio AF, Cotran RS, Jandl JH. Red cells coated with immunoglobulin G: binding and sphering by mononuclear cells in man. Science 1967; 158:1582–1585.
Schreiber AD, Frank MM. Autoimmune hemolytic anemia. In: Samter M, ed. Immunological diseases. 4th ed. Boston: Little, Brown, 1987.
Schreiber AD, Frank MM. Role of antibody and complement in the immune clearance and destruction of erythrocytes. I. In vivo effects of the IgG and IgM complement-fixing sites. J Clin Invest 1972; 51:575–582.
Silberstein LE, Berkman EM, Schreiber AD. Cold hemagglutinin disease associated with IgG cold-reactive antibody. Ann Intern Med 1987, 106:238–242.

AUTOIMMUNE LEUKOPENIA

LAURENCE A. BOXER, M.D.

NEUTROPENIA

The terms "autoimmune leukopenia" and "autoimmune neutropenia" are often used synonymously to describe conditions in which autobodies to mature neutrophils or their precursors are associated with accelerated cell destruction and a reduced circulating blood neutrophil count. Leukopenia is generally defined as a reduction in the total white cell count below 4000 cells per dl. Normal neutrophil levels should be stratified for age, race, and other factors. For whites the lower limit for normal neutrophil counts is 1000 cells per dl in infants between 2 weeks and 1 year of age; after infancy the corresponding value is 1500 cells per dl. Blacks have somewhat lower neutrophil counts, and the lower limits of normal tentatively can be considered to be 100 to 200 cells per dl less than the figures just cited for whites. These relatively low counts in blacks are probably due to a relative decrease in neutrophils in the storage compartment of the bone marrow. Individual patients may be characterized as having mild neutropenia with counts of 1000 to 1500 per dl, moderate neutropenia with counts of 300 to 1000 per dl, and severe neutropenia with counts generally below 300 per dl. This stratification is useful in predicting the risk of pyrogenic infection, since only patients with severe neutropenia have increased susceptibility to life threatening infections.

Neutropenia may accompany infections, inflammation, malignant disease, nutritional disease, hematologic disease, chemotherapy, and radiation. In many of these disorders, neutropenia is associated with varying degrees of anemia, thrombocytopenia, or both. In contrast, neutropenia may be the sole hematologic abnormality in conditions such as congenital neutropenia, drug induced neutropenia, and immune neutropenia. Clinically it is useful to classify the neutropenias pathophysiologically as disorders arising from abnormalities of bone marrow stem cell development, impaired release of neutrophils from the bone marrow reserve, abnormalities in the distribution of neutrophils between the circulating and marginating pool in the blood, and decreased survival of neutrophils in the blood. Autoimmune neutropenia can be caused by any of these mechanisms.

Eosinopenia is rarely recognized clinically, since it requires an absolute eosinophil count for its demonstration. The potential diagnostic usefulness of identifying eosinopenia occurs in limited circumstances. Eosinopenia may be produced by at least two mechanisms—acute stress with resultant stimulation of corticosteroid release or release of epinephrine or both, and acute inflammatory states. Basophilopenia, monocytopenia, and lymphopenia may accompany conditions that are associated with eosinophilopenia. In this article we discuss immunologic causes of neutropenia.

NEUTROPHIL ANTIBODY TESTING

It is well established that antineutrophil antibodies are associated with immune neutropenia. Proposed mechanisms of neutrophil destruction include direct lysis by complement binding antibodies, lymphocyte mediated neutrophil cytotoxicity, and splenic phagocytosis of opsonized neutrophils. A wide variety of neutrophil antibody assays have been used to study patients with suspected autoimmune neutropenia. Whether the assay is immunochemical or functional, all assays measure antibody on the patient's own neutrophils or indirectly in the patient's serum.

IMMUNOCHEMICAL ASSAYS

Because of its simplicity, leukoagglutination has been employed by many laboratories for the routine detection of neutrophil specific antibodies. Like hemagglutinins, IgM neutrophil antibodies can serve to cross link neutrophils into an aggregate. On the other hand, agglutination by IgG is an active process dependent on cell viability, which occurs optimally at 37° C. Unfortunately not all antineutrophil antibodies are capable of agglutinating neutrophils. The neutrophils alone have a tendency to clump, which makes assay interpretation difficult. A variety of neutrophil cytotoxic assays have been developed based on the capacity of normal neutrophils to exclude supervital dyes and to take in and retain ^{51}Cr. The presence of complement cytotoxic leukocyte antibodies alters membrane integrity and allows dye penetration into the cell, which causes staining of the cell nucleus or release of ^{51}Cr from the dying cell. Cytotoxic assays are useful but have limited applicability since not all antibodies fix complement.

Both the antiglobulin consumption test and immunofluorescence assays have been used to detect leukocyte antibodies. Their application and interpretation have been complicated by the large amounts of IgG normally associated with neutrophils. However, the use of fluorescein labeled Fab fragments has proven a reliable technique for the detection of alloantibodies and autoantibodies. Additionally, nonspecific adherence of antibodies to the neutrophils' cell surface can be prevented by treatment of neutrophils with 1 percent paraformaldehyde. Therefore indirect immunofluorescence can be used to detect surface antigens that are not affected by treatment with paraformaldehyde. Antibodies of all classes thus can be detected by immunofluorescence using class specific antiglobulins.

An efficacious probe to detect specifically antibody on the neutrophil surfaces is staphylococcal protein A. This protein, derived from *Staphylococcus aureus,* binds specifically to the Fc domain of IgG subclasses 1, 2, and 4. Following labeling of staphylococcal protein A with either ^{125}I or fluorescein, antibodies can be delineated on the neutrophil surface.

FUNCTIONAL ASSAYS

Other assays that depend on the functional characteristics of neutrophils have been employed to detect neutrophil antigens; these tests have the advantage of revealing more about the actual functional characteristics of neutrophil antigens. Examples of such tests are antiglobulin consumption, immune mediated phagocytosis, and the staphylococcal slide test.

The last test is particularly interesting because of its ease of use. Instead of using a fluorescein-antiglobulin conjugate to label antibody sensitized cells, whole staphylococci containing protein A are used. Neutrophils are isolated by allowing them to adhere to a glass slide. Following sensitization with an antiserum, staphylococci are applied. Light microscopic examination is then used to determine whether the staphylococci are adhering to the neutrophils because of the reaction between the Fc region of the neutrophil specific antibody and the protein A of the staphylococci.

Although these functional tests are not used as frequently as immunocytochemical tests, they have detected clinically significant antibody related immune mediated neutropenias. No one technique can be considered 100 percent accurate in the detection of all antigens with a particular antiserum; a combination of techniques is needed for reliable results.

There are several instances of immune mediated neutropenia arising from the suppressive effects of large granular lymphocytes on bone marrow stem cell myelopoiesis. Hyperactive suppressor cells may be responsible for neutropenia in some patients with Felty's syndrome, adults with cyclic neutropenia, and neutropenias associated with chronic lymphoproliferative disorders.

PATIENT EVALUATION

The basic approach includes a history and a physical examination with emphasis on related phenotypic abnormalities and detection of bacterial infections of the skin and mucous membranes, including gingiva and rectum, lymphadenopathy, hepatosplenomegaly, and other signs of underlying associated chronic illness. Attention then should be directed toward the frequency and dura-

tion of symptoms of drugs or toxins capable of inducing neutropenia. The family history may reveal other individuals with recurrent infection. Unexplained deaths in children less than 1 year of age and the race and ethnic group of each patient should be noted.

The duration and severity of the neutropenia greatly influence the extent of laboratory evaluation. Patients with chronic neutropenia should have white blood cell counts and differential counts twice weekly for 5 or 6 weeks in order to evaluate periodicity suggestive of cyclic neutropenia. A bone marrow aspirate and biopsy should be performed in selected patients to aid in diagnosis and assess cellularity. Additional marrow studies such as cytogenetic analysis and special staining procedures for detecting leukemia and other malignant disorders should be carried out in certain cases. Selection of further laboratory tests is dictated by the duration and severity of the neutropenia and by findings on the physical examination.

Assays for antineutrophil antibodies are helpful in detecting immune mediated destruction. Corticosteroid mobilization tests are useful in providing a rough index of storage pool sizes and predicting the probable course in patients with congenital neutropenia. The use of epinephrine to assess the marginating pool has not been valuable in defining the basis of most neutropenic states. ^{111}Indium is a convenient neutrophil label for leukokinetic studies, but its clinical utility is marginal. Employment of an in vitro bone marrow culture system using semisoft agar or liquid medium has yielded variable results, limiting its utility in evaluating the pathophysiology of congenital neutropenias. Tests designed to investigate the possibility of impaired myelopoiesis due to excessive suppressor or cytotoxic lymphocytes or serum inhibitor factors have been somewhat useful in directing potential therapies.

MANAGEMENT OF ACUTE NEUTROPENIA

Patients may become acutely ill with autoimmune neutropenia arising from the ingestion of a variety of drugs (Table 1). The management of neutropenia usually present at the time of diagnosis in patients with drug mediated neutropenia or acute leukemias or other malignant diseases, or following bone marrow suppression by chemotherapeutic drugs, differs from the approach taken in patients with chronic neutropenia. Patients with acute neutropenia may present with fever, pneumonitis, oral or anal ulcerations, cellulitis, or septicemia. Septicemia is the major hazard in any patient with acute onset neutropenia. Acute onset neutropenia despite modern antibiotics is responsible for the considerable mortality incidence in this disease. Although infections can occur at any site in the immunosuppressed patient population, they occur mostly at five or six major sites: the upper alimentary canal, lower colon and rectum, lungs, skin, and to a much lesser degree the urinary tract. Conse-

TABLE 1 Autoimmune Neutropenia and Associated Diseases

Systemic lupus erythematosus

Seropositive rheumatoid arthritis

Felty's syndrome

Immune thrombocytopenic purpura

Coombs positive autoimmune hemolytic anemia

Chronic active hepatitis

Hypogammaglobulinemia

Dysgammaglobulinemia (hyper-IgM)

Lymphoproliferative disease

Graves' disease

Hashimoto's thyroiditis

Cyclical neutropenia and T8 lymphocytosis

Immunopathic neutropenia in infants younger than 2 years of age

Infectious mononucleosis

quently the practice of initiating broad spectrum antibiotic therapy immediately following the expeditious evaluation of the patient with neutropenia in the hospital can markedly reduce the early morbidity and mortality due to infection. Marrow examination in patients with drug induced immune mediated neutropenia frequently shows reduced numbers of mature neutrophils. Recovery of marrow and increased numbers of circulating neutrophils follow discontinuation of therapy with the drug.

THERAPY FOR CHRONIC AUTOIMMUNE NEUTROPENIA

The management of chronic autoimmune neutropenia is dictated by the patient's medical history. Many adult patients with autoimmune neutropenia have associated diseases or have drug associated antibodies (see Tables 1, 2). Patients without infection or other major medical problems require no special attention. It is important not to suggest that they lead sheltered lives for fear of the acquisition of infections because this rarely occurs. In patients with more severe neutropenia with neutrophil counts below 200 to 300 per dl, infections may become an increasing problem, and the patient

TABLE 2 Drugs Associated with Immune Mediated Neutropenia

Penicillins, semisynthetic penicillin, cephalosporins

Sulfonamides

Quinidine, procainamide

Dilantin

Propylthiouracil

Chlorothiazide

Chlorpromazine

should be instructed in good oral hygiene and advised to seek immediate medical attention for chills or fever. Antibiotic therapy should be instituted promptly for infection in patients with immune neutropenias as they are encountered.

As might be expected in a syndrome with diverse causes, uncertain pathophysiology, and infrequent incidence, the proper indication for treatment of immune neutropenia is far from clear. Although controversy exists, it seems prudent to require severe or recurrent infections as well as neutropenia and reliable tests that suggest that the patient has an autoimmune disorder before undertaking specific therapy for autoimmune neutropenia.

CORTICOSTEROID THERAPY

Corticosteroid therapy has been responsible for major improvement in many patients with autoimmune neutropenia. Underlying the mechanism of action of corticosteroids is their capacity to elevate the blood count by accelerating the release of neutrophils from the storage pool in the bone marrow into the circulation and by prolonging the blood survival of neutrophils by preventing their diapedesis into tissues. These effects are seen both normally and in patients with autoimmune neutropenia.

Prolonged administration of corticosteroids may alter the rate of production of circulating antibodies and impair the removal of antibody coated neutrophils by splenic macrophages. Indeed in one study corticosteroids were found to prolong the survival of labeled neutrophils in the circulation in a patient with autoimmune neutropenia associated with systemic lupus erythematosus.

Following the administration of corticosteroids, a modest increase in the blood neutrophil count can be expected to occur within 1 to 2 weeks following the initiation of therapy. When corticosteroids are employed, they should be administered daily (e.g., 60 to 100 mg per day for an adult; 2 mg per kilogram for a child), followed in 1 month by alternate day steroid therapy at a reduced dosage, (e.g., 20 to 30 mg per day in the adult).

The paucity of response to corticosteroids in many patients described in the early literature probably relates to poorly defined autoimmune neutropenia. In vitro evidence of antineutrophil autoimmunity should be documented prior to the use of this therapeutic agent. In patients with granulated lymphocytosis associated with neutropenia in whom the neutropenia is persistent and often associated with recurrent infections, corticosteroid therapy is warranted initially.

In regard to patients with autoimmune neutropenia who have failed to benefit from corticosteroid therapy, there are several reports indicating responses with cytotoxic drugs, such as cyclophosphamide, azathioprine, and vincristine. The reports of use of these drugs indicate some responses, but the studies were not well controlled. Thus, these forms of therapy currently represent experimental approaches.

INTRAVENOUS GAMMA GLOBULIN THERAPY

Intravenous gamma globulin therapy has been used in the treatment of idiopathic thrombocytopenic purpura. It induces a significant increase in the platelet count in many cases. It is not surprising then that intravenous gamma globulin therapy has been tried in patients with immune neutropenia. Largely it has been employed in patients who continue to be plagued with neutropenia and infections and who have failed to benefit from corticosteroids. Experience with intravenous gamma globulin therapy in autoimmune neutropenia, however, is limited to only small numbers of patients. When employed, it has been administered in dosages of 500 mg per kilogram per day for 3 to 4 days.

In two patients with autoimmune neutropenia an increase in the absolute neutrophil count of more than 3000 per dl was observed within 5 days after starting therapy. Two of five patients with autoimmune neutropenia achieved complete remission after the initial treatment with intravenous doses of gamma globulin, whereas in another three patients significant improvement was achieved and maintained with maintenance intravenous doses of gamma globulin administered every other week or monthly as a single dose of 500 mg per kilogram. No adverse effect of intravenous gamma globulin therapy on neutrophil function has been observed. However, one of the major considerations in its use is the high cost of the drug.

Plasmapheresis has been employed in an uncontrolled fashion in patients with autoimmune neutropenia. This approach to remove antibodies and immune complexes remains experimental. Before plasmapheresis is attempted it would seem more rational at present to administer gamma globulin intravenously.

MANAGEMENT OF INFANTS WITH AUTOIMMUNE NEUTROPENIA

In contrast to patients over 2 years of age, children under 2 years of age who develop autoimmune neutropenia frequently associated with viral syndromes have a high likelihood of spontaneous and permanent remissions within 3 years after diagnosis. These youngsters most often do not require any form of therapy even though they remain markedly neutropenic, because they usually are fortunate to have little in the way of serious

bacterial infections. However, if youngsters under 2 years of age do develop problems with recurrent infection, it is advisable to treat them initially with corticosteroids, and if they fail therapy with the corticosteroids, administer intravenous gamma globulin therapy, which has been effective in the treatment of some of these patients.

FELTY'S SYNDROME

The approach to the treatment of patients with Felty's syndrome remains controversial. Splenectomy in the past has been the mainstay of therapy. Up to 60 percent of the patients with Felty's syndrome who undergo splenectomy sustain transient increases in neutrophil counts to more than 4000 per dl. However, following splenectomy the amount of neutrophil binding IgG in the serum in many cases remains abnormally elevated. Furthermore, it has been shown in several patients with Felty's syndrome that suppressor lymphocytes are present in the spleen. Splenectomy in Felty's syndrome may have a temporary beneficial effect on neutrophil counts, possibly related to removal of the bulk of suppressor cells. The recurrence of neutropenia several weeks after splenectomy, however, may be due to activation of suppressor cells present in other organs such as the bone marrow. It seems obvious then that other experimental approaches need to be applied in the therapy of patients with severe neutropenia and recurrent infections in Felty's syndrome. The administration of antithymocyte globulin may be one experimental approach, which should be evaluated at facilities devoted to clinical research in patients with autoimmune neutropenia. The role of splenectomy in other autoimmune disorders is even less predictable than in Felty's syndrome. For this reason splenectomy should largely be avoided in autoimmune neutropenias. If splenectomy fails in a patient with neutropenia, the patient is further predisposed to serious infections with encapsulated organisms.

SUGGESTED READING

Boxer LA. Immune neutropenias. Am J Pediatr Hematol Oncol 1981; 3:89–96.
Bussel J, et al. Reversal of neutropenia with intravenous gammaglobulin in autoimmune neutropenia of infancy. Blood 1983; 62:398–400.
McKenna RW, et al. Granulated T cell lymphocytosis with neutropenia: malignant or benign chronic lymphoproliferative disorder. Blood 1985; 66:259–266.
Webster ADP, et al. Autoimmune blood dyscrasias in five patients with hypogammaglobulinemia. Response of neutropenia to vincristine. J Clin Immunol 1981; 1:113–118.

APLASTIC ANEMIA*

EVA C. GUINAN, M.D.
DAVID G. NATHAN, M.D.

Aplastic anemia is characterized by inadequate production of blood elements in the bone marrow, resulting in peripheral pancytopenia. The epidemiologic association of multiple agents or conditions with this disorder, the numerous possible pathophysiologic mechanisms that have been invoked to explain its genesis, and the occurrence of spontaneous partial or even complete remissions make the evaluation of therapeutic options for this group of patients very difficult.

Severe aplastic anemia is generally defined as occurring in a patient who has fewer than 0.5×10^9 granulocytes per liter, a platelet count less than 20×10^9 per liter, and a reticulocyte count less than 20×10^9 per liter (or less than 1 percent corrected for hematocrit) in the setting of bone marrow biopsy demonstrating less than 25 percent cellularity. Pancytopenia that is severe but does not meet these criteria is more properly referred to as moderate aplastic or hypoplastic anemia; this distinction is extremely important in terms of understanding and interpreting the literature and in terms of establishing the prognosis and therapy for individual patients. The severity of the pancytopenia and the intervals from symptoms to diagnosis and subsequently to therapy seem to be the most reliable prognostic indicators, the former correlating inversely with outcome, whereas the latter suggests that disease that is slower in onset and tolerated by the patient for some time without therapy appears to have a somewhat better overall outcome.

The therapy of patients with aplastic anemia is composed of four parts: the careful search for etiologies that have specific therapeutic implications, delineation of a well thought out plan of blood product support, effective management of infectious complications, and initiation of therapy designed to restore adequate hematopoiesis.

ETIOLOGIC CONSIDERATIONS

Careful history taking and physical examination should be done to establish whether the patient has any stigmata of the congenital disorders linked to aplastic

anemia. The importance of this effort is illustrated in patients with Fanconi's anemia, who can be expected to have a reasonable response to androgens but not immunosuppression and who usually receive a less aggressive conditioning regimen than that commonly employed in preparation for bone marrow transplantation. A similar effort should be made to identify any environmental or drug exposure with a known relationship to aplastic anemia. Although elimination of the agent will probably not result in reconstitution of the patient's bone marrow, it is unlikely that any therapy (short of marrow transplantation) will be successful without removal of the responsible toxin.

The establishment of two other diagnoses may be of import with regard to therapy. First, the diagnosis of paroxysmal nocturnal hemoglobinuria should always be considered; diagnosis of this clonal cell disorder carries unique prognostic and therapeutic implications. Second, a cytogenetic study must be done with the bone marrow sample. Recent reports suggest that a significant proportion of patients who meet the clinical and pathologic criteria of aplastic anemia in fact have clonal cytogenetic abnormalities of the sort described in preleukemia (e.g., monosomy 7). Therapy should be influenced by that diagnosis.

BLOOD PRODUCT SUPPORT

Patients undergoing initial evaluation should be transfused sparingly; the unsensitized untransfused patient who comes to bone marrow transplantation has the best outcome. In particular, transfusion of any blood product from family members should be avoided until human leukocyte antigen (HLA) typing of the family is completed and transplantation has been excluded as a therapeutic modality.

Although blood products should always be used judiciously, the hematocrit level should be maintained in a range that allows the patient to function normally. No "spur" to bone marrow recovery is effected by keeping the patient chronically undertransfused. When possible, complete red blood cell typing should be done prior to transfusion; this proves useful if the patient subsequently develops anti-red blood cell antibodies. Washed or frozen and washed packed red blood cell products should be used in order to minimize exposure of the patient to allosensitizing leukocytes. Patients maintained on chronic red cell transfusions for a protracted time need careful attention to iron status and may benefit from chelation with desferrioxamine in order to avoid or mitigate the secondary complications of transfusional iron overload. However, thrombocytopenia may complicate the subcutaneous delivery of this drug.

Thrombocytopenia can be partially corrected by transfusion; in this case it is difficult to establish a level at which the patient should be transfused. In general, serious bleeding does not occur when the platelet count

*Study supported by grants from the National Institutes of Health and the Dyson Foundation. Dr. Guinan is an Amy Clare Potter Fellow of the Department of Medicine of The Children's Hospital.

is greater than 20×10^9 per liter. Although some patients are clinically stable at counts between 5 and 15 $\times 10^9$ per liter, others have significant skin or other organ hemorrhage. Although the best course is to assess each patient for an individual pattern of platelet consumption, response to transfusion, and bleeding diathesis, the most conservative approach would be to transfuse prophylactically in this lower range. Patients with continuing fever or infection may have increased platelet requirements. Measures should be taken to insure the best possible hemostasis and include the avoidance of all drugs with antihemostatic potential and the suppression of menses in postpubertal women. In some patients with recurrent mucosal bleeding, epsilon aminocaproic acid (0.1 g per kg orally every 6 hours) may be useful, although its use may be contraindicated in patients with underlying cardiac, hepatic, or renal disease.

As with red cells, care should be taken to minimize potential sensitization to leukocyte antigens. To this end, the utilization of single donor platelets is preferable. Patients who develop refractoriness to platelet transfusions may respond to HLA matched platelets. Patients who are not candidates for bone marrow transplantation may additionally benefit from platelets from family members.

Although granulocytes are now available from pheresed donors, transfusions of granulocytes to these chronically neutropenic patients are rarely indicated. The patient with a documented gram negative bacterial infection that persists after several days of appropriate antibiotic therapy may benefit from such support.

Transfusion therapy of any sort may result in febrile reactions, chills, and urticaria. Such reactions may be avoided successfully by premedicating with antihistamines, acetaminophen, and, if indicated, corticosteroids. Blood product support also entails exposure of the patient to a large number of viral infections, including non-A non-B hepatitis, cytomegalovirus, and human immune deficiency viruses. While better blood screening techniques are being developed and applied, patients receiving prolonged transfusional support should be monitored for the development of these secondary infectious complications.

MANAGEMENT OF INFECTIOUS COMPLICATIONS

Patients with aplastic anemia are neutropenic by definition and are generally immunosuppressed secondary to therapy. They therefore represent a fertile breeding ground for a large number of bacterial, fungal, and viral pathogens. Complete isolation of these patients when ambulatory is costly and not necessarily effective, as most infections in granulocytopenic hosts are endogenous in origin; therefore this approach is not recommended. No studies have evaluated the utility of prophylactic antibiotic therapy in this patient population.

We do not use a prophylactic regimen, believing that the possible benefits are outweighed by potential risks (e.g., further bone marrow suppression, development of resistant organisms).

Patients with fever and neutropenia must undergo an immediate and complete evaluation, including multiple cultures and radiographs as indicated, and then be started on broad spectrum intravenous antibiotic therapy. In the past we have used a semisynthetic penicillin (e.g., mezlocillin) and an aminoglycoside; recent studies suggest that derivatized cephalosporins may be used as single drugs. Persistence of fever in the absence of positive cultures at 3 to 5 days may dictate the addition of amphotericin B intravenously. Since the traditional criterion for discontinuation of antibiotic therapy (resolution of neutropenia) does not apply, patients should be followed empirically for clinical response and disappearance of laboratory or physical evidence of infection.

THERAPEUTIC OPTIONS

To date, no constellation of laboratory findings has been identified that serves to define the patients who will respond to a given therapy. One therefore is left in the unsatisfying situation of using therapies with very different potential mechanisms of action in patients in whom the particular pathophysiology is unclear, all without any indicator as to which therapy is best for an individual patient.

Nonimmunosuppressive Therapies

The most commonly used drugs to date are the androgens, in particular, 5-beta-testosterones. The mechanism of action is a direct stimulatory effect on erythroid progenitor cells and an increase in erythropoietin production. Androgens certainly affect hematopoiesis in vivo; a number of normal, pathologic, and therapeutic situations related to increases in circulating androgen levels (male puberty, Cushing's syndrome, hormonal therapy of breast cancer) result in elevations of the hematocrit level. The utility of testosterones in aplastic anemia is more difficult to support. While numerous anecdotal studies exist in the literature suggesting that there is both a survival advantage and hematologic response in patients treated with androgens versus those given supportive care alone, most of these can be criticized, particularly because of the inclusion of patients with moderate disease. Such patients may well have a response to testosterone therapy, but newer studies suggest that androgens are not useful in the therapy of most patients with severe aplastic anemia. However, for patients with moderate disease or those who have failed to benefit from all other therapies, we would initiate treatment with oxymethalone, etiocholanolone, or nandrolone decanoate at a level of 1 to 2 mg per kg intramuscularly every week or 2 to 5 mg per kg orally every day. The 17-alkylated androgens (such as oxymethalone) have the considerable advantage of oral administration in this thrombocytopenic population. Responses are usually attained within 8 to 10 weeks, and the dosage is then decreased gradually to the lowest tolerated level. If there is no response, a different preparation may be substituted.

The side effects of androgen therapy are multiple and include changes in the external genitalia of prepubertal children (including the development of pubic hair), development of amenorrhea and clitoromegaly in postpubertal females, deepening of the voice, flushing, hirsutism, and acne. In addition, exposure to androgens may hasten the rate of skeletal maturation in children, leading to short stature. There is some suggestion that concomitant treatment with corticosteroids (at oral dosages of 5 to 10 mg of prednisone daily or every other day) may blunt the latter effect. In addition, a host of liver related complications, including elevation of transaminase levels, cholestasis (including the development of bile or blood lakes), and possibly an increased potential for benign or malignant hepatic tumors, may occur.

Lithium, which has in vitro effects on hematopoietic progenitors, has been used in some patients with aplastic anemia with anecdotal success. This experience is very limited, both in scope and in degree of response.

Acyclovir, the antiviral drug, has been used with apparent success to treat a few patients with aplastic anemia. Although this experience remains anecdotal, there does exist a correlation between Epstein-Barr virus infection and subsequent development of bone marrow failure. If a patient has both a history and titers suggestive of this etiology, this approach might be indicated (while evaluation for more definitive therapy is under way).

Recombinant hematopoietic growth factors (e.g., granulocyte-macrophage colony stimulating factor) recently have become available for study in human trials. Laboratory and animal studies demonstrate the potent effects of these molecules with respect to stimulating relatively primitive hematopoietic precursor cells to proliferate and, in the case of animal trials, they hasten the recovery of peripheral blood counts to normal levels after a variety of challenges. The utility of these factors in the therapy of aplasia remains to be established. One can imagine that they may be useful in the therapy of patients with hypoplastic, if not aplastic, marrows.

Immunosuppressive Regimens

The mainstays of "immunosuppressive" treatment of aplastic anemia have been antithymocyte globulin or antilymphocyte globulin and corticosteroids. Multiple trials, randomized and nonrandomized, suggest approximately a 50 percent response to treatment with antithymocyte globulin. Failure to respond is generally predic-

tive of a poor overall outcome. The crude material is given intravenously to the hospitalized patient. Although studies have failed to identify the best possible source of material and the best dosage schedule, the literature suggests that total dosages greater than 100 mg per kg are most effective. We commonly use 15 mg per kg daily for 10 days, mixed in normal saline and administered over 4 to 6 hours. Side effects relate to hypersensitivity and serum sickness. Patients are generally premedicated with acetaminophen and antihistamines; corticosteroids, up to 40 mg per square meter per day, are added as indicated. Vigorous blood product support is necessary.

The mechanism of action of antithymocyte globulin remains unclear. It is generally assumed to be primarily immunosuppressive, although the crudity of the preparation and the difficulty in interpreting supporting data for this view raise questions regarding its mode of action. Responses may take up to 3 months to occur and are often incomplete; i.e., patients may become transfusion independent but not hematologically normal. Some responders may relapse months to years later; if retreatment with antithymocyte globulin is considered, special care must be taken to assess the patient for sensitivity and a different species source of the globulin may be indicated.

High dose bolus 6-methylprednisolone therapy has been used in some centers to good effect. The most frequently cited regimen is 20 mg per kg per day for 3 days, 10 mg per kg per day for 4 days, 5 mg per kg daily for 4 days, 2 mg per kg daily for 9 days, and 1 mg per kg daily for 10 days for a total of 30 days, followed by low dose oral prednisone therapy at 0.1 to 0.2 mg per kg per day tapered over the first year, with response incidences comparable to those seen with antithymocyte globulin. In addition, some 30 percent of nonresponders were able to be salvaged with antithymocyte globulin. We have had no responders to this therapy.

There is growing anecdotal literature suggesting that cyclosporin A may be a useful drug in the therapy of aplasia. The drug has been used in the range of 12 to 15 mg per kg daily in oral doses, aiming for trough levels between 100 and 150 μg per liter. Responses have been reported to occur as early as 1 week and as late as 8 weeks after the initiation of therapy. Side effects include renal dysfunction, hypertension, hirsutism, and hepatic dysfunction. If a response is achieved, the dosage should be decreased gradually to the lowest tolerated dosage (one can obtain a "cyclosporin effect" on an every other day schedule). No large studies of cyclosporin A in aplastic anemia are available.

Bone Marrow Transplantation

Transplantation of allogeneic marrow, if successful, is the only therapy that regularly results in reconstitution of normal hematopoiesis. Although attempts are being made to use matched unrelated or mismatched related donors, the following comments are confined to the experience with HLA matched, fully compatible marrow donors.

The overall survival of patients is 50 to 80 percent, with few therapy or disease related deaths after 2 years. The best survival is seen in previously untransfused patients because of their decreased risk of graft rejection; in this population the survival is 80 to 90 percent.

Bone marrow transplantation is an intensive therapy requiring isolation of the patient and a lengthy hospitalization. Conditioning regimens are designed to immunosuppress the host and decrease graft rejection. In general, untransfused patients are given high dosages of cyclophosphamide intravenously (200 mg per kg over 4 days). Transfused patients receive additional immunosuppression in the form of further drug or radiation therapy. Because of the ease of administration and avoidance of any possible long term side effects secondary to radiation, we have used multiagent immunosuppression consisting of rabbit antithymocyte serum, 0.2 cc per kg intravenously on days -6, -4, and -2; procarbazine, 12.5 mg per kg orally on days -7, -5, and -3; and cyclophosphamide, 50 mg per kg intravenously on days -5, -4, -3, and -2. This therapy has resulted in a graft rejection incidence of approximately 10 percent, comparable to that seen with most regimens in such patients. On day 0 the patient is given 10 cc per kg of filtered donor marrow intravenously.

Full reconstitution of hematopoiesis takes 3 to 6 weeks, during which time the patient requires vigorous blood product support. Because of the additional immunosuppression, these patients are at high risk for infections and are treated accordingly. The advent of amphotericin B, new antiviral drugs, and replacement (and prophylactic) gamma globulin therapy has improved the outcome with regard to infectious complications. The major morbidity and mortality during this interval stem from the development of graft versus host disease, presumably due to reactivity of the donor mononuclear cells to the host.

The acquisition of severe graft versus host disease is highly correlated with a poor outcome; the incidence and severity are highly correlated with age, younger patients having a much better prognosis. In addition, severe acute graft versus host disease is related to an increased risk of developing a chronic form, which results in significant sustained immunosuppression, can be debilitating, and can contribute to late bone marrow transplantation related deaths. Chronic graft versus host disease develops in approximately one third of bone marrow transplantation survivors. Continuing attempts to develop more effective prophylactic and treatment regimens for graft versus host disease should result in a better outcome for the older patient with respect to both acute and chronic forms. It is also worth noting here that patients surviving bone marrow transplantation have a significant immune deficit, which gradually improves over the first year after transplantation. During this time they require close follow-up, antibiotic prophylaxis, and often gamma globulin replacement. Optimal reimmunization schedules have not been described.

Because therapy should result in full hematopoietic recovery, bone marrow transplantation is recommended for patients under the age of 20 with a fully compatible family donor. It is generally also recommended for patients between the ages of 20 and 35. Over the age of 35 the mortality and morbidity of graft versus host disease in general outweigh the benefits of bone marrow transplantation, and patients may fare better with antithymocyte globulin or other immunosuppressive therapy. Bone marrow transplantation using unrelated matched or related mismatched marrow is still highly experimental, and its associated problems (such as a high frequency of graft rejection) are exacerbated in patients with aplastic anemia. At this time patients would be better served by existing or evolving regimens excluding bone marrow transplantation.

SUGGESTED READING

Alter BP. The bone marrow failure syndromes. In: Nathan DG, Oski FA, eds. Hematology of infancy and childhood. Philadelphia: WB Saunders, 1987: 159–241.

Alter BP, et al. Classification and aetiology of the aplastic anemias. Clin Haematol 1978; 7:431–465.

Anasetti C, et al. Marrow transplantation for severe aplastic anemia. Long-term outcome in fifty "untransfused" patients. Ann Intern Med 1986; 104:461–466.

Camitta BA, Storb R, Thomas ED. Aplastic anemia. I. Pathogenesis, diagnosis, treatment, and prognosis. N Engl J Med 1982; 306:645–652.

Camitta BA, Storb R, Thomas ED. Aplastic anemia. II. Pathogenesis, diagnosis, treatment, and prognosis. N Engl J Med 1982; 306:712–718.

Champlin R, et al. Antithymocyte globulin treatment in patients with aplastic anemia. A prospective randomized trial. N Engl J Med 1983; 308:113–118.

Gluckman E, et al. Immunosuppressive treatment of aplastic anemia as an alternative treatment for bone marrow transplantation. Semin Hematol 1984; 21:11–19.

Nathan DG. "Myelophrenia": its contribution to the management of aplastic anemia. In: Young NS, Levine AS, Humphries RK, eds. Aplastic anemia stem cell biology and advances in treatment. New York: Alan R. Liss, 1984:xxi-xxx.

Rappeport JM, Nathan DG. Acquired aplastic anemias: pathophysiology and treatment. Adv Intern Med 1982; 27:547–590.

Storb R, et al. Marrow transplantation for aplastic anemia. Semin Hematol 1984; 21:27–35.

PHAGOCYTE FUNCTION DISORDERS

PHILIP M. MURPHY, M.D.
JOHN I. GALLIN, M.D.

Disorders of phagocyte function may be classified as inherited or acquired, primary or secondary, reversible or irreversible, anomalous or clinically expressed. The inherited primary cellular defects of phagocyte function that are associated with recurrent bacterial and fungal infections are irreversible experiments of nature that have become the focus of intense scientific and clinical inquiry during the past 20 years. Despite their rarity, they merit a separate discussion of clinical management from the acquired and secondary disorders because of the type, severity, and frequency of complicating infections that dominate the clinical course. The six conditions described in Table 1 account for the majority of all patients in this group. They are chronic granulomatous disease, neutrophil specific granule deficiency, the Chédiak-Higashi syndrome, the hyperimmunoglobulin E–recurrent infection syndrome (also known as Job's syndrome), leukocyte adhesion protein deficiency (also known as Mol, LFA-1, p150, 95 deficiency), and hereditary myeloperoxidase deficiency.

The management of patients with inherited phagocyte defects principally involves the diagnosis, treatment, and prevention of pyogenic infection. In general, the inflammatory response in these patients is delayed, which can make the early localization and diagnosis of an infectious process difficult. Moreover, the response to conventional therapeutic approaches is frequently poor, prompting the design of unusually aggressive treatment strategies.

It is important to recognize that the inherited disorders of phagocyte function share certain clinical fea-

TABLE 1 Differential Features of Inherited Disorders of Phagocyte Function

Disorder	Mode(s) of Inheritance	Distinguishing Clinical Features	Cellular and Molecular Defects	Diagnosis
Chronic granulomatous diseases of childhood	X linked; autosomal recessive; autosomal dominant with incomplete penetrance	Granulomas, seborrheic dermatitis, infection with catalase + organisms, aphthous stomatitis	Absent respiratory burst due to abnormal cytochrome b_{559} dependent NADPH oxidase	NBT test; absent superoxide and H_2O_2 production by neutrophils
Hyperimmunoglobulin E–recurrent infection (Job's) syndrome	Autosomal recessive	Eczematoid or pruritic dermatitis, "cold" skin abscesses, eosinophilia, mucocutaneous candidiasis, absence of atopy, coarse facies, restrictive lung disease, scoliosis	Reduced chemotaxis in some patients, reduced suppressor T cell activity	Clinical features; serum IgE > 2000 IU/ml; high serum anti-*S. aureus* IgE; low or absent serum and salivary anti-*S. aureus* IgA
Chédiak-Higashi syndrome	Autosomal recessive	Oculocutaneous albinism, nystagmus, peripheral neuropathy, mental retardation in some patients, mild neutropenia	Reduced chemotaxis and phagolysosome fusion, increased respiratory burst activity, defective neutrophil egress from marrow	Clinical features; giant lysosomal granules in granule bearing cells
Leukocyte adhesion protein deficiency (Mol, LFA-1, p150, 95 deficiency)	Autosomal recessive, defective β-subunit gene mapped to chromosome 21	Delayed separation of umbilical cord, sustained granulocytosis	Impaired phagocytosis of iC3b coated particles, impaired neutrophil spreading and chemotaxis	Reduced phagocyte surface expression of CR3 (iC3b receptor) measured using monoclonal antibody Mol
Neutrophil specific granule deficiency	Not established	Recurrent pyogenic infection, delayed wound healing	Neutrophils lack lactoferrin, alkaline phosphatase, vitamin B_{12} binding protein; reduced chemotaxis	Clinical features; absent specific granules in Wright stained neutrophils
Myeloperoxidase deficiency	Autosomal recessive; gene mapped to chromosome 17	Clinically normal, disseminated candidiasis in patients with superimposed diabetes mellitus	Absent myeloperoxidase due to post-translational defect	Apparent absence of azurophil granules in peroxidase stained neutrophils

TABLE 2 Clinical Features Suggestive of an Inherited Disorder of Phagocyte Function

Clinical Feature	Differential Characteristics
Recurrent infections	Severe, often life threatening; slow response to appropriate antimicrobial therapy; bacterial and fungal pathogens, especially *Staphylococcus aureus*, Enterobacteriaceae, *Pseudomonas spp.*, *Hemophilus influenzae*, *Aspergillus spp.*
	Unusual bacterial pathogens, such as *Acremonium strictum*, *Pseudomonas cepacia*, *Chromobacterium violaceum*
	Suggestive infections Suppurative lymphadenitis Skin and respiratory tract infections Spontaneous visceral abscess Osteomyelitis Fungal meningitis Nonsuggestive infections Bacteremia Meningitis (typical pediatric organisms) Urinary tract infection
Chronic inflammation	Oral: periodontitis, gingivitis, aphthous stomatitis Cutaneous: pruritic, seborrheic, and eczematoid dermatitis
Disordered inflammation	Delayed and prolonged response to infection Granulomatous inflammation "Cold" skin abscesses Delayed wound healing Delayed separation of umbilical cord
Parental consanguinity Family history of phagocyte defect or recurrent infections	

tures that frequently permit a generic diagnosis in a patient presenting with infection (Table 2). Chronic oral and cutaneous inflammation together with both recurrent cutaneous and sinopulmonary infections beginning in childhood are typical clues. However, recurrent infection of skin alone or the sinopulmonary tract alone is unlikely to herald an inherited disorder of phagocyte function. In the absence of documented chronicity and recurrence, an inherited disorder of phagocyte function should be considered in cases in which a first or second infection in a child is particularly severe or unusual (such as spontaneous visceral abscess or fungal meningitis) or is poorly responsive to appropriate antimicrobial therapy, especially when the parents are consanguineous or when there is a family history of recurrent pyogenic infections.

In general, when a defect of host defense is suspected, evaluation of the complement cascade, immune function, and phagocytic cell number and function should be performed. A complete blood count with a differential, serum total hemolytic complement activity, serum immunoglobulin levels, and skin testing of delayed hypersensitivity to recall antigens together with the history and physical examination constitute a good initial screening approach that will rule out the majority of diseases associated with acquired and secondary phagocyte defects. Moreover, a diagnosis of a specific disorder of

phagocyte function sometimes can be made with high probability from this work-up. For instance, moderate neutropenia and a Wright stained peripheral blood smear that shows giant lysosomes in granule bearing cells from a patient with oculocutaneous albinism, nystagmus, and peripheral neuropathy are diagnostic of the Chédiak-Higashi syndrome. Neutrophil specific granule deficiency should be suspected in a patient with recurrent infections and delayed wound healing by the absence of granules and the presence of bilobed nuclei in neutrophils on Wright stained blood smears. A screening work-up that reveals eosinophilia and a serum IgE level greater than 2000 IU per ml in a nonatopic patient with recurrent cutaneous and sinopulmonary infections is highly suggestive of the hyperimmunoglobulin E–recurrent infection syndrome. A history of delayed separation of the umbilical cord in a patient with recurrent infections and sustained granulocytosis is highly suggestive of leukocyte adhesion protein deficiency. A child with recurrent infections with catalase positive micro-organisms and granulomatous inflammation not attributable to mycobacterial disease almost certainly has chronic granulomatous disease.

Additional studies to delineate the specific defect more precisely are not generally available in clinical laboratories and require the resources of research laboratories with a special interest in phagocyte biology.

INITIAL APPROACH TO SUSPECTED INFECTION

Since the inflammatory response to established infection is blunted in patients with these disorders, the clinical presentation may be quite indolent, tempting the clinician to ascribe the etiology of a low grade fever, unexplained malaise, and other minor symptoms to trivial self-limited causes common to pediatric practice. The consequences of this approach can be disastrous. Seemingly inconsequential local skin infections can rapidly metastasize, and areas of raging infection can remain relatively silent. Therefore, an aggressive search for the source of fever and definition of the extent of infection and inflammation should begin immediately. All symptoms, however seemingly trivial, should be exhaustively evaluated, especially when associated with fever or an elevated erythrocyte sedimentation rate.

The major challenge to the diagnosis of infection in these patients is that the usual criteria do not apply. Although on one hand inflammatory localization may be delayed, on the other hand it may be difficult to distinguish an active site of infection from chronic scarring or smoldering inflammation from a previous infection. Many of these patients have periodic flares of noninfectious gingival, periodontal, and skin disease that may mimic an infectious process. The white blood cell count is frequently not helpful: for example, patients with the Chédiak-Higashi syndrome are characteristically neutropenic and do not develop a granulocytosis when infected, whereas patients with leukocyte adhesion protein deficiency exhibit a sustained granulocytosis when well, although a further elevation can occur in response to infection. The erythrocyte sedimentation rate is enormously helpful when elevated but is not a sensitive parameter, except in chronic granulomatous disease.

Despite these daunting diagnostic difficulties, sound management principles have been developed that have been quite successful in treating infectious episodes, prolonging the infection free interval, and prolonging survival. These include the aggressive use of invasive diagnostic approaches, when necessary, to obtain material for culture from potentially infected sites, early institution of prolonged courses of antimicrobial therapy for all infectious episodes, mandatory complete drainage of all purulent and necrotic material as soon as it is recognized, the judicious use of granulocyte transfusions, local care of the skin and teeth, prophylactic intravenous antibiotic therapy for surgical and dental procedures, and in many cases, long term oral antibiotic prophylaxis.

The initial routine evaluation should include a complete physical examination, with particular attention to the skin, upper airway, and sites of previous infection. The rectal examination is particularly important in patients with leukocyte adhesion protein deficiency, since several cases of perirectal abscess have occurred. Paronychia occasionally have been complicated by osteomyelitis in patients with the hyperimmunoglobulin E–recurrent infection syndrome. Dermatitis, which is associated with many of these syndromes, often becomes superinfected with *Staphylococcus aureus,* particularly in the pubic and axillary regions. Cutaneous infections in the hyperimmunoglobulin E–recurrent infection syndrome can take the form of "cold" abscesses, which lack the usual warmth, erythema, and tenderness of a normal inflammatory response. The nares are often the site of furuncles in patients with chronic granulomatous disease.

Since localized sites of infection are frequently occult as a consequence of the disordered inflammatory response, empiric diagnostic testing may be necessary but can be targeted by knowledge of the likeliest sites of infection. In this regard, a chest radiograph is most useful. When it is normal, computed tomography of the chest occasionally has revealed small pulmonary infiltrates or subtle lymphadenopathy. Bronchoscopy or open lung biopsy is often required for microbiologic diagnosis of pneumonia or lung abscess. Pleuroscopy and mediastinoscopy have been used safely for biopsy of mediastinal and hilar lymphadenopathy.

Diagnostic imaging of the liver has revealed abscesses even in the absence of localizing signs and symptoms or abnormalities of liver function. Radionuclide imaging of bone has been similarly useful. Brain lesions, on the other hand, are infrequent and generally symptomatic, so that empiric imaging is not generally recommended. In all tissue sites where diagnostic imaging has revealed an abnormality, an attempt must be made to establish a microbiologic diagnosis by open or percutaneous biopsy or by needle aspiration. It is important to establish the residual radiologic abnormalities after resolution of an infectious or inflammatory episode as a baseline for comparison of future studies performed in the setting of a new febrile illness. In this regard, interval imaging when the patient is well can provide more accurate information, since the residual scarring may show dynamic changes as a result of ongoing fibrosis and growth in these patients. Interval pulmonary function testing also can be helpful, especially in the hyperimmunoglobulin E–recurrent infection syndrome in which the chronic consequences of pulmonary infection can be particularly severe.

Blood cultures are always performed as part of the initial diagnostic work-up, but are almost always sterile except in patients with severe leukocyte adhesion protein deficiency and in the accelerated phase of the Chédiak-Higashi syndrome (a terminal lymphoma-like condition characterized by hepatosplenomegaly, lymphadenopathy, and pancytopenia that is unresponsive to cytotoxic therapy). Bacteremia must be regarded as indicative of an underlying localized infectious source, and an appropriate diagnostic work-up should be performed. Meningitis is rare, and empiric cerebrospinal fluid culture is not recommended. Urinalysis and urine culture are routinely performed but are rarely positive. Except for the erythrocyte sedimentation rate, routine admission laboratory tests are seldom helpful in diagnosis and management. An elevated alkaline phosphatase level sometimes can be a helpful indicator of hepatic or bone infection. Serum transaminase levels are often normal in the presence of a hepatic abscess. Blind biopsy and exploratory laparotomy are not recommended as diagnostic procedures.

MEDICAL THERAPY OF FEBRILE EPISODES

The key to the successful management of febrile episodes is a rapid but thorough diagnostic work-up, aggressive and prolonged drainage of abscesses, and early institution of antimicrobial therapy. Antibiotics ideally should be withheld until a specific pathogen is identified. However, if an exhaustive diagnostic work-up is negative or if the patient is sufficiently ill, the institution of empiric antimicrobial therapy is justified. The initial choice of drug must consider the likely pathogens, the local susceptibility patterns, previous side effects in a given patient, as well as the cost.

Although a large number of different bacterial and fungal organisms have been reported to cause disease in these patients, it is worth emphasizing that penicillinase resistant, methicillin sensitive *Staphylococcus aureus* is by far the most common isolate. Unusual organisms, such as *Chromobacterium violaceum, Pseudomonas cepacia,* and *Acremonium strictum,* also can cause severe infection, particularly in chronic granulomatous disease, and should not be dismissed as contaminants or "normal flora."

When empiric coverage is necessary, we routinely give a penicillinase resistant penicillin and an aminoglycoside. A typical regimen would include oxacillin, 1 to 2 g intravenously every 4 hours, and gentamicin, 3 to 5 mg per kg daily intravenously in three divided doses. Children whose body weight is less than 40 kg are given oxacillin, 100 to 200 mg per kg per day intravenously in four to six divided doses, and gentamicin, 7.5 mg per kg per day intravenously in three divided doses. Empiric anaerobic coverage is unnecessary. Vancomycin, 40 mg per kg per day intravenously in four divided doses, is used in patients with demonstrated allergy to penicillin. This regimen is then modified if a specific microbiologic diagnosis is eventually made.

If no pathogen is isolated and fever persists, an empiric 10 to 14 day course of the initial antibiotic regimen is given and then stopped if clinical resolution has occurred, as defined by prompt defervescence, reduction of the erythrocyte sedimentation rate, and the absence of progression of inflammatory masses, if present. We find that the latter frequently persist or only very slowly resolve even when associated with a defined pathogen that has been successfully eradicated. If no pathogen was isolated and these criteria are not satisfied, further empiric diagnostic testing is indicated and antibiotic therapy is continued. Localization of an infectious process can occur during antibiotic therapy and clinical resolution may then simply require adequate drainage (see following discussion). Transfusion of normal granulocytes has been used in several cases to actually localize an infectious process.

When the clinical condition of the patient deteriorates despite these empiric measures and a specific microbiologic diagnosis is still lacking, the empiric addition of systemic antifungal therapy and, in some cases, granulocyte transfusions (to be discussed) may be indicated. Since the clinical response is generally slow, we prolong the duration of antibiotic therapy relative to similar infections in individuals without a phagocyte defect, such as surgical patients. We generally give intravenous antibiotic therapy for at least 1 week beyond the point of clinical resolution (as already defined) of cutaneous, lymphatic, and sinopulmonary infections and then switch to oral doses of an antibiotic with activity against the patient's isolate. Visceral abscesses and osteomyelitis are treated intravenously for at least 6 to 8 weeks and sometimes longer. It should be emphasized that in patients with extensive pyogenic infection, the erythrocyte sedimentation rate should decrease with successful treatment but may not actually normalize for many months. Persistent elevation is common in chronic granulomatous disease and is attributable to residual chronic inflammation; it can also result from anemia, which frequently complicates the course in patients with prolonged infection. In any case, failure of the sedimentation rate to normalize does not necessarily reflect failure to eradicate infection.

Although parenteral therapy is the safest and preferred route of administration, limited skin and upper airway infections such as cellulitis, furunculosis, sinusitis, and otitis media sometimes respond to oral dicloxacillin therapy as long as adequate drainage is established. More extensive skin and upper airway infections and limited infections which occur despite oral prophylactic therapy with antibiotics, are always treated intravenously for at least 2 weeks. Patients with the hyperimmunoglobulin E–recurrent infection syndrome who have chronic mucocutaneous candidiasis have benefited from prolonged courses of ketoconazole, 200 mg per day, without significant hepatotoxicity.

Lower respiratory symptoms, with or without a new pulmonary radiographic abnormality, are always managed with intravenous doses of antibiotics, as in established pneumonia, and invasive diagnostic procedures are performed if necessary. Bronchitis is treated with antibiotics for 1 to 2 weeks intravenously followed by 2 weeks of oral therapy. This approach is most important in the hyperimmunoglobulin E–recurrent infection syndrome in which pulmonary infection is particularly destructive, resulting in bronchiectasis, pneumatoceles, bronchopleural fistulas, scoliosis, and restrictive lung disease.

The initial choice of antibiotics in patients with suspected pulmonary infection is guided by special stains of sputum and biopsy material. For example, while awaiting the results of culture, we give a penicillinase resistant penicillin and an aminoglycoside, in the already described doses, when gram positive cocci predominate or when the initial sputum analysis is equivocal. Chloramphenicol, 50 mg per kg per day intravenously in divided doses, or a second generation cephalosporin, such as cefamandol, 150 mg per kg per day intravenously in divided doses, is given when pleomorphic gram negative coccobacilli suggestive of *Hemophilus influenzae* are seen. Ampicillin, 200 to 400 mg per kg per day intravenously in divided doses, can be substituted for chloramphenicol if the isolate is susceptible. In all cases in which aminoglycoside therapy is instituted, baseline audiometry and a creatinine clearance test should be carried out. The dosage is guided by peak and trough serum drug levels, which should be measured at least weekly.

Visceral mycosis is especially problematic in patients with chronic granulomatous disease and should be approached extremely aggressively from the onset. When a localized process is identified, extensive debridement is mandatory. In addition, we routinely give prolonged courses of amphotericin B. Patient intolerance of the multiple toxic effects of this drug often limits the total dosage that is achievable. Optimally, we deliver at least 2 g, and in some very poorly responsive cases up to 4 to 5 g, by slow intravenous infusion over several hours at a maximal rate of 1.5 mg per kg per day. We also give 5-flucytosine, 150 mg per kg per day orally in four divided doses, as well as daily granulocyte transfusions (to be discussed). We treat patients with visceral mycosis in this fashion for 3 to 4 weeks beyond the point of apparent clinical resolution. On one occasion we were forced to stop amphotericin B therapy because of drug toxicity in a patient with disseminated aspergillosis with a fungal brain abscess and persistently positive cultures, but successfully completed the course of therapy with an additional 12 months of 5-flucytosine and ketoconazole. The patient has remained well for more than 2 years.

Careful monitoring of the complete blood count and creatinine clearance is essential in patients treated with antifungal drugs. Nephrotoxicity is the major limiting side effect of amphotericin B. 5-Flucytosine is myelotoxic and renally excreted and therefore must be dose adjusted in patients with reduced renal function. This should optimally be accomplished by measuring blood levels. If this is not possible, published tables relating the creatinine clearance to a recommended dosage are available. Many patients experience severe fever and chills and occasionally become hypotensive during amphotericin B infusion. Therefore a slow initial infusion of a 1 mg test dose is given. Moreover, improved tolerance of the infusion sometimes can be achieved by gradual 10 mg daily dosage increments until the maximal daily dosage is reached. These systemic reactions can be markedly attenuated by pretreatment with meperidine, 1 mg per kg, acetaminophen, diphenhydramine, and hydrocortisone, a 125 mg intravenous bolus. Acute pulmonary infiltrates have been reported to complicate amphotericin B infusion and may be more likely to occur in patients receiving granulocyte infusions. We routinely separate the two infusions by at least 4 hours. In patients with phagocyte defects other than chronic granulomatous disease, invasive visceral fungal infections are much less common, and when they occur, granulocyte transfusions generally are not necessary.

Bulky granulomas can compress and obstruct viscera in chronic granulomatous disease. They often contract with antimicrobial therapy alone but occasionally require surgical excision. We have observed dramatic resolution of this problem in two patients treated with prednisone, 1 mg per kg per day for 2 to 3 weeks, in whom biopsy of the unresolving masses failed to reveal a pathogen. Recently we have had similarly dramatic success in a child treated with ibuprofen. A theoretical rationale exists for the steroid effect. Leukotriene B4 is an inflammatory mediator produced by phagocytic cells that has potent chemotactic activity and may not be normally metabolized by phagocytes from patients with chronic granulomatous disease. Thus, local leukotriene B4 concentrations might increase and stimulate the prolonged accumulation of additional phagocytes at the inflammatory focus. Corticosteroids block the production of leukotriene B4 in vitro.

SURGICAL THERAPY

Most infectious processes in patients with phagocyte defects slowly develop into abscess cavities. Skin abscess and suppurative lymphangitis are the most common processes requiring surgical intervention. They are usually due to infection with staphylococci and streptococci. Although multiple abscesses infected with the same organism(s) may occur in a single organ, it is unusual to see disseminated multiorgan abscesses. These collections do not resolve with medical therapy alone and should be incised, widely debrided, and drained. It is important to appreciate that the extent of infection generally exceeds the visible limits of the abscess cavity.

Lung abscess is a common complication of pneumonia, particularly in the hyperimmunoglobulin E–recurrent infection syndrome in which extension to the pleural space and sometimes to adjacent bone can also occur. The long term complications of pulmonary infection in patients with this syndrome are generally not seen in the other disorders and include restrictive lung disease resulting from scoliosis and pneumatoceles and hemoptysis resulting from areas of bronchiectasis. Surgical approaches sometimes have been useful in improving pulmonary function in these patients and are always required to establish adequate drainage from abscess cavities and to control bleeding in patients with persistent hemoptysis.

Successful treatment of liver abscess, which is seen almost exclusively in patients with chronic granulomatous disease, always requires prolonged drainage of all identifiable collections, which can be achieved in many cases by computed tomography guided catheter placement. If laparotomy and open drainage are done, precise preoperative determination of the number and location of collections is critical. Drainage often persists for weeks after defervescence has occurred so that drain removal is generally a very slow process whose pace is dictated by the rate of drainage. It is critical to maintain drain patency to avoid reinfection. This is best accomplished by frequent irrigation with 3 percent hydrogen peroxide. Intravenous antibiotic therapy is continued for 7 to 10 days after all surgical and drain wounds have closed and then is followed by prolonged oral antibiotic therapy.

Osteomyelitis, particularly of small bones of the extremities, is a problem in chronic granulomatous disease and the hyperimmunoglobulin E–recurrent infection syndrome. Again adequate debridement of all involved tissue is the mainstay of successful therapy.

Lymphadenopathy does not require surgical management unless it is suppurative. Bulky granulomatous masses occasionally may obstruct a viscus in chronic granulomatous disease and may require excision when they are refractory to medical therapy, as already outlined.

GRANULOCYTE TRANSFUSIONS

Infection in patients with chronic granulomatous disease is sometimes refractory to the approaches just outlined. We have used granulocyte transfusions with dramatic success in patients who fail to benefit from initial therapy. We also use them as initial therapy, along with appropriate antibiotics and drainage, in patients with brain abscess and visceral fungal infection who historically have had a very poor prognosis with conventional therapy. Granulocyte transfusions also can be used to localize an early infectious process when the native inflammatory response is delayed.

In our center approximately 10 billion leukocytes from non-HLA matched donors are collected by continuous flow centrifugation leukapheresis and infused within 4 hours after harvesting. Although the leukapheresis product is greatly enriched for granulocytes, 10 to 20 percent of the transfused leukocytes may be mononuclear. Because graft versus host disease is not a problem in these individuals, irradiation of the leukapheresis product is unnecessary. Platelets and erythrocytes also contaminate the product.

Patients with chronic granulomatous disease frequently lack the Kell red blood cell antigen and may become sensitized to it during transfusion. The risk of intravascular hemolysis can be minimized by carefully cross matching patient and donor for both major and minor blood group antigens prior to transfusion of all blood products, including leukapheresis products. We reduce the plasma volume, but not the number of transfused cells, in small children. Pretreatment with acetaminophen, an H_1 antihistamine, hydrocortisone, a 125 mg intravenous bolus, and meperidine, 1 mg per kg, usually attenuates the fever and chills that frequently accompany the transfusion. In patients receiving amphotericin B, the granulocyte transfusion is given at least 4 hours apart from the amphotericin B to minimize the risk of pulmonary infiltrates that may be associated with concomitant administration. With these precautions we have not had to discontinue transfusion therapy because of toxicity in any of our patients, some of whom have been treated for more than 120 days. Transfusions are maintained for 2 to 4 weeks beyond the point of clinical improvement.

It is possible to follow the fate of transfused granulocytes in these patients by measuring the production of toxic oxygen derived species, such as hydrogen peroxide and superoxide anion, by activated phagocytes from inflammatory exudates. This can be done indirectly by simply assessing the capacity of individual phagocytes incubated with phorbol myristate acetate to reduce the dye nitroblue tetrazolium, which then forms a blue-black intracellular precipitate. Phagocytes from patients with chronic granulomatous disease fail to reduce the dye. The delivery of a small percentage of competent donor cells to inflammatory foci has been associated with dramatic control of previously unresponsive infections.

LOCAL CARE

Patients with disorders of phagocyte function exhibit a variety of chronic low grade inflammatory conditions of the skin, dermal appendages, and oral cavity, which can flare and become superinfected. In several cases, osteomyelitis of underlying bone has resulted. Local care can improve patient comfort while reducing the risk of serious secondary infections.

The judicious topical use of hexachlorophene can help control eczematoid dermatitis in the hyperimmunoglobulin E–recurrent infection syndrome and seborrheic dermatitis in chronic granulomatous disease. A short course of topical steroid therapy can be helpful in cases refractory to antiseptics.

Pruritic dermatitis is a distinct condition that can be particularly problematic in the hyperimmunoglobulin E–recurrent infection syndrome, especially during the summer months. H_1 and H_2 antihistamines provide symptomatic relief for most patients. An occasional patient requires a short course of oral corticosteroid therapy (40 to 60 mg daily for 3 days with rapid tapering over 7 to 10 days) for refractory pruritus. Topical therapy consists of triamcinolone cream, 0.025 or 0.1 percent, applied to affected areas three or four times daily. For the face and groin, 1 percent hydrocortisone cream is used instead to minimize the risk of dermal atrophy. When this occurs, lubricants and moisturizing creams can be helpful.

Furunculosis and secondarily infected dermatitis generally can be treated with a short course of oral antibiotic therapy. Since *Staphylococcus aureus* is the most common organism in this context, oral doses of a penicillinase resistant penicillin, such as dicloxacillin, 250 mg every 6 hours, are most commonly used and generally are effective.

Obesity is frequently associated with dermatitis in areas of redundant skin, a situation that can be particularly problematic in patients with the Chédiak-Higashi syndrome, who can have severe peripheral neuropathy resulting in a sedentary life style and marked weight gain. Progression to frank cellulitis and skin abscess is common in these cryptic sites, since the patient may not appreciate local tenderness because of sensory neuropathy. Frequent painstaking examination of the skin is crucial in such patients. The protection of neuropathic extremities from injury is of obvious importance.

Twice daily toothbrushing with a paste prepared with 3 percent hydrogen peroxide and baking soda has been effective in controlling gingivitis and aphthous stomatitis in some patients. Biannual dental consultations should be routine. Orthodonture has been performed without infectious complications in these patients. However, all oral manipulations deemed likely to cause gingival trauma, including procedures to remove dental plaque, are covered by the prophylactic intravenous administration of antibiotics (Table 3).

Substances that may additionally impair host defenses, such as alcohol and tobacco, should be avoided. Pulmonary aspergillosis has been traced to the inhalation of contaminated marijuana or exposure to mulch in patients with chronic granulomatous disease. Patients have participated uneventfully in athletics, although caution should be exercised in the choice and level of activity to minimize the possibility of skin abrasions and lacerations, which might become infected.

PROPHYLACTIC ANTIBIOTIC THERAPY AND IMMUNIZATIONS

Limited retrospective data have consistently shown a significant reduction in the incidence and severity of infection and a very low incidence of drug side effects in patients with chronic granulomatous disease treated prophylactically with antibiotics. In some patients, however, they clearly do not work, and in others drug reactions preclude their use. The emergence of resistant organisms has not yet occurred in our patients. It is our practice to routinely administer trimethoprim and sulfamethoxazole fixed combinations (80 mg: 400 mg) in a dosage based on 4 mg per kg of the trimethoprim component twice daily in patients with chronic granulomatous disease. The complete blood count should be monitored since neutropenia and megaloblastic anemia can complicate the prolonged administration of this drug combination. Trimethoprim alone or dicloxacillin, 5 mg per kg twice daily, is given to patients with sulfa allergy. The prophylactic regimen is reinstituted after specific intravenous or oral therapy is completed for an infectious episode.

Although efficacy has been reported anecdotally with antibiotic prophylaxis for the other disorders of phagocyte function, the assembled data from small series are not impressive, so that the decision to treat or not is generally individualized on the basis of the clinical course in a particular patient. Given the small number of patients involved and the fact that their care is decen-

TABLE 3 Antibiotic Prophylaxis for Patients with Inherited Disorders of Phagocyte Function and Recurrent Infections Undergoing Surgical or Dental Procedures

Drug	Dose		Timing
	Adult*	Pediatric	
Standard regimen			
Oxacillin	2 g IV	50 mg/kg IV	1 hour pre
plus			8 hours post and
Gentamicin	1.5 mg/kg IV or IM	3 mg/kg IV or IM	16 hours post
Substitutions for oxacillin			
Vancomycin (if allergic to penicillin)	0.5–1.0 g IV	20 mg/kg IV	Same as standard regimen
Dicloxacillin (if IV administration is not possible†)	2 g PO 500 mg PO	25 mg/kg PO 12.5 mg/kg PO	1 hour pre q6h for 8 doses

* Adult dosing regimens are applied to children weighing greater than 40 kg.
† Gentamicin, in the doses indicated for the standard regimen, are coadministered intramuscularly.
Modified from Buescher ES, Gallin JI. Current therapy in hematology–oncology 1983–1984. Toronto: BC Decker, 1983.

tralized, it is unlikely that a more specific recommendation will soon be available.

Patients with the hyperimmunoglobulin E–recurrent infection syndrome who have problematic mucocutaneous candidiasis have been maintained on long term courses of ketoconazole, 200 mg daily, with good results and minimal side effects.

We routinely give prophylactic antibiotic therapy prior to surgical and dental procedures, as outlined in Table 3. Patients with phagocyte defects also should receive the usual series of pediatric immunizations. There is no evidence that these patients have more frequent or more severe viral infections.

THERAPY DIRECTED AT THE UNDERLYING CELLULAR DEFECT

Currently there is no specific treatment for the underlying cellular defect that can be generally recommended in any of these diseases. Several drugs, such as levamisole (an antihelminth and immunomodulator) and ascorbic acid, have improved the function of neutrophils from patients with chemotactic defects in vitro, but in vivo efficacy generally has been lacking. The efficacy of high dose vitamin C therapy (8 to 10 g per day) in the Chédiak-Higashi syndrome, chronic granulomatous disease, and the hyperimmunoglobulin E–recurrent infection syndrome has been reported in a few patients, although gastritis was a limiting complication. As bone marrow transplantation becomes increasingly successful, there will be an increased impetus to apply it to patients with inherited disorders of phagocyte function. The experience to date in only a few patients with chronic granulomatous disease, the Chédiak-Higashi syndrome, and leukocyte adhesion protein deficiency generally has been disappointing. Since the aggressive management approach already outlined has been successful in prolonging survival in patients with these disorders, the risk of bone marrow transplantation as a general approach is currently unacceptable.

Recently the genes for multiple immunomodulatory proteins and colony stimulating factors have been cloned and in some cases expressed in large quantities in prokaryotic cells. Pure recombinant proteins, such as gamma interferon, cachectin, and GM-CSF, known to enhance phagocyte function in vitro are now available and eventually may find a role in the treatment of infected patients with phagocyte disorders.

The ideal approach to therapy in patients with inherited disorders would be the identification and correction of the underlying genetic defect. In this regard there is hope that the recent identification of a gene that is missing or abnormal in patients with chronic granulomatous disease will enable investigators to pursue a rational approach in finding a specific cure for this disease.

Genetic counseling should be offered to families of all patients with inherited phagocyte defects. Prenatal diagnosis of chronic granulomatous disease by the analysis of granulocytes from fetal blood has been reported and is theoretically possible for other disorders of phagocyte function. If specific genetic probes can be developed for these diseases, accurate prenatal diagnosis through the detection of restriction fragment length polymorphisms in DNA should be possible and could be accomplished by amniocentesis.

SUGGESTED READING

Anderson DC, et al. The severe and moderate phenotypes of heritable Mac-1, LFA-1 deficiency: their quantitative definition and relation to leukocyte dysfunction and clinical features. J Infect Dis 1985; 152:668–689.

Buescher ES, Gallin JI. Leukocyte transfusions in chronic granulomatous disease. N Engl J Med 1982; 307:800–803.

Donabedian H, Gallin JI. The hyperimmunoglobulin E recurrent infection (Job's) syndrome. Medicine 1983; 62:195–208.

Gallin JI, Buescher ES, Seligmann BE, Nath J, Gaither T, Katz P. Recent advances in chronic granulomatous disease. Ann Intern Med 1983; 99:657–674.

Gallin JI, Fletcher MP, Seligmann BE, Hoffstein S, Cehrs K, Mounessa N. Human neutrophil-specific granule deficiency: a model to assess the role of neutrophil-specific granules in the evolution of the inflammatory response. Blood 1982; 59:1317–1329.

COMMON VARIABLE IMMUNODEFICIENCY

REBECCA H. BUCKLEY, M.D.

Common variable immunodeficiency is a term that encompasses two different categories in the latest revision of the World Health Organization's primary immunodeficiency diseases classification. The categories share the feature of variable decreases in multiple immunoglobulin isotypes despite normal or low numbers of surface immunoglobulin bearing B lymphocytes. They differ in whether there is a predominant antibody or cellular immunodeficiency. For each type a variety of presumed pathogeneses have been postulated, including intrinsic B cell defects, decreased numbers of B or T cells, activated suppressor T cells, and autoantibodies to B or T cells. The primary biologic errors are unknown. Terms formerly used to refer to these defects include idiopathic late onset (or "acquired") hypogammaglobulinemia and congenital non-X linked (or sporadic) hypogammaglobulinemia. Although these defects have been considered to be acquired, there are few documentations of true "acquisitions" of immunoglobulin deficiency, and considerable evidence has been presented to support the view that genetic mechanisms are involved.

These defects are distinct from X linked agammaglobulinemia, which is characterized by a near absence of blood B cells and normal numbers of bone marrow pre-B cells; however, the immunoglobulin deficiency can be just as profound in common variable immunodeficiency as in X linked agammaglobulinemia. Males and females are affected with equal frequencies. Common variable immunodeficiency disorders are also to be distinguished from hypogammaglobulinemia due to transcobalamin II deficiency (correctable by intramuscular injections of vitamin B_{12}), from that due to protein losing states, and from that secondary to multiple myeloma or chronic lymphocytic leukemia. In protein losing enteropathy or states of renal protein loss, antibody synthesis proceeds normally, so that replacement therapy is not indicated. Indeed attempts at replacement are usually futile, as the IgG administered is also lost.

Because they lack the major heat stable opsonin of body fluids, patients with common variable immunodeficiency are susceptible to infections with high grade extracellular encapsulated bacterial pathogens. Most commonly these include *Haemophilus influenzae, Streptococcus pneumoniae,* group A streptococci, or *Staphylococcus aureus.* A majority of such patients have histories of chronic or recurrent pyogenic infections involving the upper and lower respiratory tracts. Bronchiectasis develops in approximately one third of the patients, often before diagnosis of the immunodeficiency is made. Septicemia and meningitis are also problems prior to initiation of replacement therapy. Much less frequently, patients with predominantly cellular common variable immunodeficiency have had pulmonary infections with opportunistic mycobacterial, fungal, and parasitic agents (for example, *Pneumocystis carinii*). In addition, there is a high incidence of gastrointestinal problems in patients with these defects. These include diarrhea secondary to infestation with *Giardia lamblia,* bacterial overgrowth, lactose or gluten intolerance, steatorrhea, or autoantibodies against gut epithelial antigens; pernicious anemia, usually associated with atrophic gastritis, achlorhydria, and absence of intrinsic factor; and gallbladder disease, such as cholelithiasis or cholangitis. The pernicious anemia may occur at any age and is not associated with easily demonstrable antibodies to parietal cells or to intrinsic factor. The diarrhea is often accompanied by jejunal villous atrophy or nodular follicular lymphoid hyperplasia of the bowel.

Lymphoid hyperplasia is also manifest as splenomegaly, which occurs in 25 to 30 percent of such patients and can result in hematologic evidence of hypersplenism. Pseudolymphoma and lymphoid interstitial pneumonia are also relatively common. As with other primary immunodeficiency disorders, there is a high incidence of lymphoreticular malignant disease, particularly in females in the fifth or sixth decade of life. Finally, because of the tendency of such patients to develop autoimmune reactions, there is an increased incidence of arthritis, thyroid disease, alopecia areata, and keratoconjunctivitis.

THERAPEUTIC APPROACHES

In the past, therapeutic modalities have consisted primarily of intramuscular immune serum globulin replacement and antimicrobial therapy. However, during the past two decades intravenous infusions of whole normal plasma and various experimentally modified Cohn fraction II preparations have been tried as alternatives. Nevertheless, until 1981 only immune serum globulin for intramuscular use was available commercially. With the marketing of one form of immune globulin intravenous preparation in that year and of others more recently, major changes have occurred in gamma globulin replacement therapy. There undoubtedly will be other revisions as additional preparations become available and as the body of information concerning optimal use of intravenous immune globulin therapy grows.

Intramuscular Administration of Immune Serum Globulin

Immune serum globulin for intramuscular administration is prepared from outdated blood bank or volunteer plasma by the ethanol fractionation method of Cohn and is supplied in solutions containing 14.5 to 16.5 g per 100 ml of IgG. Although the latter constitutes 95 to 99 percent of the protein, varying quantities of IgA, IgM, IgD, IgE, albumin, B1C, and transferrin are also present. The small quantities of immunoglobulin other than IgG are probably inconsequential from a beneficial clinical standpoint. However, patients with selective IgA deficiency or common variable immunodeficiency who have anti-IgA antibodies may have life threatening anaphylactic reactions to the IgA present. Neither hepatitis virus nor human immunodeficiency virus has been transmitted by immune serum globulin injections, suggesting that the antibodies present in such preparations protect against these diseases, that the responsible agents are eliminated by the separation procedures, or that the initial ethanol treatment inactivates them. Such preparations have been shown to aggregate and fragment and, as a consequence, to demonstrate anticomplementary activity, which can cause anaphylactoid reactions if they are given intravenously. The half-life of IgG in such preparations ranges from 17.5 to 22.1 days, with a mean of 19.8 days in normal subjects. It is usually longer in agammaglobulinemic subjects, although the presence of active bacterial infection may result in a shortening of the half-life in such patients.

There are a number of problems with intramuscular immune serum globulin therapy: The quantity that can be administered is limited by the muscle mass available, such injections are painful, there can be local digestion by muscle enzymes, abscess formation and sciatic nerve injury have been reported, and anaphylactoid reactions can occur if the intravascular space is inadvertently entered. For all these reasons major efforts were made to develop alternatives, including plasma therapy and various intravenous immune globulin preparations.

Normal Human Plasma

There are several reasons why normal human plasma would be ideal therapy for severe humoral immunodeficiency diseases: First, antibodies of all five immunoglobulin isotypes can be provided in significant quantities. Second, such intravenous infusions are far less painful than intramuscular immune serum globulin injections and thus have greater patient acceptability. Third, adverse reactions are few. Finally, higher serum immunoglobulin concentrations can be more readily achieved than with intramuscular immune serum globulin injections. Ten milliliters of plasma per kilogram of body weight provides approximately 100 mg per kg of immune serum globulin. Moreover, the donor can be immunized to provide higher titers of some antibodies than can be achieved with pooled gamma globulin.

The disadvantages include the following: (1) There is potential danger of transmitting hepatitis B, non-A, non-B hepatitis, or human immunodeficiency virus; (2)

an available regular donor is required, as random blood bank plasma increases these risk; (3) it provides a narrower range of antibody specificities, since it is derived from a single donor; (4) there is risk of graft versus host disease in infants with severe T cell defects from immunocompetent cells in the plasma; (5) volume overload can be a problem in some patients; and (6) it is inconvenient or impractical to perform plasmapheresis on a regular basis in some clinical settings. The risk of hepatitis B or human immunodeficiency virus transmission can be greatly reduced by careful donor selection, but transmission of non-A, non-B hepatitis remains an uncontrollable risk. The danger of graft versus host disease can be avoided either by carefully removing all cellular elements, by freezing the plasma, or by irradiating it sufficiently (with 3000 rad) to destroy the graft versus host disease potential of the immunocompetent cells.

Immune Globulin Intravenous Preparations

In my opinion intravenous immune globulin preparations clearly constitute the preferred form of therapy. There are several advantages to the administration of gamma globulin by the intravenous route: Much larger doses can be given than would be possible by the intramuscular route, the action is more rapid, there is no loss due to local proteolysis, and the therapy is far less painful. For nearly 3 decades there has been considerable interest in the development of gamma globulin preparations free of aggregates and anticomplementary activity so that they can be given safely by the intravenous route. Several approaches have been successful.

The two methods used in preparing currently available preparations in the United States include incubation at a low pH for varying periods of time and ion exchange chromatography. Both Sandoglobulin (Sandoz) and Gamimune N (Cutter) are prepared by the low pH method, and Gammagard (Travenol) is made by ion exchange chromatography. Each lot of these preparations is prepared from a pool of plasma from 2000 to 10,000 donors, each of whom also has been previously screened for antibodies to hepatitis viruses and human immunodeficiency virus. Antibody activities appear to be comparable in all three preparations, and the IgG molecules in all have retained good Fc function. The only clinically important difference is that there is much less IgA and IgE in Gammagard than in the other two products.

All have been tested in carefully supervised clinical trials. I have personally used five different intravenous immune globulin preparations and all appeared to be clinically safe and effective. Although only one preparation has undergone a controlled clinical trial to evaluate efficacy, it appears that a number of intravenous immune globulin preparations will prove to be both safe and efficacious.

Antimicrobial and Other Nonspecific Therapy

Probably because it is impossible to replace the major host defense component of external secretions, secretory IgA, a majority of patients with common variable immunodeficiency experience chronic or recurrent infections of mucous membrane surfaces (ears, sinuses, lungs, gastrointestinal tract) despite gamma globulin therapy. Even if enriched preparations of IgA were to become available for intramuscular or intravenous administration, the body has no mechanism for transporting IgA molecules from those compartments onto mucous membrane surfaces. Complications of chronic upper and lower respiratory tract infections, such as sinusitis and bronchiectasis, and chronic diarrhea account for most of the morbidity seen in these conditions. Thus, antibiotic therapy is frequently required for control of such infections.

Because of a predominance of *H. influenzae* organisms in sputum and other external secretions of such patients, antimicrobial drugs effective against these organisms are preferred. I find ampicillin (or amoxicillin) or trimethoprim and sulfamethoxazole to be effective in most patients. These antibiotics are used either for specific infections at full therapeutic dosages or for prolonged periods at lower dosages in patients with bronchiectasis or persistent pyogenic infections. If they are used for prolonged periods, I find it helpful to alternate between the two types of antibiotics, usually on a monthly or bimonthly basis. It is important to emphasize that they are given in addition to gamma globulin replacement. For patients who become infected with beta lactamase positive *H. influenzae,* cefaclor (Ceclor) or ampicillin with potassium clavulanate (Augmentin) may be given. I have also found chloromycetin to be an effective drug in that situation, particularly if the patient shows signs of acute or progressive chronic infection, despite long term antimicrobial therapy. Ampicillin or amoxicillin is preferable to trimethoprim and sulfamethoxazole if there is concurrent infection with *S. pneumoniae* or group A beta hemolytic streptococcal organisms. Tetracycline is not very useful for long term therapy in these patients. Staphylococcal infections are less common; cultures are helpful in alerting to a need for antistaphylococcal drugs. Percussion and postural drainage on a twice daily basis are also helpful adjuncts to therapy in patients with bronchiectasis.

Occasionally patients with common variable immunodeficiency may develop interstitial pneumonia due to *P. carinii.* This is prevented by long term therapy with trimethoprim and sulfamethoxazole. If Pneumocystis pneumonia does occur, it usually responds to high dose therapy with that drug or to pentamidine isethionate. Patients with these defects may also develop tuberculosis or fungal infections of the lung, but these are far less common than those due to high grade bacterial pathogens. Nevertheless resistant gram negative or opportunistic infections should be suspected in patients

with these defects who do not respond to the drugs just listed.

Patients with chronic diarrhea may also benefit from antibiotic therapy, particularly when they have persistent infections with Salmonella or Shigella, but also occasionally when there is an overgrowth of normal intestinal organisms. Most commonly, however, the diarrhea is associated with *G. lamblia* infestation. The latter should be treated with quinacrine hydrochloride (Atabrine) at a dosage of 6 mg per kg per day, not to exceed 300 mg per day, in three divided doses orally for 5 days. Alternatively (as a second choice) metronidazole (Flagyl) may be used in three divided doses totaling 15 mg per kg per day (not to exceed 750 mg) for 5 days; the latter would also be effective against infections with *Clostridium difficile.*

For patients with pernicious anemia, life-time parenteral therapy with vitamin B_{12} is usually required.

DOSAGE OF GAMMA GLOBULIN

For many years after the first agammaglobulinemic patient was treated with gamma globulin, the recommended dosage of intramuscular immune serum globulin for the treatment of humoral immunodeficiency was 100 mg per kg per month (0.6 to 0.7 ml per kg per month), after a loading dose of two to three times that amount. Those doses necessarily required the administration of large volumes by the intramuscular route, resulting in great discomfort to the recipient. It is well to point out that the dosages recommended were selected empirically. Although Janeway and Rosen reported that the 100 mg per kg per month dosage resulted in serum levels of approximately 200 mg per dl soon after administration in most of their patients, in my experience IgG concentrations are much lower than this for most of the month in patients given 100 mg per kg per month. Mean trough serum IgG concentrations of my agammaglobulinemic patients treated with that dosage of immune serum globulin were generally less than 100 mg per dl, and peak concentrations did not exceed 150 mg per dl. More important, there was wide variation from patient to patient in the serum IgG concentrations achieved, despite administration of a uniform per kilogram dosage.

These shortcomings pointed up the need for investigations to determine the optimal dosage. Because of volume limitations with intramuscular immune serum globulin therapy, however, new dosing is being investigated almost entirely with intravenous immune globulin preparations. Work to date indicates that there is considerable variability in the half-life of IgG from patient to patient, suggesting that a uniform dose may not always be appropriate. In studies I did in which 400 mg per kg per month of immune globulin therapy was given intravenously to a number of patients with common variable immunodeficiency, most had trough serum IgG concentrations of 200 to 400 mg per dl 4 weeks later. It is entirely possible that controlled studies will show dosages of this magnitude to be far more appropriate. However, it is again important to emphasize that the ideal dosage is not known and that, in all likelihood, it will not be a uniform one for all patients. In patients with severe or chronic bacterial infections, even higher dosages or more frequent administration may be needed.

ADVERSE EFFECTS OF GAMMA GLOBULIN THERAPY

Adverse Effects of Intramuscular Therapy with Immune Serum Globulin and Normal Human Plasma

Adverse effects of intramuscular therapy with immune serum globulin and normal human plasma have been summarized under the discussion of immune serum globulin and plasma therapy.

Adverse Reactions to Intravenous Immune Globulin Therapy

Reactions to intravenous infusions of unmodified immune serum globulin have been known for some time to be more frequent and more severe in patients with antibody deficiency syndromes or with acute infections than in normal individuals, for reasons that are not clear. The same is true with the new intravenous immune globulin preparations, but fortunately the overall frequency is much lower. It has been postulated that these reactions are secondary to inflammatory reactions caused by the union of antibodies with free antigen in the patient's circulation, since they occur most frequently in newly treated, infected, or infrequently and inadequately treated patients. Symptoms and signs of such reactions most often include back or abdominal pain, nausea, and vomiting within the first 30 minutes, and chills, fever, and fatigue beginning at the end of the infusion and continuing for several hours afterward. Most of these adverse effects can be prevented by slowing the initial rate of infusion or by pretreatment with aspirin. The frequency and severity of these reactions diminish after infection, particularly of the lungs, has been brought under control by long term antibiotic therapy and regular intravenous immune globulin therapy for a few months. On the basis of experience with high dose gamma globulin treatment in idiopathic thrombocytopenic purpura, there appear to be few or no adverse effects from dosages as high as 500 mg per kg per day given on 5 successive days. True anaphylactic reactions have been rare except in patients with anti-IgA antibodies.

Adverse Effects of Gamma Globulin Therapy in Patients with Anti-IgA Antibodies

As already noted, systemic anaphylactic reactions to immune serum globulin, plasma, and intravenous immune globulin therapy have been noted in patients with common variable agammaglobulinemia who have antibodies to IgA. Symptoms are those of a classic IgE mediated anaphylactic reaction, in contrast to those observed with intravenous immune globulin therapy in patients without anti-IgA antibodies. They appear seconds to minutes after the injections or infusions and include one or more of the following: flushing, facial swelling, pruritus, dyspnea, cyanosis, anxiety, nausea, vomiting, malaise, hypotension, loss of consciousness, and death. The treatment of such reactions is the immediate administration of epinephrine, oxygen, and antihistamines and the intravenous administration of fluids and corticosteroids.

I have evaluated and treated three patients with common variable agammaglobulinemia who have had anaphylactic reactions to IgA and who have high titers of IgG class specific anti-IgA antibodies. In addition, I have recently demonstrated the presence of IgE anti-IgA antibodies in these patients. Initially I used IgA deficient plasma provided from clinically normal donors by the American Red Cross. However, one patient developed non-A, non-B hepatitis while receiving such infusions. It is important to point out that only the ion exchange prepared intravenous immune globulin (Gammagard) contains almost no detectable IgA (less than $1.5 \mu g$ per ml in most lots). I have used this preparation without reactions in the treatment of these three patients with common variable immunodeficiency who have had nearly fatal anaphylactic reactions to intramuscular gamma globulin therapy, plasma infusions, or intravenous immune globulin preparations not prepared by ion exchange chromatography. The unusual feature in these patients is that, although they had no detectable serum IgA, they also had very low concentrations of IgG and IgM, yet were still able to produce both IgG and IgE anti-IgA antibodies. These experiences clearly demonstrate that anti-IgA antibodies may exist in immunodeficient patients other than those with typical selective IgA deficiency. Thus, it is imperative that this possibility be investigated prior to beginning replacement therapy in any patient with no serum IgA, even though concentrations of the other two classes may be abnormally low. The American Red Cross can test for IgG antibodies to IgA, but it is highly probable that it is the IgE antibodies to IgA that cause most of these anaphylactic reactions.

SUGGESTED READING

Buckley RH. Primary immunodeficiency diseases. In: Wyngaarden JB, Smith LG, eds. Cecil textbook of medicine. 18th ed. Philadelphia: WB Saunders, 1988, 1855.

Buckley RH. Gamma globulin replacement. Clin Immunol Allergy 1985; 5:141–158.

Burks AW, Sampson HA, Buckley RH. Anaphylactic reactions following gamma globulin administration in patients with hypogammaglobulinemia. Detection of IgE antibodies to IgA. N Engl J Med 1986; 314:560–564.

Report of a World Health Organization Scientific Group. Primary immunodeficiency diseases. Clin Immunol Immunopathol 1986; 40:166.

Stiehm ER, Ashida E, Kim KS, Winston DJ, Haas A, Gale RP. Intravenous immunoglobulins as therapeutic agents. Ann Intern Med 1987; 107:367–382.

SEVERE COMBINED IMMUNODEFICIENCY DISEASE

RAIF S. GEHA, M.D.

Severe combined immunodeficiency disease (SCID) is a syndrome that comprises a group of heterogeneous disorders affecting the functional integrity of T and B lymphocytes. The syndrome is present in infants with no circulating lymphocytes as well as in those with normal numbers of T and B lymphocytes. In some of these children the T cells are of maternal origin. As a rule, patients lack all aspects of T cell immunity and show an absence of or very poor in vitro proliferative response to phytohemagglutinin. Rarely a mixed lymphocyte response or phytohemagglutinin induced proliferative response may be present. Profound hypogammaglobulinemia and failure of specific antibody formation are common. In exceptional cases there are normal levels of all classes of circulating immunoglobulins and normal levels of IgM or monoclonal immunoglobulin production, but specific antibody responses are absent.

Most patients with combined immunodeficiency disease present between 2 and 6 months of age with failure to thrive, recurrent infections, thrush and pneumonia usually contributed to by *Pneumocystis carinii,* and diarrhea. The disease exists in both X linked and autosomal recessive forms. The male to female ratio is 3:1 or 4:1. If untreated, most infants die before 12 months of age.

Briefly, SCID may result from the absence of the appropriate lymphoid precursors, the absence of the appropriate microenvironment for differentiation, or intrinsic cellular defects, which despite normal differentiation cause lymphocytes to be functionally effete. Many patients with SCID have normal numbers of B lymphocytes, and some of the patients appear to have abnormalities of T cell differentiation alone.

The major microenvironment for T cell development is the thymus. There is probably a complex sequence of events responsible for T cell differentiation. Defects in thymic epithelial cell function, defects in receptors for thymic hormones, abnormal trafficking patterns, and potential inhibitors may account for the observed heterogeneity for SCID. In one group of patients (approximately 15 percent of those with SCID) an associated absence of the purine enzyme adenosine deaminase has been described. In a very few patients the purine enzyme nucleoside phosphorylase is deficient.

GENERAL THERAPEUTIC CONSIDERATIONS

Adequate caloric and fluid intake and appropriate antibiotic therapy are the mainstays of the supportive therapeutic program. Although gamma globulin is usually given, it is of limited value because of the nature of many of the infections suffered by these patients.

These patients are highly susceptible to the development of acute graft versus host disease (GVHD) after the administration of blood or blood products containing immunocompetent cells or bone marrow transplantation. Administration of as little as 5 ml of blood to these children has resulted in death from acute GVHD. Acute GVHD reactions are characterized by a maculopapular rash, which usually begins on the face and spreads to involve the entire body; fever; diarrhea; splenomegaly; hepatic dysfunction; occasionally eosinophilia; and, if the reaction is severe and unchecked, death. To avoid this problem, blood or blood products should be irradiated to inactivate immunocompetent cells, or frozen red cells should be used.

RECONSTITUTION THERAPY IN SCID

Correction of the immune deficiency in SCID may take one of two forms: reconstitution therapy or replacement therapy. Reconstitution therapy implies the provision of self-renewing precursor cells, which, following engraftment, will be immunocompetent. Thus, these functional lymphocytes would be of donor origin.

Bone Marrow Transplantation

Successful reconstitution of immune function in patients with SCID has been achieved following bone marrow transplantation in more than 80 patients.

Genotypically Identical Donors. The majority of successful transplants have been from HLA-A, -B, and -D genotypically identical sibling donors. Several instances of reconstitution have followed transplants from genotypically identical family members other than siblings.

Overall, approximately 60 percent of the patients receiving a genotypically identical transplant survive beyond 1 to 2 years; the longest survival is now 16 years. The reasons for some of the failures are unclear, but in many cases intercurrent infections are a major limiting factor. Some defects (for example, intrathymic defects) may not be responsive to simple provision of lymphoid precursor cells. For successful transplants, a single intravenous infusion of 5×10^7 nucleated marrow cells per kilogram of body weight is often sufficient, although as few as 5×10^6 cells have been used. Pretransplant immunosuppressive therapy is generally not required. Although acute GVHD in the post-transplant period is not unusual, it is most often self-limited and rarely fatal in this group. Therefore, drugs to prevent or combat GVHD are not generally used. When used, treatment consists of either methotrexate given at the earliest signs of GVHD or in vivo administration of pan T cell monoclonal antibody.

Engraftment usually is observed in 14 to 21 days, with an increase in numbers and function of T lymphocytes and the appearance of immunoglobulins. This is paralleled by improvement in general well being as evidenced by weight gain and resolution of infections. As a rule, functional T lymphocytes are donor in origin, whereas B lymphocyte function may be derived from recipient as well as donor cells. Engraftment is restricted to the lymphoid cells. Hematopoietic stem cells remain of recipient origin, although transient red cell chimerism has been observed.

Phenotypically Identical Donors. Successful transplants have been achieved only rarely using phenotypically identical donors, and then only from related rather than unrelated donors. Overall, GVHD has been most severe and often fatal in this group. With partial matching between donor and recipient, the MLC or HLA-Dr locus is more important in the prevention of GVHD than the HLA-A or -B locus. Recent experience suggests that depletion of mature T cells from the bone marrow inoculum (to be discussed) enhances survival in this group.

Nonidentical Donors. Severe and often fatal GVHD has regularly followed transplantation from a histoincompatible donor, usually a haploidentical parent. Early attempts to remove immunocompetent T cells from the bone marrow inoculum to prevent these consequences were based on cell separation procedures by physical means, suiciding with radioisotope, or use of heterologous anti-T cell antisera. Each of these has been generally unsuccessful in avoiding GVHD or permitting lymphoid engraftment.

Two new approaches have resulted in successful reconstitution of haploidentical marrow. The first approach is based on the selective removal of T lymphocytes on lectin (soybean agglutinin) columns. The second approach is to utilize specific monoclonal antibodies directed against T cell antigens in the treatment of the bone marrow inoculum prior to transplant, and GVHD in the post-transplant period. The monoclonal antibodies are used in conjunction with rabbit complement to kill the T cells. Alternatively the bone marrow is treated with $(Fab')_2$ fragments of monoclonal antibody conjugated to ricin. The latter procedure has the advantage of not requiring repeated washes of the bone marrow cell suspension. The recipient is treated with lymphocytotoxic drugs (for example, antilymphocytic serum and cyclophosphamide, 50 mg per kg per day for 4 days) prior to transplant. In both approaches lymphoid engraftment is slow, with T cell function taking as long as 8 months to 1 year to become detectable. Recovery of B cell function, when it occurs, is further delayed. To date about 20 children have received T cell depleted haploidentical marrow. One third of them have survived beyond 6 to 12 months. In children with SCID haploidentical bone marrow stable chimerism of red cells and monocytes has been observed. In most of these children the B cells and monocytes are of recipient origin, whereas the T cells are always of donor origin. In a few children receiving very heavy cytotoxic therapy, B as well as T cells and in some cases monocytes are of donor origin.

Fetal Liver Transplantation

Fetal liver was considered as a possible source to replace missing or defective lymphoid stem cells. The lack of histocompatibility and the risk of GVHD require the use of cells from fetuses of less than 11 to 13 weeks' gestation.

In the majority of cases, lymphoid engraftment was not achieved; in some, GVHD was observed, indicating that immunocompetent T cells were transplanted. In those with engraftment, including those who received both fetal liver and fetal thymus together, immune function was very limited. In those with normal immune function, the donor derived T cells recognize antigen in association with HLA antigens of the recipient.

REPLACEMENT THERAPY IN SCID

Replacement therapy in SCID implies the provision of a missing cell, factor, and enzyme, which could lead to the functional differentiation of host lymphocytes.

Thymus Tissue

Fetal thymus transplants can be considered as reconstructive therapy. Fetal thymus initially was used in an attempt to replace defective thymus tissue in patients with SCID, especially when a histocompatible donor was not available. Fetal tissue of less than 12 weeks' gestation is implanted in a pouch created within an accessible muscle bundle (such as the rectus abdominis).

In rare cases immune reconstitution has been achieved, and several instances of mild to severe GVHD have been reported. In virtually all cases in which benefit has been observed, the T lymphocytes have been donor in origin, and immunity, if present, has been exclusively T cell and short-lived.

Despite histoincompatibility, GVHD is rarely seen. The responses of patients to such transplants have been extremely variable. In many, increased numbers of circulating T lymphocytes of host origin are observed 6 to 8 weeks following transplant. They are often of immature phenotype, short-lived, and marginally functional. In others, sustained production of host T cells is maintained, but full functional integrity is rarely, if ever, achieved. There have been no documented cases in which fetal thymus has provided a source of functional thymus epithelium, leading to differentiation of host T cells. The acquisition of B cell function has also been very variable. Of particular concern has been the striking incidence of the development of B cell lymphomas after epithelial cell transplants. Whether this reflects transmission of virus (such as the Epstein-Barr virus) or the lack of immunoregulation is uncertain at present.

Thymus Derived Factors

There is considerable evidence that the later stages of T cell differentiation are susceptible to cell-free thymus derived factors. Several laboratories have identified and in some cases partially purified substances from the thymus that affect immune responsiveness. Among the factors isolated from the thymus, the best characterized are thymopoietin and a group of peptides contained in the calf thymus extract, thymosin. Few patients with SCID show any demonstrable response to these factors in vitro. Similarly, in vivo trials with these preparations to replace missing "hormones" have been without benefit clinically and have not induced T cell immunocompetence.

Enzyme Replacement

As discussed, approximately 15 percent of the patients with SCID have an associated absence of the enzyme adenosine deaminase. Following the in vitro observation that exogenous adenosine deaminase improved the responsiveness of SCID T cells to phytohemagglutinin, replacement therapy with irradiated erythrocytes as a source of enzyme has been attempted. Regular transfusions with erythrocytes have significantly corrected the metabolic abnormalities, but improvement in lymphocyte numbers, and particularly lymphocyte function, has been the exception. Recently the gene for the human adenosine deaminase enzyme has been successfully cloned. This opens the possibility of genetic reconstruction in adenosine deaminase deficient patients with SCID.

SUGGESTED READING

Buckley RH, Schiff SE, Sampson AA, Schiff RI, Market ML, Knutsen AP, Hershfield MS, Huang AT, Mickey GH, Ward FE. Development of immunity in human severe primary T cell deficiency following haploidentical bone marrow stem cell transplantation. J Immunol 1986; 136:2398–2407.

Friedrich W, Goldmann SF, Ebell W, Blutters-Sawatzki R, Gaedecke G, Raghavachar A, Peter HH, Belohradsky B, Kreth W, Kubanek B, Kleihauer E. Severe combined immunodeficiency: treatment by bone marrow transplantation in 15 infants using HLA haploidentical donors. Eur J Pediatr 1985; 144:125–130.

Levey RH, Klemperer MR, Gelfane EI, Sanderson A, Batchelor JR, Rosen FS. Bone marrow transplantation in severe combined immunodeficiency syndrome. Lancet 1971; 2:571–575.

Reinherz E, Geha R, Rappaport JM, Wilson M, Penta AC, Hussey RE, Fitzgerald KA, Daley JF, Levine H, Rosen FS, Schlossman SF. Reconstitution after transplantation with T lymphocyte depleted HLA haplotype mismatched bone marrow for severe combined immunodeficiency. Proc Natl Acad Sci USA 1982; 79:6047–6051.

Reisner Y, Kapoor N, Kirkpatrick D, Pollack MS, Cunningham-Rundles C, Dupont B, Hodes HZ, Good RA, O'Reilly RJ. Transplantation for severe combined immunodeficiency with HLA-A, B, D, DR incompatible parental marrow cells fractionated by soybean agglutinin and sheep red blood cells. Blood 1983; 61:341–348.

Rosen FS. The primary immunodeficiencies and serum complement defects. In: Nathan DG, Oski FA, eds. Hematology of infancy and childhood. Philadelphia: WB Saunders, 1981:866.

CONGENITAL IMMUNODEFICIENCY DISEASES

ALEXANDER R. LAWTON, M.D.

Inherited diseases that impair host defense capabilities include deficiencies in numbers or function of lymphocytes, phagocytic cells, or proteins of the complement system. This discussion is confined to the primary immunodeficiency diseases, which are disorders of lymphocyte differentiation. These rare disorders have been classified by a Scientific Group of the World Health Organization into three groups: diseases associated predominantly with defects in antibody production, those in which both antibody production and cell mediated immunity are impaired, and a group in which immunodeficiency is associated with some other condition. The classification is far from perfect, reflecting continued ignorance of the pathogenesis of most of these diseases.

Antibody deficiency states predispose to recurrent infections with encapsulated bacteria, particularly *Hemophilus influenzae, Streptococcus pneumoniae,* and *Streptococcus pyogenes.* The response of patients with acute systemic infections to appropriate antibiotic therapy is usually not different from that of normal persons. However, recurrent infections of the upper and lower respiratory tract eventually lead to tissue damage predisposing to chronic bronchitis, bronchiectasis, sinusitis, and otitis media, which are difficult to treat adequately. In these situations the pyogenic bacteria are frequently replaced by nontypable *H. influenzae,* staphylococci, and enteric bacteria.

With a few prominent exceptions, viral or fungal infections are not a particular threat to patients with antibody deficiency. Although the course of the childhood exanthems in hypogammaglobulinemic children is similar to that in normal children, permanent immunity may not develop. It might be predicted that failure to produce antibodies to the many respiratory viruses would lead to a higher incidence of recurrence of infections caused by these agents. In practice, the passive immunization provided by treatment with exogenous immunoglobulin makes the frequency of virus infections no higher than expected in normal persons.

There are important exceptions to these generalizations about susceptibility to virus infections. A subgroup of agammaglobulinemic patients have a high risk of developing a chronic progressive encephalomyelitis caused by enteric viruses, particularly echovirus and poliomyelitis. Disseminated enterovirus infection may closely resemble dermatomyositis. Hepatitis B virus also may also cause fulminant and frequently fatal infections in these patients. Patients at risk for the development of chronic enterovirus encephalitis or the dermatomyositis-like illness appear to be those who lack B lymphocytes. Most reported patients have been males with X linked agammaglobulinemia, in whom genesis of B lymphocytes is blocked at the pre-B cell stage. This suggests that B lymphocytes may have a role in host defense independent of their function in antibody production.

Pneumocystis carinii pneumonia is most commonly associated with defective T lymphocyte function, but occasionally is seen as the presenting infection in patients with antibody deficiency. Septic arthritis involving multiple large joints due to *Ureaplasma urealyticum* has occurred in several patients; both ureaplasmas and mycoplasmas may cause respiratory or urinary tract infections.

Patients with severe defects of T cell function usually develop multiple opportunistic viral, fungal, bacterial, and protozoan infections shortly after birth. For many of these infections no curative treatment is available. Death occurs during infancy or early childhood unless T cell function can be restored.

THERAPEUTIC APPROACHES

The principles for the treatment of infections occurring in immunodeficient patients do not differ from those in any other patient. Adequate specimens for culture should be obtained whenever possible. Patients with known or suspected T cell deficiencies who develop acute febrile illness should be treated early and aggressively with combinations of antibiotics given intravenously, with the presumption that they may have multiple organism septicemia caused by enteric flora and perhaps staphylococci. Febrile patients with hypogammaglobulinemia should be evaluated frequently and carefully for signs of bacterial infection, but it is not necessary to treat every such illness with antibiotics.

ANTIBODY DEFICIENCY DISORDERS

From the early 1960s to 1981, replacement therapy for hypogammaglobulinemia could be accomplished only by intramuscular injections of gamma globulins (Cohn fraction II). The recommended dosage of 100 mg per kg monthly was empirical and was limited by the volume that could be tolerated by intramuscular injection. Since 1981 several preparations of chemically or physically modified immunoglobulins suitable for intravenous administration have been marketed. These have proven to be safe, with a reaction incidence considerably less than that occurring with intramuscularly administered preparations, and effective. The main factor limiting the intravenous dosage of immunoglobulin is its considerable expense. An average adult dosage of 200 mg per kg, the lowest used for monthly maintenance in most centers, costs approximately $600 (wholesale, not including costs for administration).

The optimal intravenous dosage of immunoglobulin has not yet been established. Acute pneumonias, meningitis, and septicemic infections generally have been well controlled by intramuscular injections of 100 mg per kg and are clearly well controlled by intravenous dosages of 200 mg per kg of immunoglobulin. It is not yet clear whether higher dosages, 400 to 800 mg per kg (or even the dosage necessary to maintain serum IgG concentrations at 5 mg per ml or higher), will significantly ameliorate chronic sinusitis, otitis media, and bronchitis that have not been responsive to low dosage immunoglobulin therapy. Many agammaglobulinemic children diagnosed early and treated optimally with intramuscular immunoglobulin therapy never have acute pneumonia but nevertheless have developed chronic bronchopulmonary disease. Whether this problem is preventable by early high dosage intravenous immunoglobulin therapy is not certain. Some preliminary studies suggest that patients with intractable sinopulmonary disease do considerably better when immunoglobulin levels are maintained within the normal range.

The most important unresolved question about intravenous immunoglobulin therapy for agammaglobulinemia concerns prevention of chronic enterovirus meningoencephalitis. This disease is probably becoming the most common cause of death in boys with X linked agammaglobulinemia. High intravenous doses of immunoglobulin selected for high titers of antibody to the specific viral agent, given both intravenously and intracerebrally, have produced clinical remission and clearance of virus from the cerebrospinal fluid in some patients, but most have eventually relapsed. Prevention probably can be achieved by adequate intravenous doses of immunoglobulin; determination of the required dose is of the utmost importance.

Intravenous Treatment with Immunoglobulin

The most difficult aspect of the intravenous use of immunoglobulin is the decision about whom to treat. Patients with severe panhypogammaglobulinemia (less than 2 mg per ml of IgG), deficiency of IgG and IgA with normal or elevated IgM levels, or combined immunodeficiency obviously require treatment. Patients with isolated deficiency of IgA and infants with transient hypogammaglobulinemia usually are not benefited, and may be harmed, by treatment. The "gray area" occurs in patients in whom serum concentrations of IgG are moderately decreased, and especially those having selective deficiencies of IgG subclasses.

Because IgG1 is the major class of IgG, selective deficiency of this immunoglobulin is almost always associated with a low value for the total IgG concentration. Deficiency of IgG2, in contrast, infrequently occurs in patients with normal or only mildly decreased concentrations of IgG. IgA deficiency may or may not be present. There is no question that many patients with selective IgG2 deficiency have recurrent infections with encapsulated bacteria and will benefit from intravenous immunoglobulin therapy. This condition is easy to diagnose; because normal concentrations of IgG2 are relatively high, significant deficiency is easily detectable.

Deficiencies of IgG3 and IgG4 are much more difficult to ascertain, for several reasons. First, concentrations of these subclasses are low and variable, both in the population and from time to time in the same patient. Second, quantification is difficult, and results obtained from commercial laboratories may not be reliable. Third, there is no convincing evidence that these immunoglobulins have a special role in host defense that cannot be served by another immunoglobulin class.

Rarely patients with relatively normal concentrations of IgG have severe deficits in specific antibody production. These include boys with the Wiskott-Aldrich syndrome, who have a defect in antibody responses to carbohydrate antigens, some patients with ataxia telangiectasia, and patients with the Nezelof's syndrome. Intravenous immunoglobulin treatment would be expected to benefit only patients who have chronic and recurrent bacterial sinopulmonary disease and in whom defects in specific antibody production are demonstrable.

The decision to treat a patient falling into the "gray area" with regard to IgG concentrations should be based on a history of recurrent bacterial infections and evidence of inability to produce specific antibodies. Such evidence is usually obtained by immunizing with commercial vaccines and measuring the responses 1 to 2 weeks later. A "trial" of immunoglobulin therapy often does more harm than good. The effects of this sort of therapy can be measured only over a period of months to years and are therefore difficult to evaluate. Parents and patients may easily become convinced that their health, or even life, depends upon continued treatment. In my experience weaning from intravenous immunoglobulin therapy can be as difficult as weaning from corticosteroids.

In our clinic most patients receive monthly dosages of 200 mg per kg. Gamimune N and Sandoglobulin are chemically similar preparations of intact IgG prepared at a low pH and stabilized with maltose or sucrose. The major difference is in packaging. Gamimune is supplied as a liquid in units of 10, 50, and 100 ml of 5 percent IgG, whereas Sandoglobulin is lyophilized in 1, 3, or 6 g quantities, which are reconstituted with saline to make either 3 or 6 percent protein solutions. Gammagard, the newest intravenously administered immunoglobulin product, is purified by ultrafiltration and ion exchange chromatography and has a neutral pH. This preparation contains very small amounts of IgA (less than 10 μg per ml) and has been used safely in a patient who developed anaphylaxis following infusion of other preparations, owing to the presence of IgE antibodies to

IgA. Gammagard is supplied lyophilized in 2.5 or 5 g quantities.

All products are derived from similar large plasma pools. To my knowledge, none has been associated with transmission of viral disease. The measured half-lifes are similar. Except for the rare patient who might react to the small amounts of IgA present in Gamimune N and Sandoglobulin, the preparations are equivalent, and the choice can be made on the basis of cost.

We carefully follow the administration instructions in the package insets. Side effects are minimal if the infusion is begun slowly (about 0.5 ml per kg per hour). The maximal recommended infusion rate is 4 ml per kg per hour. Flushing, sensations of chest tightness, and back pain occur sometimes with high infusion rates and disappear when the rate is decreased. Pretreatment with a small dose of aspirin seems to lessen the frequency of discomfort during infusions. Trials of home administration are being conducted at several centers, attesting to the generally excellent tolerance to intravenous infusion of these immunoglobulin preparations.

We generally obtain a preinfusion IgG concentration 3 to 4 months after initiation of treatment, a time at which equilibrium should be established. The half-life of infused IgG may vary markedly from patient to patient; the main reason for this check is to detect patients in whom the half-life is inordinately short. An IgG concentration less than 100 mg per dl would necessitate an increase in dose. In most patients taking 200 mg per kg, nadir levels are maintained in the 200 to 400 mg per dl range. We are much more concerned, at least for the present, with clinical response than with IgG concentrations. Patients continuing to have symptoms of chronic bronchitis or bronchiectasis probably should receive a higher dose.

Other Therapy

Many agammaglobulinemic patients continue to suffer from chronic and recurrent infections of the respiratory mucosal surfaces, particularly otitis media, sinusitis, and bronchitis. This presumably reflects the failure to replace secretory antibodies, largely secretory IgA. The organisms most frequently responsible for acute and chronic infections have been mentioned earlier. Our group frequently treats problem patients with rotating 2 week courses of ampicillin and trimethoprim-sulfamethoxazole (5 to 10 mg per kg of trimethoprim), particularly during the winter months. Whenever possible, antibiotic therapy should be guided by isolation of the organisms and determination of sensitivity to antibiotics. As already mentioned, preliminary data suggest that these problem patients may improve significantly on high dose intravenous immunoglobulin therapy.

I am convinced that patients with chronic productive cough, regardless of whether they have demonstrable bronchiectasis, benefit from regular postural drain-

age. Parents or spouses of patients are taught the technique of chest percussion and drainage by respiratory therapists and are encouraged to do about 20 minutes of therapy on arising and just before bedtime. Using the analogy of the role of brushing the teeth in preventing dental caries, I urge my patients to continue this therapy even when they are well. A few minutes in a hot shower seems to increase the effectiveness of postural drainage. Treatment with antihistamines or vasoconstrictors should be avoided.

Patients with panhypogammaglobulinemia, deficiency of IgG and IgA, or isolated deficiency of IgA appear to be considerably more susceptible to chronic enteritis due to *Giardia lamblia* than normal children. Cryptosporidium infection has also been described. We attempt to identify Giardia by stool examination in patients with persistent diarrhea, but often treat empirically with metronizadole, 25 mg per kg per day for 5 days, even if cysts are not seen.

The question of immunizations is frequently raised by physicians caring for immunodeficient patients. The passive immunization received by patients given intravenous immunoglobulin therapy probably affords protection from all the diseases for which vaccines are currently available. There is no advantage to be gained from administering any of the live attenuated virus vaccines to any agammaglobulinemic patient, and there is clearly a risk associated with the polio vaccine. As mentioned earlier, there are several reports of vaccine related poliomyelitis in boys with X linked agammaglobulinemia. Although I know of no evidence that T cell immunity in the absence of antibody formation is protective, immunization of agammaglobulinemic children with killed polio (Salk) vaccine seems reasonable and is safe. There is no point in immunizing with diphtheria or tetanus toxoids or with the newly introduced carbohydrate vaccines of *H. influenzae*, pneumococcus, or meningococcus, because stimulating T cells with these vaccines is not relevant. We do not advocate the use of influenza vaccine, because intravenous immunoglobulin therapy seems to afford considerable passive protection.

Hypogammaglobulinemic patients with normal cell mediated immunity are not at increased risk from varicella and probably will not develop the disease if they are being treated with intravenous immunoglobulin therapy.

The problem of chronic enteroviral meningoencephalitis in agammaglobulinemic patients is discussed in a recent review by McKinney et al. A combination of high dose monthly intravenous immunoglobulin treatment and intermittent infusions of immunoglobulin directly into the cerebrospinal fluid via an indwelling intraventricular catheter has produced long remissions in a few patients. Patient sera should be monitored periodically for neutralizing antibody to the causative enterovirus, if one has been isolated. Ideally the preinfusion titer should be 1:4 or higher. For intraventricular infusions, products with a pH near neutral (Gammagard) may be tolerated better, although other products have been used with only minor side effects. The titer should be 1:16 or higher. Daily or twice daily exchange infusions of increasing volumes up to 10 ml should be given until the lumbar spinal fluid is normal and viral cultures from both lumbar and ventricular spinal fluid are persistently negative.

Since this complication occurs almost exclusively in patients lacking circulating B lymphocytes (most commonly, boys with X linked agammaglobulinemia), I believe that high dosage (400 mg per kg) intravenous immunoglobulin therapy should begin in this group as soon as the diagnosis is made. Prevention is probably more attainable, and certainly more cost effective, than successful treatment.

COMBINED IMMUNODEFICIENCY

The severe combined immunodeficiencies are a heterogeneous group of diseases, which differ in inheritance patterns, lymphocyte phenotypes, and molecular pathogenesis. These diseases have in common the absence of both humoral and cell mediated immune functions, leading inexorably to death from multiple viral, bacterial, and fungal infections before 2 years of age. Considering the differences in molecular etiology, it is remarkable that most if not all patients with severe combined immunodeficiency can be cured by transplantation of bone marrow derived stem cells.

The first successful restoration of immune function by bone marrow transplantation in a patient with severe combined immunodeficiency was reported in 1968. For many years this therapy was available for only a small proportion of patients, because the requirement for complete matching at the major histocompatibility locus limited donors to HLA identical siblings. Introduction of two techniques for the removal of mature T cells from marrow has now made this therapy available for all patients with severe combined immunodeficiency. Since T cell depleted marrow does not cause fatal graft versus host disease despite a major histocompatibility difference, haploidentical transplants, usually from parent to child, are now feasible. One of the methods for T cell removal utilizes complement dependent lysis of T cells by monoclonal antibodies. The second method involves depletion of T cells by rosetting with sheep erythrocytes followed by agglutination with soy lectin. Although the latter method appears crude by comparison, it apparently avoids a major complication. Several patients receiving transplants of haploidentical marrow depleted of T cells by monoclonal antibodies have developed fatal Epstein-Barr virus induced B cell lymphomas of donor origin. It is speculated that removal of virtually all T cells from the marrow may permit the outgrowth of donor-derived transformed B cells.

Haploidentical marrow transplantation has produced partial or complete restoration of immune cells and function in patients with X linked or autosomal recessive severe combined immunodeficiency as well as in those with adenosine deaminase deficiency. The first mentioned group generally have had normal or nearly normal numbers of B lymphocytes, but few if any T cells. Although this phenotype suggests a defect in the thymic microenvironment, the regular appearance of donor derived T cells following transplantation of T depleted marrow indicates that this is not correct.

In comparison with transplantation of unfractionated major histocompatibility (MHC) identical marrow, the kinetics of restoration of T and B cell populations following transplantation with T depleted marrow are leisurely. Donor cells may be detectable by 4 to 6 weeks, but normal numbers are rarely achieved before 3 months.

These diseases are rare and their treatment is complicated and time consuming. A successful clinical outcome and maximal accrual of knowledge are most likely to occur in centers doing several transplant procedures each year. For these reasons many pediatric immunologists, including me, have elected to refer patients with newly diagnosed severe combined immunodeficiency to one of the several centers with active research programs in bone marrow transplantation. Rather than describing the techniques for definitive therapy, I will focus on early recognition and the supportive therapy during the pretransplant period.

Infants with severe combined immunodeficiency become ill within days to weeks after birth with diarrhea, cough and tachypnea, chronic infections of mucous membranes and diaper area with Candida albicans, and failure to gain weight. The diagnosis usually can be made by the demonstration of lymphopenia by the white blood cell count and differential. The minority of patients with these clinical manifestations with normal numbers of circulating lymphocytes prove to have T lymphopenia if appropriate marker studies are done. Concentrations of IgM and IgA are usually very low. T cell functional studies are usually done, but the abnormally low results are predictable in the T lymphocytopenic patient.

Following diagnosis, patients should be placed in protective isolation and treated vigorously with intravenous antibiotic therapy if bacterial infection is suspected. Prophylactic therapy for Pneumocystis carinii pneumonia should be instituted with trimethoprim-sulfamethoxazole at a dosage of 5 to 10 mg per kg of trimethoprim. If pneumocystis pneumonia is present, the dosage should be doubled. Neutropenia may develop with high dosages of this drug and may be counteracted by the administration of folinic acid. Mucocutaneous candidiasis should be treated with ketoconazole, because no response to topical therapy can be expected. Infections with herpes or varicella virus should be treated with acyclovir.

Nearly all patients with severe combined immunodeficiency have intractable diarrhea. A variety of enteroviruses or rotavirus may be demonstrated in the stool. Pseudomembranous colitis due to the toxin of Clostridium difficile may be present; if so, treatment with oral doses of vancomycin is indicated. There is no specific therapy for viral gastroenteritis, but institution of high dosage intravenous immunoglobulin therapy may produce some amelioration and possibly prevent dissemination. Nutritional support is vital. Early institution of total parenteral nutrition through an indwelling central catheter is usually warranted, despite the risk of catheter related infections.

Except for intravenous immunoglobulin infusions, infusion of blood products should be avoided if possible. These patients are susceptible to fatal graft versus host disease, which may be induced by small numbers of T lymphocytes present in packed whole blood red cells, platelets, or even fresh plasma. Moreover, any of these products may transmit viruses, such as cytomegalovirus, Epstein-Barr virus, and hepatitis and human immunodeficiency viruses. If blood products are necessary, all (except intravenous immunoglobulin preparations) should be irradiated with 5000 R before administration. Erythrocyte transfusions should utilize glycerol-frozen cells, since the washing process eliminates plasma and most leukocytes. Even frozen cells should be irradiated, however.

OTHER CONGENITAL IMMUNODEFICIENCIES

The DiGeorge syndrome is being recognized with increased frequency, largely as a result of improved techniques for diagnosis and early correction of major anomalies of the heart and great vessels. It has been our experience that most patients with this syndrome do not have major problems with host defense capabilities. We have seen several infants with fewer than 5 percent T lymphocytes at initial evaluation who within a period of a few months have developed normal T cell numbers and functions. Other immunologists have had similar experiences. It is our practice to follow patients for several months with serial evaluations of T cell numbers, functions, and clinical status. Independent of the initial degree of T lymphopenia, those with increasing T cell numbers can be expected to do well without any immunologic treatment. It is important to note that these observations cast doubt on the efficacy of thymus transplantation for this condition, since it is apparent that recovery is common even in the ''complete'' DiGeorge syndrome. The precautions concerning blood transfusions discussed earlier for patients with combined immunodeficiency should be followed in all patients with the DiGeorge's syndrome. Also we do not administer live viral vaccines to these children.

A minority of patients develop the clinical signs of T cell immunodeficiency, primarily chronic viral and fungal infections. One of our patients had parainfluenza virus type III pneumonia at 6 months, which persisted for 9 months, finally causing her death. Several courses of therapy with ribavirin produced only short term im-

provement. Neither treatment with Thymopentin (TP-5) nor transplantation with cultured thymus epithelium had any effect on her clinical status or immunologic function. Unfortunately we are currently unable to distinguish patients who will do poorly before infectious problems begin.

The immune deficiency of ataxia-telangiectasia is variable; many patients have no significant problems with infections, whereas others have serious bacterial sinopulmonary infections. Among the latter group some are deficient in IgG2 as well as IgA and may benefit from intravenous immunoglobulin treatment. There is no definitive therapy for this disease.

Boys with the Wiskott-Aldrich syndrome also vary considerably with regard to infectious problems as well as bleeding episodes. Transplantation with HLA matched bone marrow from sibling donors has resulted in restoration of hematologic and immunologic normalcy in several patients. Haploidentical marrow transplantation may be applicable to this group, but this approach is complicated by the need for immunosuppression in order to achieve engraftment. Splenectomy, coupled with prophylactic antibiotic therapy, has been advocated in patients with severe bleeding problems.

Other Therapies

A number of immunomodulatory drugs have been used in patients with mild to moderate deficiencies of cell mediated immunity. These include transfer factor, thymosin, Thymopentin, levamisole, interferon, and others. Despite reports of clinical and immunologic improvement in some patients, none has been shown to be effective in an adequate controlled trial. The experience gained by the treatment of large numbers of patients with AIDS will likely show which, if any, of these or similar drugs might be useful in patients with partial immunodeficiencies.

I thank my colleagues, Larry B. Vogler, M.D., and Donna S. Hummell, M.D., for their helpful comments.

SUGGESTED READING

Buckley RH, Schiff SE, Sampson HA, Schiff RI, Markert ML, Knutsen AP, Hershfield MS, Huang AT, Mickey GH, Ward FE. Development of immunity in human severe primary T cell deficiency following haploidentical bone marrow stem cell transplantation. J Immunol 1986; 136:2398–2407.

McKinney RE Jr, Katz SL, Wilfert CM. Chronic enteroviral meningoencephalitis in agammaglobulinemic patients. Rev Infect Dis 1987; 9:334–356.

Roifman CM, Rao CP, Lederman HM, Lavi S, Quinn P, Gelfand EW. Increased susceptibility to mycoplasma infection in patients with hypogammaglobulinemia. Am J Med 1986; 80:590–594.

Rosen FS, et al. Primary immunodeficiency diseases. Report of a World Health Organization scientific group. Clin Immunol Immunopathol 1986; 40:166–196.

Shearer WT, et al. Epstein-Barr virus-associated B-cell proliferations of diverse clonal origins after bone marrow transplantation in a 12-year-old patient with severe combined immunodeficiency. N Engl J Med 1985; 312:1151–1159.

Stiehm ER, Chin TW, Haas A, Peerless AG. Infectious complications of the primary immunodeficiencies. Clin Immunol Immunopathol 1986; 40:69–86.

HYPERIMMUNOGLOBULIN E SYNDROME

PAUL G. QUIE, M.D.
KIRAN K. BELANI, M.D.

Patients with hyperimmunoglobulin E–recurrent infection (Job's) syndrome characteristically present with recurrent serious bacterial infections of the skin and otobronchosinopulmonary infections early in life. Eosinophilia and markedly elevated serum IgE levels are found during immunologic evaluation. Additional characteristics of the syndrome include coarse facies, chronic eczematoid dermatitis, and mucocutaneous candidiasis.

The skin infections are frequently "cold" subcutaneous abscesses (20 percent of all infectious episodes) caused by *Staphylococcus aureus,* the most common bacterial pathogen in this syndrome. The abscesses are called "cold" because classic signs and symptoms of inflammation (heat, redness, pain) are often muted, but this is not a universal finding. Other important sites of infection include the middle and external ear canal, salivary glands, mastoid processes, gingiva, pharynx, sinuses, bronchi, and lungs. Septicemia and central nervous system infections are exceptionally rare.

S. aureus is the most common pathogen, accounting for approximately 60 percent of all infections in patients followed by us and at the National Institutes of Health. *H. influenzae* is recovered in 10 percent of all infectious episodes. In addition, 50 percent of our patients have chronic mucocutaneous candidiasis. Important but infrequent pathogens are *Streptococcus pneumoniae, Pseudomonas aeruginosa, Klebsiella pneumoniae, Cryptococcus neoformans, Aspergillus fumigatis,* and herpes simplex virus.

In addition to increased serum IgE levels, other immunologic abnormalities include elevated levels of anti-*S. aureus,* anti-*Candida albicans,* IgE antibodies in serum, and total IgD and recently a deficit of salivary total IgA and of both serum and salivary anti-*S. aureus* IgA levels. Deficiency in IgA antibodies may contribute to susceptibility, since 75 percent of all infections in patients with the hyperimmunoglobulin E syndrome involve organs in which secretory IgA may play an important role in host defense. Defective neutrophil chemotactic responsiveness is a variable finding possibly related to suppressive factors released in excessive amounts from mononuclear cells. In addition, abnormal suppressor T cell numbers and function, deficiencies of proliferative responses to various antigens, and delayed hypersensitivity responses have been reported.

Noninfectious clinical problems encountered include vernal conjunctivitis, recurrent keratoconjunctivitis, episodic asymptomatic noninflammatory oligoarticular arthritis, and severe scoliosis. Cranial synostosis, osteoporosis, osteogenesis imperfecta tarda, and lymphoma have been reported.

THERAPEUTIC ALTERNATIVES

Two therapeutic approaches are valuable in patients with the hyperimmunoglobulin E syndrome. The first is aggressive management of acute infections and antibiotic prophylaxis with conventional drugs to prevent staphylococcal and other infections. The second is persistent therapy of the skin and mucous membranes, such as antimycotic therapy for mucocutaneous candidiasis and topical treatment of eczematoid dermatitis. A third approach is therapy with immunomodulators directed toward stimulation of the immune function, which has not proven beneficial in controlled trials and is not recommended.

SURGICAL THERAPY

Indications for surgical management are abscess lesions obstructing the airway, deep organ abscesses that do not respond to aggressive antimicrobial therapy, persistent pneumatoceles, and bronchopleural fistulas.

MANAGEMENT OF ACUTE INFECTIONS

Careful evaluation of minor complaints is mandatory, especially with regard to the lungs, where *S. aureus* pneumonia with abscess formation may evolve with minimal early symptoms. Diagnosis of an acute infection is often delayed owing to the muted inflammatory response. To identify the site of infection, extensive radiologic and other investigations are often necessary. Gallium scanning and computed tomographic scanning are necessary supplements to routine roentgenography for the location of abscesses. The basic principles of management are especially important in patients with the hyperimmunoglobulin E syndrome, i.e., identification of causative agents, drainage of localized pus, and aggressive intravenous antibiotic therapy with higher doses and for a more extended duration than in the normal host.

Subcutaneous and other abscesses generally develop slowly and become dangerously large before patients seek medical attention. Typically abscesses are minimally red, warm, or tender; however, hot and tender lesions also may develop in these patients. Pending identification of pathogen(s), therapy may be initiated with a penicillanase resistant antistaphylococcal penicillin and an aminoglycoside. The surgical approach should be influenced by the knowledge that the amount of infected tissue is almost always greater than it appears. Drainage may have to be maintained for prolonged periods (3 to 4 weeks).

RESPIRATORY TRACT INFECTIONS

Aggressive management also applies to abscesses involving the tonsils, salivary glands, and lymph nodes. Otitis media and sinusitis may be treated empirically with oral therapy with antistaphylococcal drugs but with close follow-up since chronic mastoiditis may develop.

In one case retropharyngeal abscesses in a mother and several years later in her daughter required incision and drainage to relieve upper airway obstruction (authors' experience).

The lungs are frequent sites of infection and can be the source of great morbidity. For a patient presenting with mild pulmonary complaints (even without fever), chest roentgenography, a complete blood count with a differential, and Gram staining and culture of sputum are mandatory. An erythrocyte sedimentation rate can be useful when baseline values are known, but nearly normal values are frequent in conjunction with a significant infection. It is often difficult to rule out localized pneumonitis in a patient with chronic pulmonary scarring. In these cases we act conservatively and institute treatment for pneumonia. Initial drug therapy is chosen on the basis of sputum Gram staining, but includes an aminoglycoside (gentamicin or tobramycin) and a penicillinase resistant penicillin if gram positive cocci (presumably *S. aureus*) are seen or if the Gram stain findings are equivocal.

Intravenous antibiotic therapy is continued for at least 2 weeks and is followed by 2 weeks of oral antibiotic therapy (Table 1). The abnormal inflammatory response in patients with the hyperimmunoglobulin E syndrome contributes to a delay in the appearance of radiographic abnormalities even in clinically significant infections. Therefore patients with clinically apparent acute bronchitis are treated with parenteral doses of antibiotics for 1 to 2 weeks, followed by 2 weeks of oral antibiotic therapy. This aggressive approach is necessary because bronchiectasis, lung abscess, and pneumatocele are such frequent complications. Patients who are infected with *S. aureus* and allergic to penicillin often can be treated with a cephalosporin (e.g., cephalothin), recognizing the possibility of cross sensitivity between these classes of antibiotics. Alternative antibiotic drugs include vancomycin, clindamycin, and erythromycin. Cefuroxime can be administered as an alternative to chloramphenicol for *H. influenzae* infections.

Pulmonary abscess, enlarging or recurringly infected pneumatocele, and the presence of a bronchopleural fistula following resolution of *S. aureus* pneumonia are indications for surgical resection. Severe scoliosis may develop following lung resection, especially in children, and may further compromise lung function. Periodic pulmonary function tests are useful.

Other infections that deserve mention are cellulitis and osteomyelitis. Osteomyelitis should be treated with parenteral antibiotic therapy for 6 to 8 weeks followed by 6 months of appropriate antibiotic therapy by the oral route. Cellulitis should be treated with parenteral doses of antibiotics for 2 weeks followed by 2 weeks of oral antibiotic therapy. Herpetic whitlow should be treated with topical acyclovir therapy for 2 weeks.

PROPHYLAXIS

The long term management of patients with the hyperimmunoglobulin E syndrome includes prevention of recurrent infections, but prophylaxis against infection is still a controversial topic. We have been impressed that antistaphylococcal antibiotics have decreased the frequency of serious staphylococcal infections in these patients. Therefore we suggest daily treatment with trimethoprim-sulfamethoxazole or dicloxacillin.

Prophylactic antibiotic therapy is not effective in all patients, however, and a prospective double blind study is clearly needed.

Antibiotics should be used routinely prior to dental and elective surgical procedures.

MANAGEMENT OF ASSOCIATED PROBLEMS

Oral thrush and episodic Candida vaginitis occur in patients with the hyperimmunoglobulin E syndrome independent of concurrent antibiotic therapy. Candida esophagitis has not been a major problem. Prolonged

TABLE 1 Management of Hyperimmunoglobulin E Syndrome: Preferred Approach

	Adult Dose	Pediatric Dose
1. Prophylaxis		
Trimethoprim-sulfamethoxazole	PO one tab b.i.d.	PO 1 tsp b.i.d.
Dicloxacillin	PO 500 mg b.i.d.	PO 25–50 mg/kg/d b.i.d.
Ketoconazole	PO 200 mg/d q.d.	PO 5–10 mg/kg/d q.d.
2. Acute Infections		
A. Penicillinase resistant penicillins		
Nafcillin	IV 1–1.5 g q4h	IV 50–100 mg/kg/d q6h
Methicillin	IV 1–2 g q4h	IV 150–200 mg/kg/d q6h
Dicloxacillin	PO 500 mg q6h	PO 25–50 mg/kg/d q6h
B. Aminoglycosides		
Gentamicin	IV 3–5 mg/kg/d q8h	IV 5–7.5 mg/kg/d q8h
Tobramycin	IV 3–5 mg/kd/d q8h	IV 5–75. mg/kd/d q8h
C. Cephalosporin		
Cephalothin	IV 1–2 g q6h	IV 75–125 mg/kg/d q6h
Cefuroxime	IV 1–1.5 g q8h	IV 75–150 mg/kg/d q8h
D. Miscellaneous therapy		
Vancomycin	IV 500 mg q6h	IV 40 mg/kg/d q6h
Chloramphenicol	IV 50 mg/kg/d q6h	IV 50–75 mg/kg/d q6h
E. Antifungal drugs		
Amphotericin B	IV 1 mg/kd/day q.d.	IV 0.5–1.0 mg/kd/d
Ketoconazole	PO 200 mg/kg/d	PO 5–10 mg/kg/d

oral administration of ketoconazole effectively alleviates the symptoms of mucocutaneous candidiasis and is relatively free of serious side effects. Serious fungal infections are rare, although isolated cases of cryptococcal esophagitis and meningitis, mediastinal Candida granuloma, pulmonary aspergillosis, and ileocecal histoplasmosis have been reported. These illnesses require treatment with intravenous amphotericin B therapy.

Pruritic dermatitis is a frequent problem in patients with the hyperimmunoglobulin E syndrome, and topical doses of steroids combined with oral doses of antihistamines are effective. Systemic steroid therapy is best avoided in these patients; fortunately there is usually a satisfactory response to topical therapy. Frequent applications of 0.025 or 0.1 percent triamcinolone is usually sufficient. The face and groin are treated with 1 percent hydrocortisone to prevent thinning of the skin in these areas. Baths with dilute solutions of Hibiclens, pHisohex, or Betadine are beneficial for impetiginous rashes. Topical therapy with antibacterial drugs tends to be irritating, and any of the topically applied drugs may exacerbate the dermatitis in sensitive patients and are not recommended.

Vernal conjunctivitis and keratoconjunctivitis may result in corneal ulceration and scarring and require ophthalmologic consultation.

Patients with the hyperimmunoglobulin E syndrome have an increased incidence of oral ulcerations or gingivitis and require rigorous oral hygiene. Toothbrushing with a paste of 3 percent hydrogen peroxide and baking soda is recommended.

IMMUNOMODULATORS

Therapy with immunomodulators, whose efficacies remain unproved, has become popular during the last decade. Levamisole (an anthelmintic) was shown to normalize in vitro neutrophil chemotaxis in the hyperimmunoglobulin E syndrome and was claimed anecdotally to help several patients. Unfortunately this drug was found to be inferior to placebo in a double blind randomized clinical trial. Transfer factor (an incompletely defined substance derived from mononuclear cell cultures) has been used in the hyperimmunoglobulin E syndrome with anecdotal reports of clinical efficacy. However, transfer factor has not been tested in a rigorous fashion in this disease, and in one patient recurrent therapy with high dose transfer factor led to further immunosuppression. Therefore, transfer factor has generally fallen from favor.

High dose ascorbic acid therapy (8 to 10 g daily) has been reported to correct the in vitro chemotactic defect in some patients with the Chédiak-Higashi syndrome and may help some patients with the hyperimmunoglobulin E syndrome, but this application has not been adequately tested. Gamma globulin therapy has also been ineffective in the hyperimmunoglobulin E syndrome. These early clinical observations have been strengthened by a recent report of normal levels of anti-*S. aureus* IgG and elevated levels of anti-*S. aureus* IgM in this syndrome. The recent report of anti-*S. aureus* IgA deficiency is not an indication for parenteral immunoglobulin therapy because parenterally administered IgA does not reach mucosal surfaces.

Antihistamine therapy (a combination of H_1 and H_2 blockade) has been proposed, since histamine interferes with leukocyte function in vitro and elevated plasma histamine values have been reported in some but not most patients with the hyperimmunoglobulin E syndrome. It is possible that local tissue histamine levels may be elevated sufficiently to interfere with leukocyte function without causing a detectable rise in plasma or urinary histamine values, and antihistamine therapy, although unproved, may benefit certain patients. The effect of cimetidine on the metabolism of other drugs (e.g., theophylline) must be considered.

COMPLICATIONS OF THERAPY

Lobectomy is frequently necessary for pneumatoceles, and loss of pulmonary function is a major complication of therapy. We believe that pneumatoceles are preventable with aggressive diagnosis and treatment of staphylococcal pneumonia. Scoliosis may be another complication of lobectomy, and surgical correction of scoliosis is difficult in patients with a propensity toward cutaneous or subcutaneous *S. aureus* infections.

Adverse reactions to antibiotics have been minor and restricted to maculopapular rashes and gastrointestinal disturbances. Leukopenia associated with trimethoprim-sulfamethoxazole, neutropenia following nafcillin therapy, and pseudomembranous colitis following clindamycin therapy have been reversible when the drugs were discontinued. Ketoconazole has been associated with nausea, vomiting, and pruritus, but we have not had to discontinue therapy. Transient elevation of the serum transaminase or alkaline phosphatase level and hepatitis have been reported. Ketoconazole should not be recommended if pregnancy is anticipated.

SUGGESTED READING

Butrus SI, Leung DYM, Gellis S, Baum J, Kenyon KR, Abelson MB. Vernal conjunctivitis in the hyperimmunoglobulin E syndrome. Ophthalmology 1984; 91:1213–1216.

Donabedian H, Gallin JI. The hyperimmunoglobulin E–recurrent infection (Job's) syndrome. A review of the NIH experience and the literature. Medicine 1983; 62:195–207.

Dreskin SC, Goldsmith PK, Gallin JI. Immunoglobulins in the hyperimmunoglobulin E and recurrent infection (Job's) syndrome. Deficiency of anti-*Staphylococcus aureus* immunoglobulin A. J Clin Invest 1985; 75:26–34.

Hill HR, Quie PG, Pabot HR, Ochs HD, Clarke RA, Klebanoff S, Wedgewood RJ. Defect in neutrophil granulocyte chemotaxis in Job's syndrome of recurrent "cold" staphylococcal abscesses. Lancet 1974; 2:617–619.

Merten DF, Buckley RH, Pratt PC. Hyperimmunoglobulin E syndrome—radiographic observations. Radiology 1979; 132:71–78.

Schopfer K, Baerlocher K, Price P, Krech U, Quie PG, Douglas SD. Staphylococcal IgE antibodies, hyperimmunoglobulinemia E and *Staphylococcus aureus* infections. N Engl J Med 1979; 300:835–838.

AMYLOIDOSIS*

MARTHA SKINNER, M.D.
ALAN S. COHEN, M.D.

The treatment of amyloidosis has been limited because of an incomplete knowledge of its biochemical nature and pathogenesis. In the past few years it has become clear that amyloid is the broad term for a protein that takes on a unique configuration when it is deposited in tissue and that multiple biochemical forms as well as clinical syndromes exist. With these more precise definitions, the current treatment program has evolved.

The common denominator of the various forms of amyloid are the appearance of green birefringence on polarization microscopy after Congo red staining, the electron microscopic display of nonbranching fibrils, and the cross beta pattern visible on x-ray diffraction. The physicochemical phenomena that lead the different proteins to this final common amyloid fibril pathway are far less understood than the nature of the individual amyloid proteins, and probably represent the major unknown problem whose elucidation would lead to the resolution of already established amyloid disease.

Although there may be generally applicable principles in amyloid therapy, it is likely that from the view of prevention of the accumulation of these different proteins, multiple approaches may be needed.

*Study supported by grants from the U.S. Public Health Service, NIAMDD (AM 04599 and AM07014), the General Clinical Research Centers Branch of the Division of Research Resources, National Institutes of Health (RR 533), the Multipurpose Arthritis Center, the National Institutes of Health (AM 20613), and the Arthritis Foundation.

TABLE 1 Differentiation of Amyloid Type

	Primary (AL)	Secondary (AA)	Hereditary (AF)	Hemodialysis (AH)
History	No underlying disease	Chronic inflammation	Family history	On dialysis many years
Physical examination	Macroglossia	Associated with underlying disease	Scalloped pupil, neuropathy, carpal tunnel syndrome, vitreous opacities	Carpal tunnel syndrome
Laboratory studies	Increased plasma cells in bone marrow; M component in serum	Elevated SAA protein in serum	Decreased prealbumin in serum	Elevated beta-2 microglobulin
Potassium permanganate–Congo red staining of biopsy specimen	Resistant	Sensitive	Resistant	Sensitive
Immunohistochemical reaction of biopsy specimen	Not diagnostic	Positive reaction with anti-AA antiserum	Positive reaction with anti-prealbumin antiserum	Positive reaction with antibeta-2 microglobulin antiserum
Tissue isolation of fibrils	Light chains	AA protein	Prealbumin	Beta-2 microglobulin

DIAGNOSIS

To treat any disorder properly, the diagnosis must be firmly established. A wide variety of clinical symptoms may lead the physician to suspect a diagnosis of systemic amyloidosis; however, its actual prevalence is low. The diagnosis must be made by tissue biopsy in which a specimen is stained with Congo red and examined in polarized light. Abdominal fat aspiration has become the screening biopsy method of choice because of its ease in performance and lack of risk to the patient. If the abdominal fat analysis is negative, a more invasive biopsy may need to be undertaken. Once the diagnosis is established, the amyloid disease is classified according to type by a number of parameters, including the history, physical examination, laboratory studies, and special staining of biopsy material (Table 1). The systemic types include AL (primary or immunoglobulin related), AA (secondary or reactive), AF (hereditary or prealbumin related), and AH (associated with hemodialysis) amyloidosis. Localized types associated with endocrine organs, aging, or particular areas of the body also exist.

The patient's history can lead one to suspect primary amyloidosis if there is no history of preceding illness, or one may suspect secondary amyloidosis if chronic inflammation has been present, or the hereditary form if there is a family history of amyloidosis. The history, however, in our experience is often complicated and not always clear enough to define the biochemical type of disease present. The physical examination is important but likewise not diagnostic as to the type. It may show an enlarged liver and spleen in both primary and secondary amyloidosis, neuropathy in both primary and hereditary amyloidosis, and severe cardiac involvement in primary and hereditary types as well. However, two physical findings are more suggestive in the determination of type; they are macroglossia in primary amyloidosis and a scalloped pupil in hereditary amyloidosis (familial amyloid polyneuropathy).

No single laboratory test is in itself diagnostic of amyloid disease, including those that measure the amyloid fibril precursor protein. A serum monoclonal gammopathy is found in about 75 percent of the patients with primary (AL) amyloidosis, but its presence is not diagnostic, for a number of other conditions may be characterized by serum M components. Likewise an elevated serum amyloid A (SAA) protein level does not predict, or may not even always be found in, secondary (AA) amyloidosis. SAA concentrations in normal individuals are less than 1 μg per ml and in patients with AA amyloidosis have been normal to very high (0.6 to 100 μg per ml). SAA is an acute phase protein, and an elevated concentration is simply an indication of inflammation or cell necrosis. Similarly, although a lowered prealbumin level has been shown to be present in individuals with hereditary (AF) amyloidosis, it is not sufficiently depressed below normal values to be diagnostic in any one individual.

The biochemical classification of amyloid type can be determined to some extent on the basis of biopsy material. Paraffin embedded tissue sections can be treated with potassium permanganate prior to Congo red staining. If the amyloid fibrils are of the secondary (AA) type, they are "sensitive" by this test; i.e., they lose their capacity to stain with Congo red after treatment with potassium permanganate. Both primary (AL) and hereditary (AF) fibril types are "resistant," or retain their capacity to stain with Congo red after potassium permanganate treatment.

To differentiate the AL and AF fibril types one must perform immunohistochemical staining with specific antisera to prealbumin. This procedure identifies the hereditary (AF) amyloid fibril type. The immunohistochemical staining procedure can also confirm the identity of (AA) amyloid fibrils with an antibody specific for AA protein, but this procedure is available only in research laboratories. There is no specific antibody for AL amyloid fibrils, and biochemical classification is inferred by the lack of reaction to antibodies specific for the other types. In the hemodialysis associated (AH) type, the fibrils are "sensitive" in the potassium permanganate–Congo red staining procedure and by reactive immunohistochemical staining with antiserum to beta-2 microglobulin. When enough biopsy material is available, definitive identification of the amyloid type can be made by fibril isolation from the tissue followed by sequence analysis of the isolated protein. This requires a relatively large piece of unfixed biopsy material or, more frequently, autopsy tissue.

TREATMENT

There is as yet no adequate specific therapy for any form of established amyloid disease. A number of therapeutic interventions have been tried, and two were found to be helpful after being used in large series of patients. In addition, supportive measures directed at the specific problems associated with amyloidosis have increased the length of life and made life more comfortable for many individuals. For all patients it is important that the amyloid type be clearly defined biochemically at the outset. This information aids in determining the prognosis and in addressing family concerns regarding heredity and planning for eventual supportive therapies.

In primary (AL) amyloidosis the two therapeutic interventions most frequently used have been colchicine and melphalan combined with prednisone (Table 2). In clinical trials both colchicine and melphalan have been shown to prolong survival two to three times that in control patients given no treatment. Because primary amyloidosis is a plasma cell dyscrasia, the use of chemotherapeutic drugs has a logical basis. However, since it is not a true malignant disease, there has been some reluctance to subject patients with AL amyloidosis to the bone marrow suppression risks of chemotherapy. In addition, the long term risk of developing leukemia now approaches 11 percent for patients who have received large amounts of melphalan and who survive long enough (3 or more years). Nevertheless the large series of Kyle and coworkers and several single case reports have shown that in some patients treated with melphalan, there is improvement in measurable clinical parameters, i.e., urine protein excretion, hepatomegaly, bone marrow plasmacytosis, and monoclonal gammopathy.

The recommended dosage for melphalan has been 0.15 to 0.25 mg per kg per day with prednisone, 1.5 to 2.0 mg per kg per day. Both drugs are given for 4 days and the treatment repeated every 6 weeks. We recommend that treatment be discontinued after 1 year to maintain the total dosage of melphalan at less than 600 mg, at which level the risk of leukemia is minimal. This seems to be a reasonable approach, because many of the long term survivors with the AL form who have shown measurable improvement received only 1 year or less of therapy. A blood count must be obtained at midcycle and prior to the next course of therapy; the dosage of melphalan is altered accordingly.

The other therapeutic option for AL amyloidosis is treatment with colchicine. The rationale for this treatment is no more precisely defined, but in a large clinical trial it proved to be effective in improving survival. Colchicine is known to affect mitosis, to disrupt microtubule organization, and to potentially interfere with microtubule cell function. Owing to the presumed participation of the macrophage in the pathogenesis of AA amyloidosis, and the concept that in AL amyloid the immunoglobulin is processed by the macrophage prior to its tissue deposition, it seems reasonable to suspect that it might alter or delay fibril formation or deposition in AL amyloid. The recommended dosage of colchicine is 0.6 mg twice daily, with a reduction to 0.6 mg daily if gastrointestinal side effects occur.

Other major therapies that have been used for the treatment of amyloidosis include ascorbic acid, dimethyl sulfoxide, penicillamine, and cytoxan. Most of these therapies have been reported in single case studies and definitive benefit from therapy has been unconvincing.

Supportive measures relating to the treatment of involved organ systems are of the utmost importance, particularly since there is not yet a definitive major therapy. AL amyloidosis affects all organ systems to some degree, but is often marked in the cardiac, renal, autonomic nervous, and gastrointestinal systems. Each patient presents a unique set of symptoms and degree of organ involvement, and a supportive program for treatment must be individualized. Some guidelines for this treatment that have been helpful are presented in Table 2.

The degree of organ involvement should be measured by appropriate noninvasive tests prior to instituting therapy. In fact, even if a patient has no symptoms in a particular organ system, a number of tests are warranted to note whether asymptomatic involvement is present. Assessment of the heart by an electrocardiogram, an echocardiogram, and 24 hour Holter monitoring and the kidneys by function tests and a 24 hour urine protein analysis are important parts of the management for all patients. In some patients the gastrointestinal system should be examined by x-ray studies, a gastric emptying scan, and tests for malabsorption.

After the organ system involvement has been identified, the treatment program is symptomatic according to the physiologic problem presented. For example, the congestive heart failure of AL amyloidosis usually is due to a constrictive cardiomyopathy and is best treated with moderate salt restriction and vigorous diuretic therapy. The use of digitalis is not indicated. In fact, both digitalis and calcium channel blocking drugs have been

TABLE 2   Treatment for Primary (AL) Amyloidosis

Major therapy options:

Pharmacologic Therapy
1. Melphalan 0.15–0.25 mg/kg/day × 4 days
   Prednisone 1.5–2.0 mg/kg/day × 4 days
      Repeat administration every 6 weeks for 1 year with dosage changes according to CBC results
2. Colchicine 0.6 mg bid
      May be given as the major therapy alone or in combination with the above, omitting it on the days melphalan and prednisone are given

Supportive therapy (generally applicable to systemic amyloid of AL, AA, or AF types):

Organ System	Symptom	Treatment
Cardiac	Congestive failure	Salt restriction of 1–2 g/day (unless patient also has orthostatic hypotension)
		Diuretics
	Heart block	Pacemaker
Renal	Nephrotic syndrome	Salt restriction of 1–2 g/day
		Elastic stockings for edema
		Dietary increase of protein to 1.5 g/kg body weight
	Renal failure	Dialysis (chronic ambulatory peritoneal dialysis or hemodialysis)
Autonomic nervous	Orthostatic hypotension	Increase salt to at least 6 g/day (need to evaluate cardiac and renal systems first)
		Elastic stockings
		9-alpha-fluorohydrocortisone (Florinef)
	Gastric atony	Small frequent feedings (6/day) low in fat
		Metoclopramide hydrochloride (Reglan; use with caution if patient also has orthostatic hypotension)
		Jejunostomy tube for commercially prepared formula feeding
Gastrointestinal	Diarrhea	Dietary changes
		Medium chain triglyceride oil supplements of 60 ml/day
		Low fat diet of 40 g or less
		Medications
		Tetracycline
		Diphenoxylate hydrochloride with atropine (Lomotil)
		Psyllium hydrophilic muciloid (Metamucil)
		Total parenteral nutrition
	Macroglossia	Maintain airway
		Hemiglossectomy
Peripheral nervous	Neuropathy	Physical therapy
		Medications
		Amitriptyline
		Carbamazepine (Tegretol)
Hematologic	Intracutaneous bleeding	Avoid trauma
	Factor X deficiency	Splenectomy

shown to bind to amyloid fibrils, and their use has been associated with sudden death. Thus, unless a nonamyloid cardiac problem occurs coincidentally, their routine use is not recommended.

Major amyloid involvement of the kidneys poses another set of problems, with the nephrotic syndrome often associated with massive proteinuria, edema, and a low serum albumin concentration. Patients should be encouraged to increase the dietary protein to 1.5 g per kg body weight in an attempt to replace urinary protein loss and raise the serum albumin concentration. It is recommended that 80 percent of this protein be of high biologic value (meat, milk) and that, if necessary, the salt restriction be liberalized to make this diet palatable. The total caloric intake should be 30 to 50 cal per kg per day. Albumin infusions have been helpful, but because they are of very temporary benefit, they are not recommended. Rest periods during the day with the legs elevated and the use of elastic stockings decrease peripheral edema. If renal failure occurs, long term ambulatory peritoneal dialysis and hemodialysis are options for therapy, and both have been successful. Since amyloid involvement of many organ systems is often present, kidney transplantation is usually not considered, although it is not contraindicated.

Symptoms relating to the autonomic nervous system are the most difficult to treat. Orthostatic hypotension is treated initially by increasing the salt in the diet to 6 g per day or more and use of elastic stockings of the fitted antigravity type. Patients are also encouraged to stand up slowly and may be given 9-alpha-fluorohydrocortisone with some benefit. Symptoms of always feeling full and occasionally vomiting may represent gastric atony. If this is confirmed by a gastric emptying scan, treatment should start with small frequent feedings that are low in fat. Metoclopramide hydrochloride can be tried, but this drug may make orthostasis worse and should be used with caution. A surgically placed jejunostomy tube for enteral formula feeding may be lifesaving in providing adequate nutritional support in patients with gastric atony and can be used in place of or to supplement the oral intake.

Other supportive therapies in AL amyloidosis include changes in the dietary fat content or a trial of medications that slow the bowel or add bulk to combat diarrhea. Total parenteral nutrition is used as a last resort. Macroglossia has been a difficult problem to manage. Surgical intervention may be needed to maintain an airway or for cosmetic reasons if the tongue becomes so massive that the mouth cannot be closed.

Peripheral sensory neuropathy is mild in AL amyloidosis, and symptoms of pain disappear as the neuropathy worsens. Tranquilizing or antiseizure medications are helpful. Physical therapy is important in maintaining muscle mass and preventing contractures if motor neuropathy occurs.

Symptoms associated with bleeding can be mild or can constitute a serious hematologic emergency. Those of a mild nature include intracutaneous bleeding, for which there is no specific therapy other than avoiding trauma; intracutaneous bleeding is presumed to be due to the increased friability of small blood vessels with amyloid fibril deposits within their walls and is not a hematologic abnormality. Serious bleeding can occur with factor deficiencies, most commonly factor X, but all calcium dependent clotting factors can be deficient. This is believed to be the result of the affinity of anionic amyloid fibril deposits for clotting factors (as well as other proteins) and their removal from plasma by absorption onto the fibril deposit. It is important to assess the clotting status prior to all surgical procedures. In emergency bleeding situations patients can be given commercial clotting factor preparations. In a few patients with splenomegaly, removal of the spleen has corrected the factor deficiency, perhaps by removing a large deposit of amyloid fibrils.

In AA amyloidosis the major therapy depends on the underlying inflammatory or infectious disease (Table 3). The suppression or elimination of infection is of the utmost importance. Colchicine is the major therapy for patients with familial Mediterranean fever and is also used in AA amyloidosis due to other causes along with the major therapy appropriate for the underlying inflammation. If the disease is a form of arthritis, treatment with nonsteroidal anti-inflammatory drugs along with rest and exercises is appropriate. In addition a remittive drug should be given to completely suppress the underlying inflammation. If the patient has proteinuria (very common in AA amyloidosis), gold salts and D-penicillamine are not recommended, but methotrexate could be considered. It is not clear whether prednisone accelerates amyloid fibril deposition within tissues. Along with therapy it is wise to monitor the serum SAA level; it is a more accurate measure of inflammation than the sedi-

TABLE 3   Treatment for Secondary (AA) Amyloidosis

Major therapy:

   1 Aggressive treatment of underlying inflammatory disease with monitoring of SAA level on a regular basis

   2 Surgical excision of infectious process when feasible, i.e., lung lobectomy for bronchiectasis, bone resection for osteomyelitis, colectomy for chronic ulcerative colitis

   3 Colchicine 0.6 mg bid

Supportive therapy (in addition to that outlined for AL amyloid):

Organ System	Symptom	Treatment
Renal	Renal failure	Avoid nonsteroidal anti-inflammatory drugs; if necessary use Aspirin or Clinoril
		Dialysis
		Kidney transplant should be considered

mentation rate, especially when the patient has the nephrotic syndrome.

If the underlying disease is an infection, surgical excision may be feasible, particularly if medical therapy has been ineffective. Usually after AA amyloidosis develops (it generally takes years), there is some urgency to resolve the infection. Surgical excision has been used with success in patients requiring partial pulmonary lobectomy for bronchiectasis, resection of bone affected with osteomyelitis, colectomy for chronic ulcerative colitis, and tooth extractions for dental abscesses. When surgery can be applied to remove a source of infection, it stops the progression of amyloid disease. In some patients who have already developed the nephrotic syndrome, progression of renal disease may continue.

Supportive therapy follows the recommendations given for AL amyloidosis when it is necessary. Because organ involvement with amyloidosis is usually considerably less, the need for supportive therapy is minimal. Renal involvement, however, is frequently present, and progression to renal failure occurs even when optimal therapy is given for the underlying disease. In these patients kidney transplantation should be strongly considered, for reports have shown that patients do well and in AA amyloidosis the survival is fairly long.

In hereditary (AF) amyloidosis the deposition of amyloid fibrils occurs because of a genetic variant structure of the protein prealbumin. No treatment has been defined that specifically interferes with or slows this process, and because patients with this condition survive 10 to 20 years, therapeutic benefit is difficult to measure. Colchicine has been given at a dosage of 0.6 mg twice daily because of its potential capacity to delay fibril processing noted earlier and its lack of toxicity. Supportive measures for the treatment of peripheral neuropathy, autonomic neuropathy, and diarrhea are frequently needed. They are used as outlined in Table 2 for AL amyloidosis. In addition, genetic counseling regarding the autosomal dominant nature of the genetic defect and the identification of ''at risk'' family members who are carriers of the trait can be offered. It is likely that technologic advances in genetic engineering will have more to offer for this form of amyloidosis in the future.

Amyloid associated with hemodialysis (AH) is a result of an excessively high serum level of beta-2 microglobulin, which is not filtered out by the cuprophan dialysis membrane. Normal levels of beta-2 microglobulin are less than 4 mg per liter, whereas in patients treated with hemodialysis, levels are from 45 to 189 mg per liter. It takes years of dialysis (usually 10 or more) for this type of amyloid to develop, and it forms in synovial membranes surrounding large joints (hips,

shoulders, wrists) with erosive lesions within adjacent bones. Only rarely have amyloid deposits of the same biochemical composition been found in other tissues. Effective treatment will likely require a change in dialysis membrane that allows filtration of the 11,000 dalton protein, beta-2 microglobulin. It is reported that patients given hemodialysis with an AN 69 membrane, which currently has limited use in Europe, have beta-2 microglobulin levels consistently lower by 50 to 60 percent. It is known that in chronic ambulatory peritoneal dialysis the beta-2 levels are elevated to a lesser extent (range, 17 to 79 mg per liter) than in hemodialysis. It may be that patients given chronic ambulatory peritoneal dialysis will not get AH amyloidosis or that a longer time with dialysis treatment will be necessary for it to develop.

Localized amyloid deposits occasionally pose the need for surgical excision. These are most commonly located in the tracheobronchial tree, the urinary bladder, or the conjunctiva. The biochemical composition of this form of amyloid is not yet known. Biopsy staining patterns have always shown it to be potassium permanganate resistant, and immunohistochemical tests indicate that it is negative with antisera to AA protein and prealbumin. In patients suspected of having localized amyloidosis it is important to rule out a systemic form. If the amyloid deposit is localized, the treatment is usually observation. Enlargement of the amyloid deposit may take place; however, spreading to another site has never occurred. Local excision may be necessary to correct respiratory obstruction or for cosmetic purposes. Laser resection is usually used for respiratory tract lesions because it minimizes of the danger of excessive bleeding.

SUGGESTED READING

Cohen AS, Rubinow A, Anderson JJ, Skinner M, Mason JH, Libbey C, Kayne H. Survival of patients with primary (AL) amyloidosis: cases treated with colchicine from 1976–1983 compared with cases seen in previous years 1961–1973. Am J Med 1987; 82:1182–1190.

Cohen AS, Skinner M. The diagnosis of amyloid. In: Cohen AS, ed. Laboratory diagnostic procedures in the rheumatic diseases. 3rd ed. New York: Grune & Stratton, 1985; 377.

Kyle RA, Greipp PR. Primary systemic amyloidosis: comparison of melphalan and prednisone versus placebo. Blood 1978; 52:818–827.

Kyle RA, Greipp PR, Garton JP, Gertz MA. Primary systemic amyloidosis: comparison of melphalan/prednisone versus colchicine. Am J Med 1985; 79:708–716.

Zemer D, Pras M, Sohar E, Modan M, Cabili S, Gafni J. Colchicine in the prevention and treatment of the amyloidosis of familial Mediterranean fever. N Engl J Med 1986; 314:1001–1005.

HASHIMOTO'S THYROIDITIS*

KENNETH D. BURMAN, M.D., Col. M.C.

Hashimoto's disease is a complex autoimmune disease in which perturbations of T and B lymphocytes result in the production of antithyroglobulin and antimicrosomal antibodies. It is presently speculated that hypothyroidism in this condition results from the interaction of antimicrosomal antibodies with thyroid peroxidase enzymes, thus inhibiting the generation of thyroxine (T_4) and triiodothyronine (T_3) and resulting in a compensatory increase in thyroid stimulating hormone (TSH) production and thyroidal enlargement. Despite this proposed scheme, most authorities believe that the precise temporal and pathophysiologic relationship between antithyroid antibodies and thyroidal enlargement or destruction is not yet completely understood.

Clinically, the diagnosis of Hashimoto's disease is documented by the presence in serum of high titers of antithyroglobulin or antimicrosomal antibodies or by cytologic or histologic study of a thyroid tissue sample that is characterized by lymphocytic infiltration, and perhaps germinal centers, with occasional macrophages or plasma cells. Thyroid follicles may be decreased in number and colloid accumulation may be scant; numerous large oxyphilic thyrocytes and inflammatory giant cells are usually present. Patients with Hashimoto's disease may be clinically euthyroid, hypothyroid, or even rarely hyperthyroid, and the thyroid gland may be normal in size, enlarged, or even not palpable. The specific goals of therapy usually are restoration of euthyroidism, when appropriate, and suppression of growth of an enlarged thyroid gland.

INTERPRETATION OF THYROID FUNCTION TESTS

The thyroid hormones, T_3 and T_4, circulate in serum bound to either albumin, thyroxine binding globulin, or prealbumin; only about 0.3 percent of the T_3 and 0.03 percent of the T_4 are unbound and thus available for binding to tissues. The serum TSH level, in a sensitive assay, is elevated in primary hypothyroidism and undetectable in thyrotoxicosis. The serum T_3 level by radioimmunoassay may be normal in many patients with hypothyroidism, but the serum T_4 level is usually decreased. Systemic illness of any nature may alter thyroid function test results, usually causing decreased serum T_4 and T_3 levels by radioimmunoassay and elevated resin T_3 uptake; these characteristic findings reflect the diminished binding of iodothyronines to serum proteins and also decreased serum T_4 to T_3 conversion. In this circumstance, as well as in healthy patients, the resin T_3 uptake does not reflect function but indicates the number of T_3 or T_4 binding sites available. In most laboratories a decrease in the number of binding sites is associated with low serum T_4 and T_3 radioimmunoassay levels and increased resin T_3 uptake; an increase in available binding sites is usually reflected by elevated serum T_4 and T_3 radioimmunoassay levels and by a decreased resin T_3 uptake.

Conditions that may elevate the number of thyroid hormone binding sites include estrogen administration, pregnancy, and birth control pills, and conditions that may decrease the number of binding sites include systemic illnesses, testosterone or glucocorticoid administration, and the nephrotic syndrome. A patient may also be born with decreased or increased thyroid hormone binding proteins. The typical alterations in T_4, T_3 radioimmunoassay, and resin T_3 uptake levels must be borne in mind in the interpretation of thyroid function test results in hypothyroid patients who also have other systemic illnesses. In general, a concordant change in T_4 and resin T_3 uptake levels suggests a bona fide alteration in thyroid function, and a discordant change suggests a binding abnormality. Of course, primary hypothyroidism also can occur in a patient who has decreased binding, in which case the T_4 level would be low, the resin T_3 uptake normal or elevated, and the TSH level increased; the serum TSH level is expected to be normal if there is a binding abnormality alone.

The proper interpretation of thyroid function tests relies on an understanding of the concept that the "normal range" is relative; not only can persons with normal thyroid function have abnormal serum T_4 levels, but an individual with abnormal thyroid function may have a normal serum T_4 level. Our interpretation of these tests is simplified by virtue of the fact that homeostatic mechanisms elevate the TSH level when insufficient T_4 or T_3 reaches the tissues. Thus, great importance is placed on T_4, T_3 radioimmunoassay, resin T_3 uptake, and especially TSH levels in the evaluation of a hypothyroid patient.

PRIMARY HYPOTHYROIDISM

Normally, in a 70 kg person, the thyroid gland secretes about 130 nmoles (100 μg) of T_4 daily. The total T_3 production is about 50 nmoles (32 μg); about 85 percent of this T_3 production is from peripheral T_4 conversion, and only about 15 percent is derived directly from thyroidal secretion. Serum T_4 and T_3 circulate

*The opinions or assertions contained herein are the private views of the author and are not to be construed as official or as reflecting the views of the Department of the Army or the Department of Defense.

bound to three proteins (thyroxine binding prealbumin, thyroxine binding globulin, and albumin), and, as noted earlier, only about 0.03 percent of T_4 and 0.3 percent of T_3 are bound and thus available to enter tissues to mediate biologic action. Serum TSH levels, as measured by a highly sensitive assay, are normally about 0.5 to 3.5 μU per ml and are elevated in patients with primary hypothyroidism. Therefore, a typical patient with primary hypothyroidism would have clinical symptoms that are consistent, decreased serum T_4 and T_3 radioimmunoassay and resin T_3 uptake levels, and an elevated TSH value. Consistent symptoms include cold intolerance, fatigue, constipation, slow speech, bradycardia, and decreased body temperature. Dry skin, loss of body hair, and hoarse voice may be present, and rarely patients may have pericardial or pleural effusions.

In such a patient synthetic levothyroxine (LT_4) usually should be used for treatment. The replacement dosage is about 1.7 μg per kg per day, which usually means 0.1 to 0.2 mg daily. The goal of therapy in this circumstance is a serum T_4 level between 6 and 12 μg per dl and a T_3 level between 120 and 180 ng per dl in a clinically euthyroid asymptomatic patient. The TSH value should be between 0.5 and 3.5 μU per ml when LT_4 is administered for the treatment of hypothyroidism.

In the treatment of hypothyroid subjects it is most prudent to institute levothyroxine therapy in a gradual manner. Gradual restoration of euthyroidism is mandatory if the patient has accompanying atherosclerosis, known coronary artery disease, or angina. It may be useful to obtain an electrocardiogram in these patients prior to and during therapy.

A typical gradual regimen might be to administer 25 μg of LT_4 daily for 2 weeks and 50 μg daily for the next 2 weeks and then to increase the maintenance dosage to 75 μg daily. The patient continues with this daily dosage for 4 to 6 weeks and returns at that time for a repeat examination and thyroid function tests. If further increases are needed, they then can be instituted gradually. A patient must be receiving a given daily dosage of LT_4 for 4 to 6 weeks before blood tests represent an accurate assessment of the presumed biologic effect. After this close observation, patients receiving levothyroxine therapy for the treatment of primary hypothyroidism should be monitored with clinical examination and serum T_4, resin T_3 uptake, and TSH values about every 6 to 12 months. Patients who have autoimmune hypothyroidism are at higher risk for other autoimmune disorders and should be questioned about symptoms relevant to adrenal insufficiency, panhypopituitarism, systemic lupus erythematosus, rheumatoid arthritis, and scleroderma. Every patient with the diagnosis of hypothyroidism should have the serum TSH level measured, and in the case of primary hypothyroidism it should be elevated. If the patient has clinical hypothyroidism with decreased serum T_4 and resin T_3 uptake levels and a normal or low TSH level, secondary hypothyroidism should be suspected and a pituitary computed tomographic scan should be obtained.

SUBCLINICAL PRIMARY HYPOTHYROIDISM

Subclinical, latent, or biochemical hypothyroidism occurs when a patient does not have specific or notable signs or symptoms of hypothyroidism, and the serum T_4 and T_3 levels are within the normal range but the TSH concentration is mildly elevated, perhaps 5 to 15 μU per ml. Subclinical hypothyroidism is most frequent in elderly patients. This circumstance illustrates the clinical conundrum of whether to institute treatment with levothyroxine or simply to follow the patient at regular intervals. There is no simple answer to this problem.

I recommend a thorough history and physical examination, trying to elicit signs or symptoms related to hypothyroidism; I also measure the serum antithyroglobulin and antimicrosomal thyroid antibody levels. It is generally believed that the higher the antibody titer, the more likely it is that such cases will evolve into overt hypothyroidism. If there are specific symptoms or findings on physical examination that might be related to hypothyroidism, I consider instituting levothyroxine therapy. The presence of high titers of antithyroid antibodies makes me follow the patient more closely and consider levothyroxine therapy more strongly. Therapy is instituted with the full understanding and cooperation of the patient; the same precautions already noted with regard to gradual institution of therapy apply in these circumstances. Consideration also should be given to whether the patient has permanent primary hypothyroidism or whether the event may be transient, such as subacute thyroiditis or postpartum thyroiditis. Care should be taken to insure that the diagnosis of permanent primary hypothyroidism is correct prior to prescribing lifelong levothyroxine therapy.

HASHIMOTO'S DISEASE WITH AN ENLARGED THYROID GLAND

Some patients with Hashimoto's disease have an enlarged thyroid gland, which usually coexists with either euthyroidism or hypothyroidism. When a patient is hypothyroid, the guidelines already noted apply, except that careful attention must be given to whether the thyroid gland has areas of decreased function on radioisotopic scanning. If such areas exist and correspond to palpable nodules, an aspiration biopsy may be indicated. If the biopsy findings are indicative of malignancy, surgery may be advised, taking into consideration the general state of the patient. If the biopsy findings are benign and the nodular area is "cold" or hypofunctioning by scan, evaluation of the nodule's response to levothyroxine therapy is indicated. If the nodule does not decrease in size over several months, surgery should be considered. It must be kept in mind, however, that we are discussing only patients with known Hashimoto's disease, supported by either a high titer of antithyroid antibodies or a diagnostic aspiration. In this setting a nodular thyroid gland would be expected as an integral part of the disease process. Nevertheless it is still possible for a "cold" nodule to appear in a patient with Hashimoto's disease, and although it would be unusual, the possible co-occurrence of carcinoma should not be overlooked. The more usual circumstance is for the nodular enlargement to represent lymphocytic infiltration and fibrosis as a result of Hashimoto's disease; unnecessary surgery in this situation should be avoided. Growth of a nodule, lymphadenopathy in or around the thyroid gland, and symptoms of hoarseness, dysphagia, or pain may suggest a malignant process, since these findings usually do not occur in an uncomplicated routine case of Hashimoto's disease.

In a patient with Hashimoto's disease, generalized thyroid enlargement may occur in conjunction with a euthyroid state. If the patient does not have symptoms suggestive of rapid growth of the thyroid gland, such as dysphagia, hoarseness, or pain (in which case biopsy and surgery may be indicated), and if the patient is euthyroid clinically and chemically, levothyroxine therapy for suppression is usually indicated, with application of the precautions already noted. After stabilization, the patient is followed every 6 to 12 months with periodic examinations and thyroid function tests. The rationale for treating a patient with an enlarged thyroid gland with levothyroxine is based on the belief that levothyroxine suppression inhibits further growth or, perhaps, even shrinks the gland by inhibiting TSH secretion. Although this general course is followed by most clinicians, there are few definitive studies assessing this approach in patients with Hashimoto's disease.

"HASHITOXICOSIS"

"Hashitoxicosis" is an uncommon entity in which a patient has the usual manifestations of Hashimoto's disease, such as elevated antimicrosomal or antithyroglobulin antibody titers and an enlarged firm thyroid gland, yet displays clinical and biochemical evidence of hyperthyroidism, with elevated serum T_4 and T_3 and increased 24 hour radioactive iodine uptake. When it is documented that such a patient does not have other forms of thyrotoxicosis such as postpartum or subacute thyroiditis, appropriate treatment is indicated.

The pathophysiology of this hybrid entity between Hashimoto's disease and Graves' disease is unknown, but strikes at the basic causes of these two diseases. Some clinicians believe that Graves' disease and Hashimoto's disease represent different manifestations of the same or similar defects, presumably B cell escape from regulation, which then allows production of antithyroid antibodies. In some cases the antithyroglobulin and antimicrosomal antibodies predominate, resulting in clinical manifestations known as Hashimoto's disease, whereas in other circumstances the predominant antibodies are

directed against the TSH receptor, and the clinical entity is Graves' disease. "Hashitoxicosis," or more accurately, the coexistence of Graves' disease and Hashimoto's disease, has not been adequately studied in order to document its natural history, the frequency of serum anti-TSH receptor antibodies, or the response to therapy.

With these reservations noted, when I encounter such a patient, I attempt to discern whether other factors (e.g., iodide ingestion, a recent history of childbirth) may be precipitating the thyrotoxicosis. If, for example, the thyrotoxicosis has occurred several weeks after a study in which radiographic contrast agents were used, I might believe that the patient has iodide induced thyrotoxicosis, and definitive therapy such as ^{131}I ablation or thyroidectomy should be avoided. I would treat such a patient with beta blocking drugs (e.g., Atenolol, 50 to 100 mg daily) and antithyroid drugs (propylthiouracil, 100 mg three times daily, or methimazole, 10 mg three times daily) for several months to induce euthyroidism. At the end of that time I would discontinue these drugs to determine whether thyrotoxicosis recurs. In the case of recurrent thyrotoxicosis or a clear case of Hashimoto's thyroiditis at presentation, I still render the patient euthyroid with beta blocking drugs and antithyroid drugs, but when euthyroidism is restored, I discuss definitive management (i.e., surgery or ^{131}I) with the patient. For Graves' disease I prefer ^{131}I as therapy if the patient is over 25 to 30 years old, and I usually prefer surgical therapy if the patient is younger. "Hashitoxicosis" is a much rarer entity, but the same guidelines probably apply. Some clinicians also consider long term antithyroid drug treatment in an effort to induce a remission.

I would emphasize that individual patient preference should be given major consideration in this cooperative decision; the desirable goal of both these treatments is permanent hypothyroidism, and the patient then can be treated with levothyroxine replacement. Obviously ^{131}I therapy should not be given to a female patient who is or may shortly become pregnant. Further details regarding indications, methods, and objectives of the approaches can be obtained from recent references.

PREGNANCY

Hashimoto's disease with hypothyroidism can be treated during pregnancy with levothyroxine therapy. Because estrogens increase thyroxine binding globulin concentrations and binding capacity, the total serum T_4 and T_3 radioimmunoassay values may rise, but the resin T_3 uptake value decreases. A serum T_4 level between 8 and 18 μg per dl in most assays and a serum T_3 level between 120 and 240 ng per dl may be considered normal. These elevated total T_4 and T_3 radioimmunoassay values, as compared to the case in nonpregnant patients, are simply due to increases in binding proteins, and free hormone levels are expected to be normal and the patients clinically euthyroid. The dose of levothyroxine required is not believed to change significantly during pregnancy, and the rise in the serum T_4 level is expected and does not signify per se that the dose must be changed. Careful examination of the patient and evaluation of the laboratory tests will indicate whether modifications in therapy are needed. Occasionally it may be necessary to measure the free T_4 level directly.

POSTPARTUM THYROIDITIS

Postpartum thyroiditis is a recently recognized clinical syndrome in which alterations in thyroid function occur within the first year after delivery. This entity is very common, occurring in perhaps 5 to 8 percent of all women who have delivered babies. This syndrome may be characterized by transient hypothyroidism or hyperthyroidism, but a principal hallmark of the disease is that thyroid function evolves from one clinical state to another. Presentation at about 4 months post partum with hyperthyroidism, with evolution to hypothyroidism at 8 months and euthyroidism at 12 months, would be a common course. The clinician must be careful not to treat one clinical manifestation with definitive therapy (i.e., ^{131}I or surgery), since the natural history is so varied and the disease is usually transient. It is preferable to treat the clinical manifestations (e.g., with a beta blocker) when the patient is thyrotoxic, but then to consider withdrawing the drugs later to determine whether normal endogenous thyroid gland function has returned.

Because of its varied course and presentation, definitive treatment guidelines cannot be given. Rather the general advice to treat symptoms with short term therapy is prudent. To make matters even more complex, however, a small percentage of patients with postpartum thyroiditis have permanent hypothyroidism or permanent thyrotoxicosis. There is no method or test available to predict or detect such patients, and continued follow-up is mandatory. The cause of postpartum thyrotoxicosis is not known, but it does seem that such patients frequently have elevated serum titers of antithyroglobulin or antimicrosomal antibodies. The presence of anti-TSH receptor antibodies would be unusual and might signify the occurrence of permanent thyrotoxicosis, although further studies assessing these factors in postpartum thyroiditis are required.

LYMPHOMA

Primary thyroid lymphoma is a serious life threatening disorder that should be diagnosed as early as possible. This disease can arise in an otherwise normal gland, but it is now known that Hashimoto's disease predisposes to the development of thyroid lymphoma.

There are no laboratory parameters that can help assess the likelihood that this disease will occur in a patient with Hashimoto's disease, although recent growth of the thyroid gland, pain in the neck, hoarseness, dyspnea, dysphagia, and the presence of lymphadenopathy proximal to the thyroid gland may all suggest that a thyroid lymphoma has arisen. The likelihood that a patient with Hashimoto's disease will develop thyroid lymphoma is not known to be related to the thyroid antibody titer or the size of the gland. Although thyroid lymphomas occur much more frequently in patients with Hashimoto's disease, the chance that an individual patient with Hashimoto's disease will develop thyroid lymphoma is still slight.

Aspiration biopsies of a suspected lymphomatous gland may be helpful if the infiltrating lymphocytes are found to be especially immature and if there are few plasma cells and Hürthle cells. However, in many cases the customary infiltrating lymphocytes and plasma cells that occur with Hashimoto's disease alone make it difficult to distinguish Hashimoto's disease from lymphoma. Surgical thyroidectomy or removal and examination of involved lymph nodes may be required for the correct diagnosis. Laboratory and radiographic studies to assess lymphoma elsewhere in the body are indicated either before surgery if the suspicion of thyroid lymphoma is high or after surgery for staging purposes. External radiation and chemotherapy are further customary treatment modalities used after the diagnosis is established.

THYROID MEDICATION

For either hypothyroidism or goiter suppression, levothyroxine is the drug of choice. The rationale for its use is that the half-life of T_4 is about 7 days, and this medication can be ingested only once daily. If the drug is taken in this manner, serum T_4 and T_3 levels are stable and thus give an accurate estimate of the dose ingested and absorbed. Further, when exogenous levothyroxine is given, the T_4 is converted to T_3, the more biologically active hormone, at a rate determined by the body's own homeostatic mechanism. The maintenance levothyroxine dose is about 1.7 μg per kg per day.

Cytomel (L-triiodothyronine, LT_3) should not be given for the long term treatment of hypothyroidism or for goiter suppression, because the half-life is only about 24 to 30 hours and therefore the pills must be ingested several times daily. Further, the serum levels after Cytomel administration fluctuate widely, for example, starting at an undetectable level prior to the morning T_3 dose (since the effects of the previous evening's dose are dissipated owing to its short half-life) and rising to several hundred ng per dl several hours after T_3 ingestion. These fluctuations result in a variable T_3 effect throughout the day and also may aggravate angina pectoris or arrhythmias in susceptible patients. Serum T_4

and T_3 levels cannot be used to help assess the adequacy of therapy when a patient is receiving T_3 but are helpful when T_4 is given. Other preparations such as LT_4-LT_3 mixtures and crude powdered thyroid gland should not be used for many of the same reasons.

CHILDREN

Hashimoto's disease with hypothyroidism can occur in children, and the plan already noted regarding diagnosis and treatment applies. In children a further consideration is the long term potentially adverse effects of hypothyroidism on growth. The recommended maintenance T_4 dosage in children is either 3 μg per kg of body weight per day or 100 μg per square meter. Therapy in a severely hypothyroid child should be initiated with a half-maintenance dosage for 1 to 2 weeks to help minimize adverse effects, such as tachycardia. Careful monitoring for the adequacy of therapy is critical, attention being given to growth curves, clinical examination, and thyroid function tests. Excessive T_4 dosage and resultant hyperthyroidism also should be avoided. The goal is serum T_4 and T_3 radioimmunoassay levels in the upper half of the normal range and a serum TSH level that is normal. Although in neonates with hypothyroidism the capacity of T_4 to suppress the pituitary secretion of TSH may be defective, thus diminishing the usefulness of the serum TSH level as an effective monitor, children with Hashimoto's disease and hypothyroidism are expected to have normal feedback regulation while taking T_4.

THERAPEUTIC GOALS

The main objectives of therapy are to render a hypothyroid patient clinically and chemically euthyroid with normal serum T_4, T_3 radioimmunoassay, and TSH levels or, when treating a patient with a goiter, to suppress the serum TSH to undetectable levels while maintaining a normal or only slightly elevated T_4 level, a normal serum T_3 level, and clinical euthyroidism.

A guideline for daily LT_4 dosage is 1.7 μg per kg of body weight for replacement and 2.1 μg per kg of body weight for suppression. The serum T_4 level may be slightly elevated (perhaps as high as 14 μg per dl) when a person is ingesting exogenous thyroid hormone, and yet if the serum T_3 level is normal and the patient is clinically euthyroid, the dosage may be considered appropriate. A detectable serum TSH level in a supersensitive assay may indicate that pituitary suppression has not been achieved.

Occasionally thyrotropin-releasing hormone may be indicated. Following 200 to 500 μg of thyrotropin-releasing hormone given intravenously, normally there is a rise (usually at least a doubling) of the TSH level at 15 and 30 minutes; adequate suppression is indicated by undetectable basal values that do not rise after injection. Of course, this test cannot be used to distinguish a T_4 dosage that is excessive and causing clinical overt thyrotoxicosis from an appropriately suppressive dosage. The clinical examination and history give important information regarding the appropriateness of the dosage and, of course, serum T_4 and T_3 radioimmunoassay levels are also helpful. Symptoms suggestive of mild thyrotoxicosis (e.g., tachycardia, fine hand tremor, nervousness, and rapid return of reflexes) may suggest an excessive T_4 dosage; there are no diagnostic laboratory tests that can accurately reflect the excessive thyroid hormone levels presented to the tissues. When treating a patient for goiter suppression, finding the exogenous LT_4 dosage just sufficient to suppress TSH yet maintain normal laboratory test results and clinical parameters is the goal. Thyroid function tests can be effectively interpreted only at about 4 to 6 weeks after alteration of the dosage.

TOXICITY

Each patient's response to excess thyroid hormone ingestion varies with dose and duration of therapy as well as individual patient characteristics. Most commonly palpitations, nervousness, anxiety, insomnia, heat intolerance, tremors, diarrhea, or menstrual irregularities are noted. Cardiac manifestations such as the presence or aggravation of angina pectoris, arrhythmia, or congestive heart failure may predominate when a patient has underlying atherosclerosis or coronary artery disease.

DRUG INTERACTIONS

Thyroid hormones should be administered with caution to patients who also are taking tricyclic antidepressants, adrenergic agonists, or oral anticoagulant therapy, since they may potentiate the action of these drugs. Cholestyramine can bind T_4 in the gastrointestinal tract and thus decrease its absorption; ingestion of these two drugs must be separated by at least 2 hours. Exogenous thyroid hormone administration to hypothyroid subjects may alter the biologic half-life of other drugs, and their doses must be carefully considered after a hypothyroid patient has become euthyroid.

SURGERY

Thyroidectomy is only rarely indicated or required in Hashimoto's disease and would be considered when there are palpable hypofunctioning nodules in the thyroid gland that are not suppressed with 1 to 3 months of thyroxine therapy or nodules that are found to be enlarged at a follow-up examination; when there are palpably enlarged lymph nodes surrounding the thyroid gland that are considered clinically significant; or when aspiration biopsy of the thyroid or surrounding lymph nodes is diagnostic or suggestive of cancer or lymphoma. Many coincident factors are also considered, including the presence of clinical symptoms (dysphagia, pain, and dyspnea) suggesting progressive thyroid enlargement. Aspiration biopsy findings consistent with uncomplicated Hashimoto's disease may be difficult to discriminate from the subtle features suggesting lymphomatous involvement.

DISEASES THAT MAY BE ASSOCIATED WITH HYPOTHYROIDISM

Hashimoto's disease may occur in association with other autoimmune diseases, including adrenocortical insufficiency, myasthenia gravis, systemic lupus erythematosus, scleroderma, and pernicious anemia. The pathophysiologic mechanism by which these autoimmune disorders occur together is unknown. The clinical courses of these diseases, as compared to that of Hashimoto's disease, may vary, with either disease occurring initially and either disease being more severe. A clinical history to detect the development of another autoimmune disease is taken during each visit of a patient with Hashimoto's disease. Examination of the patient also includes a search for orthostatic hypotension and increased skin and buccal mucosa pigmentation, each a manifestation of adrenal insufficiency. If there is sufficient clinical suspicion, a 24 hour urinary free cortisol level should be obtained; if it is decreased, an adrenocorticotropic hormone (ACTH) stimulation test

should be performed. Some clinicians prefer to use the ACTH stimulation test as the initial screening test, rather than a 24 hour urinary free cortisol test.

In this test 25 units of synthetic ACTH is administered intravenously, a serum cortisol level being obtained immediately prior to ACTH injection and again 30 and 60 minutes later. A normal adrenal response is a basal serum cortisol level between 5 and 20 μg per dl (between 7:00 and 10:00 AM), which at least doubles after ACTH injection. Some authorities consider a post-ACTH serum cortisol level greater than 20 μg per dl also to be indicative of a normal response. Depending on the clinical circumstances and the degree of suspicion of adrenal insufficiency, either hydrocortisone therapy can be started when the ACTH response is clearly low or a longer ACTH infusion can be given to confirm the diagnosis. Clinical suspicion of the coexistence of one of the other autoimmune diseases should be confirmed by appropriate laboratory data.

SUGGESTED READING

Ahmann AJ, Burman KD. The role of T lymphocytes in autoimmune thyroid disease. Endocrinol Metab Clin North Am 1987; 16:287.
Burman KD, Baker JR Jr. Immune mechanisms in Graves' disease. Endocr Rev 1985; 6:183–232.
Graham GD, Burman KD. Radioiodine treatment of Graves' disease: an assessment of its potential risks. Ann Intern Med 1986; 105:901.
Hamburger JI, Miller JM, Kini SR. Lymphoma of the thyroid. Ann Intern Med 1983; 99:685–693.
Hennessey JV, Evaul JE, Tseng Y-C, Burman KD, Wartofsky L. L-thyroxine dosage: a re-evaluation of therapy with contemporary preparations. Ann Intern Med 1986; 105:11.
Wartofsky L, Burman KD. Alterations in thyroid patients with systemic illness: the "euthyroid sick syndrome." Endocr Rev 1982; 3:164–217.
Weetman AP, McGregor AM. Autoimmune thyroid disease: developments in our understanding. Endocr Rev 1984; 5:309–355.

INSULIN ALLERGY AND RESISTANCE

BARRY J. GOLDSTEIN, M.D., Ph.D.
C. RONALD KAHN, M.D.

INSULIN ALLERGY

Allergic reactions to insulin have been observed since pancreatic extracts of this protein were used to treat diabetes. The spectrum of immunologic reactions to insulin involves both cellular and humoral immunity, causing local as well as systemic reactions (Table 1). In recent years a movement toward the use of more purified (monocomponent) porcine insulin or human insulin produced by recombinant DNA or semisynthetic methods has reduced the incidence of insulin allergic reactions. Many patients, however, continue to receive mixed beef-pork insulin. The antigenicity of insulin arises from denaturation of the tertiary structure (a problem with human insulin preparations), the variation in peptide sequence that occurs in different animal insulins, and other components that are present in various formulations of insulin, including zinc, protamine, proinsulin and its intermediates, and other pancreatic hormone contaminants. Some insulin formulations, such as ultra-

TABLE 1 Allergic Reactions to Insulin

Local reactions
    Local erythema, induration, pruritus
    Biphasic subcutaneous reactions
    Local delayed reaction
    Lipoatrophy

Systemic reactions
    Generalized urticaria
    Angioedema with variable features of anaphylaxis
    Serum sickness with generalized lymphadenopathy
    Immunologic insulin resistance

lente, are available only as the more antigenic beef insulin. Studies have shown that certain histocompatibility antigens (HLA-B7, DR2, and DR3) may be associated with allergic reactions to insulin in diabetic patients, suggesting a genetic predisposition. Up to 50 percent of the patients with insulin allergy also give a history of allergy to other drugs, particularly penicillin.

Local Reactions

The most common clinical manifestations of insulin allergy are local erythema and swelling, which may be accompanied by mild pain or itching at the injection site. Occurring in 5 to 15 percent of the patients soon after the initiation of insulin therapy, these reactions are likely to be due to IgE mediated immediate hypersensitivity. In most cases the local reaction subsides within a few weeks despite continued therapy. The patient's injection technique should be carefully reviewed to determine whether an error in administration of insulin is causing a local irritation that is not actually immune mediated. If necessary, small doses of antihistamines can be given systemically or even mixed in the same syringe with insulin prior to subcutaneous injection. The dose of insulin may also be divided among several injection sites to reduce the magnitude of the local response. Switching to a more purified insulin preparation (purified pork or human insulin) has been effective in further reducing the local allergic reaction in up to 70 percent of affected patients.

Other local reactions include a biphasic subcutaneous response and delayed local reactions. Biphasic reactions occur at the injection site 4 to 6 hours following an initial wheal and flare reaction. These may be managed as the more typical local immediate type reaction and are likely to be due to IgE antibody. Local delayed reactions of the Arthus type and also delayed hypersensitivity have been described. The latter may be ameliorated by changing insulin preparations, and in some patients zinc-free insulin is necessary.

Lipoatrophy and lipohypertrophy are local changes in the amount of subcutaneous fat at insulin injection sites. Lipohypertrophy is due to increased lipid accumulation in adipose cells, probably as a result of local pharmacologic doses of injected insulin. Careful rotation of injection sites is often helpful in this condition. Lipoatrophy, on the other hand, may represent a form of immunologic reaction, since many patients have had previous allergic responses to insulin. Improvement at lipoatrophic sites may be achieved by switching to a more purified form of insulin and injecting into the circumference of the atrophic areas. Local steroid injections may also reduce the lipoatrophy if monocomponent or human insulin does not succeed.

Systemic Reactions

Systemic allergic reactions to insulin are uncommon, occurring in far less than 0.1 percent of the patients. Possible immediate manifestations include generalized urticaria, angioedema (with or without respiratory compromise and shock), laryngeal edema, and other signs of anaphylaxis. Treatment of the acute episode of anaphylaxis is standard. A significant fraction of patients with systemic reactions to insulin have a history of interrupted insulin therapy at some time in the past. As a preventive measure, in situations in which transient insulin therapy is planned (e.g., gestational diabetes or type II diabetes requiring insulin therapy for control during an intercurrent illness or surgery), the least antigenic insulin (purified pork or human) should be used. This may reduce the incidence of subsequent severe reactions, although even human insulin has caused clinically significant allergic reactions as well as the formation of IgG and IgE antibodies.

A local reaction at the injection site helps to confirm insulin as the etiologic factor in the systemic reaction. Assay of serum IgE antibody to insulin may not be helpful, since many insulin treated patients have measurable levels and do not manifest a clinically significant allergy. Insulin skin tests would be expected to be positive in affected patients, but 40 to 50 percent of all insulin treated individuals have been reported to have positive intradermal skin test reactivity. In practice, the suspicion of a systemic allergic reaction to insulin is based on clinical findings and not laboratory tests. Skin testing of various insulin formulations may help in selecting the type of insulin to which the patient is least sensitive. A key factor in determining the management of a patient who has had a systemic reaction to insulin is whether the insulin therapy has been discontinued for any length of time. If insulin is required for metabolic control, a patient receiving daily therapy should continue insulin therapy, but the dosage should be reduced to one third or one sixth of the dosage that caused the reaction. The insulin dosage can be increased daily by several units to the level required for optimal metabolic control. If a reaction does occur, the dosage should be reduced to a previously tolerated level and then raised by smaller increments once again.

If insulin therapy has been discontinued for several days to weeks following a reaction, the patient may be exquisitely sensitive to additional antigenic challenge. It is important to assess whether diet, weight loss, or oral hypoglycemic therapy may be effective in a noninsulin requiring patient before proceeding with desensitization. If further therapy with insulin is indicated, desensitization is required.

The desenitization procedure should be done in the hospital with emergency measures available to treat anaphylaxis. Intradermal skin testing should be performed first to determine the least antigenic insulin species for the patient. Drugs that mask or modify allergic responses (e.g., glucocorticoids or antihistamines) should not be taken. A typical desensitization schedule, as proposed by Galloway and Bressler, is shown in Table 2. Such procedures have been successful in about 75 percent of the cases. A kit containing materials for desenitization is available on request from the Eli Lilly Company.

Once desensitization has been performed, it is important to maintain this state by continued daily injections of insulin. In the unusual event that this procedure fails, the patient may be treated with glucocorticoids or less antigenic insulin preparations. Sulfated insulin, which is commercially available in Canada but not in the United States, is particularly valuable in such patients.

A rare systemic reaction consisting of serum sickness, generalized adenopathy, and a high insulin requirement due to anti-insulin IgG and immune complexes with insulin in the serum has been described in one

TABLE 3   Causes of Insulin Resistance

Nonimmunologic causes
  Obesity
  Stress
  Infection
  Pregnancy
  Excessive counterinsulin hormones
  Genetic alterations in insulin action
    Type A syndrome with acanthosis nigricans
    Lipoatrophic diabetes
    Leprechaunism

Immunologic causes
  Anti-insulin antibodies
  Anti-insulin receptor antibodies
    Type B syndrome
    Ataxia telangiectasia

patient. This unusual syndrome responded to prednisone therapy.

INSULIN RESISTANCE

Insulin resistance is considered to be present whenever normal amounts of insulin elicit less than a normal biologic response. Since the average rate of secretion of endogenous insulin is between 0.3 and 0.6 unit per kg of body weight per day, any patient receiving more than 1 unit per kg of body weight daily has some degree of insulin resistance. Clinically most patients are not considered to have significant insulin resistance until the daily dosage exceeds 200 units or, in children, 2 units per kg of body weight. The causes of insulin resistance are summarized in Table 3.

Nonimmunologic Causes of Insulin Resistance

In evaluating insulin resistant patients, it is important to assess common reasons for rising insulin requirements, including poor compliance with a dietary regimen, associated conditions such as obesity, stress, or infection, and excessive counterinsulin hormones, including glucocorticoids in Cushing's syndrome, catecholamines in pheochromocytoma, growth hormone in acromegaly, and pregnancy. The type A syndrome is a rare, possibly genetic disorder of insulin receptors that affects young women and includes insulin resistance, acanthosis nigricans, polycystic ovaries, and features of virilization. Insulin requirements are moderate to extremely elevated (up to 48,000 units per day). When treating these patients, a rapid increase in the insulin dosage is necessary but may not be successful even at

TABLE 2   Rapid Desensitization Schedule for Insulin Allergy*

Time (hours)	Insulin Dose (units)	Route of Administration
0	1/1000	Intradermal
½	1/500	Intradermal
1	1/250	Subcutaneous
1½	1/100	Subcutaneous
2	1/50	Subcutaneous
2½	1/25	Subcutaneous
3	1/10	Subcutaneous
3½	1/5	Subcutaneous
4	1/2	Subcutaneous
4½	1	Subcutaneous
5	2	Subcutaneous
5½	4	Subcutaneous
6	8	Subcutaneous

Followed by 2 to 10 units every 4 to 6 hours for next 24 to 36 hours before switching to lente or other insulins.

* Adapted from Galloway JD, Bressler R. Insulin treatment in diabetes. Med Clin North Am 1978; 62:663–680.

massive levels. Leprechaunism and lipoatrophic diabetes are rare syndromes that occur in childhood and have associated insulin resistance, possibly as a result of insulin receptor abnormalities.

Immunologic Insulin Resistance

Insulin resistance also may arise from antibodies to insulin or to the insulin receptor. The type B syndrome of insulin resistance and acanthosis nigricans usually affects older women and is characterized by the presence of anti-insulin receptor antibodies and other autoimmune (lupus-like) features. A fraction of these patients have a spontaneous remission of diabetes over a 2 to 3 year period. Other patients have required immunosuppressive therapy with prednisone (60 to 80 mg per day) or cyclophosphamide (1 mg per kg per day).

Insulin resistance due to the development of high titer IgG anti-insulin antibodies is rare, occurring in only 0.01 percent of all insulin treated diabetic patients. The diagnosis is suspected in an insulin treated patient with a rising insulin requirement in whom other causes of insulin resistance have been ruled out. Common clinical features include intermittent insulin therapy in the past, prior allergic reactions to insulin, and the use of less purified beef or pork insulins. Since almost all patients receiving insulin, especially less purified forms, develop some anti-insulin antibodies within a few months, confirmation of anti-insulin IgG as the cause of insulin resistance requires a quantitative measurement of antibody in a competitive protein binding assay. In noninsulin resistant patients, the concentration of antibody is low and rarely exceeds a binding capacity of 5 units (200 μg) of insulin per liter of plasma. Most patients with clinically significant insulin resistance due to anti-insulin IgG have substantially higher binding capacities.

The simplest initial treatment is to switch to a highly purified pork or human insulin. Since these insulins bind to pre-existing antibodies with lower affinity, they may provide adequate diabetic control in up to 50 percent of the patients. Additional control is gained later as the antibody titer falls in the presence of the weaker immunogenic challenge. It should be kept in mind,

however, that immunologic insulin resistance tends to be a self-limited disorder that spontaneously remits in about 60 percent of the patients within 6 months. Other less immunogenic insulins that may be used include fish insulin, desalanine pork insulin (in which the single amino acid different from human insulin has been removed), and sulfated insulin. Although sulfated insulin has half the biologic activity of regular insulin on a weight basis, on the average a patient with immunologic insulin resistance initially requires only 15 percent of the previous insulin dosage. As the antigenic stimulus is removed and antibody titers fall, the patient must be monitored for further reductions in insulin dosage in order to avoid hypoglycemia.

Glucocorticoids may be required to treat immunologic insulin resistance when the other maneuvers described are not successful. The patient should be started on a moderately high dosage of prednisone (60 to 80 mg per day) and watched carefully for a therapeutic response, which typically occurs within several days. A decreased insulin requirement is expected in up to 75 percent of the patients. Since individual responses are not easily predicted, patients need to be monitored for worsening of hyperglycemia (due to the counterinsulin effects of prednisone) as well as the possibility of a precipitous fall in the blood glucose level and the insulin requirement if antibody titers fall rapidly. After an initial response, the prednisone dosage should be tapered and discontinued over 2 to 3 weeks. Cytotoxic drugs such as cyclophosphamide and 6-mercaptopurine have been used occasionally. However, since alternate therapies are available and the condition is usually self-limited, such aggressive therapy is rarely, if ever, warranted.

SUGGESTED READING

Galloway JA, Bressler R. Insulin treatment in diabetes. Med Clin North Am 1978; 62:663–680.
Grammer L. Insulin allergy. Clin Rev Allergy 1986; 4:189–200.
Kahn CR, Rosenthal AS. Immunologic reactions to insulin: insulin allergy, insulin resistance and the autoimmune insulin syndrome. Diabetes Care 1979; 2:283–295.
Wiles PG, Guy R Watkins SM, Reeves WG. Allergy to purified bovine, porcine, and human insulins. Br Med J 1983; 287:531.

CHRONIC MUCOCUTANEOUS CANDIDIASIS

PETER G. SOHNLE, M.D.

Chronic mucocutaneous candidiasis is an uncommon disorder characterized by persistent and recurrent infections of the skin, nails, and mucous membranes by *Candida albicans*. Whereas this organism is part of the normal flora in the gastrointestinal tract of most humans, it usually does not cause infections without a significant predisposing factor. In normal persons such factors generally are present for only short periods, and the resulting candidiasis is self-limited. In chronic mucocutaneous candidiasis, however, the infections persist for years unless treated appropriately. Deep Candida infections are rare in chronic mucocutaneous candidiasis, indicating that the mechanisms that prevent invasion are intact in these patients.

Chronic mucocutaneous candidiasis may present in infants as oral thrush or as a Candida diaper rash. In older children or adults the infection may present as scalp lesions, thrush, or nail infections. Oral thrush and Candida vaginitis are common in patients with chronic mucocutaneous candidiasis. The esophagus is sometimes involved, but further visceral extension is rare. The skin infections in chronic mucocutaneous candidiasis are generally red, raised, hyperkeratotic lesions that usually are not painful. The scalp is often involved and may show thick hyperkeratotic scales. Epidermal neutrophilic microabscesses, which are characteristic of acute cutaneous candidiasis, are rare among the lesions of chronic mucocutaneous candidiasis. Nail involvement causes severe dystrophic changes with chronic swelling of the distal phalanx and marked thickening, distortion, and fragmentation of the nails themselves. The oral thrush and Candida vaginitis of chronic mucocutaneous candidiasis closely resemble acute Candida infections of mucous membranes in other patients, except that they are more chronic. The oral lesions are usually painful and tender.

There are a number of other disorders associated with chronic mucocutaneous candidiasis. Most prominent among these are the endocrinopathies, particularly hypoadrenalism, hypoparathyroidism, hypothyroidism, ovarian insufficiency, and diabetes mellitus. The combination of chronic superficial candidiasis and endocrine hypofunction has been termed the "Candida endocrinopathy syndrome." Patients with chronic mucocutaneous candidiasis also may have a number of other associated abnormalities, including alopecia totalis, vitiligo, malabsorption, chronic hepatitis, dysplasia of the dental enamel, congenital thymic dysplasia, thymomas, and other kinds of infections. The major immunologic abnormality in patients with chronic mucocuta-

neous candidiasis is a deficiency of cell mediated immune responses to Candida antigens. However, some of the patients also have defects in phagocytic cell function that may be associated with repeated pyogenic infections. Still others appear to be normal immunologically.

TREATMENT

The superficial infections of chronic mucocutaneous candidiasis are chronic and can be very disfiguring, although generally not life threatening. Before ketoconazole became available, the treatment of this condition was extremely difficult. Although the administration of amphotericin B generally produced rapid clearance of the skin lesions, relapses usually occurred. Ketoconazole, an orally administered imidazole drug, represented a major advance in the treatment of chronic mucocutaneous candidiasis because it could be given in maintenance dosages for long periods. Even so, this drug does have some significant toxic effects, and the treatment of chronic mucocutaneous candidiasis therefore is still not entirely satisfactory.

The initial evaluation of patients with chronic superficial Candida infections is important because some of the other conditions associated with these infections can be very serious. In very young children presenting with chronic mucocutaneous candidiasis, the possibility of thymic deficiency should be entertained. Endocrinopathies also should be considered in patients with chronic mucocutaneous candidiasis, particularly in those who present as children. Endocrine dysfunction, including life threatening adrenal crises, can develop after presentation of the Candida infections. Therefore, patients with chronic mucocutaneous candidiasis need to be followed carefully for the signs and symptoms of abnormal endocrine function. Patients who present with chronic mucocutaneous candidiasis as adults should be evaluated for the presence of a thymoma. Also, because chronic oral candidiasis occurs commonly in the acquired immunodeficiency syndrome (AIDS), patients presenting with this form of the infection should be questioned to see whether they belong to one of the risk groups for AIDS and also should be tested for antibody to the human immunodeficiency virus. Other patients with chronic mucocutaneous candidiasis probably deserve at least a minimal evaluation of immunologic function, including delayed hypersensitivity skin tests to Candida antigen and other common antigens, and enumeration of T lymphocytes and lymphocyte subsets.

Systemic Therapy

In patients with chronic mucocutaneous candidiasis limited to the mucous membranes local antifungal therapy may be tried first. However, those with skin or nail infections generally do not respond to topical drug therapy and need systemic therapy from the outset. Ketoconazole is now the major form of treatment for chronic mucocutaneous candidiasis. These patients are clearly predisposed to recurrences of infections after treatment, presumably because of the underlying immunologic dysfunction. Therefore, maintenance therapy is usually required.

Ketoconazole is a member of the imidazole class, which also includes clotrimazole, tioconazole, econazole, and miconazole. Ketoconazole is soluble in acidic aqueous solutions and therefore can be absorbed if given orally to persons with normal gastric acidity. The mechanism of action of this drug is to produce increased membrane permeability of the organism by suppressing its synthesis of sterols (particularly ergosterol) and other membrane lipids. Inhibition of germ tube formation by Candida yeast at ketoconazole concentrations of as little as 0.01 μg per ml is another important effect of this drug.

The usual initiating daily dosage of ketoconazole in an adult is a single 200 mg tablet taken orally. In children over 2 years of age, a reasonable dosage is approximately 3 mg per kg. There is not sufficient information to justify use of this drug in children under 2 years of age. It is metabolized in the liver and excreted in an inactive form in the bile, with a small amount also found in the urine. Because plasma levels are not significantly affected by decreased renal or hepatic function, the ketoconazole dosage does not have to be adjusted for these conditions. In addition, neither peritoneal dialysis nor hemodialysis removes the drug to a significant degree. Ketoconazole concentrates in sebum and thus is particularly useful in the treatment of cutaneous fungal infections, including chronic mucocutaneous candidiasis.

Ketoconazole requires normal gastric acidity for dissolution and absorption. Therefore, if the patient is also receiving antacids, anticholinergics, or H_2 blockers, they should be given at least 2 hours after ketoconazole is taken. If the patient has achlorhydria, the ketoconazole tablet can be dissolved in 4 ml of 0.2 N hydrochloric acid, which then should be ingested through a drinking straw to avoid contact with the teeth. Occasional patients may need an increase in dosage to control the superficial Candida infection or associated chronic dermatophytosis. On the other hand, it may be worthwhile periodically to try to lower the dosage or even to discontinue the drug, because a small number of patients have remained in remission after treatment was discontinued. In most such cases, however, the infections recur, although the patient should respond to retreatment.

There are some toxic effects associated with the use of ketoconazole. Indeed a few patients may not be able to tolerate it and some other therapeutic regimen will have to be used. Whereas nausea and vomiting are among the most frequent adverse effects reported with this drug, they occur in a dose dependent fashion and are less common at the dosage of 200 mg per day

usually given for chronic mucocutaneous candidiasis. Ketoconazole occasionally has been associated with severe hepatic toxicity, and some fatalities have occurred. Asymptomatic elevation of the serum transaminase level occurs in about 2 to 5 percent of the patients and can progress to symptomatic hepatic toxicity in a much smaller percentage of patients. Most, but not all, of these cases occur within 3 months after starting therapy with the drug. The patient should be told to report signs or symptoms of liver dysfunction, including unusual fatigue, anorexia, nausea or vomiting, jaundice, dark urine, or pale stools, so that appropriate biochemical tests can be done. Other complications of treatment that may occur are various hypersensitivity reactions and interference with the synthesis of steroid hormones. A temporary dose dependent depression of the serum testosterone level and the adrenocorticotropic hormone stimulated cortisol response has been seen with the use of this drug, as has gynecomastia. Oligospermia has been seen with very high doses in investigational studies.

Because the lesions of chronic mucocutaneous candidiasis are visible, the effect of therapy can be followed easily. In this regard, a careful assessment of the initial extent of the infections should be recorded in the patient's record so that the effectiveness of the treatment regimen, or the occurrence of relapses, can be recognized. In particular, the extent of oral candidiasis, the number of nails involved, and the size and location of skin lesions should be recorded. Because the oral lesions are usually painful, improvement can be judged by a reduction in symptoms as well as by disappearance of the white plaques. The initial sign of improvement in an affected nail is a small rim of normal appearing nail at the base. Skin lesions generally become less inflamed and shrink if the treatment is going well.

Some patients cannot be maintained on ketoconazole therapy because of intolerance or ineffectiveness of this drug. Intravenous therapy with amphotericin B may be used in these patients to clear the superficial infections. However, a number of patients were treated with this drug before ketoconazole became available, and in most of these the infections recurred after good initial clearing. Therefore, some adjunctive therapy, either with systemic or topical therapy with a different antifungal drug or by some form of immunologic reconstitution, may be needed after treatment with amphotericin B. This drug also has serious toxic effects, some of which occur in almost every treated patient. Therefore, it is indicated more for patients with deep or systemic mycoses rather than superficial infections, and its use is justified in only a small number of cases of chronic mucocutaneous candidiasis.

Amphotericin B is a member of the polyene class of antifungal drugs. As its name suggests, it has seven conjugated double bonds, forming part of a large ring structure. Combining of the drug with sterols, primarily ergosterol, in the fungal cell membrane is the principal mechanism of action of drugs in this class. There is also a recent report suggesting that active oxygen species produced through the reaction of amphotericin B with oxygen may be responsible for some of the drug's antifungal activity. The commercially available preparation of amphotericin B contains desoxycholate to produce a colloidal suspension of the drug. The vials should be reconstituted in distilled water or dextrose solutions because the addition of an electrolyte causes aggregation of the colloidal solution. Amphotericin B does not have to be protected from light under the usual infusion conditions. The drug is excreted to only a minor extent in either urine or bile, and blood levels are not affected by either hepatic or renal failure.

Therapy with amphotericin B should be initiated with a 1 mg test dose, which is given over a 30 minute period. If the patient tolerates the test dose, larger dosages then can be given. Since chronic mucocutaneous candidiasis is not a rapidly progressive condition, the dosage of amphotericin B can be increased slowly as a way of reducing the immediate reactions to the infusions. These include fever, chills, nausea, vomiting, headache, and sometimes hypotension or dyspnea. After the initial infusion, the dosage can be increased by 5 mg per day until approximately 0.5 mg per kg is being given daily or every other day. The addition of 25 to 50 mg of hydrocortisone to the amphotericin B solution may reduce the severity of immediate reactions to the infusions. It also may be necessary to premedicate the patient with aspirin or acetaminophen, diphenhydramine, and perhaps an antinausea drug. A total dosage of about 1.0 g is usually adequate to cause clearance of the infections, although in some cases oral candidiasis may not clear completely. Renal dysfunction is the most important toxic effect of amphotericin B and is usually manifested by a reduction in the glomerular filtration rate with a resulting elevation in the serum creatinine level. Renal function almost always improves with cessation of therapy, and the dosage can be adjusted according to the creatinine level, which should be kept below 3.0 mg per dl. Some of the other important toxic effects that can occur are phlebitis at the infusion site, hypokalemia, renal tubular acidosis, weight loss, anemia, and thrombocytopenia. The response to amphotericin B therapy can be evaluated as already discussed for ketoconazole.

There are some alternative drugs presently available for the treatment of chronic mucocutaneous candidiasis, but they have limited usefulness at present. Miconazole is an imidazole that can be given intravenously but is rather difficult to administer and probably has no advantage over ketoconazole. Flucytosine is the fluorine analogue of cytosine. It was developed originally as an antitumor drug and was later found to have antifungal effects. It is converted by deamination in the fungus to 5-fluorouracil, which then interferes with DNA synthesis by the organism. Because the development of drug resistance during therapy is a major problem with this drug, it probably is not useful for the treatment of chronic mucocutaneous candidiasis. Itraconazole, a drug in the triazole class, is undergoing clinical trials at present and has shown promise for the treatment of superficial fungal infections.

Topical Therapy

Nystatin is a polyene antibiotic with a structure very similar to that of amphotericin B. It is not absorbed orally and is useful mainly for topical therapy. Available preparations include creams or ointments for cutaneous use, oral suspensions, and vaginal suppositories. Vaginal tablets, containing 100,000 units per tablet, are inserted by an applicator high into the vagina once or twice daily for 14 days. The oral nystatin suspension (100,000 units per ml) can be taken in a dose of 5 ml to be swished around in the mouth and then swallowed, four times per day.

Clotrimazole is an imidazole that has good activity against Candida, but it also has significant in vivo toxicity, which limits its effectiveness as systemic therapy. However, this drug is very effective when used topically. It is probably more effective than nystatin for the treatment of oral candidiasis. The drug is available as 10 mg troches, which can be used orally five times per day. Also available are vaginal creams and 100 mg vaginal tablets.

Immunologic Therapy

Deficiencies in cell mediated immunity to Candida antigens appear to contribute significantly to the high incidence of relapse after antifungal therapy in patients with chronic mucocutaneous candidiasis. Therefore, immunologic reconstitution has been attempted as a way to prolong remissions after initial clearance of the lesions with amphotericin B treatment. The most satisfactory results have been obtained using dialyzable transfer factor, which is an extract of lymphocytes from normal persons who manifest delayed hypersensitivity to Candida on skin testing. However, because the preparation and administration of transfer factor are cumbersome, this type of treatment remains experimental at present. Other forms of immunologic reconstitution, particularly in individuals who have chronic mucocutaneous candidiasis as a manifestation of thymic deficiency, are also experimental at the present time. For the usual patient with chronic mucocutaneous candidiasis, maintenance therapy with ketoconazole is probably a more reasonable approach. However, if better methods can be developed for restoring immune responses in these patients, this approach may prove superior to the administration of potentially toxic antifungal drugs for the prolonged periods necessary in the treatment of chronic mucocutaneous candidiasis.

SUGGESTED READING

Graybill JR, Herndon JH, Kniker WT, Levine HB. Ketoconazole treatment of chronic mucocutaneous candidiasis. Arch Dermatol 1980; 116:1137–1141.

Horsburgh CR, Kirkpatrick CH. Long-term therapy of chronic mucocutaneous candidiasis with ketoconazole: experience with twenty-one patients. Am J Med 1983; 74:23–29.

Kauffman CA, Shea MJ, Frame PT. Invasive fungal infections in patients with chronic mucocutaneous candidiasis. Arch Intern Med 1981; 141:1076–1078.

Kirkpatrick CH, Rich RR, Bennett JE. Chronic mucocutaneous candidiasis: model-building in cellular immunity. Ann Intern Med 1971; 74:955–978.

Kirkpatrick CH, Sohnle PG. Chronic mucocutaneous candidiasis. In: Safai B, Good RA, eds. Immunodermatology. New York: Plenum Press, 1981:495–514.

IMMUNOLOGICALLY MEDIATED NEPHRITIC RENAL DISEASE*

MARC J. SADOVNIC, M.D.
WARREN K. BOLTON, M.D.

Glomerulonephritis has been attributed to glomerular deposition of preformed circulating immune complexes, in situ immune complex formation, antibodies against glomerular basement membrane, or antibody independent mechanisms involving cell mediated immunity. Despite a variety of animal models and continued clinical investigations, a thorough understanding of the immunopathology of these diseases and efficacy of treatment with corticosteroids, other immunosuppressive drugs, plasmapheresis, anticoagulants, and antiplatelet drugs are lacking.

Table 1 lists the nephritic diseases thought to be immunologically mediated. Many are covered in other articles in this book. Here we consider IgA mesangial nephropathy, nephritis associated with infection, and idiopathic hematuria. The prognosis in these entities is generally favorable with the control of hypertension and fluid overload and the eradication of infection. Treatment specifically directed toward the nephritis is enthusiastically recommended only with the biopsy proven clinicopathologic entity of rapidly progressive glomerulonephritis. Chronic progressive disease may be treated in some centers.

MESANGIAL NEPHROPATHY

Diffuse mesangial IgA deposits have been described in a variety of conditions—celiac disease, dermatitis herpetiformis, alcoholic and other liver disease, and certain neoplasms. Occasionally there is acute reversible or, rarely, progressive deterioration in renal function. Circulating IgA immune complexes resulting from increased mucosal permeability to a variety of antigens, decreased reticuloendothelial system function, or increased IgA synthesis is thought to contribute to the glomerulonephritis. Elevated serum IgA levels are present in a majority of patients, as is positive immunofluorescence for IgA in skin arterioles. Other syndromes characterized by isolated or combined deposits of IgM, Clq, or C3 may be associated with mesangial proliferative glomerulonephritis. The prognosis is good unless heavy proteinuria, hypertension, glomerular sclerosis, or crescents are present. Some of these cases, especially with C3 deposits, may represent resolving postinfectious glomerulonephritis.

Treatment

No specific therapy is indicated unless the nephrotic syndrome is present. In this case, therapy as for minimal change disease may be effective (see chapter *Immunologically Mediated Nephrotic Renal Disease*). Patients with progressive disease may be treated with aspirin and dipyridamole and a low protein diet. Those with this histologic picture, numerous crescents, and rapidly progressive glomerulonephritis are probably better considered to have variants of acute crescentic glomerulonephritis.

BERGER'S DISEASE

Berger's disease accounts for over 10 percent of the biopsy proven cases of primary glomerular disease. The typical presentation is macroscopic hematuria, often within days after the onset of an upper respiratory tract infection ("synpharyngitis") without the latent period associated with poststreptococcal glomerulonephritis. There is a tendency to recurrence, a male preponderance, and a peak incidence in the second through fourth decades. Reversible decreases in renal function may be associated with gross hematuria. Rapidly progressive glomerulonephritis is uncommon, although crescents are

*This work was supported in part by U.S. Public Health Service grant DK 32530 from the National Institute of Diabetes and Digestive and Kidney Diseases.

TABLE 1 Immunologically Mediated Nephritic Diseases

Type	Characteristic Renal Biopsy Findings*	Other Characteristic Features	Treatment
Berger's disease	FGN—mesangial IgA†	Increased serum IgA and positive arteriolar immunofluorescence for IgA on skin biopsy specimens	None unless rapidly progressive GN
		Serum complement levels usually normal	Consider ASA, dipyridamole, diet
Henoch-Schönlein purpura	FGN—mesangial IgA and fibrinogen†	Same as in Berger's disease; also rash, arthralgias, GI symptoms	None or prednisone as for Berger's disease
Poststreptococcal GN	Exudative DPGN—subepithelial humps, C3*	Increased antibody titers to streptococcal antigens, hypocomplementemia	Symptomatic. None unless rapidly GN
Other infection associated GN	F or DPGN, F embolic—humps, C3*	Positive blood or other cultures; hypocomplementemia, serologic evidence of infection	Eradicate infection and remove prosthetic devices
Idiopathic hematuria	Variable, often FGN—mesangial IgM, C3, C1q, or no deposits	Proteinuria absent to moderate	None
Allergic interstitial nephritis	Interstitial inflammatory cell infiltrates	Variable, including fever, eosinophilia, eosinophiluria, hematuria	See chapter *Acute Interstitial Nephritis*
Membranoproliferative GN	Membranoproliferative GN—C3, glomerular basement membrane splitting†	Hypocomplementemia	See chapter *Immunologically Mediated Nephrotic Renal Disease*
Rapidly progressive GN	Crescentic disease—no deposits, granular deposits, or antiglomerular basement membrane antibodies	Circulating antiglomerular basement membrane antibodies in some cases	See chapter *Goodpasture's Syndrome* on rapidly progressive GN
Systemic lupus erythematosus	Variable, including F and DPGN, membranous nephropathy—C1q immunoglobulins*	Positive ANA, anti-DNA, hypocomplementemia	See chapter *Lupus Nephritis*
Systemic vasculitis	Variable—F and DPGN, tuft ischemia, crescents	Multisystem involvement	See chapter *Systemic Vasculitis*
Wegener's granulomatosis	F necrotizing GN, tuft ischemia crescentic GN	Upper and lower respiratory tract involvement	See chapter *Systemic Vasculitis*

* F, focal. D, diffuse. P, proliferative. GN, glomerulonephritis.
† Occasionally may have epithelial crescents.

often noted in biopsy specimens. The pathologic changes on light microscopy are variable, with both diffuse and focal lesions. There is an increase in the mesangial matrix or cellularity with diffuse positive immunofluorescence for IgA. The prognosis, initially believed to be excellent, has been revised with the accumulation of long term data showing a tendency toward hypertension and progressive renal insufficiency in perhaps 20 to 30 percent of the patients.

Treatment

There are few data available to support the use of any specific therapy. Effective blood pressure control, prevention and treatment of infection, and a general approach to management of the patient are obvious. Although phenytoin lowers serum IgA levels, in con-

trolled trials it did not affect the clinical or pathologic course of the disease. Cyclophosphamide and anticoagulants have been used according to anecdotal reports with some success, and plasmapheresis is successful in removing circulating immune complexes. Any long term benefits remain to be shown. Tetracycline treatment has resulted in a decrease in the urinary red cell count in treated patients compared to controls but without an associated change in renal function. Corticosteroids have been reported to be effective in the nephrotic syndrome with IgA deposits in normotensive patients with normal renal function. Those with mesangial changes with segmental sclerosis and proliferation or hypertension with crescents do not appear to respond to corticosteroids.

Our own approach to therapy for Berger's disease is supportive care with specific attention to blood pressure control. In patients with glomerulosclerosis or progressive disease, we utilize a regimen of aspirin, 325 mg twice a day, and dipyridamole, 75 mg three times a day. Patients with severe progressive disease are also given a low protein diet on the assumption that this will decrease intraglomerular pressure and retard progression of the disease. Patients with the nephrotic syndrome are treated with prednisone, 1 mg per kg per day, as we would treat minimal change disease. In patients who have a clinical course of rapidly progressive glomerulonephritis, we utilize pulse methylprednisolone therapy. Methylprednisolone, 30 mg per kg of body weight to a maximal total dosage of 3 g, is administered intravenously over exactly 20 minutes every other day for 3 days. The patient needs to be volume repleted and must not take diuretics before or after the pulse therapy. We monitor the blood pressure, and in patients with a history of cardiac arrhythmias we also use a cardiac monitor. Forty-eight hours after the third dose of methylprednisolone, oral alternate day prednisone therapy, 2 mg per kg for 2 weeks, is begun, followed by administration of 1.75 mg per kg for 1 month and 1.5 mg per kg for 3 months, with progressive decreases as previously described to cover approximately 5 years of therapy. The oral alternate day prednisone dosages are adjusted to 75 percent of these dosage levels for patients who are 60 years old and older. In those who have not responded by 10 weeks, the dosage is tapered rapidly and patients are supported on dialysis with transplantation.

IgA nephropathy is known to recur in patients with renal allografts. Nonetheless the reappearance of IgA nephropathy is not associated with an excessive loss of the graft. Therefore, renal transplantation should be considered in patients with Berger's nephritis and is not a contraindication to allografting.

HENOCH-SCHÖNLEIN PURPURA

Henoch-Schönlein purpura is characterized by leukocytoclastic vasculitic nonthrombocytopenic purpura, usually of the buttocks and lower extremities. Other systemic manifestations may include nephritis with clinical and pathologic features indistinguishable from those of Berger's disease, a nondeforming arthritis, and abdominal pain secondary to vasculitic gut involvement. The peak incidence occurs in children under 5 years of age, although the disorder has been reported uncommonly in adults. Renal involvement is inconsistent and is most commonly evident as hematuria, which may be macroscopic. Proteinuria may reach nephrotic levels. Oliguria with progressive renal failure is rare but occurs. In some patients there is a history of a food allergy, an insect bite, or a synpharyngitic upper respiratory infection. Male preponderance is less sharply defined than in Berger's disease, and there tends to be a history of resolution and recurrence after the initial episode. Renal biopsy is rarely necessary but may be of value if the initial skin lesions are not evident, or may be used to justify therapy when the clinical picture suggests rapidly progressive glomerulonephritis.

Treatment

A dramatic decrease in the systemic manifestations of Henoch-Schönlein purpura can be effected with prednisone. The joint and gastrointestinal symptoms respond best; it has not been proven that skin and renal lesions respond.

Some investigators have used cytotoxic and anticoagulant drugs in combination or alone. Chlorambucil, cyclophosphamide, and dipyridamole have been used with the claim that fewer patients progress to renal failure when treated with these drugs and that the interval between the onset of nephropathy and renal failure is longer. However, there are no controlled trials to prove the benefit of any type of therapy in nephritis. In patients with the clinical course of rapidly progressive glomerulonephritis and with significant crescents (more than 20 percent of the glomeruli), we treat with the regimen described for rapidly progressive glomerulonephritis in Berger's disease, i.e., pulse methylprednisolone therapy followed by alternate day prednisone therapy. Until prospective controlled trials are available, it seems appropriate to treat the systemic manifestations of Henoch-Schönlein purpura with prednisone. If an acute nephritic course is present with rapid progression, the patient should be treated as for rapidly progressive glomerulonephritis. We treat slowly progressive disease with evidence of chronicity with aspirin-dipyridamole or diet modification as for Berger's disease.

Although Henoch-Schönlein purpura has been reported to recur in renal allografts, this is an unusual event and should not preclude the use of transplantation as a therapeutic option in patients who sustain progression of the underlying disease to uremia.

GLOMERULONEPHRITIS ASSOCIATED WITH INFECTION

Poststreptococcal Glomerulonephritis

Poststreptococcal glomerulonephritis follows pharyngitis or pyoderma caused by group A beta-hemolytic nephritogenic strains of Streptococcus. This occurs after a latent period of 1 to 3 weeks. The clinical presentation is variable, with hematuria reaching macroscopic proportions in a majority of patients. Proteinuria is typically less than 2 g per day but may reach the nephrotic range, especially in adults. Hypertension is present in half the patients and is usually mild. Fluid retention associated with edema is common and may progress to ascites (less often pulmonary edema). Oliguria and uncommonly anuria may be present, and mild azotemia is frequent. There is a nephritic urinary sediment and a characteristic course with resolution or a decrease in clinical abnormalities within 6 weeks after presentation. There is often evidence of circulating immune complexes. Total hemolytic complement (CH_{50}) and C3 levels are reduced in a majority of patients. Continued reduction in the serum complement level for more than 8 weeks, especially with unrelenting nephritis, should raise the possibility of other types of hypocomplementemic glomerulonephritis, including membranoproliferative glomerulonephritis, other infection associated glomerulonephritis, lupus nephritis, or essential cryoglobulinemia. Renal biopsy is usually not necessary for diagnosis but is useful in verifying the diagnosis in patients following a protracted course or in establishing progression to crescentic rapidly progressive glomerulonephritis in a minority of patients.

The prognosis is favorable with restoration of normal renal function, although chronic and progressive renal insufficiency may occur in patients with persistent oliguria or nephrotic proteinuria or in those with biopsy evidence of crescentic disease. Adults have more severe disease and are more likely to have a chronic course. Microscopic hematuria and mild proteinuria may persist for over 1 year and do not affect the prognosis.

Treatment

Patients with postinfectious nephritis usually can be treated by supportive measures alone. Since the hallmark of the disease is salt and water retention, patients should be given a low sodium (2 g) diet and fluid restriction should be imposed. The blood pressure should be controlled with antihypertensive medications. Patients with documented streptococcal infections should receive appropriate antibiotics, not to prevent progression of renal disease, which is unassociated with treatment, but to prevent spread of the infection. In children with clinical evidence of rapidly progressive glomerulonephritis, the course is generally favorable, with spontaneous recovery. It is our practice, however, to treat with pulse methylprednisolone adults who are oligoanuric and who have significant numbers of crescents. The regimen followed is that already described for Berger's disease.

Bacterial Endocarditis

Mild azotemia with urinary abnormalities primarily consisting of microscopic hematuria and mild proteinuria is often seen with subacute and chronic bacterial endocarditis. Most often there are other stigmata of endocarditis. The serum complement level is typically depressed, and there is laboratory evidence of circulating immune complexes. Renal biopsy is often unnecessary but when performed shows diffuse proliferative, focal proliferative, or focal necrotizing glomerulonephritis. Rarely there is crescentic glomerulonephritis. Interstitial infiltrates are often seen and may be a direct consequence of endocarditis or may be associated with antibiotics used in treatment. Bland and septic valvular emboli with renal infarction and abscess formation, acute tubular necrosis from hypotension secondary to valvular lesions, or nephrotoxic antibiotics may also cause renal dysfunction.

Treatment

Treatment is directed at eradicating infection, correcting hemodynamic compromise, and minimizing antibiotic associated renal injury. Renal function often returns to premorbid levels, although occasionally azotemia may persist if it is associated with severe glomerular injury. Immunosuppressive drugs and plasmapheresis have been reported to be helpful in rare cases of crescentic disease associated with infective endocarditis.

Shunt Nephritis

Infection is a common complication of ventriculoatrial and ventriculoperitoneal cerebrospinal fluid shunts inserted to relieve hydrocephalus. This is most often manifested by persistent fever. Blood cultures may be negative, but cultures of shunt fluid are diagnostic. Renal deposition of circulating immune complexes with prolonged infection leads to a hypocomplementemic glomerulonephritis as in bacterial endocarditis. There is a decreased tendency toward anemia and splenomegaly compared to bacterial endocarditis but an increased incidence of heavy proteinuria approaching the nephrotic range in approximately 25 percent of the cases. Nephritis also has been reported with an infected peritoneovenous Le Veen shunt. Hematuria is most often microscopic, but gross hematuria does occur. Membranoproliferative glomerulonephritis has been reported most often on renal biopsy, although diffuse proliferative or mesangial glomerulonephritis with IgM, IgA, and C3 deposits is also seen.

Treatment

The systemic administration of antibiotics to clear shunt infections is seldom successful. There are several reports of synergistic combinations of antibiotics that have eradicated shunt infections with subsequent improvement in glomerulonephritis, but generally systemic antibiotic therapy is not efficacious. Direct instillation of antibiotics into the cerebrospinal fluid by an indwelling ventricular reservoir is more successful in clearing central nervous system infections. However, the most successful and most predictable treatment is removal of the infected ventricular jugular shunt combined with systemic antibiotic therapy and then shunt replacement when the patient is no longer infected.

Renal function often returns to normal with reso-.
lution of urinary abnormalities after adequate therapy.
However, severe renal involvement may not resolve.
Treatment of the nephrotic syndrome with corticosteroids or immunosuppressive drugs should be considered only after shunt removal and appropriate antibiotic therapy.

Other Infections Associated with Glomerulonephritis

Diffuse proliferative, focal proliferative, and crescentic glomerulonephritis have been described with a
variety of bacterial, fungal, viral, protozoal, and helminthic infections, including visceral abdominal abscess, syphilis, typhoid fever, histoplasmosis, infectious
mononucleosis, quartan and falciparum malaria, and
trichinosis. Treatment should be directed at eradicating
infection if possible. In most cases recovery of renal
function is complete.

IDIOPATHIC HEMATURIA

The syndrome of idiopathic hematuria is characterized by recurrent or persistent hematuria without evidence of lower urinary tract, systemic, or secondary
glomerular disease. Proteinuria is absent or mild to
moderate. Renal biopsy findings are variable and may
reveal unsuspected evidence supporting hereditofamilial,
infectious, or vasculitic etiologies. Focal and segmental
proliferative glomerulonephritis, often with mesangial
IgM deposits, without clear evidence of other primary
or secondary glomerulonephritis is a common finding.
If proteinuria is less than 1 g per day, the prognosis is
favorable and biopsy is unnecessary. With more significant proteinuria or progressive renal insufficiency, a
biopsy should be carried out to rule out treatable forms
of glomerulonephritis.

TIMING OF THERAPY

Since it is not clear that therapy is indicated or has
a beneficial effect in most of these diseases, personal
judgment must play a major role in the decision to treat.
Our approach is to diagnose and treat rapidly progressive
glomerulonephritis as soon as possible, on an emergency
basis. Patients with the nephrotic syndrome may be
given therapy electively, and measures to address chronic
progressive disease are usually begun when the serum
creatinine level is about 2.0 mg per dl or higher. We
do not give pulse therapy to patients with rapidly progressive glomerulonephritis who are hypercatabolic or
febrile until the etiology of those states has been clarified. In all cases the patient's understanding and agreement are part of the decision making process.

MECHANISMS OF ACTION

The exact mechanism of these various therapeutic
interventions are unknown. Aspirin and dipyridamole
normalize platelet survival, decrease adhesiveness, presumably diminish deposition of glomerular platelet antigens, and may affect efferent glomerular arteriolar
tone. Steroids and cytotoxic drugs affect both antibody
and cellular immune systems at multiple points as well
as the reticuloendothelial system. Low protein diets
presumably decrease glomerular flow, filtration, and
intraglomerular pressure.

SIDE EFFECTS AND COMPLICATIONS OF THERAPY

Aspirin and dipyridamole occasionally cause bleeding complications. These are usually mild, consisting of
subcutaneous hemorrhage and nose bleeds. Occasionally
they may be more serious and necessitate cessation of
therapy. Pulse therapy is associated with a metallic taste,
flushing, and occasional arthralgias, myalgias, and psy-
chotropic effects. Arrhythmias and hypotension may
occur in patients with pre-existing heart disease or those
who are volume depleted. Alternate day prednisone
therapy causes few side effects compared to daily steroid
therapy—chemical diabetes, weight gain, a cushingoid
facies, hirsutism, cataracts, and rarely aseptic necrosis
of the hip.

SUGGESTED READING

Arze RS, Rashid H, Morley R, Ward MK, Kerr DNS. Shunt nephritis:
report of two cases and review of the literature. Clin Nephrol 1983;
19:48–53.
Austin HA III, Balow JE. Henoch-Schönlein nephritis: prognostic
features and the challenge of therapy. Am J Kidney Dis 1983;
2:512–520.
Bolton WK. The role of cell mediated immunity in the pathogenesis
of glomerulonephritis. Plasma Ther Transfus Technol 1984; 5:415–
430.
Clarkson AR, Woodroffe AJ. Therapeutic perspectives in mesangial
IgA nephropathy. Contr Nephrol 1984; 40:187–194.
Pardo V, Berian MG, Levi DF, Strauss J. Benign primary hematuria:
clinicopathologic study of 65 patients. Am J Med 1979; 67:817–
822.
Rouzar MA, Logan JL, Ogden DA, Graham AR. Immunosuppressive
therapy and plasmapheresis in rapidly progressive glomerulonephritis associated with bacterial endocarditis. Am J Kidney Dis
1986; 7:428–433.

THERAPEUTIC APPROACH TO RENAL TRANSPLANTATION

ALAN B. LEICHTMAN, M.D.
TERRY B. STROM, M.D.

Transplantation is firmly established as the preferred treatment for patients suffering from end stage renal disease. Nonetheless no consensus has developed about how to achieve optimal immunosuppression, and many individual centers, employing different protocols, report excellent graft and patient survival.

Immunologic considerations, including antirejection therapy, at Boston's Beth Israel Hospital, are organized around five general principles. The first is careful patient preparation and selection of the best available human leukocyte antigen (HLA) match. The second is a biologic approach to immunosuppressive therapy similar to that employed in chemotherapy; several drugs are used simultaneously, each of which is directed at a different cellular activation mechanism. Such a strategy allows various drugs to work synergistically, using each drug at lower doses and thereby limiting the toxicity of each drug while increasing the total immunosuppressive effect. The third principle is that higher doses or more immunosuppressive drugs are required to gain early engraftment and to treat established rejection than are needed to maintain immunosuppression in the long term, "almost" tolerant host. In other words intensive "induction" and modest "maintenance" treatment protocols are used. Next is careful investigation of each episode of post-transplant renal dysfunction, in the realization that most of the common causes of graft dysfunction, including rejection, cyclosporine toxicity, and acute renal failure, can, and frequently do, coexist. Successful therapy therefore often involves several simultaneous therapeutic maneuvers. Finally, the appropriate dosage reduction or withdrawal of an immunosuppressive drug, when that drug's toxicity exceeds its therapeutic benefit, is as necessary to overall patient survival as proper initiation of immunosuppression is to graft survival. We will discuss only the first three principles and the specific usage of each immunosuppressive drug.

Immunologic damage to renal allografts is mediated by both humoral and cellular mechanisms. Acute humoral rejection results in a vasculitic catastrophe, occurring when kidneys are transplanted into hosts bearing preformed cytotoxic antibodies targeted against ABO or HLA-A, -B, or -C associated antigens present in the transplanted organ. Chronic humoral rejection also principally targets the graft endothelium and typically leads to clinically "silent," but inexorable, late graft loss. In either event, and despite the application of many different therapeutic strategies, including cytotoxic drugs in combination with plasma exchange, humoral rejection is essentially refractory to available antirejection medications and is best treated by prevention through accurate tissue typing. If diffuse fixed vascular lesions are present, recognition should lead to the appropriate withdrawal of immunosuppressive therapy to protect such patients from overimmunosuppression, which often occurs when full doses of immunosuppressive drugs are used in metabolically impaired azotemic patients. Cellular rejection, on the other hand, is much more readily treated.

Both cellular and chronic humoral rejection pathways are initiated by activation of a small population of recipient antidonor T lymphocyte clones that recognize donor histocompatibility antigens present in the graft. T cell activation requires multiple signals—interaction between T cells, accessory cells, and their products, e.g., interleukin 1 and of course graft antigens. These events in turn lead to elaboration of interleukin-2 receptors on the surface of activated T lymphocytes and release of interleukin-2 by activated T cells. Interaction between interleukin-2 and its cellular receptor is the signal for DNA synthesis, DNA replication, and clonal proliferation of activated interleukin-2 receptor bearing T cells, and for the release of other lymphokines that activate B cells and macrophages and also recruit these cells into the graft.

PRETRANSPLANT PATIENT PREPARATION

Potential recipients of cadaver donor renal transplants receive a minimum of three random blood transfusions. Although transfusion was a powerful adjunct to transplant therapy in the era when HLA-DR typing and cyclosporine were not generally available, the short term benefits of transfusion on 1 and 2 year graft survival have recently been more difficult to demonstrate in the cyclosporine era.

There is even less agreement concerning the role of donor specific transfusions for recipients of one-haplotype matched living related donor renal transplants. One-haplotype matched recipients treated with cyclosporine enjoy the same general 90 percent 1 year allograft survival demonstrated in azathioprine treated patients following donor specific transfusion. Moreover, donor specific transfusion is associated with a 10 to 30 percent incidence of deleterious sensitization of the donor against donor class I HLA molecules. Since these sensitized patients cannot be subjected to transplantation with the transfusion donor, we no longer employ donor specific transfusion.

ABO typing and cross matches between recent and historic recipient serum and donor T and B cells are obtained to exclude the presence of preformed recipient antidonor class I HLA cytotoxic antibodies capable of precipitating acute humoral rejection. Mixed lymphocyte cultures require 5 to 6 days to perform and thus cannot be employed for pretransplant testing for cadaveric donors because the limit of safe ex vivo organ preservation is 72 hours; however, mixed lymphocyte cultures are used in transplantation from living related donors to aid in typing of class II HLA antigens. Finally, after taking into consideration the compatibility of a cadaveric kidney in the patients on the transplant list who are most in need and most difficult to match, e.g., the existence of multiple preformed anti-HLA antibodies, the best available match is obtained.

THERAPY DESIGNED TO PREVENT REJECTION

Antirejection protocols at Boston's Beth Israel Hospital are aimed at interrupting four consecutive stages in lymphocyte activation pathway leading to allograft rejection. First, patient selection is undertaken utilizing HLA matching to minimize histoincompatibility antigenicity between donor and recipient. Next our basic immunosuppressive protocol employs three drugs, each directed at a separate discrete site in the T cell activation cascade. Prednisone is used from the time of transplantation, because corticosteroids used prior to or at the time of accessory cell activation block transcription of interleukin-1 encoding messenger RNA, thereby preventing delivery of the interleukin-1 signal involved in primary T lymphocyte activation. Cyclosporine, on the other hand, blocks transcription of interleukin-2 encoding messenger RNA and other lymphokine genes, thus depriving activated T cells of the stimulation necessary to sustain activation and initiate DNA synthesis requisite for cell activation and clonal expansion. Finally, azathioprine, an antimetabolite, the nitroimidazole derivative of 6-mercaptopurine, is used to inhibit both DNA and RNA synthesis. Therefore, azathioprine blocks cellular proliferation of the T lymphocytes that manage to "slip past" the more proximal hurdles to the T cell activation process imposed by steroids and cyclosporine.

We use the same basic protocol for both living donor and cadaver donor renal transplants. On the evening before or on the day of surgery, immunosuppression is initiated with cyclosporine (8 mg per kg per day orally, or one third of this dosage intravenously), azathioprine (2 mg per kg per day orally or intravenously), and prednisone (30 mg per day or its equivalent intravenously). Many cadaver organ recipients sustain a period of acute renal failure as the graft recovers from the perils of ex vivo preservation. Because of the difficulties associated with the use of cyclosporine (a potent nephrotoxin) in patients experiencing post-transplant acute renal failure, the cyclosporine dosage is halved in the absence of early post-transplant diuresis and reduced by increments of 50 to 100 mg, beginning with the third

postoperative week, in almost every patient. The azathioprine dosage is matched to the white count, with 50 percent reductions for patients whose total white counts fall below 5000 per cubic mm and temporary cessation of azathioprine therapy for patients whose white counts drop below 3000 per cubic mm. Most patients are maintained with azathioprine at dosages of 75 to 125 mg per day. Prednisone therapy is continued at a dosage of 30 mg per day for 1 month, reduced to 20 mg per day over the following 6 weeks, and then slowly decreased to 10 to 20 mg every other day over the course of the following year.

In experimental animals the successful introduction of an immunosuppressed state results in suppressor cell induction, graft tolerance, and the opportunity for drastic reductions in immunosuppressive therapy. Although tolerance has not been achieved in clinical practice, by 1 year after transplantation the immunosuppressive regimens in most patients have been greatly reduced in an individualized manner. At this time prednisone dosages generally range between 10 mg per day and 10 mg every other day, azathioprine between 1 and 2 mg per kg per day, and cyclosporine between 2 and 4 mg per kg per day. The actual dosage of each drug may be higher or lower, depending on the clinical course in the patient.

Individuals with end stage renal disease are particularly vulnerable to a number of drug toxic effects. Many such patients suffer from hypertension, diabetes mellitus, osteopenia, and osteomalacia, all of which frequently are aggravated by steroid treatment. Indeed pre-existent bone disease in steroid treated hosts may lead to aseptic necrosis of long bones, especially at the femoral head. Pediatric patients with renal disease already suffer from growth retardation, although the rate of growth usually increases after transplantation despite steroid use. Steroids also predispose to infection, delayed wound healing, cataracts, and perhaps psychiatric disturbances and peptic ulcer disease. For these reasons great care is taken to reduce the steroid dosage in the first post-transplant year.

Azathioprine, an antimetabolite, frequently results in reversible dose dependent leukopenia. Thrombocytopenia, megaloblastic anemia, and cholestatic jaundice may also occur. Azathioprine therapy is associated with an increased incidence of lymphomas of all types and skin cancers, especially of the squamous cell variety. The azathioprine dosage must be decreased by two thirds or more in patients who are simultaneously treated with allopurinol, which blocks oxidation of the active azathioprine metabolite, 6-mercaptopurine. Indeed we rarely use the potentially lethal combination of allopurinol and azathioprine.

Perversely, the principle target of cyclosporine toxicity is the kidney itself. Nephrotoxicity can occur at any time following transplantation. Although the early reversible form of toxicity leads to decreased renal blood flow due to vasoconstriction, failure to reduce nephrotoxic dosages promptly eventually results in interstitial fibrosis, glomerulosclerosis, and permanently impaired graft function. Cyclosporine is strongly lipophilic; therefore, measured drug levels correlate rather poorly with toxicity, and there is much overlap between levels in patients suffering from rejection and in those who are cyclosporine toxic. Cyclosporine, a nephrotoxin itself, potentiates renal injury caused by other nephrotoxic drugs. Patients with acute renal failure in the immediate transplant period are especially vulnerable to cyclosporine. It should be reiterated that acute renal failure, rejection, and cyclosporine toxicity may coexist in any combination. Nonrenal complications of cyclosporine therapy include hyperbilirubinemia, elevations in the bone specific fraction of alkaline phosphatase, hirsutism, and tremor.

Infection with cytomegalovirus resulting in fever and graft dysfunction occurs frequently during the second and third post-transplant months. Such patients are gravely immunodeficient and at high risk for the development of secondary superinfections. A recent multihospital trial in Boston indicates that prophylactic treatment of anticytomegalovirus antibody negative graft recipients receiving organs from anticytomegalovirus positive individuals with human serum containing high titers of anticytomegalovirus antibodies is extraordinarily effective in reducing the dreaded complications of active cytomegalovirus disease in transplantation recipients. Prophylaxis with trimethoprim sulfa should be instituted in patients with active cytomegalovirus disease, and azathioprine and cyclosporine therapy should be reduced or discontinued. Prednisone administration should be maintained but at a low level. This withdrawal of immunosuppression is potentially lifesaving, and we believe that rejection is rare during active cytomegalovirus infection. This belief is based on study of renal biopsy material in patients with active cytomegalovirus disease and graft dysfunction. Graft function returns to normal as the viral disease abates.

THERAPY DESIGNED TO TREAT ESTABLISHED REJECTION

Prednisone, cyclosporine, and azathioprine are effective in the prophylaxis of acute cellular rejection because each blocks various facets of T lymphocyte activation. Their proximal sites of activity, however, render low dose prednisone, cyclosporine, and azathioprine therapy ineffective in blocking the activity of already activated T cells and thus relatively incapable of abrogating an already established acute rejection reaction. Treatment of established rejection requires the use of drugs that act against already fully activated T cells. Three such drugs—high doses of corticosteroids, antithymocyte globulin, and OKT3, a murine monoclonal antibody recognizing a component of the human T3 complex—are thus held in reserve as therapies for the treatment rather than the prophylaxis of acute cellular rejection.

More than two thirds of acute cellular rejections respond to corticosteroid boluses. Typically these rejections are characterized by a dense infiltration of T cells in the medullary regions of the graft. We treat first, and frequently second, rejection episodes with 1 g of methylprednisolone intravenously daily for 3 consecutive days. The mechanism by which corticosteroids act to reduce the density of inflammatory infiltration in a rejecting allograft has not been fully elucidated; however, release of interleukin-1 by already activated accessory cells is blocked by high dose steroid therapy at the post-transcriptional level and T cell trafficking patterns are altered.

The T3 complex comprises a trio of proteins that are noncovalently associated with the two chains of the T cell receptor for antigen. This complex is expressed on the surface of all functionally competent T lymphocytes. Binding of OKT3 results in modulation of the entire antigen receptor–T3 complex from the T cell surface. Hence, OKT3 treated T cells lose their antigen receptor proteins and literally become blinded to the presence of the allograft; thus rejection abates. OKT3 therapy is more effective in the treatment of cellular rejection than corticosteroids. More than 90 percent of first rejections and a high percentage of second rejections respond to OKT3 therapy. Many corticosteroid insensitive cellular rejections are sensitive to OKT3 therapy.

Patients are skin tested with 0.1 ml of a 1 μg per ml solution of OKT3 prior to administration of the first dose. OKT3 then is given as a daily 5 mg intravenous bolus for 10 to 20 consecutive days. The first and sometimes the second dose are associated with the release of lymphokines from the targeted T cells; the consequences of lymphokine release are the development of fever, chills, dyspnea, chest pressure, wheezing, tremor, and nausea. Severe pulmonary edema is noted in hypervolemic patients as the first dose of OKT3 causes a ''capillary leak'' syndrome. Because of these troublesome symptoms, we reserve OKT3 therapy for steroid insensitive rejection episodes. Subsequent doses are well tolerated. Seventy-five percent of the patients develop IgG or IgM anti-idiotype or anti-isotype antibodies against OKT3. Cyclophosphamide, 400 mg intravenously, on days 7, 10, and 13, is employed to limit the frequency and delay the onset of occurrence of these anti-OKT3 antibodies. OKT3 is not efficacious in patients who have developed anti-idiotypic antibodies against OKT3.

Antithymocyte globulin is a polyclonal antibody preparation derived form animals immunized with human lymphocytes. The antibodies are directed against multiple formed elements, primarily against lymphocytes, present in human blood. More than 80 percent of steroid resistant first rejection episodes respond to antithymocyte globulin. Patients are skin tested with 0.1 ml of a 1:1000 dilution of antithymocyte globulin prior to administration of the first dose and pretreated before each dose with diphenhydramine and steroids. Antithymocyte globulin, at a dosage of 10 to 15 mg per kg, is administered by slow intravenous infusion over 4 to 8 hours for 10 to 14 days. Adverse reactions include anaphylaxis, hemolysis, thrombocytopenia, neutopenia, dyspnea, chills, fever, hypotension, chemical phlebitis, pruritus, serum sickness, and chest, flank, and back pain. Unlike the situation with OKT3, the severity of anaphylactoid side effects can increase with subsequent doses. Frank anaphylaxis can occur at any time during treatment. Our usage of antithymocyte globulin has decreased because OKT3 is less toxic than antithymocyte globulin and comparably effective in reversing rejection.

We rarely treat a patient for more than three early rejection episodes in the early post-transplant period, since third and fourth rejections tend to be vasculitic forms of rejection, which are therapeutically resistant, and the risks to the patient from zealous immunosuppression are, by that point, unacceptably high.

ALTERNATIVE APPROACHES

A number of other centers have adopted an alternative approach to antirejection prophylaxis. They administer Minnesota antilymphoblast globulin, a polyclonal antibody antithymocyte globulin-like preparation, along with prednisone and azathioprine in the immediate post-transplant period. An immunosuppressive umbrella is established that enables engraftment without the use of cyclosporine in the critical early post-transplant days during which time the graft is highly sensitive to cyclosporine's nephrotoxic effects. Cyclosporine treatment is not initiated until after the serum creatinine level has fallen below 3.0 mg per dl, at which point, after a brief overlap period, antilymphoblast globulin therapy is withdrawn. Kidney allografts undergoing acute renal failure are thereby spared the additional nephrotoxic effects of cyclosporine until the renal failure has resolved, and any incipient rejection episode is treated by the use of what we view as essentially antirejection strategies to induce immunosuppression. This ''sequential'' therapy has proven quite effective, with overall 1 year survival incidences for cadaver renal donor grafts in excess of 85 to 90 percent, the same incidence achieved in the best matched (zero HLA-B, DR mismatches) cadaver renal donor recipients treated with cyclosporine and prednisone alone. An analogous trial, with favorable early results, in which OKT3 is substituted for antithymocyte globulin is under way.

NEW THERAPIES

The interleukin-2 receptor is expressed transiently on the surface of activated T cells and small populations of macrophages and B cells, but not by resting or memory T lymphocytes. Drugs targeted at interleukin-2

receptor bearing cells either in the immediate post-transplant period or during episodes of acute cellular rejection offer the potential for destroying only those T lymphocytes destined to be responsible for a rejection reaction. With cessation of such therapy, the remainder of the immune system should remain intact to pursue its ordinary surveillance functions.

Two such drugs are under development. Phase 1 testing of anti-TAC, a murine monoclonal antibody against the human interleukin-2 receptor, is being successfully completed at the Beth Israel and Brigham and Women's Hospitals in Boston. A similar anti-interleukin-2 receptor monoclonal antibody has been employed in France in patients not receiving cyclosporine for the first 10 days after transplantation. Similar antibodies, administered as single agents for the first 10 post-transplant days only, have permitted indefinite survival of approximately 60 percent of heterotropic cardiac allografts in rats and mice. Although tolerance has not been achieved in clinical practice, immunologic graft failure has not yet been noted in any of the first 40 recipients prophylactically administered 10 to 20 mg per day of these anti-interleukin-2 receptor antibodies for 10 days.

Of potentially even more interest, however, is the successful fusion of the human interleukin-2 gene with a gene encoding a truncated diphtheria toxin related protein and the subsequent expression of a novel interleukin-2 toxin chimeric protein. The truncated diphtheria toxin related protein potently inhibits protein synthesis but on its own is incapable of binding to mammalian cells. Interleukin-2, on the other hand, undergoes receptor mediated endocytosis following interaction with its receptor, and thus interleukin-2 both delivers and restricts the chimera to its intended site of activity within the cytosol of the activated lymphocyte. This chimera effectively destroys activated T lymphocytes and interleukin-2 receptor bearing tumor lines in vitro while sparing resting T cells and interleukin-2 receptor negative tumor lines. It has also abrogated, in delayed type hypersensitivity in vivo, a T cell mediated immune reaction, similar in many ways to rejection. The potential value of these two anti-interleukin-2 receptor directed therapies to transplantation is of immense interest to our unit.

SUGGESTED READING

Leichtman AB, Goldszer RC, Strom TB, Tilney NL. Acute renal failure associated with renal transplantation. In: Brenner BM, Lazarus JM, eds. Acute renal failure. Philadelphia: WB Saunders, 1987.
Morris PJ, ed. Kidney transplantation. London: Grune & Stratton, 1984.
Opelz G. Correlation of HLA matching with kidney graft survival in patients with or without cyclosporin treatment. Transplantation 1985; 40:240–243.
Ortho Multicenter Transplant Study Group. A randomized clinical trial of OKT3 monoclonal antibody for acute rejection of cadaveric renal transplants. N Engl J Med 1985; 313:337–342.

Strom TB: Toward more selective therapies to block graft rejection. AKF Nephrol Letter 1987; 4:13.

Taube DH, Williams DG, Hartley B, Rudge CJ, Neild GH, Cameron JS, Ogg CS, Welsh KI. Differentiation between allograft rejection and cyclosporine nephrotoxicity in renal-transplant recipients. Lancet 1985; 2:172–174.

ACQUIRED IMMUNO-DEFICIENCY SYNDROME

ROBERT WALKER, M.D.
H. CLIFFORD LANE, M.D.
ANTHONY S. FAUCI, M.D.

EPIDEMIOLOGY AND INCIDENCE

The acquired immunodeficiency syndrome (AIDS) was first described as a new disease in 1981. The syndrome consists of the occurrence of life threatening opportunistic infections or unusual neoplasms or both in previously healthy individuals. The majority of cases occur in homosexual or bisexual men (73 percent), intravenous drug abusers (16 percent), individuals in both groups (8 percent), hemophiliacs (1 percent), and the heterosexual partners of affected individuals (4 percent). In 1983 the virus responsible for causing AIDS was first isolated, and is now called human immunodeficiency virus (HIV; formerly lymphadenopathy associated virus [LAV] or human T cell lymphotropic virus, type 3 [HTLV-III]). HIV belongs to a family of RNA viruses called retroviruses and contains the RNA dependent DNA polymerase, reverse transcriptase. This virus is responsible for the progressive destruction of the T4 lymphocyte population, a critical component of the immune system with important regulatory functions. The destruction of this T cell subset leads in time to an immunodeficiency state clinically characterized by the occurrence of unusual infections and cancers.

In addition to AIDS a variety of conditions are currently recognized in individuals infected with HIV. The Centers for Disease Control has recently reclassified the spectrum of HIV infection into four groups (Table 1). Group I consists of patients in the stage of acute HIV infection, which has been characterized as resembling infectious mononucleosis with fever, skin rash, and arthralgias. In group II are individuals who are asymptomatic and otherwise healthy but test positive for the antibody to HIV by enzyme linked immuno-absorbent assay (ELISA) and Western blot assay of serum. Long term follow-up studies indicate that 20 to 40 percent of asymptomatic seropositive individuals may go on to develop AIDS over a 6 year period. In group III are individuals who have persistent generalized lymphadenopathy, defined as two or more extrainguinal sites of lymphadenopathy present for more than 3 months. These people are very similar to the group II patients prognostically and immunologically. In group IV are the more severely ill HIV positive individuals, groups IVc and IVd constituting the classic definition of AIDS.

As of January 1988, over 50,000 cases of AIDS in the United States had been reported to the Centers for Disease Control. Current estimates are that between 1 and 2 million people in the United States are infected with HIV.

OPPORTUNISTIC INFECTIONS

Opportunistic infections that have been reported to occur in patients with AIDS are listed in Table 2. The most common nonviral opportunistic infection in AIDS is *Pneumocystis carinii* pneumonia (PCP), seen in approximately 60 percent of the patients. Although the most common presentation in this illness is fever, cough, shortness of breath, and abnormal chest x-ray findings, patients may present with an indolent picture with fever as the only manifestation. In the setting of fever of unknown origin, gallium scanning may be helpful in identifying the lung as the site of inflammation. Bronchoscopy with bronchoalveolar lavage and biopsy is usually adequate to establish a diagnosis of PCP, yielding positive results in over 90 percent of the cases.

TABLE 1 CDC Classification Scheme for HIV Infection

Group I	Acute infection
Group II	Asymptomatic infection
Group III	Persistent generalized lymphadenopathy
Group IV	Other disease
Subgroup A	Constitutional disease
Subgroup B	Neurologic disease
Subgroup C	Secondary infectious diseases
Category C1	Specified secondary infectious diseases listed in CDC surveillance definition for AIDS
Category C2	Other specified secondary infectious diseases
Subgroup D	Secondary cancers
Subgroup E	Other conditions

TABLE 2 Typical Infections in Patients with AIDS

Pneumocystis carinii pneumonia

Disseminated *Mycobacterium avium* complex

Cryptococcus neoformans meningitis

Disseminated *Mycobacterium tuberculosis*

Candida albicans esophagitis and thrush

Disseminated cytomegalovirus infection

Progressive herpes simplex virus infection (particularly perianal)

Toxoplasma gondii infection (particularly central nervous system)

Cryptosporidia enteritis

Salmonella typhimurium bacteremia

Sputum examination for pneumocysts by an experienced examiner may establish the diagnosis in some cases, thereby avoiding the need for an invasive procedure. However, this test is not uniformly reliable, and a negative result does not rule out the diagnosis.

The treatment of PCP consists of either trimethoprim-sulfamethoxazole (20 mg per kg per day of trimethoprim and 100 mg per kg per day of sulfamethoxazole) divided into four oral or intravenous doses per day, or pentamidine isethionate (4 mg per kg per day) as a single daily intravenous dose. Although the recommended duration of therapy for this disease is 14 to 21 days, we have often found this to be inadequate in the treatment of patients with AIDS. Accordingly we repeat the bronchoalveolar lavage in our patients after 21 days of therapy if clinically indicated to look for persistent organisms. If organisms are present, the patient undergoes an additional 2 to 3 weeks of therapy followed by repeat lavage and continued therapy, if organisms remain and symptoms persist. Current research efforts are directed at examining the value of the aerosolized administration of pentamidine and other therapeutic drugs, including dapsone and the dihydrofolate reductase inhibitor trimetrexate in the treatment of PCP.

A striking feature of trimethoprim-sulfamethoxazole therapy in this patient group has been an extraordinarily high incidence of adverse drug reactions, predominantly hypersensitivity and skin rashes (30 percent) or leukopenia (30 percent). These reactions have been noted in patients taking both therapeutic and prophylactic doses of the drug. Accordingly we do not routinely use trimethoprim-sulfamethoxazole prophylaxis, reserving that therapy for acute infection. Recent anecdotes have advocated the use of aerosolized pentamidine as a prophylactic measure; its efficacy is currently under study.

The herpesvirus family gives rise to several clinical problems in patients with AIDS. Herpes simplex may cause severe erosive mucocutaneous disease in either oral or anal regions and cutaneous lesions, especially of the digits in the form of herpetic whitlow. These are usually responsive to intravenous treatment with acyclovir (5 mg per kg every 8 hours for 7 days). Although the disease is apt to recur following the cessation of therapy, oral doses of acyclovir may help to prevent relapses. Herpes zoster infection may present as either dermatomal or disseminated disease. In contrast to the situation with herpes simplex, the efficacy of acyclovir in herpes zoster is unclear. We currently reserve it for the patient with widespread cutaneous or disseminated disease and use a high dose intravenous regimen (5 mg per kg every 4 hours).

The third member of the herpesvirus family, cytomegalovirus, is a common isolate from the blood, urine, and sputum of patients with AIDS. In addition to causing a necrotizing retinitis leading to progressive irreversible blindness, cytomegalovirus may cause pneumonitis, esophagitis, and colitis. At autopsy patients are often noted to have diffuse organ involvement with cytomegalovirus, and this virus may be one of the leading causes of death in AIDS. Dihydroxypropoxymethylguanine (5 mg per kg twice daily for 2 to 3 weeks), an experimental drug that is structurally similar to acyclovir, may have a temporizing effect on organ dysfunction due to cytomegalovirus; however, long term maintenance therapy (6 mg per kg per day, 5 days of the week) is required to reduce the incidence of relapses.

Fungal infections play a prominent role in patients with AIDS. The two most common fungal infections are oral or esophageal candidiasis and cryptococcal meningitis. Oral candidiasis usually can be managed with either oral nystatin therapy (500,000 units every 4 hours), clotrimazole lozenges (one troche every 4 hours), or oral ketoconazole therapy (100 to 200 mg every 12 hours). Candida esophagitis may also be treated with oral doses of ketoconazole (200 mg every 12 hours for 14 days). Because Candida esophagitis can cause life threatening complications, such as perforations and hemorrhage, some prefer to treat it with low dosage amphotericin B therapy (0.3 mg per kg per day intravenously for 7 to 10 days). Cryptococcal infection may present as disseminated disease or may be confined to the central nervous system. We generally treat these patients with amphotericin B (0.6 mg per kg per day intravenously for 6 weeks). In the patient who has difficulty tolerating this dosage of amphotericin, flucytosine (125 mg per kg per day orally) may be added to the regimen and the dosage of amphotericin cut in half. In patients with cryptococcal disease the response to therapy is usually poor, relapses being common.

Mycobacterium avium-intracellulare is a common environmental contaminant that has been known rarely to cause invasive lung disease in immunocompromised patients. For reasons that are not understood, this atypical Mycobacterium commonly causes a disseminated infection in patients with AIDS and may be isolated from bone marrow, liver, lung, spleen, and blood. Investigational compounds such as ansamycin and clofazamine often show good in vitro activity against *Mycobacterium avium-intracellulare* infection, but their safety or efficacy in chemotherapeutic regimens has not been established. At the present time no successful therapy exists for infections caused by this organism.

Toxoplasmosis most commonly presents in patients with AIDS as a cerebral mass lesion or as an encephalitic syndrome. Serologic testing may not be useful for diagnosis owing to the inability of most patients with AIDS to mount a de novo serologic response following antigenic exposure. Thus, the diagnosis depends upon demonstration of the tachyzoite in tissue sections or a high index of suspicion based on the clinical setting. Therapy consists of sulfadiazine (1 g orally every 6 hours) and pyrimethamine (a 75 mg loading dose followed by 25 mg every 24 hours orally). These drugs have been effective in limiting the progression of toxoplasmosis in some but not all patients with AIDS. Since these drugs are static and not cidal agents, therapy probably should be continued indefinitely. Unfortunately bone marrow toxicity usually limits the continuous long term use of these drugs.

A syndrome of diarrhea and wasting has been described in patients with AIDS. Occasionally routine pathogens (*Giardia lamblia, Entamoeba histolytica,* Shigella, and Salmonella species) are isolated from the stool and infections can be treated. More commonly no pathogen is isolated and the treatment becomes symptomatic. Tincture of opium, diphenoxylate, and cholestyramine have been tried with varying degrees of success. Cryptosporidiosis, an animal protozoan disease that on rare occasion has caused self-limiting diarrhea in healthy humans with animal exposure, has been reported as one cause of severe diarrhea in patients with AIDS. No effective therapy exists for infection by this organism.

NEOPLASTIC DISEASES

The two neoplastic diseases reported to occur in patients with AIDS are Kaposi's sarcoma and non-Hodgkin's lymphoma. Kaposi's sarcoma is a malignant neoplasm manifested primarily by multiple vascular nodules in the skin and other organs. The disease is multifocal, with courses ranging from indolent, with only skin manifestations, to fulminant, with extensive visceral involvement. At present approximately 10 percent of all patients with AIDS develop Kaposi's sarcoma. There is no universally accepted therapy for Kaposi's sarcoma in patients with AIDS. Single agent or combination chemotherapy has been successful in reducing the tumor burden in certain patients. Unfortunately these drugs do nothing for the underlying HIV infection or immune defect, which presumably predisposes the patients to develop the neoplasm. Furthermore, courses of chemotherapy may be complicated by opportunistic infections. Radiation, both gamma and electron beam, has also been an effective form of palliative therapy for both

cutaneous and visceral disease. It should be mentioned that patients with AIDS have been noted to have a high incidence of side effects, such as radiation mucositis, following standard treatment regimens. Trials of innovative therapeutic agents are currently under way in these patients. The use of alpha interferon has been successful in inducing complete remissions in at least 10 percent and partial remissions in 20 to 40 percent of AIDS patients with Kaposi's sarcoma, particularly those with high T4 counts (over 300 per cubic millimeter). In some patients this has been accompanied by improvement in immune function and decreased viremia. Further studies are needed before this drug can be recommended as standard therapy for this disease.

An increased incidence of lymphoma, especially central nervous system lymphoma, has been noted in this patient group. These tumors are almost always resistant to conventional and modified chemotherapeutic regimens. Therapy for this entity, as well as therapy for Kaposi's sarcoma, is best given in consultation with an oncologist.

ANTIVIRAL THERAPY

A number of drugs have been shown to have in vitro activity against HIV, and many of these are currently being tested in clinical trials. To date, only 3'-azido-3'-deoxythymidine (AZT, Retrovir, or Zidovudine), a dideoxynucleoside, has been shown to benefit certain patients with AIDS and AIDS related complex (ARC) in controlled clinical studies. AZT is believed to inhibit viral replication by acting as a chain terminator in the DNA synthesis involved in reverse transcription.

In a phase II trial AZT was shown to prolong survival (compared to placebo) in patients with AIDS who previously had recovered from an episode of PCP. Additionally AZT prolonged survival in patients with late stage ARC. However, AZT did not cure these patients of the HIV infection nor did it result in sustained improvement in immune function as measured by T4 counts. In early 1987 the Food and Drug Administration licensed AZT for the treatment of patients with AIDS who had recovered from PCP and for HIV-infected patients with systemic symptoms and T4 counts less than 200 cells per cubic millimeter (dosage: 200 mg orally every 4 hours).

AZT is generally well tolerated; however, it does have the potential for causing significant toxicity. Bone marrow suppression, usually anemia or granulocytopenia, occurs in at least 20 percent of the patients and may require either interruption of therapy or dose modification. In our experience a drop in the hemoglobin level to values less than 10 g per dl occurred at an average of 6 weeks after starting AZT but may be seen as early as 3 weeks. Keeping in mind that complications of iron overload may occur after approximately 100 units of blood, we attempt to maintain our patients' hemoglobin levels above 10 g per dl and accept a transfusion requirement of 2 units of packed red cells every 28 days. If a patient exceeds this level, we reduce the dosage of AZT to 100 mg every 4 hours and expect a reduction in the transfusion requirement approximately 6 weeks later. A further dosage reduction to 50 mg every 4 hours may decrease transfusion dependence in patients who remain severely anemic with the 100 mg dosage.

Many patients receiving AZT develop a peripheral macrocytosis with a mean corpuscular volume in excess of 115 cubic microns. Although it is important to exclude vitamin B_{12} and folate deficiencies, AZT may be the only explanation for this finding. Generally patients demonstrating macrocytosis do not develop transfusion-requiring anemia, while patients with only minor changes in the mean corpuscular volume have a greater likelihood of becoming transfusion dependent. We have examined bone marrow specimens in a number of patients taking AZT who have required transfusions, and each specimen revealed pure red cell aplasia or hypoplasia.

Granulocytopenia occurs less frequently than anemia and usually reverses more rapidly once AZT therapy is stopped or the dosage is reduced. If the total neutrophil count (polymorphonuclear leukocytes plus band forms) falls below 750 cells per cubic millimeter, we reduce the AZT dosage by half. If the total neutrophil count falls below 500 cells per cubic millimeter, we discontinue AZT, wait until the total neutrophil count exceeds 1000 cells per cu mm, and then resume AZT therapy at half the previous dosage.

Because of the potential for hematologic toxicity, patients starting AZT therapy should have routine complete blood counts with differential counts performed weekly for at least 6 weeks and, if stable, every 2 weeks thereafter. For a patient manifesting granulocytopenia, this test should be carried out even more often so that profound neutropenia is detected early.

Other side effects of AZT include mild headaches, nausea, dyspepsia, and dysgeusia. These are usually so mild as not to require treatment or dosage modification and generally subside after the first few weeks of therapy.

Although no other antiviral drugs for the treatment of HIV infection have been proven to be effective, numerous clinical trials are in progress with a variety of single drug and combination regimens. Two other dideoxynucleosides, 2', 3'-dideoxyadenosine and 2', 3'-dideoxycytidine, as well as other drugs, including alpha interferon, ribavirin, foscarnet, and HPA-23, are being evaluated. Other strategies employing the coadministration of two antiviral drugs, such as AZT and acyclovir, or employing the sequential administration of multiple antiviral drugs akin to cancer chemotherapy, will be the focus of future studies.

Major efforts are under way to prevent and treat HIV infection. Although AZT represents an important advance, future therapies will need to address both the immune defects and retroviral infection in order to prevent the inexorable complications seen in AIDS patients and other HIV infected individuals.

SUGGESTED READING

DeVita VT Jr, Broder S, Fauci AS, Kovacs JS, Chabner BA. Developmental therapeutics and the acquired immunodeficiency syndrome. Ann Intern Med 1987; 106:568–581.

Fauci AS, Masur H, Gelmann EP, Markham PD, Hahn BH, Lane HC. The acquired immunodeficiency syndrome: an update. Ann Intern Med 1985; 102:800–813.

Fischl MA, Rickmare DD, Greco MH, et al. The efficacy of azidothymidine in the treatment of patients with AIDS and AIDS related complex: a double-blind, placebo controlled trial. N Eng J Med 1987; 317:185–191.

Gallo RC. The AIDS virus. Sci Am 1987; 256:47–56.

Kovacs JS, Masur H. Opportunistic infections. In: Gallin JI, Fauci AS, eds. Advances in host defense mechanisms: Volume 5. Acquired immunodeficiency syndrome. New York: Raven Press, 1985:35.

Lane HC, Fauci AS. Immunologic abnormalities in the acquired immunodeficiency syndrome. Ann Rev Immunol 1985; 3:477–500.

A

Acetylcholine receptors, in myasthenia gravis, 231
Acquired immunodeficiency syndrome, 331, 343–346
  antiviral therapy, 345–346
  epidemiology, 343
  incidence, 343
  neoplastic disease with, 345
  opportunistic infections with, 343–345
Acute interstitial nephritis, 198
  biopsy in, 199
  corticosteroids in, 199–201
  drug induced, 198–199
  hypersensitivity triad in, 198–199
Acyclovir, 191, 346
  in aplastic anemia, 291
Additives, in drug reactions, 78–79
Adrenergic agents
  aerosol solutions, 32
  in asthma, 23, 27–28
  in childhood asthma, 32–36
  in exercise-induced asthma, 40
  in status asthmaticus, 45–46, 47
Adrenocorticotropic hormone (ACTH)
  in multiple sclerosis, 228–229
  stimulation test, 327
Agammaglobulinemia, 308, 310–311
  immunoglobulin therapy, 309
Air pollution, 48–52
Airway obstruction
  with anaphylaxis, 95–96
  with drug reactions, 80
Allergic disease, universal reactor, 51
Allergic rhinitis, 1–5
  avoidance in, 2
  classification, 1
  immunotherapy, 5
  pharmacotherapy, 2–5
  sprays/washes in, 4
  therapy, 1–5
Allergic rhinitis (perennial), 8–21
  airborne allergen control, 13
  avoidance in, 12–13, 15–16
  desensitization in, 11–12
  drug therapy, 9–12, 16–19
  immunotherapy, 19
  noninhaled allergens, 13
  patient assessment, 14–15
  saline solutions in, 17
  surgery in, 19–20
5-Aminosalicylic acid, in ulcerative colitis/ Crohn's disease, 243–244
Amphotericin B, in chronic mucocutaneous candidiasis, 332–333
Amyloidosis, 316–321
  AA (secondary), 317, 318, 320, 321
  AF (hereditary), 317, 321
  AH (hemodialysis), 317, 318, 321

AL (primary), 317, 318, 320, 321
  classification, 317–318
  colchicine in, 318, 320, 321
  diagnosis, 317–318
  melphalan in, 318
  prednisone in, 318
  SAA (serum amyloid A), 317
  treatment, 318–321
Anaphylactoid reaction, 98–99
Anaphylaxis, 91–98
  airway obstruction with, 95–96
  angioedema with, 97
  antihistamines in, 97
  avoidance of, 97
  biphasic, 96–97
  cardiac function with, 95
  cholinergic, 100
  classification, 91–92
  clinical manifestations, 92, 98
  cricothyrotomy in, 96
  cryptogenic, 98–100
  death from, 92–93
  desensitization with, 97–98
  diagnosis, 93
  differential diagnosis, 98–99
  with drug reactions, 78, 79, 80
  emergency treatment, 99–100
  endocrine factor, 99
  epinephrine in, 94–95
  exercise induced, 41, 99–100
  in food sensitivity, 57
  hypotension with, 95
  with insect sting sensitivity, 82–83, 87, 88
  management, 93–97
  nonimmunological risk factors, 93
  patient assessment, 93–94
  with penicillin sensitivity, 69
  pulmonary function in, 96
  recurrent, 99
  recurrent idiopathic, 98–100
  theophylline in, 96
  treatment, 79
  urticaria with, 97
Androgen therapy
  in aplastic anemia, 290–291
  in hereditary angioedema, 67–68
Anemia. See Aplastic anemia; Autoimmune hemolytic anemia
Angioedema
  acute attack therapy, 66–67
  with anaphylaxis, 97
  androgen therapy, 67–68
  C1 INH in, 66–68
  maintenance therapy, 67–68
  prophylactic therapy, 67
  vibratory, 65
Angiotensin converting enzyme inhibitors, in nephrotic syndrome, 194–195
Animal exposure allergy, 5–7, 12

clinical manifestations, 6
  diagnosis, 6
  immunotherapy, 7
  pathophysiology, 6
  treatment, 6–7
Ankylosing spondylitis, 130–135
  corticosteroids in, 134
  diagnosis, 130–131
  drug management, 132–134
  extra-articular disease, 134
  genetic factor, 131
  immunosuppressive agents in, 134
  irradiation in, 134
  nonsteroidal anti-inflammatory agents in, 132–133
  patient education, 134
  physical measures, 132
  surgery for, 134
  therapy, 131–134
  therapy side effects, 133–134
Antibiotics
  in common variable immunodeficiency, 303
  in perennial allergic rhinitis, 18–19
  in phagocyte function disorders, 296–297, 299–300
  in rheumatic fever prevention, 258–260
  in ulcerative colitis/Crohn's disease, 245
Antibody deficiency disorders, 308–311
  immunoglobulin therapy, 308–310
  infection management, 310–311
Anticholinergics, in asthma, 24
Antidiarrheals, in ulcerative colitis/Crohn's disease, 245
Antierythrocyte antibodies, 280
Antifungals
  in allergic bronchopulmonary aspergillosis, 221
  in phagocyte function disorders, 297
Antiglobulin consumption test, 285
Anti-glomerular basement membrane antibody, 209–212
Antihistamines
  in allergic rhinitis, 2
  in anaphylaxis, 97
  in atopic dermatitis, 181
  in contact dermatitis, 185
  in cutaneous vasculitis, 156–157
  in perennial allergic rhinitis, 9, 16–17
  in urticaria, 60–61, 62–65
Anti-inflammatory agents, in rheumatoid arthritis, 108–109
Antimalarials, in systemic lupus erythematosus, 104
Antimitochondrial antibody test, in primary biliary cirrhosis, 254
Antirheumatic therapy, 260–261
Antispasmodics, in ulcerative colitis/Crohn's disease, 245
Antistreptococcal vaccine, in acute

rheumatic fever, 262
Anti-TAC, 342
Antithymocyte globulin, in aplastic
  anemia, 291
Aortitis, with Cogan's syndrome, 171–172
Aplastic anemia, 289–292
  acyclovir in, 291
  androgen therapy, 290–291
  antithymocyte globulin in, 291
  blood product support, 289–290
  bone marrow transplantation, 291–292
  corticosteroids in, 291
  cyclosporin A in, 291
  etiology, 289
  immunosuppression in, 291
  infection management, 290
  lithium in, 291
  recombinant hematopoietic growth
    factors, 291
  therapeutic options, 290–292
Aquagenic urticaria, 65
Arteriography, in Takayasu's arteritis,
  161–162
Arteritis, in Behçet's syndrome, 168
Aspergillosis. *See* Bronchopulmonary
  aspergillosis
Aspergillus fumigatus, 220
Aspirin
  in pericarditis, 269–270
  in postcardiac injury syndrome,
    264–265
Aspirin sensitivity
  with asthma and rhinosinusitus, 36–39
  corticosteroids in, 37–38
  cross reactions, 37
  emergency management, 37
  treatment, 37–39
Asthma, 21–25
  atopy/atopic state in, 21
  avoidance in, 22–23
  food induced, 22
  immunotherapy in, 25
  mast cell stabilizers in, 24
  occupational, 22
  pharmacotherapy, 23–25
  with rhinosinusitus in aspirin sensitivity,
    36–39
Asthma (adult), 25–31
  acute mild, 26–27
  acute moderate, 27
  acute severe, 27
  chronic mild, 25–26
  chronic moderate, 26
  chronic severe, 26
  complications, 27–29
  patient support, 29, 31
  pharmacotherapy, 26–29
  in pregnancy, 28–29
Asthma (childhood), 31–36
  acute attacks, 31–33
  adrenergic agonists in, 32–36
  allergy management, 34
  bronchodilators in, 32–36
  corticosteroids in, 33, 36
  home treatment, 36
  hospitalization for, 32–33
  respiratory failure with, 33
  sinusitis with, 34
  status asthmaticus, 32–33
Asthma (exercise-induced), 39–41
  adrenergic agents in, 40
  cromolyn in, 40
Asthma (sulfite induced), 42–44
  attack prevention, 43–44

reaction treatment, 44
Ataxia-telangiectasia, 312
Atopic dermatitis, 177–182
  acute flares management, 178–180
  allergy management, 181–182
  antihistamines in, 181
  corticosteroids in, 178–180, 181
  ketoconazole in, 181
  maintenance therapy, 180–181
  management principles, 177–178
  pathophysiology, 177–178
  phototherapy, 181
  psychological support, 182
  systemic therapy, 181
Autoimmune hemolytic anemia, 280–284
  cephalothin induced, 282
  danazol in, 284
  drug induced, 281–282
  gamma globulin in, 284
  glucocorticoids in, 282
  hapten type, 281
  IgG antibodies in, 281
  IgM antibodies in, 280–281
  immunosuppressive agents in, 283–284
  α-methyldopa type, 281–282
  penicillin induced, 281
  plasmapheresis in, 284
  quinidine induced, 281
  splenectomy in, 283
  therapy, 282–284
  transfusion therapy, 284
Autoimmune leukopenia, 285–288
  functional assays, 286
  immunochemical assay, 285–286
  neutrophil antibody testing, 285
  patient evaluation, 286
Autoimmune neutropenia, 285
  acute, 286–287
  chronic, 287
  corticosteroids in, 287–288
  gamma globulin in, 288
  in infants, 288
Azathioprine, 345–346
  in autoimmune uveitis, 237
  in bullous pemphigoid, 189–190
  in chronic active hepatitis, 252, 253
  in dermatomyositis-polymyositis, 143
  in Goodpasture's syndrome, 210–211
  in idiopathic thrombocytopenic
    purpura, 279
  in lupus nephritis, 207
  in multiple sclerosis, 229
  in myasthenia gravis, 234
  in myocarditis, 273
  in pemphigus vulgaris, 187–188
  in postcardiac injury syndrome, 267
  in primary biliary cirrhosis, 256–257
  in rheumatoid arthritis, 112
  in systemic vasculitis, 152
  in Takayasu's arteritis, 164
  in temporal arteritis, 160
  in ulcerative colitis/Crohn's disease, 245

B

Bacterial endocarditis, glomerulonephritis
  and, 337
Beclomethasone dipropionate, in allergic
  rhinits, 4, 11, 18
Behçet's syndrome, 165–170
  central nervous system involvement,
    167–168
  chlorambucil in, 167–169, 170
  clinical features, 165–166

colchicine in, 166–167
corticosteroids in, 166, 167–169
cutaneous vasculitis with, 167
cyclophosphamide in, 168
cyclosporine in, 169–170
dapsone in, 166
gastrointestinal involvement, 168
immunosuppressive therapy, 168–169
indomethacin in, 167
joint involvement, 167
levamisole in, 166
mucocutaneous involvement, 166–167
phlebitis/arteritis in, 168
prednisone in, 168
thalidomide in, 166
therapeutic approach, 166–170
treatment evaluation, 170
uveitis with, 167
Berger's disease, 197–198, 334–336
Beta-lactam antibiotic sensitivity, 68–76
Biliary cirrhosis (primary), 254–258
  clinical/laboratory features, 254
  colchicine in, 257
  complications management, 255–256
  diagnosis, 255
  immunosuppressive therapy in, 256–257
  liver biopsy in, 255
  liver transplantation in, 257–258
  penicillamine in, 257
  prognosis, 255
  staging, 255
Bone marrow transplantation
  in aplastic anemia, 291–292
  in severe combined immunodeficiency
    disease, 305–306, 311
Bronchodilators
  in childhood asthma, 32–36
  in status asthmaticus, 45–46, 47
Bronchopulmonary aspergillosis (allergic),
  220–222
  allergen immunotherapy in, 222
  corticosteroids in, 221–222
  with cystic fibrosis, 222
  serum immunoglobulins in, 220–222
Building materials, in chemical sensitivity,
  49–50
Bullous pemphigoid, 189–190
  corticosteroids in, 189–190
  immunosuppressive agents in, 189–190

C

C3b receptors, 281
Caldwell-Luc procedure, 20
Candida albicans, 331
Candidiasis. *See* Chronic mucocutaneous
  candidiasis
Captopril
  in pemphigus induction, 188
  in Takayasu's arteritis, 165
Cardiac function
  with anaphylaxis, 95
  with drug reactions, 80–81
  in mixed connective tissue disease,
    147–148
  with Reiter's syndrome, 122
  in scleroderma, 138
Cardiac injury. *See* Postcardiac injury
  syndrome
Cardiac tamponade, with pericarditis,
  71–72
Central nervous system
  with Behçet's syndrome, 167–168
  in Sjögren's syndrome, 129

Cephalosporin sensitivity, 72–73
 desensitization in, 73–75
 penicillin cross-sensitivity, 72–73
Cephalothin, in autoimmune hemolytic
 anemia, 282
Chemical sensitivity, 48–52
 body load factor, 50–51
 chemical challenge in, 50
 emotional factor, 51
 olfaction in, 51–52
 protocol approach, 50
 sensory tolerance and, 52
 universal reactor, 51
Children
 asthma in, 31–36
 food sensitivity, 52–56
Chlorambucil
 in autoimmune hemolytic anemia, 284
 in autoimmune uveitis, 238
 in Behçet's syndrome, 167, 168–169,
  170
 in glomerular disease, 196
 in primary biliary cirrhosis, 257
 in sarcoidosis, 227
 in systemic vasculitis, 152
Cholinergic urticaria, 63
Chronic mucocutaneous candidiasis,
 331–334
 amphotericin B in, 332–333
 clotrimazole in, 333
 immunologic therapy, 333
 ketoconazole in, 315, 316, 331, 332
 systemic therapy, 331–333
 topical therapy, 333
 treatment, 331–333
Cimetidine hydrochloride, 61
C1 INH, 66–68
Clotrimazole, in chronic mucocutaneous
 candidiasis, 333
Cogan's syndrome, 170–173
 aortitis/vasculitis in, 171–172
 corticosteroids in, 171–172
 cyclophosphamide in, 172
 drug side effects, 172
 with interstitial keratitis, 171
 therapeutic approach, 171–172
 vestibuloauditory dysfunction in, 171
Colchicine
 in amyloidosis, 318, 320, 321
 in Behçet's syndrome, 166–167
 in primary biliary cirrhosis, 257
Cold hemagglutin disease, 280–281
Cold urticaria, 63–64
Common variable immunodeficiency,
 301–305
 adverse effects of gamma globulin
  therapy, 304
 anti-IgA antibodies in, 304
 antimicrobials in, 303
 immune serum globulin in, 301–304
 intravenous immune globulin in, 302,
  304
 normal human plasma in, 302
Coombs' test, 281, 282
Complement C1 INH, 66–68
Congenital immunodeficiency diseases,
 308–313
Conjunctiva
 in erythema multiforme, 241
 ocular pemphigoid, 241
Conjunctivitis (allergic)
 drug induced, 239
 giant papillary, 239
 with hay fever, 240

vernal keratoconjunctivitis, 239–240
Connective tissue. See Mixed connective
 tissue disease
Constrictive pericarditis, with postcardiac
 injury syndrome, 268
Contact dermatitis, 182–186
 antihistamines in, 185
 corticosteroids in, 184–185
 cream bases in, 183
 physical agents in, 186
 topical therapy, 184–186
 water avoidance, 183–184
 water role in, 182–184
 wet dressings/soaks, 183
Cornea, herpes simplex infections, 241
Corneal graft rejection, 241–242
Corneal infiltrates
 inferior peripheral, 240–241
 melting with, 241
Corticosteroids. See also specific
  compounds
 acute interstitial nephritis, 199–201
 in acute rheumatic fever, 260–261
 in allergic bronchopulmonary
  aspergillosis, 221–222
 in allergic rhinitis, 4
 in anaphylaxis, 96–97
 in ankylosing spondylitis, 134
 in aplastic anemia, 291
 in aspirin sensitivity, 37–38
 in asthma, 24, 28–29
 in atopic dermatitis, 178–180, 181
 in autoimmune neutropenia, 287–288
 in autoimmune uveitis, 235–237
 in Behçet's syndrome, 166–169
 in bullous pemphigoid, 189–190
 in childhood asthma, 33, 36
 in chronic active hepatitis, 251–252, 253
 in Cogan's syndrome, 171, 172
 in contact dermatitis, 184–185
 in dermatomyositis-polymyositis, 140,
  141–142
 in erythema multiforme, 191
 in glomerular disease, 196–197
 in Goodpasture's syndrome, 210–211
 in herpes gestationis, 176–177
 in hypersensitivity pneumonitis,
  213–214
 in idiopathic pulmonary fibrosis, 218
 in idiopathic thrombocytopenic purpura,
  276–280
 in lupus nephritis, 206
 in mixed connective tissue disease, 148
 in multiple sclerosis, 228–229
 in myasthenia gravis, 233–234
 in myocarditis, 273
 in pemphigus vulgaris, 187
 in perennial allergic rhinitis, 11, 17–18
 in pericarditis, 271
 in postcardiac injury syndrome, 266,
  267
 in primary biliary cirrhosis, 256
 in Reiter's syndrome, 124
 in renal transplant rejection, 203
 in rheumatoid arthritis, 119
 in sarcoidosis, 223–227
 side effects, 172
 in status asthmaticus, 46
 in systemic lupus erythematosus,
  103–104
 in systemic vasculitis, 150–154
 in Takayasu's arteritis, 162–164
 in temporal arteritis, 157–160
 in ulcerative colitis/Crohn's disease,

244–245
CREST syndrome, 135, 136
Cricothyrotomy, in anaphylaxis, 96
Crohn's disease, 242–251
 drug therapy, 243–246, 249
 extragastrointestinal disorders with, 250
 fistula formation in, 249–250
 intestinal obstruction with, 248–249
 management, 248–250
 nutritional management, 243, 249
 patient education, 243
 perianal disease in, 249–250
 pregnancy with, 250
 surgery in, 249
Cromolyn sodium
 in allergic rhinitis, 4
 in asthma, 24
 in exercise-induced asthma, 40
 in perennial allergic rhinitis, 10–12, 17
Cutaneous disorders
 with mixed connective tissue disease,
  146
 in scleroderma, 136
Cutaneous necrotizing venulitis, 155–156
Cutaneous sicca, with Sjögren's syndrome,
 127
Cyclo-oxygenase inhibitors, 37
Cyclophosphamide
 in autoimmune hemolytic anemia,
  283–284
 in autoimmune uveitis, 238
 in Behçet's syndrome, 168
 in bullous pemphigoid, 189–190
 in Cogan's syndrome, 172
 in dermatomyositis-polymyositis,
  143–144
 in glomerular disease, 196
 in Goodpasture's syndrome, 210–211
 in idiopathic pulmonary fibrosis, 218
 in idiopathic thrombocytopenic purpura,
  279
 in lupus nephritis, 207
 in multiple sclerosis, 229–230
 in myocarditis, 273
 in pemphigus vulgaris, 187–188
 in postcardiac injury syndrome, 267–268
 in rheumatoid arthritis, 112
 in sarcoidosis, 227
 side effects, 172
 in systemic vasculitis, 150–154
 in Takayasu's arteritis, 164
 in temporal arteritis, 160–161
Cyclosporine
 in autoimmune uveitis, 238
 in Behçet's syndrome, 169–170
Cyclosporin A
 in aplastic anemia, 291
 in dermatomyositis-polymyositis, 144
 in rheumatoid arthritis, 113
 side effects, 172
 in systemic vasculitis, 153
 in temporal arteritis, 161
Cystic fibrosis, allergic bronchopulmonary
 aspergillosis in, 222
Cytomel, 325
Cytotoxic agents
 in dermatomyositis-polymyositis,
  142–144
 in myocarditis, 273–274
 in Reiter's syndrome, 124
 in rheumatoid arthritis, 111–112
 in systemic vasculitis, 152
 in Takayasu's arteritis, 164
 in temporal arteritis, 160–161

D

Danazol
  in autoimmune hemolytic anemia, 284
  in idiopathic thrombocytopenic purpura,
    278–279
Dapsone
  in Behçet's syndrome, 166
  in dermatitis herpetiformis, 173–175
  in pregnancy, 175
Deafness, with Cogan's syndrome, 171
Decongestants
  in allergic rhinitis, 3–4
  in perennial allergic rhinitis, 9–10,
    16–17
Dermatitis herpetiformis, 173–176
  dapsone therapy, 173–175
  dietary management, 175
  histology, 173
  sulfapyridine in, 175
Dermatomyositis, 140–144
  alternative therapies, 144
  corticosteroids in, 140, 141–142
  cytotoxic agents in, 142–144
  immunosuppressive agents in, 140
  therapy, 140–144
Dermographism, 63
Desensitization
  in anaphylaxis, 97–98
  in beta-lactam antibiotic sensitivity,
    73–75
  in drug reactions, 79
  in insulin allergy, 329
Dialysis, in Goodpasture's syndrome, 211
DiGeorge syndrome, 312
Disodium cromoglycate, in perennial
  allergic rhinitis, 10–11
Downes respiratory scoring system, 33
Dressler's syndrome, 263
Drug reaction, 77–81
  anaphylaxis with, 78, 79, 80
  classification, 79–81
  desensitization in, 79
  diagnosis, 77–78
  to drug additives, 78–79
  glucocorticoids in, 81
  immune mediated classification, 77
  prevention, 77–78
  recurrence prevention, 81
Dust mites, 12

E

Edema, with nephrotic syndrome, 194
ELISA test, 69, 71
  in chemical sensitivity, 51
  in childhood asthma, 34
Emotional factor
  in chemical sensitivity, 51
  in childhood asthma, 34
Endocrine factor, in anaphylaxis, 99
Environmental chemicals, 48–52
Eosinopenia, 285
Epinephrine, in anaphylaxis, 94–95
Episcleritis, 242
Equine ATG, in renal transplant rejection,
  204
Erythema multiforme, 190–192
  continuous, 191
  corticosteroids in, 191
  Herpesvirus hominus infection and, 191
  patient evaluation, 190
  prevention, 191
  therapeutic alternatives, 191

Erythromycin, in rheumatic fever
  prevention, 259
Esophageal stricture, with scleroderma,
  137
Exercise
  anaphylaxis induction, 41, 99–100
  asthma induction, 39–41
Eyelid dermatitis, 239

F

Fc receptors, 281
Felty's syndrome, 288
Flunisolide, in allergic rhinitis, 4, 11, 18
Food sulfite sources, 43
Food sensitivity (adult), 56–59
  anaphylaxis in, 57
  controversies, 58–59
  dietary management, 57
  drug therapy, 57–59
  food animal sources, 59
  food plant sources, 58
  nonimmunologic mechanisms, 56
  therapy, 56–58
Food sensitivity (childhood), 52–56
  diagnosis, 52–54
  evaluation protocol, 53–54
  food challenge in, 53, 54
  treatment, 54–55
Fungi, 12–13

G

Gamma globulin
  in autoimmune hemolytic anemia, 284
  in autoimmune neutropenia, 288
  in idiopathic thrombocytopenic purpura,
    276–277, 279, 280
Gastrointestinal disorders
  in mixed connective tissue disease, 147
  with scleroderma, 137
Genetic factor
  in ankylosing spondylitis, 131
  in hereditary angioedema, 66
  in immunodeficiency disease, 308–312
  in phagocyte function disorders,
    293–294, 300
Glomerular disease
  corticosteroids in, 196–197
  cytotoxic agents in, 196
  minimal change disease, 196
Glomerulonephritis, 196–197
  with bacterial endocarditis, 337
  membranoproliferative, 197
  poststreptococcal, 336–337
Glomerulosclerosis, 196–197
Glucocorticoids. *See also specific agents*
  in autoimmune hemolytic anemia, 282
  in drug reactions, 81
  in insulin resistance, 330
Gluten sensitivity enteropathy, 173, 175
Gold therapy, in rheumatoid arthritis, 110,
  118
Goodpasture's syndrome, 209–212
  diagnosis, 209
  dialysis in, 211
  immunosuppressive agents in, 210–211
  patient monitoring, 211–212
  plasma exchange therapy in, 210–211
  respiratory support in, 211
  therapeutic rationale, 209–210
  treatment, 210–212
Graft versus host disease, 305
Granulocyte-macrophage colony

stimulating factor, 291
Granulocyte transfusion, in phagocyte
  function disorders, 298

H

Hashimoto's thyroiditis, 322–327
  associated diseases, 327
  in children, 326
  drug interaction in, 326
  hypothyroidism with, 322–323
  postpartum thyroiditis with, 325
  pregnancy with, 324–325
  surgery in, 326–327
  therapeutic goals, 326
  thyroid enlargement with, 323–324
  thyroid function tests in, 322
  thyroid lymphoma with, 325
  thyroid medication in, 325–326
  toxicity in, 326
Hashitoxicosis, 324
Heat urticaria, 65
Hematuria, idiopathic, 338
Henoch-Schönlein purpura, 336
Hepatitis (Chronic active), 251–254
  complications, 253
  immunosuppressive therapy, 251–252,
    253
  remission criteria, 252–253
  results, 252–253
  treatment criteria, 251
  treatment regimens, 251–252
Herpes gestationis, 176–177
  corticosteroids in, 176–177
Herpesvirus hominus infection, 191
HLA antigens, in dermatitis herpetiformis,
  173
Hydrocephalus, shunt nephritis with, 337
Hydrochloroquine, in rheumatoid arthritis,
  109, 118–119
Hypercoagulability, in nephrotic
  syndrome, 196
Hyperimmunoglobulin E syndrome,
  313–316
  antibiotic prophylaxis, 314
  associated disorders management,
    314–315
  immunomodulators in, 315–316
  infection management, 313–314
  respiratory tract infection in, 314
  surgical therapy, 313
  therapy complications, 316
Hyperlipidemia, in nephrotic syndrome,
  195–196
Hypersensitivity pneumonitis, 212–214
  corticosteroids in, 213–214
  environmental controls in, 212–213
  therapeutic approach, 212
Hypogammaglobulinemia, 308–310
  immunoglobulin therapy, 308–309
Hypotension
  with anaphylaxis, 95
  with drug reactions, 80
Hypothyroidism, with Hashimoto's
  thyroiditis, 322–323

I

Ibuprofen
  in pericarditis, 269–270
  in postcardiac injury syndrome, 265
Idiopathic pulmonary fibrosis, 214–220
  biopsy in, 215–216
  blood examination, 216

bronchoalveolar lavage in, 217
diagnosis, 215
imaging techniques in, 217
immunosuppressive therapy in, 217–219
patient monitoring, 219
staging disease activity, 216–217
therapy, 217–219
Idiopathic thrombocytopenic purpura,
274–280
acute childhood, 276–277
chronic, 277–279
corticosteroids in, 276–280
danazol in, 278–279
diagnosis, 275
gamma globulin therapy, 276–277, 279,
280
immunosuppressive therapy, 279
pathophysiology, 275
plasma exchange in, 277
platelet transfusion in, 277, 278
in pregnancy, 279–280
serology, 276
splenectomy in, 277, 278
symptomatology, 274–275
treatment, 276–279
vincristine in, 279
IgA nephropathy, 197–198, 334–336
Immune globulin, intravenous
preparations, 302, 304
Immune serum globulin, in common
variable immunodeficiency, 301–304
Immunizations, in phagocyte function
disorders, 299–300
Immunoassay (in vitro)
in insect sting sensitivity, 82, 85, 87–88
in penicillin sensitivity, 69, 71
Immunodeficiency. See Common variable
immunodeficiency; Congenital
immunodeficiency disease; Severe
combined immunodeficiency disease
Immunofluorescence assay, 285–286
Immunoglobulin E, in allergic
bronchopulomonary aspergillosis,
220–222
Immunoglobulin G, in allergic
bronchopulmonary aspergillosis,
220–222
Immunoglobulin G antibody, in autoimmune hemolytic anemia, 281
Immunoglobulin M antibody, in homolytic
anemia, 280–281
Immunoglobulin therapy
in agammaglobulinemia, 309
in antibody deficiency disorders,
308–310
in hypogammaglobulinemia, 308–309
intravenous, 309–310
in panhypogammaglobulinemia, 309
Immunology, of mixed connective tissue
disease, 145
Immunodulators, in hyperimmunoglobulin
E syndrome, 315–316
Immunosuppressive agents. See also
specific drugs
in ankylosing spondylitis, 134
in Behçet's syndrome, 168–169
in dermatomyositis-polymyositis, 140
in Sjögren's syndrome, 129–130
in systemic lupus erythematosus, 104
in ulcerative colitis/Crohn's disease, 245
Immunotherapy
in allergic rhinitis, 5
in animal exposure allergy, 7

in asthma, 25
in chronic mucocutaneous candidiasis,
333
in insect sting sensitivity, 83–86, 88–91
in perennial allergic rhinitis, 19
Indomethacin
in ankylosing spondylitis, 132–133
in Behçet's syndrome, 167
in pericarditis, 270–271
in postcardiac injury syndrome, 265–266
in Reiter's syndrome, 122–123
Inflammatory myocarditis, 268–274
Insect sting sensitivity (adult), 81–86
anaphylaxis with, 82–83, 88
diagnosis, 82
skin tests in, 82
therapy, 82–86
venom immunotherapy, 83–86
Insect sting sensitivity (childhood), 87–91
anaphylaxis with, 87
avoidance in, 88
diagnosis, 87–88
immunoassay in, 82, 85, 87–88
medical therapy, 88
reaction types, 87
therapy, 88–91
venom immunotherapy, 88–91
Insulin allergy, 327–329
densitization in, 329
local reactions, 328
system reactions, 328–329
Insulin resistance, 329–330
glucocorticoids in, 330
immunologic, 330
nonimmunologic causes, 329–330
Interferon, in multiple sclerosis, 229
Interleukin-2 receptor, 342
Ipratropium bromide, in perennial allergic
rhinitis, 11, 17

J

Joint disorders
with Behçet's syndrome, 167
with mixed connective tissue disease,
146
Job's syndrome, 313

K

Keratitis (interstitial), with Cogan's
syndrome, 171
Keratoconjunctivitis
phlyctenular, 241
vernal, 239–240
Keratoconjunctivitis sicca, 240
with Sjögren's syndrome, 126–127
Ketoconazole
in atopic dermatitis, 181
in chronic mucocutaneous candidiasis,
315, 316, 331, 332, 333
Ketotifen, 24–25
Kidney function, in mixed connective
tissue disease, 148
Kidney disease,
with scleroderma, 138
with Sjögren's syndrome, 128
Kidney transplant. See Renal transplant
Koebner phenomenon, 191

L

Leukoagglutination, 285
Leukopenia, See Autoimmune leukopenia
Levamisole, in Behçet's syndrome, 166

Levothyroxine, in Hashimoto's thyroiditis
325–326
Linear IgA dermatosis, 173
Lithium, in aplastic anemia, 291
Liver transplantation
in primary biliary cirrhosis, 257–258
in severe combined immunodeficiency
disease, 306
Lupus erythematosus. See Systemic lupus
erythematosus
Lupus nephritis, 204–208
clinical vs pathological features,
204–205
end stage renal failure in, 208
experimental therapies, 208
immunosuppressive agents in, 206–208
plasmapheresis in, 208
treatment, 206–208
treatment criteria, 205–206
Lymphoma, with Sjögren's syndrome, 130
Lymphoplasmapheresis, in systemic
vasculitis, 153

M

Marie-Strümpell arthritis. See Ankylosing
spondylitis
Melphalan, in amyloidosis, 318
6-Mercaptopurine, in ulcerative
colitis/Crohn's disease, 245
Mesangial nephropathy, 334
Methotrexate
in bullous pemphigoid, 189–190
in dermatomyositis-polymyositis, 143
in pemphigus vulgaris, 187–188
in rheumatoid arthritis, 111–112,
119–120
α-Methyldopa, in autoimmune hemolytic
anemia, 281–282
Methyl prednisolone
in acute interstitial nephritis, 200
in aplastic anemia, 291
in dermatomyositis-polymyositis, 144
in lupus nephritis, 206, 207
in postcardiac injury syndrome, 267
in pericardial tamponade, 272
in temporal arteritis, 159–160
Methylxanthines, in asthma, 23
Mixed connective tissue disease, 145–148
cardiac involvement, 147–148
clinical features, 145
constitutional symptoms, 145–146
corticosteroids in, 148
gastrointestinal involvement, 147
immunologic features, 145
joint involvement, 146
kidney involvement, 148
muscle involvement, 146–147
pulmonary involvement, 147
Raynaud's phenomenon with, 146
skin involvement, 146
treatment, 145–148
Mucocutaneous disorders
with Behçet's syndrome, 166–167
with Reiter's syndrome, 122
Multiple sclerosis, 228–230
ACTH therapy, 228–229
acute attack, 228–229
attack reduction therapy, 229
azathioprine in, 229
corticosteroids in, 228–229
cyclophosphamide in, 229–230
interferon in, 229
progressive disease management,

229–230
symptom control, 230
Muscle disorders, in mixed connective
tissue disease, 146–147
Musculoskeletal disorders, with
scleroderma, 137–138
Musculoskeletal syndrome, with Sjögren's
syndrome, 129
Myasthenia gravis, 231–235
acetylcholine receptors in, 231
cholinesterase inhibitors in, 231–232
corticosteroids in, 233–234
crisis, 234–235
immunosuppressive agents in, 234
neonatal, 235
plasmapheresis in, 234
thymectomy in, 232–233
thyroid disease with, 231
Myocarditis
activity restriction in, 273
corticosteroids in, 273
cytotoxic agents in, 273–274
inflammatory, 268–274
pericarditis differentiation, 268–269
therapy, 269, 270
Myopericarditis, 272–274

N

Nasal polyps, in aspirin sensitivity, 38
Nedocromil sodium, in asthma, 25
Nephritis. *See* Acute interstitial nephritis;
Lupus nephritis
Nephrotic syndrome, 192–196
angiotensin converting enzyme inhibitors
in, 194–195
biochemical disturbances, 193–194
biopsy in, 193
edema management, 194
etiology, 192
hypercoagulability management, 196
hyperlipidemia in, 195–196
nutritional management, 194–195
proteinuria management, 194–195
Neurologic disorders, in mixed connective
tissue disease, 148
Neutropenia. *See* Autoimmune neutropenia
Neutrophil antibody testing, 285
Nonsteroidal anti-inflammatory agents
in ankylosing spondylitis, 132–133
cross-reaction with aspirin, 37
in Reiter's syndrome, 122
in rheumatoid arthritis, 107–108,
117–118
in systemic lupus erythematosus,
102–103
Normal human plasma, in common
variable immunodeficiency, 302
Nystatin, in chronic mucocutaneous
candidiasis, 333

O

Occupational factor
in animal exposure allergy, 5, 7
in asthma, 22
in chemical sensitivity, 48, 49
Occupational therapy, in rheumatoid
arthritis, 115–116
Ocular disorders
with Reiter's syndrome, 122
with Sjögren's syndrome, 126–127
Ocular pemphigoid, 241
OKT3 monoclonal antibody, for renal

transplant rejection, 203–204
Olfaction, in chemical sensitivity, 51–52
Oral disorders, with Sjögren's syndrome,
127

P

Pain, with drug reactions, 80
Panhypogammaglobulinemia, 310
immunoglobulin therapy, 309
Pemphigus, 186–189
drug-induced, 188
Pemphigus foliaceus, 188
Pemphigus vulgaris, 186–188
corticosteroids in, 187
cytotoxic agents in, 187–188
Penicillamine
in pemphigus induction, 188
in primary biliary cirrhosis, 257
in rheumatoid arthritis, 110–111, 119
in scleroderma, 139
Penicillin
in autoimmune hemolytic anemia, 281
in rheumatic fever prevention, 258–260
Penicillin sensitivity, 68–76
anaphylaxis from, 69
cephalosporin cross-sensitivity, 72–73
desensitization in, 73–75
non-IgE mediated reactions, 75–76
patient evaluation, 69–72
to semisynthetic penicillin, 71–72
skin testing, 69–71, 72
in vitro immunoassay, 69
Pericardiac injury syndrome, cytotoxic
therapy in, 267
Pericardiocentesis, in postcardiac injury
syndrome, 266–267
Pericarditis
aspirin/ibuprofen therapy, 269–270
constrictive, 272
corticosteroids in, 271
indomethacin in, 270–271
myocarditis differentiation, 268–269
recurrent, 272
with tamponade, 271–272
therapy, 269–272
Peripheral vascular defects, with
anaphylaxis, 95
Phagocyte function disorders, 293–300
antibiotics in, 296–297, 299–300
antifungal agents in, 297
cellular defect factor, 300
clinical features, 293–294
febrile episodes management, 296–297
granulocyte transfusions in, 298
infection factor, 295–296
inherited, 293–294, 300
mucocutaneous disorders management,
298–299
prophylactic antibiotic therapy, 299–300
surgical therapy, 297–298
Phenylbutazone
in ankylosing spondylitis, 132–134
in Reiter's syndrome, 122–124
Phlebitis, in Behçet's syndrome, 168
Phototherapy, in atopic dermatitis, 181
Physical allergy, urticaria, 61
Physical therapy
in ankylosing spondylitis, 132
in rheumatoid arthritis, 115–116
Plasma exchange therapy
in Goodpasture's syndrome, 210–211
in idiopathic thrombocytopenic purpura,
277

Plasmapheresis
in autoimmune hemolytic anemia, 284
in dermatomyositis-polymyositis, 144
in lupus nephritis, 208
in myasthenia gravis, 234
in rheumatoid arthritis, 113
in systemic lupus erythematosus, 104
in systemic vasculitis, 153
Platelet transfusion, in idiopathic
thrombocytopenic purpura, 277, 278
Pneumonitis. *See* Hypersensitivity
pneumonitis
Polymyositis, 140–144
alternative therapies, 144
corticosteroids in, 140–142
cytotoxic agents in, 142–144
immunosuppressive agents in, 140
therapy, 140–144
Postcardiac injury syndrome, 263–268
anticoagulation therapy with, 265
aspirin therapy, 264–265
complications management, 266–267
constrictive pericarditis in, 268
corticosteroids in, 266, 267
ibuprofen in, 265
indomethacin in, 265–266
patient evaluation, 263–264
pericardiocentesis in, 266–267
recurrences, 264–267
treatment regimens, 264
Postmyocardial infarction syndrome, 263
Postpartum thyroiditis, 325
Postpericardiotomy syndrome, 263
Prednisone
in acute interstitial nephritis, 200
in acute rheumatic fever, 261
in amyloidosis, 318
in aplastic anemia, 291
in aspergillosis, 221, 222
in asthma, 24, 28, 36
in atopic dermatitis, 181
in autoimmune hemolytic anemia, 282
in autoimmune uveitis, 237
in Behçet's syndrome, 166–168
in bullous pemphigoid, 189
in Cogan's syndrome, 171
in contact dermatitis, 184
in dermatomyositis/polymyositis,
141–142
in erythema multiforme, 191
in glomerulonephritis, 196
in idiopathic pulmonary fibrosis, 218
in idiopathic thrombocytopenic purpura,
276, 278, 280
in inflammatory myocarditis, 271
in insulin resistance, 330
in juvenile rheumatoid arthritis, 119
in lupus nephritis, 206, 207
in mixed connective tissue disease,
146–147
in multiple sclerosis, 229
in myasthenia gravis, 233–234
in myocarditis, 273
in pemphigus, 187
in postcardiac injury syndrome, 266,
267
in rheumatoid arthritis, 112
in sarcoidosis, 226
in systemic lupus erythematosus, 103
in systemic vasculitis, 150, 151–152
in Takayasu's arteritis, 164
in temporal arteritis, 158–159

Pregnancy
  with asthma, 28–29
  dapsone therapy in, 175
  Hashimoto's thyroiditis with, 324–325
  herpes gestationis with, 176–177
  idiopathic thrombocytopenic purpura
    and, 279–280
  systemic lupus erythematosus with, 105
  ulcerative colitis/Crohn's disease with,
    250
Proteinuria, in nephrotic syndrome,
  194–195
Pruritus, with drug reactions, 80
Public health, sulfite-induced asthma,
  42–43
Pulmonary fibrosis. *See* Idiopathic
  pulmonary fibrosis
Pulmonary function
  in anaphylaxis, 96
  in mixed connective tissue disease, 147
  with Reiter's syndrome, 122
  with scleroderma, 138
  with Sjögren's syndrome, 128
Pyridostigmine, in myasthenia gravis,
  231–232

Q

Quinidine, in autoimmune hemolytic
  anemia, 281

R

Radiation synovectomy, in rheumatoid
  arthritis, 112–113
Radiation therapy
  in ankylosing spondylitis, 134
  in rheumatoid arthritis, 113
RAST test, 69, 71, 82, 85, 87–88
Raynaud's phenomenon
  in mixed connective tissue disease, 146
  with scleroderma, 135, 136
Recombinant hematopoietic growth
  factors, in aplastic anemia, 291
Reiter's syndrome, 121–124
  antibiotics, in 124
  articular disorders with, 121
  cardiac disease with, 122
  clinical manifestations, 121
  corticosteroids in, 124
  cytotoxic agents in, 124
  diagnosis, 121
  mucocutaneous lesions with, 122
  nonsteroidal anti-inflammatory agents in,
    122–124
  ocular disorders with, 122
  patient education, 121–122
  periarticular disorders with, 122
  pulmonary disease with, 122
Renal disease, immunologically mediated,
  nephritic, 334–338
Renal transplant, 339–343
  patient preparation, 339–340
  rejection management, 341–342
  rejection prevention, 340
Renal transplant rejection, 201–204
  acute, 202
  cellular elements in, 201–202
  chronic, 203
  equine ATG in, 204
  humoral elements, 201–202
  hyperacute, 202
  maintenance immunosuppressive
    therapy, 201

OKT3 monoclonal antibody therapy,
    203–204
  renal biopsy in, 202–203, 204
  steroid pulse therapy, 203
Respiratory failure, in childhood asthma,
  33
Respiratory support, in Goodpasture's
  syndrome, 211
Rheumatic fever (acute), 258–262
  activity rebounds, 261–262
  antibiotics in prevention, 258–260
  antirheumatic therapy, 260–261
  antistreptococcal vaccine in, 262
  carditis management, 261
  continuing management, 262
  corticosteroids in, 260–261
  general management, 260
  primary prevention, 258
  prognosis, 262
  salicylates in, 260–261
Rheumatoid arthritis, 106–114
  "burn out" with, 114
  cytotoxic agents in, 111–112
  early aggressive disease, 113
  experimental therapy, 112–113
  family considerations, 107
  generalized fatigue/aching with, 114
  gold therapy, 110
  hydroxychloroquine in, 109
  injectable steroids in, 112
  management planning, 106–107
  night pain with, 113
  nonsteroidal anti-inflammatory agents in,
    107–108
  patient discouragement, 113
  penicillamine in, 110–111
  physical measures, 107
  salicylates in, 107–108
  single inflamed/dominant joint in, 114
  slow acting anti-inflammatory agents in,
    108–109
  social considerations, 107
  surgery for, 112
  therapy failures, 113–114
Rheumatoid arthritis (juvenile), 115–120
  classification, 115, 116
  complications, 116–117
  corticosteroids in, 119
  general measures, 115
  gold therapy in, 118
  hydroxychloroquine in, 118–119
  methotrexate in, 119–120
  nonsteroidal anti-inflammatory agents
    in, 117–118
  occupational therapy in, 115–116
  penicillamine in, 119
  physiotherapy in, 115–116
  slow-acting antirheumatic agents in, 118
  surgical management, 120
Rhinitis medicamentosa, 17
Rhinosinusitis, with asthma in aspirin
  sensitivity, 36–39

S

Salicylates
  in acute rheumatic fever, 260–261
  in rheumatoid arthritis, 107–108
Sarcoidosis, 223–227
  corticosteroids in, 223–227
  cytotoxic agents in, 227
  nonsteroidal therapy, 224
  staging in, 225–226

therapy results, 226–227
  therapy vs no therapy, 223–224
Scleritis, 242
Scleroderma, 135–140
  cardiac function with, 138
  CREST features, 135, 136
  drug therapy, 139
  gastrointestinal dysmotility, 137
  musculoskeletal disorders with, 137–138
  penicillamine in, 139
  pulmonary function with, 138
  Raynaud's phenomenon with, 135, 136
  renal crisis with, 138
  Sjögren's syndrome with, 138
  skin care in, 136
  vascular disorders with, 136
Severe combined immunodeficiency
    disease, 305–307, 311–312
  bone marrow transplantation in,
    305–306, 311
  enzyme replacement in, 307
  fetal liver transplantation in, 306
  infection management, 311–312
  thymus derived factors in, 307
  thymus tissue transplant in, 307
Shunt nephritis, 337–338
Sick building syndrome, 49–50
Sinusitis, in asthmatic children, 34
Sjögren's syndrome, 125–130, 240
  glandular disease management, 126–128
  immunosuppressive therapy with,
    129–130
  lymphoma with, 130
  management principles, 125–126
  musculoskeletal syndrome with, 129
  organ specific disease with, 128
  with scleroderma, 138
  systemic disease with, 128–130
Skin tests
  in insect sting sensitivity, 82
  in penicillin allergy, 69–71, 72
Solar urticaria, 64–65
Splenectomy
  in autoimmune hemolytic anemia, 283
  in idiopathic thrombocytopenic purpura,
    277, 278
  in systemic lupus erythematosus, 105
Staphylococcal protein A, 286
Staphylococcal slide test, 286
Status asthmaticus, 44–48
  adrenergic agents in, 45–46, 47
  bronchodilator in, 45–46, 47
  in children, 32–33
  corticosteroids in, 46
  death from, 45, 47
  pathophysiology, 44–45
  therapy, 45
  toxic reactions in, 46–47
  ventilatory support in, 47
Steroid pulse therapy, in renal transplant
  rejection, 203
Sulfadiazine, in rheumatic fever
  prevention, 259
Sulfapyridine, in dermatitis herpetiformis,
  175
Sulfasalazine, in ulcerative colitis/Crohn's
  disease, 243–244
Sulfites
  asthma induction, 42–44
  food sources, 43
  medication sources, 44
  public health aspects, 42
Sympathomimetics, in asthma, 23

Systemic lupus erythematosus, 101–105
  antimalarials in, 104
  corticosteroids in, 103–104
  disease activity, 101–102
  drug therapy, 102–104
  immunosuppressive agents in, 104
  medical management, 101
  nonsteroidal anti-inflammatory drugs in,
    102–103
  patient education, 101
  plasmapheresis in, 104
  pregnancy with, 105
  splenectomy in, 105
  thrombocytopenia with, 105
Systemic sclerosis. *See* Scleroderma

T

T cell deficiency, 308, 312
Takayasu's arteritis, 161–165
  ancillary therapy, 165
  anti-inflammatory therapy, 164
  arteriography in, 161–162
  "burnt out" stage, 163
  captopril in, 165
  corticosteroids in, 162–164
  cytotoxic agents in, 164
  diagnosis, 161–162
  with inflammatory disease, 162–163
  surgery in, 165
  therapeutic approach, 162–165
Temporal arteritis, 157–161
  alternative therapy, 160–161
  corticosteroids in, 157–160
  cytotoxic agents in, 160–161
  diagnosis, 157
  morbidity with corticosteroid therapy,
    158, 159–160
  therapy, 157–161
Thalidomide, in Behçet's syndrome, 166
Theophylline
  in anaphylaxis, 96
  in asthma, 23, 28
Thrombocytopenia, with systemic lupus
  erythematosus, 105
Thrombocytopenic purpura. *See* Idiopathic
  thrombocytopenic purpura
Thymectomy, in myasthenia gravis,
  232–233
Thymus derived factors, in severe
  combined immunodeficiency disease,
  307
Thymus tissue transplant, in severe
  combined immunodeficiency disease,
  307
Thyroid disease, with myasthenia gravis,
  231

Thyroid enlargement, with Hashimoto's
  thyroiditis, 323–324
Thyroid function tests, in Hashimoto's
  thyroiditis, 322
Thyroid lymphoma, 325
Thyroiditis, postpartum, 325
Thyroxine, in Hashimoto's thyroiditis,
  325–326
Toxic megacolon, 247
Transfusion
  in aplastic anemia, 289–290
  in autoimmune hemolytic anemia, 284
L-triiodothyronine, 325–326

U

Ulcerative colitis, 242–251
  cancer surveillance in, 247–248
  in childhood/adolescence, 250–251
  drug therapy, 243–246
  dysplasia with, 247–248
  extragastrointestinal disorders with, 250
  long term management, 247–248
  nutritional management, 243
  patient education, 243
  pregnancy with, 250
  surgery in, 248
Ulcerative colitis (acute)
  mild to moderate, 246
  severe fulminant, 246–247
  toxic megacolon, 247
Universal reactor, 51
  olfaction and, 51–52
Urticaria
  with anaphylaxis, 97
  exercise-induced, 41–42
Urticaria (chronic), 60–62
  ancillary drug therapy, 61
  antihistamines in, 60–61
  therapeutic approach, 60–62
  therapy evaluation, 61–62
Urticaria (physical), 61, 62–65
  antihistamines in, 62–65
  aquagenic, 65
  cholinergic, 63
  classification, 62
  cold induced, 63–64
  delayed pressure, 64
  dermographism, 63
  localized heat, 65
  solar, 64–65
Uveitis, with Behçet's syndrome, 167
Uveitis (autoimmune), 235–238
  alkylating drugs in, 238
  azathioprine in, 237
  cyclosporine in, 238

  periocular corticosteroid therapy,
    236–237
  surgery in, 238
  systemic corticosteroid therapy, 237
  topical corticosteroids in, 236

V

Vaginitis sicca, with Sjögren's syndrome,
  127–128
Vascular disorders, with scleroderma, 136
Vasculitis
  with Cogan's syndrome, 171–172
  with Sjögren's syndrome, 128–129
  syndromes classification, 149
Vasculitis (cutaneous), 155–157
  antihistamines in, 156–157
  with Behçet's syndrome, 167
  clinical features, 155–156
  distinctive lesions, 156
  laboratory findings, 156
  therapy, 156–157
Vasculitis (systemic), 149–155
  with antigen stimulus, 150
  bolus corticosteroid-cyclophosphamide
    therapy, 152–153
  cyclophosphamide-prednisone therapy,
    150–154
  cyclosporin A in, 153
  cytotoxic agents in, 152
  lymphoplasmapheresis in, 153
  miscellaneous therapy, 153
  plasmapheresis in, 153
  primary systemic/multisystem
    syndromes, 150–153
  therapeutic approach, 149–153
  therapy complications, 153
  with underlying disease, 150
Venom immunotherapy, 83–86, 88–91
  adverse reactions, 84–85
  cessation of, 86
  mechanism of, 83
  method, 84
  monitoring, 85
  patient selection, 83, 88–89
  reactions, 90–91
  treatment failures, 91
Ventilatory support, in status asthmaticus,
  47
Vibratory angioedema, 65
Vincristine, in idiopathic
  thrombocytopenic purpura, 279

X

Xerostomia, with Sjögren's syndrome, 127